Silymarin puzzle

Silymarin puzzle

From basic science to practical applications in human and veterinary medicine and nutrition

Peter F. Surai
Anton Surai

Wageningen Academic
Publishers

The Library of Congress Cataloging-in-Publication Data is available online at https://catalog.loc.gov

EAN: 9789086863914
e-EAN: 9789086869442
ISBN: 978-90-8686-391-4
e-ISBN: 978-90-8686-944-2
DOI: 10.3920/978-90-8686-944-2

First published, 2023

Dedications

To Helen, Katie, Ingrida, Aiste, Oscar,
Arthur, Henry and Gareth
who gave us an inspiration for writing this book.

Preface

In the quest for an ideal human diet, it was identified that vegetables and fruit contain high concentrations of polyphenolic compounds, which could be responsible for their health-promoting properties. Therefore, for the last 30 years polyphenols were in the centre of research work worldwide. Among polyphenols silymarin (SM), an extract from a medicinal plant *Silybum Marianum*, also known as milk thistle, has a special place, having been used in human medicine for the management of liver diseases since ancient times. This topic has received tremendous attention in recent years, with more than 2500 peer-reviewed research papers with 'silymarin or its derivatives' in paper title or more than 4500 papers with the same words in abstracts found in the PubMed database with more than 800/1500 papers published in the last 5 years alone.

Accumulating scientific evidence indicates that SM is characterised by a wide range of protective pharmacological activities, including: hepatoprotective, neuroprotective, anti-diabetic, cardio-protective, anti-inflammatory, immune-modulatory, anti-viral, anti-cancer and anti-toxic/chemo-preventive activities. They were well proven in various *in vitro* and *in vivo* model systems, but clinical trials with SM have been rather disappointing. There is a range of publications showing positive effects of SM in poultry and farm animal nutrition. Molecular mechanisms of protective action of SM have for many years been related to its antioxidant activities, however, recent evidence indicates that direct antioxidant activity of this compound in animals and human is of minor importance, if any. Indeed, protective effects of SM in many disease states are still, to a large extent, enigmatic.

However, until now there has been no single monograph addressing major questions related to SM chemistry, biochemistry and practical applications.

Therefore, the aim of this comprehensive monograph is to address the following:

1. Recent view on general antioxidant defence network and roles of polyphenolics, as most fashionable natural antioxidants.
2. Molecular mechanisms of protective SM action including mitochondria preservation/stabilisation and decreased ROS production, vitagene modulation and improved stress adaptation, Nrf2 activation and additional synthesis of a range of antioxidants and redox homeostasis maintenance, NF-κB and pro-inflammatory cytokine down-regulation leading to anti-inflammatory action, oestrogen receptor (ER) regulation, modulation of PPAR and other transcription factors, etc.
3. SM application in human diseases, including hepatoprotection, neuroprotection, anti-diabetic, anti-arthritis and other protective activities.
4. Immunomodulating, anti-inflammatory, anti-toxic protective activities of SM.
5. Practical applications of SM in poultry and animal industry with special emphases on its protective roles in gut health maintenance.

The book contains 19 chapters with a comprehensive recent reference list related to each subject described. All chapters are connected to each other with an aim to show

SM importance from basic science to practical applications in human and veterinary medicine and nutrition with a special attention to molecular mechanisms of SM action.

The book is intended to be of practical importance to medical scientists, including medical doctors, pharmacists, consultants, etc. as well as to poultry/animal scientists, poultry producers, nutritionists and vets, as well as students of medical, biological and agricultural backgrounds. It can also be of interest for researchers in areas related to physiology, biochemistry, nutrition and veterinary medicine.

Peter F. Surai and Anton Surai

About the authors

Dr Peter Surai started his studies at Kharkov University, Ukraine, where he obtained his PhD and DSc in biochemistry studying effects of antioxidants on poultry. Later he became Professor of Human Physiology. In 1994 he moved to Scotland to continue his antioxidant related research and in 2000 he was promoted to Professor of Nutritional Biochemistry at the Scottish Agricultural College. Recently he was awarded Honorary Professorships in 7 universities in various countries, including UK, Hungary, Bulgaria, Russia and Ukraine. He has more than 900 research publications, including 360 papers in peer-reviewed journals, 17 books and 57 chapters in various books. In 1999 he received the prestigious John Logie Baird Award for Innovation for the development of 'super-eggs' and, in 2000, The World's Poultry Science Association Award for Research in recognition of an outstanding contribution to the development of the poultry industry. He successfully transferred the vitagene concept of stress adaptation from medical sciences into poultry and animal sciences. For the last 20 years he has been lecturing all over the world visiting more than 70 countries.

Anton Surai graduated with Bachelor's degree in Biochemistry and Pharmacology from the Strathclyde University (Glasgow, UK) and has almost 20 years of practical experience within the feed industry, supplying pig and poultry sectors worldwide. Having obtained his MBA from the Open University in the UK in 2009, he has focused on improving economic efficiency in pig and poultry production through developing novel approaches to deal with commercially-relevant stresses. In particular, he was the first to introduce vitagene concept into poultry and pig industries. His major interests focus on understanding biological/physiological limits of highly productive poultry and pigs, with specific emphases on gut health and development and feed utilisation. Recently he has been involved in further development of technologies of supplying chickens and pigs with vitagene-modulating mixtures to mobilise their internal resources in order to overcome stresses, reducing loss in productive and reproductive performance.

Table of contents

Part III. Silymarin in immunity, inflammation and gut health

Part IV. Practical applications of silymarin in clinical practice

Part V. Practical applications of silymarin in poultry/animal industry

Abbreviations

6-OHDA	6-hydroxydopamine
6PGDH	6-phosphogluconate dehydrogenase
Ab	antibody
ABC	transporters adenosine triphosphate Binding Cassette transporters
ABCG2	breast cancer resistance protein, also known as BCRP
AChE	acetylcholinesterase
AD	Alzheimer's disease
AF	aflatoxin
AGEs	advanced glycation end products
AgNPs	silver nanoparticles
AhR	aryl hydrocarbon receptor
AIA	adjuvant-induced arthritis
Akt	serine/threonine kinase
ALP	alkaline phosphatase
ALT	alanine transaminase
AMPK	5′-adenosine monophosphate-activated protein kinase
AO	antioxidant
AP-1	transcription factor
APAP	acetaminophen
APC	antigen presenting cells
APP	amyloid precursor protein
ARE	antioxidant response element
AST	aspartate aminotransferase
ATF	activating transcription factor
ATM	ataxia-telangiectasia-mutated
ATR	ataxia-telangiectasia and Rad 3-related
B(a)P	benzo[a]pyrene
Bcl-2	B-cell lymphoma 2
BCR	B-cell receptor
BD	basal diet
BHA	butylated hydroxyanisole
BHT	butylated hydroxytoluene
BMI	body mass index
BNIP3	BCL2 Interacting Protein 3
BW	body weight
C/EBPα	CCAAT enhancer binding protein α
CA	carbonic anhydrase
CAT	catalase
c/EBPβ	CCAAT-enhancer-binding protein beta
CoQ	coenzyme Q
COX-2	cyclooxygenase-2
CP	cyclophosphamide
CREB	cAMP responsive element binding protein
CRP	C-reactive protein

CS	cisplatin
CTL	cytotoxic T-cell
CUL3	cullin 3 protein
CUMS	chronic unpredictable mild stress
CVD	cardiovascular diseases
DASH	dietary Approach to Stop Hypertension
DC	dendritic cells
DDI	drug-drug interactions
DDR	DNA damage response
DGA	Dietary Guidelines for Americans
DHA	docosahexaenoic acid
DMH	1,2-di-methylhydrazine
DON	deoxynivalenol
DOX	doxorubicin
Drp1	dynamin-related protein 1
EGCG	epigallocatechin gallate
eNOS	endothelial nitric oxide synthase
ER	endoplasmic reticulum
ERβ	oestrogen receptor β
ERR	oestrogen-related receptor
ESR	energy stress response
ETC	electron transport chain
FABP4	fatty acid-binding protein 4
FB1	Fumonisin B1
FBG	fasting blood glucose
FCR	feed conversion ratio
FLHS	fatty-liver haemorrhagic syndrome
FOXO	forkhead box O, a transcription factor
FXR	Farnesoid-X activated receptors
G6PD	glucose 6-phosphate dehydrogenase
GAPDH	glyceraldehyde 3-phosphate dehydrogenase
GCL	glutamate cysteine ligase
GGT	gamma-glutamyl transferase
GIT	gastrointestinal tract
GP	grape pomace
GPx	glutathione peroxidase
GR	glutathione reductase
Grx	glutaredoxin
GSE	grape seed extract
GSH	reduced glutathione
GSSG	oxidised glutathione
GST	glutathione S-transferase
HCV	hepatitis C virus
HEI	Healthy Eating Index
HFD	high-fat diet-fed
HIF	hypoxia-inducible transcription factor

HISR	hypoxia-induced stress response
HO-1	heme oxygenase 1
HSF	heat shock factor
HSP	heat shock protein
i.p.	intraperitoneal
i.v.	intravenous
I/R	ischemia/reperfusion
IBV	infectious bronchitis virus
IDH2	isocitrate dehydrogenase 2
IFN	interferon
Ig	immunoglobulin
IGF-1	insulin-like growth factor 1
IKK	IκB kinase
IκB	inhibitor of κB
IL	interleukin
IL-2R	interleukin 2 receptor
INH	isoniazid
iNOS	inducible nitric oxide synthase
Insig-1	insulin induced gene-1
IR	insulin resistance
IRE1	inositol-requiring enzyme 1
ISR	inflammatory stress response
Keap1	Kelch-like-ECH-associated protein 1
LC	L-Carnitine
LC-MS/MS	liquid chromatography with tandem mass spectrometry
LDLR	LDL receptor
LOOH	lipid hydroperoxide
LPS	lipopolysaccharide
MAO	monoamine oxidase
MAPK	mitogen-activated protein kinase
MASI	melasma
MCD diet	methionine- and choline-deficient diet
MDA	malondialdehyde
MDR	multidrug resistance
MEF2A	myocyte enhancer factor 2
MHC	major histocompatibility complex
MIA	mono-iodoacetate
MIND	Mediterranean-DASH diet Intervention for Neurodegenerative Delay
miRNAs	microRNAs
MITF	microphthalmia-associated transcription factor
MMP3	matrix metalloproteinase-3
MPO	myeloperoxidase
MPs	macrophages
MPTP	1-methyl-4-phenyl-1,2,3,6-tetrahydropyridine
MRP1	multidrug resistance-associated protein 1, also known as ABCC1
Msr	methionine sulfoxide reductase

MT	milk thistle
mtDNA	mitochondrial DNA
MTS	milk thistle seeds
MTX	methotrexate
Mtx	mycotoxins
NASH	non-alcoholic steatohepatitis
NAFLD	non-alcoholic fatty liver disease
NFIL3	nuclear factor interleukin (IL)-3 regulated
NF-κβ	nuclear factor kappa-light-chain-enhancer of activated B cells
NF-κBp65	nuclear factor kappa-B p65 subunit
NK cells	natural killer cells
NKT cells	natural killer T cells
NLRP3	NOD-like receptor protein 3
NLRs	NOD (nucleotide-binding oligomerization-domain protein) like receptors
Nox4	NADPH Oxidase 4
NQO1	NAD(P)H quinone oxidoreductase-1
Nrf2	nuclear factor erythroid-2 related factor 2;
NSR	nutritional stress response
OA	osteoarthritis
OATPs	organic anion-transporting polypeptides
OTA	ochratoxin A
p53	tumour protein P53,
PAAC	partial abdominal aortic constriction
PAFAs	polyunsaturated fatty acids
PAMPs	pathogen-associated molecular patterns
PBMC	peripheral blood mononuclear cells
Peg-IFN	pegylated interferon
PD	Parkinson's disease
PERK	PKR-like ER kinase
PFA	plant feed additives
PGC1α	peroxisome proliferator-activated receptor-γ co-activator 1α
PGE2	prostaglandin E2
P-gp	P-glycoprotein, also known as ABCB1 or MDR1 P-gp
PHA	phytohemagglutinin
PKA	protein kinase A
PKC	protein kinase C
PLD	Paleolithic diet
PPARs	peroxisome proliferator-activated receptors
PPRE	peroxisome proliferator response element
PQ	paraquat
Prx	peroxiredoxin (thioredoxin peroxidase)
PRR	pattern recognition receptors
Prx	peroxiredoxins
PXR	pregnane X receptor
PZA	pyrazinamide

RA	rheumatoid arthritis
RBV	ribavirin
RCR	respiratory control ratio
RCTs	randomised controlled clinical trials
RIF	rifampicin
RNS	reactive nitrogen species
RONS	reactive oxygen and nitrogen species
ROS	reactive oxygen species
SAPK	stress-activated p38 and JNK MAPK (SAPK)
SB	silybin/silibinin
SFN	sulforaphane
SIRT	sirtuin
SM	silymarin
SNc	substantia nigra pars copmacta
SNP	sodium nitroprusside
SOD	superoxide dismutase
SR	stress response
Srx	Sulfiredoxin
SREBP	sterol regulatory element binding protein
STAT	signal transducer and activator of transcription
STZ	streptozotocin
T2D	type 2 diabetes
TAA	thioacetamide
TAU	taurine
TBARS	thiobarbituric acid reactive substances
TC	tea catechins
TCA	tricarboxylic acid
TCR	T-cell receptor
TD	tibial dyschondroplasia
Tfh cells	T follicular helper cells
TGF	transforming growth factor
Th cells	T helper cells
TMD	Traditional Mediterranean diet
Tmem cells	T memory cells
TNF-α	tumour necrosis factor alpha
Treg cells	T regulatory cells
Trx	reduced thioredoxin
TrxR	thioredoxin reductase
TXNIP	thioredoxin interacting protein
UCP	uncoupling proteins
UPR	unfolded protein response
XO	xanthine oxidase
Zen	zearalenone

Part I.
From optimal diet to optimal health

Necessity is the mother of invention

Chapter 1
A search for ideal diets, the case of polyphenols

Diets cures more than the lancet

Peter F. Surai[1-6] and Anton Surai[7]*
[1]Vitagene and Health Research Centre, Bristol, UK; [2]Department of Microbiology and Biochemistry, Faculty of Veterinary Medicine, Trakia University, Stara Zagora, Bulgaria; [3]Department of Animal Nutrition, Faculty of Agricultural and Environmental Sciences, Szent Istvan University, Hungary; [4]Saint-Petersburg State Academy of Veterinary Medicine, St. Petersburg, Russia; [5]Sumy National Agrarian University, Sumy, Ukraine [6]Odessa National Academy of Food Technologies, Odessa, Ukraine; [7]Healthy Food Services, Bristol, UK
psurai@feedfood.co.uk

Abstract

In the scientific literature several so called 'ideal diets' have received substantial attention over the past decades. First of all, these are Mediterranean, Japanese and Hunter-gatherer diets. The Mediterranean diet is associated with decreased rates of various diseases and based on green and yellow vegetables, fruits, grains and olive oil, has a protective effect against development of atherosclerosis. The Japanese diet reflects the highest life expectancy, and the Hunter-gatherer diet is based on a nutrient consumption similar to our ancestors during human evolution. In addition, currently, three basic dietary healthy patterns: MedDiet, Dietary Approach to Stop Hypertension (DASH), and Mediterranean-DASH diet Intervention for Neurodegenerative Delay (MIND) have been developed and tested. The aforementioned diets are different in composition, but they have some similarities in terms of low saturated fat and high levels of naturally occurring antioxidants, including polyphenolics and the last 20-30 years could be called a 'polyphenolic era'. There is abundant data obtained from laboratory and farm animal models related to the biological and pharmacological effects of various plant extracts containing high concentrations of polyphenols. However, there are several important points which to some extent restrict wide usage of polyphenol-rich plant extracts in medical practise and animal/poultry nutrition. It is impossible to guarantee the composition of the extract. Flavonoid/polyphenol concentration and composition would depend on many factors including conditions of plant growth (soil composition, fertilisation, temperature, humidity, etc.), extraction procedure, extract storage conditions, etc. Main polyphenols in plant extracts are characterised, but there could be many other undetected and uncharacterised compounds possessing biological activities. Low bioavailability of most polyphenols makes it difficult to explain molecular mechanisms of their biological activity. Most *in vitro* research showing various benefits of polyphenolic compounds used their concentrations which much higher those achievable in biological tissues. Direct AO action of polyphenols, including silymarin, is most likely not the case in animal cells, but their regulatory effects of various transcription factors (e.g. NF-κB and Nrf2) and vitagenes are of great importance in maintaining redox

DOI:10.3920/978-90-8686-944-2_001,

balance in various tissues/cells. Polyphenol interactions with other nutrients and drugs are not fully addressed at the moment and need more attention. Clearly there is a need for further research in this exciting area.

Keywords: ideal diets, polyphenols, silymarin, antioxidants, oxidative stress

1.1 Introduction

It is well appreciated that poor diet and low levels of physical activity are among major risk factors for various diseases, including cardiovascular diseases, cancer, type-2 diabetes and obesity, while the number of deaths associated with poor diet (e.g. low fruit and vegetable intake, high energy-dense food intake) and low levels of physical activity has significantly increased for the last decade (Lobczowska *et al.*, 2022). Hippocrates' observations on the relation between health and food choices began discussions about the factors that determine our health many centuries ago. However, during the past three decades it has become obvious that while our lifestyle, including diet, stress, smoking, medical attention, exercise and genetics, is a major determinant of our health status it is diet that has the pivotal role. The effect of nutrition on human health has received tremendous attention and traditional medical teaching that diet and nutrients play only limited roles in human health is being revised. In most developed countries nutritional practice has changed the focus from combating nutrient deficiencies to addressing nutrient requirements for maintaining good health throughout the life. It thus appears that one of the most fascinating ideas in human nutrition is that selected foods and their components can improve physical or mental performance or decrease disease risk. Thus, beyond meeting nutrition needs, diet may modulate various body functions and may play beneficial or detrimental roles in maintaining our health. For example, dietary factors are considered to be major contributors to the leading causes of death of Americans, namely coronary heart disease and certain types of cancer. Epidemiological findings, supported by animal studies, have led to recommendations that people should consume at least two servings of fruit and three servings of vegetable daily in addition to at least two servings of fish weekly. While findings and reports such as these have had an impact on the type and quantity of the food that many of us eat most adults in developed countries fall well short of meeting healthy eating guidelines (Surai, 2002). The aim of the present chapter is a critical analysis of achievements and misconceptions related to polyphenol physiological actions in human and animals/poultry with a specific emphasis to their antioxidant-related properties *in vivo* as a way to antioxidant systems modulation.

1.2 What are ideal diets?

In the scientific literature three major so called 'ideal diets' have received substantial attention over the past decades. They are Mediterranean, Japanese and Hunter-gatherer diets (Table 1.1). The Mediterranean diet is associated with decreased rates of various diseases. For example, this diet, based on green and yellow vegetables, fruits, grains

Table 1.1. Some characteristics of ideal diets (adapted from Surai, 2002).

Mediterranean	Japanese	Hunter-gatherer
High consumption of legumes and cereals, fruits and vegetables	High consumption of soya, seaweeds, raw fish and rice	High consumption of many different parts of plants and animals, high in fibre
Moderate consumption of milk and dairy products and alcohol	Moderate consumption of salt	Arachidonic acid and DHA are major PUFAs
Low consumption of meat and meat products	Low consumption of fat and sugar	Low in saturated feed, low n-6/n-3 ratio
Variable amount of olive oil, some fish, cheese and nuts, little sugar		It does not include cereals, milk, refined sugar, salt or alcohol

and olive oil, has a protective effect against development of atherosclerosis. The Japanese diet reflects the highest life expectancy, and the Hunter-gatherer diet is based on a nutrient consumption similar to our ancestors during human evolution. These three diets are different in composition, but they have some similarities in terms of low saturated fat and high levels of naturally occurring antioxidants.

1.2.1 Hunter-gatherer/Paleolithic diet

The evolution of humans is connected with a lifestyle of hunting and gathering. The food sources (animal and plant) remained basically the same during the evolution, but the proportions of foods, preferences, preparations and the attainability substantially changed. It has been suggested that the nutritional patterns of Paleolithic humans influenced genetic evolution during the time period within which defining characteristics of contemporary humans were selected. Because the human genome has not changed much since the beginnings of agriculture, genetically, humans remain adapted for a Paleolithic dietary regimen (for a review see Surai, 2002). Such diets were based mainly on wild game, fish, and uncultivated plant foods.

In comparison to Paleolithic man, today our diet is characterised by a substantial increase in some substances and a decrease in other nutrients (Table 1.2). For example, in comparison to the Paleolithic period, current diets contain substantially decreased levels of natural antioxidants. In the history of mankind, anthropology shows that humans were gatherers of fruits and vegetables for their daily nutritional needs. This tradition has changed dramatically with the development of agricultural industries. Furthermore, the relocation of people from rural areas to cities also decreased fruit and vegetable consumption. Therefore, in contrast to our ancestors who used to eat a variety of various wild plants in large amounts, today's diet includes a limited number of plants, consumed in limited amounts, and as a result is comparatively poor in food-derived antioxidant compounds. In general, it seems likely that the Paleolithic diet contained quite high concentrations of various antioxidants.

Table 1.2. Comparison of modern and Paleolithic diets (adapted from Surai, 2002).

Modern diet in comparison to Paleolithic one is characterised by	
Increased	**Decreased**
Energy content	Energy expenditure
Saturated fat	Omega-3 PUFA
Omega-6 PUFA	Complex carbohydrate
Trans fatty acids	Fibre
Cereal grains	Fruits and vegetables
Sodium	Animal protein
Saccharose	Antioxidant
Lactose	Phytochemicals
Alcohol	Potassium and calcium
Dairy products	Vitamins

An inverse association between the Paleolithic diet (PLD) and cardiovascular risk factors was shown (De la O *et al.*, 2021; Ghaedi *et al.*, 2019). In a recent systematic review and meta-analysis based on data presented in 120 research papers evaluating the effects of the PLD in patients with metabolic disorders it was found a significant reduction in the PLD group *versus* control group in important health-related clinical parameters/biomarkers (Sohouli *et al.*, 2022):

- insulin resistance;
- fasting insulin;
- total cholesterol;
- triglycerides;
- low-density lipoprotein cholesterol;
- blood pressure; and
- C-reactive protein levels.

Of note, recently it has been suggested that the PLD may have cardiovascular benefits in participants from a Mediterranean country (De la O *et al.*, 2022). The main advantage of the described diet is an evolutionary adaptation of the human digestive system to most of those nutrients. This means that high efficiency of assimilation from the diet and distribution in the body could be a driving force in health promoting properties of various compounds, including antioxidants and phytochemicals.

1.2.2 Mediterranean diet

In the early 1950s in Naples very low incidence of coronary heart disease was associated with a specific diet, which later was called the 'good Mediterranean diet'. That diet was mainly vegetarian and differed from American and northern European diets in that it was characterised by decreased amounts of meat and dairy products and included fruit for dessert (for a review see Surai, 2002). That observation led to subsequent research in the Seven Countries Study. At the end of the 1950s that study was designed to investigate the relations between diet and cardiovascular diseases. The comparison was made between Finland, Greece, Italy, Japan, The Netherlands, US, and Yugoslavia. The study published in 1975 provided important information on national differences in diet preferences. For example, in Finland the intake of milk, potatoes, edible fats, and sugar products was very high. A similar but lower intake pattern was observed in The Netherlands. Fruit, meat, and pastry consumption was high in the US; cereal and alcoholic drink consumption was high in Italy; and bread consumption was high in Yugoslavians except for those in Belgrade. In Greece the intake of olive oil and fruit was high, and the Japanese cohorts were characterised by a high consumption of fish, rice, and soy products. Therefore, interest in the Mediterranean diet began more than 45 years ago, when the results of the famous Seven Countries Study were published. The term Mediterranean diet is associated with dietary patterns found in olive growing areas of the Mediterranean region and described in the 1960s. It was argued that there is no single ideal Mediterranean diet since there are important differences in the food habits of the Mediterranean countries having different diets, religions and cultures. As a result, their diets differ in many nutrients. The Greek version of the Mediterranean diet is dominated by the consumption of olive oil and by high consumption of vegetables and fruits. In general, there are several variants of the Mediterranean diet, but some common components can be identified (Table 1.1). Growing evidence demonstrates that the Mediterranean diet is beneficial to health with the stronger evidence for coronary heart disease, but with possible application to some forms of cancer. For example, Mediterranean diet adherence was shown to be inversely associated with risk of overweight and/or obesity as well as 5-y weight gain (Lotfi *et al.*, 2022). Traditional Mediterranean diet (TMD) was reported to reduce the incidence of infant morbidity and contributes to the disappearance of inflammatory and recurrent diseases (Calatayud-Sáez *et al.*, 2022). Similarly, a positive correlation of Mediterranean diet adherence with health-related quality of life in children and adolescents has been reported (Romero-Robles *et al.*, 2022). Interestingly, patients with metabolic syndrome with high adherence to the Mediterranean dietary pattern were characterised by less altered by disease anthropometric parameters, blood biochemical profile, and better oxidative and inflammatory status (Quetglas-Llabrés *et al.*, 2022). Mediterranean diet was found to be associated with reduced incidence of gestational diabetes mellitus and gestational weight gain (Zhang *et al.*, 2022). Among middle-aged and older Hispanic or Latino adults Mediterranean diet was reported to be associated with better cognitive performance and decreased 7-year learning and memory decline (Moustafa *et al.*, 2022). The inverse association was also found between adherence to the Mediterranean diet and the risk of hepatic steatosis (Lampignano *et al.*, 2022).

To explain the beneficial effects of the diet the antioxidant properties of several plant foods in the Mediterranean diet were postulated to be critical mediators of the beneficial effects of this diet. Antioxidants represent a common element in the components of the Mediterranean diets. In particular, wild edible greens frequently eaten in rural Greece in the form of salads and pies contain very high quantities of flavonoids. While there is no direct evidence that these antioxidants are the main players in the benefits of the Mediterranean diet, indirect evidence from epidemiological data and the increasing understanding of their mechanisms of action suggest that antioxidants may play a major role. Therefore, from the data presented above important conclusions can be drawn about an important role for natural antioxidants in the healthy image of the Mediterranean diet. Unfortunately, today this diet is changing under the strong influence of Western culture.

1.2.3 Japanese diet

The traditional Japanese diet has attracted the attention of many researchers since it is beneficial for preventing ischaemic heart disease and certain types of cancers. Japanese dietary habits were directly related to the lower the BMI and cholesterol levels, as well as mortality rate from coronary heart disease with the higher the average life expectancy among the Japanese (Mori *et al.*, 2022). A recent meta-analysis of prospective cohort studies based on data presented in 58 research papers, confirmed that the Japanese-style diet and characteristic Japanese foods may reduce CVD mortality (Shirota *et al.*, 2022). Furthermore, adherence to a traditional Japanese diet was reported to be inversely associated with cognitive decline with ageing (Saji *et al.*, 2022). It has been shown that this diet, containing little fat but enriched in complex carbohydrates and n-3 fatty acids of marine origin, may be related to the low atherogenic index in rural areas in the Okayama Prefecture in Japan (for a review see Surai, 2002). Main characteristic features of this diet are the low level of fat and low calorific content. A wide variety of marine products, including seaweeds and root vegetables, make this diet different from others. After analysing 39 papers devoted to the Japanese diet it was concluded that major three characteristics of the Japanese diets are soybeans/soybean-derived products, seafood and vegetables and they followed by rice and miso soup (Suzuki *et al.*, 2018). Thus, the dietary habits of the Japanese have made possible a high n-3 PUFA intake within a low-fat regimen. Among the Japanese, flavonoids and isoflavones originating from soya related products are the main components among non-nutrient phytochemicals with antioxidant potential in the diet and their high consumption may contribute to the low incidence of coronary heart disease in Japanese women. Isoflavones have a limited distribution in nature, and, for practical purposes, soy foods are the only nutritionally relevant dietary source of these phytochemicals. Seaweeds in the Japanese diet provide substantial amounts of various antioxidant compounds. Plants consumed by humans contain thousands of phenolic compounds. Among them the effects of dietary polyphenols are of great current interest due to their antioxidant, anti-inflammatory and possible anticarcinogenic activities. Therefore, similarly to two other 'ideal' diets the Japanese diet contains quite high levels of phytochemicals possessing antioxidant activity, which, in combination with n-3 fatty acids, could have health promoting properties.

Internationalisation of food and a fashion for fast food make it difficult to preserve the typical Japanese or Mediterranean diets. The main conclusion which can be made from the analysis of the 'ideal' diets is that natural antioxidants are among major players in these diets. Recent research on phytochemicals has changed the view on dietary factors affecting our health. In particular, it seems likely that there are hundreds of such factors and now we are dealing just with the tip of the iceberg. However, emerging information can help us to understand and to some extent explain a beneficial effect of various vegetables and fruits in our diet.

1.2.4 Other healthy diets

In addition, currently, three basic dietary healthy patterns: MedDiet, Dietary Approach to Stop Hypertension (DASH), and Mediterranean-DASH diet Intervention for Neurodegenerative Delay (MIND) have been developed and tested (Klimova *et al.*, 2020). In fact, the MedDiet pattern is characterised by fruits, vegetables, whole grains, olive oil, fish, nuts, legumes, moderate wine consumption, low consumption of processed foods, dairy products, red meat, and vegetable oils. This diet is rich in antioxidants, including anthocyanins, flavonoids and catechins, vitamins and minerals (Klimova *et al.*, 2020). The DASH diet is rich in fruits, vegetables, fish, whole-cereal products and low-fat dairy products and this dietary pattern is characterised by reduction of foods high in saturated fat and sugar. The MIND diet includes the 10 brain-healthy food groups such as green leafy vegetables, other vegetables, nuts, berries, beans, whole grains, seafood, poultry, olive oil, and wine and the five unhealthy food groups (red meats, butter and stick margarine, cheese, pastries, and sweets, and fried/fast food; Klimova *et al.*, 2020). The results of a review of the clinical trials/studies confirmed that all three dietary patterns have positive effect on cognitive performance among healthy seniors (Klimova *et al.*, 2020). These three dietary pattens are also rich in fruits and vegetables. The list of healthy diets can be continued and also include Healthy Nordic Diet, an adaptation of the Mediterranean, DASH, and other health-promoting diets into a regionally tailored dietary pattern by using traditional, local Nordic foods. This dietary pattern includes green leafy vegetables, other vegetables, fruits, fish and seafood, potatoes, berries, whole grains, nuts, low-fat dairy products, rapeseed, sunflower, and/or soya oils and limited intake of fresh red meat and sugar (Cena and Calder, 2020). The authors also include in the list Traditional Asian Diets including Traditional Korean and Chinese diets, in addition to the aforementioned Japanese diet. Similar to previously mentioned healthy diets, the Traditional Asian diets also include a great variety of polyphenol-rich foods.

The Healthy Eating Index (HEI) shows if a set of foods aligns with the Dietary Guidelines for Americans (DGA). Therefore, according to DGA healthy eating pattern includes (Krebs-Smith *et al.*, 2018):

- fruits, especially whole fruit;
- vegetables from all subgroups;
- grains with at least half been whole grains;
- fat-free or low fat dairy;
- protein foods, including animal (seafood, lean meats and poultry, eggs) and plant (legumes, nuts, seeds and soy products) sources;
- oils.

Again, fruits and vegetables, rich sources of polyphenols, are at the top of the list of the DGA. There is a convincing evidence of protective associations of participants' adherence to Mediterranean diet, to HEI and DASH with specific non-communicable diseases outcomes, including mortality, cardiovascular disease, type 2 diabetes, and total cancer (Miller *et al.*, 2020). Therefore, there is a growing scientific evidence that regular consumption of fruits and vegetables is beneficial for human health. It is noteworthy that recently the association between dietary patterns and changes in intrinsic capacity over 3 years in Japanese older adult has been studied and the results indicated that adherence to the 'fruits and vegetables' and 'protein-rich' (animal-based protein in particular) dietary patterns were associated with greater intrinsic capacity. In a great contrast, adherence to the 'sugar and fat' dietary pattern was associated with decreased intrinsic capacity. Similarly, in older adults from the Melbourne Collaborative Cohort Study with a 11.7-year of follow up, adherence to the 'fruit' pattern was positively associated with successful aging (Yeung *et al.*, 2021). However, there is no consensus on the nutrients obtained from fruits and vegetables, as a part of the diet responsible for health promotion. Initially it was suggested that vitamin E was responsible for health promoting properties of healthy diets, however, clinical trials did not confirm an idea that increased vitamin E consumption can improve health status. The same was true for carotenoids promotion as health-enhancing nutrients. Similar to vitamin E, carotenoids failed to prove their health-promoting properties in clinical trials. The next nutrients to be tested were polyphenolics and the last 20-30 years could be called a 'polyphenolic era'.

1.3 What are polyphenols?

Polyphenols constitute one of the most extensive groups of chemicals in the plant kingdom and more than 8,000 such compounds have been isolated and described. All these polyphenols are found in plants, esterified with glucose and other carbohydrates (glycosides), or as free aglycones. Polyphenols isolated from fruits, vegetables, green and black teas, herbs, roots, spices, propolis, beer and red wine are extensively researched for health-promoting potential (Szliszka and Krol, 2011). Numerous studies have demonstrated the beneficial effects of polyphenol-rich foods (Egert and Rimbach, 2011; McCullough *et al.*, 2012). Accumulating evidence indicates therapeutical potential of polyphenols as therapeutic agents that could help to alleviate the non-communicable diseases burden (Rana *et al.*, 2022). This includes protective effects of polyphenols in:

- cardiovascular diseases (Bachheti *et al.*, 2022; Bianchi *et al.*, 2022) including atherosclerosis (Zheng *et al.*, 2022) and Ischemic Stroke (Liu *et al.*, 2022);
- neurodegenerative diseases (Sahebnasagh *et al.*, 2022), including Alzheimer's Disease (Sharifi-Rad *et al.*, 2022);
- Type-2 diabetes mellitus (Chen *et al.*, 2022; Menezes *et al.*, 2022);
- metabolic syndrome (Wang *et al.*, 2022);
- oral diseases and infections (Cheng *et al.*, 2022);
- kidney diseases (Ashkar *et al.*, 2022);
- cancer (Hao *et al.*, 2022; Li *et al.*, 2022; Vladu *et al.*, 2022; Zheng *et al.*, 2022);
- aging (Lee *et al.*, 2022).

It was suggested that polyphenols play an important role in improving human (and animal) health, particularly gut health, via promoting the abundance of favourable bacteria and protozoa and suppressing harmful bacteria, exhibiting prebiotic activities (Santhiravel *et al.*, 2022). However, the molecular mechanisms of polyphenol effects on gut microbiota need further investigations (Si *et al.*, 2021), and available evidence does not support the modulating effects of polyphenols on of the gut microbiota as a main mechanism of their action (Freitas *et al.*, 2022).

However, positive associations between flavonoids intake and antioxidant defences *in vivo* (Duthie and Morrice, 2012) and human health (Jin *et al.*, 2012) are not always the case. There are two main basic questions related to polyphenols which urgently require answers. Firstly, it is necessary to understand processes of polyphenol absorption and metabolism in the body, including assessment of their availability and metabolism by gut microbiota. Generally speaking, most of polyphenolic compounds are poorly absorbed in the gut and their concentrations in the target tissues are comparatively low. Secondly, more research should be conducted to understand molecular mechanisms of polyphenol action in the biological system. Initially, antioxidant properties of flavonoids attracted a substantial attention and generated a range of publications. However, recent, more comprehensive, studies indicate that direct antioxidant properties of polyphenol compounds are not major players in their mode of action. Nevertheless, a range of flavonoid-based products have been developed and marketed for human and some feed additives were designed for animals including poultry. Even there were attempts in animal production to claim a possible replacement of traditional vitamin E supplementation with various plant extracts possessing antioxidant activities *in vitro* (Surai, 2014).

1.4 Antioxidant activities of polyphenols

Plant polyphenols can be divided into two major groups, flavonoids and non-flavonoids (Stagos *et al.*, 2012; Table 1.3; Figure 1.1).

Flavonoids make up the largest and the most important single group of polyphenols, and they share a common flavan core formed with 15 carbon atoms, and this class can be subdivided into several subgroups, including flavanols, flavonols, anthocyanidins, flavones, flavanones and isoflavonoids. However, laboratory and epidemiologic studies have focused on six flavonoid subgroups: flavones, flavonols, flavan-3-ols (catechins), procyanidins, flavanones and isoflavones (Theodoratou *et al.*, 2007). The non-flavonoids contain an aromatic ring with one or more hydroxyl group and are represented by stilbene, phenolic acids, saponin and some other polyphenols. In nature, polyphenols are synthesised by plants for their defence against infection and provide protective effects against stress such as ultraviolet light, pathogens and physical damage (Robbins, 2003). Polyphenols identified in some foods are shown in Table 1.4.

Table 1.3. A simplified classification of natural polyphenols (adapted from Surai, 2014).

Group	Class	Sub-class	Compounds
Flavonoids	Anthocyanins		aurantinidin, cyanidin, delphinidin, europinidin, luteolinidin, pelargonidin, malvidin, peonidin, petunidin, rosinidin, etc.
	Flavonols		3-hydroxyflavone, azaleatin, fisetin, galangin, gossypetin, kaempferide, kaempferol, isorhamnetin, morin, myricetin, natsudaidain, pachypodol, quercetin, rhamnazin, rhamnetin, etc.
	Flavones		apigenin, luteolin, tangeritin, chrysin, 6-hydroxyflavone, baicalein, scutellarein, wogonin, diosmin, flavoxate, etc.
	Flavanones		butin, eriodictyol, hesperetin, hesperidin, homoeriodictyol, isosakuranetin, naringenin, naringin, pinocembrin, poncirin, sakuranetin, sakuranin, sterubin, etc.
	Isoflavonoids	Isoflavones	genistein, daidzein, lonchocarpane, laxiflorane, etc.
		Isoflavanes	equol, etc.
	Flavanols	Monomers	catechin, epicatechin (EC), epigallocatechin (EGC), epicatechin gallate (ECG), epigallocatechin gallate (EGCG), epiafzelechin, fisetinidol, guibourtinidol, mesquitol, robinetinidol, etc.
		Oligomers and polymers	theaflavins, thearubigins, condensed tannins, proanthocyanidins etc.
Non-flavonoids	Phenolic acids	Derivatives of cinnamic acid	p-coumaric acid, caffeic acid, chlorogenic acid, ferulic acid, sinapic acid, etc.
		Derivatives of benzoic acid	gallic acid, gentisic acid, protocatechuic acid, syringic acid, vanillic acid, etc.
	Lignans		pinoresinol, podophyllotoxin, steganacin, etc.
	Stilbenes		resveratrol analogues, etc.

Initially, molecular mechanisms of polyphenol health-promoting properties were related to their antioxidant properties. This assumption seemed to be supported by numerous model studies *in vitro* (Andriantsitohaina *et al.*, 2012). Flavonoids can prevent injury caused by free radicals by the following mechanisms (Prochazkova *et al.*, 2011):

- direct scavenging of reactive oxygen species (ROS);
- activation of antioxidant enzymes;
- metal chelating activity;
- reduction of α-tocopheryl radicals;
- inhibition of oxidases;
- mitigation of oxidative stress caused by nitric oxide;
- increase in uric acid levels;
- increase in antioxidant properties of low molecular antioxidants.

However, despite the vast amount of research, the direct antioxidant effects have been questioned (Hu, 2011; Surai, 2014):

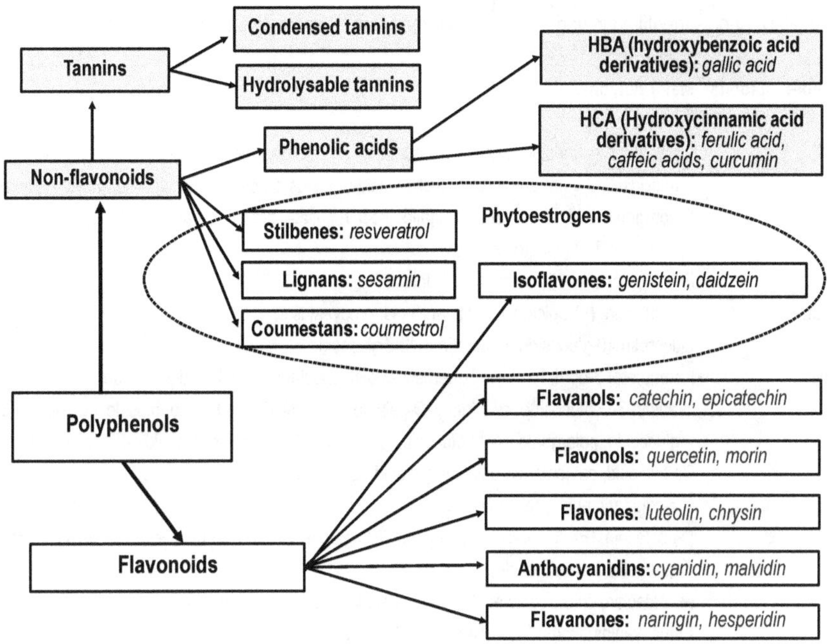

Figure 1.1. Polyphenol classification (adapted from Manach *et al.*, 2004; Si *et al.*, 2021; Surai, 2014; Vauzour, 2012).

1. Data with model systems cannot simply be translated to the *in vivo* situation (Schewe *et al.*, 2008). Many *in vitro*/cell culture studies on the antioxidant activity of phytochemicals employed relatively high concentrations (often in the 10-100 μM range) of the test compounds. It should be mentioned that the average concentration of most plant polyphenols in plasma rarely exceeds 1 μM in healthy subjects. For example, human plasma levels ranged from 0.072 to 5 μM when polyphenol intake ranged from 6.4 to 1,000 mg/day (Scalbert and Williamson, 2000), while catechin levels in plasma plateau at 1.0 and 0.3 μM after ingestion of five cups of green and black tea respectively (Skibola and Smith, 2000). Similarly, achievable plasma concentrations of resveratrol, curcumin, quercetin, genistein and daidzein were 2.15, 1.6, 1.5, 1.26 and 0.76 μM, respectively (Bisht *et al.*, 2010).
2. The effect of polyphenols in physiologically relevant concentrations would be relatively limited when taking into account concentrations of other antioxidants in plasma, including vitamin C (26.1-84.6 μM), vitamin E (20-30 μM), albumin and urate (several hundred μM) (Hu, 2011). Given a total antioxidant value in plasma of over 1,000 μM, a minimum concentration of 20-50 μM additional antioxidant from dietary sources would be required to make a significant contribution to systemic antioxidant capacity (Halliwell *et al.*, 2005). This is unlikely to occur, as even high intakes of dietary polyphenols typically result in unconjugated serum levels of up to 1 μM. Similar situation could be found in chickens where antioxidant

Table 1.4. Polyphenols identified in various foods (adapted from Bianchi *et al.*, 2022; Si *et al.*, 2021).

Polyphenol-rich foods	Major polyphenols in the food
Wine	Caffeic acid, caftaric acid, catechin, coumaric-O-hexoside, epicatechin, gallic acid, gentisic acid, malvidin 3-O-glucoside, protocatechuic acid-O-hexoside, protocatechuic acid, p-hydroxybenzoic acid
Green tea	Chlorogenic acid, epicatechin, epigallocatechin gallate, proanthocyanidin B2, quercetin-3-O-galactoside
Coffee	Flavonoids, phenolic acids, secoiridoids
Cocoa beans	(+)-catechin, (−)-epicatechin, flavan-3-ols, procyanidins
Onions	Quercetin-40-glucoside, quercetin-3,40-diglucoside
Cabbage	Kaempferol 3-di(tri, feruloyldi, quercetin-3-disinapoyl-triglucoside-7-diglucoside
Beans	cyanidin-3-O-glucoside, cyanidin-3-O-galactoside, cyanidin-3-O-sambubioside, delphinidin-3-O-glucoside, pelargonidin-3-O-glucoside, malvidin-3-O-glucoside, petunidin-3-O-glucoside
Barley	Caffeic acid, catechin, cereals, ellagic acid, ferulic acid, gallic acid, isoscoparin-2'-O-glucoside, p-coumaric acid, procyanidin B2
Nut	(+)-catechin, (−)-epicatechin, naringenin-7-O-glucoside, procatechuic acid, p-hydroxybenzoic acid, quercetin-3-O-rutinoside,
Apples	(+)-catechin, chlorogenic acid, (−)-epicatechin, procyanidin, quercetin,
Grape	Anthocyanins, flavan-3-ols, flavonols, stilbenes
Strawberry	Cyanidin, ellagic acid derivatives, glycosides of quercetin, kaempferol, taxifolin 3-O-arabinoside, peonidin, pelargonidin
Blueberry	Anthocyanins, flavonols, flavan-3-ols, resveratrol, phenolic acids
Cherry	Anthocyanins, hydroxycinnamic acids, flavonoids

concentrations in plasma are in the same range (vitamin C: 61-66 μM; Howard and Constamble, 1958; McKee *et al.*, 1997; vitamin E: 13-15 μM, Surai, 2002; and total antioxidant value in plasma could vary from 336.9 μM, Brenes *et al.*, 2008; up to 740-830 μM, Willemsen *et al.*, 2011).

3. It is still unclear whether polyphenols have any direct antioxidant effects *in vivo*, although they might be capable of exerting such effects within the gastrointestinal tract, where polyphenols may come into direct contact before absorption and metabolism (Surai, 2018; Surai and Fisinin, 2015, Surai *et al.*, 2004).
4. Although flavonoids display potent antioxidant activity *in vitro*, the bioactive forms of flavonoids *in vivo* are not those forms found in plants (i.e. flavonoid glycosides) due to their extensive biotransformation in the small intestine and hepatic metabolism on absorption (Prochazkova *et al.*, 2011). Therefore, metabolic modifications occurring *in vivo* may substantially influence the antioxidant activity of dietary flavonoids.
5. Flavonoids are typical xenobiotics for animals and humans, metabolised as such and rapidly removed from the circulation (Natella *et al.*, 2002).
6. In many cases of *in vitro* studies of polyphenols in cell cultures ROS production can occur by chemical reactions in the culture media with H_2O_2 generation in

cell culture media, giving false results on the flavonoid effects reflecting effects of degradation products, not intact polyphenols (Halliwell, 2014, 2018).

Emerging findings suggest a large number of potential mechanisms of action of polyphenols in preventing disease, which may be beyond their conventional antioxidant activities (Rodrigo *et al.*, 2011). Therefore, it seems likely that direct antioxidant activity is not a major mechanism for benefits of flavonoids on endothelial function, atherosclerosis and cardiovascular disease risk (Hodgson, 2008), as inhibition of atherosclerosis in animal models is not associated with substantial change in oxidative damage. On the other hand, there is consistent data indicating that flavonoids can enhance nitric oxide status and improve endothelial function, which may be, at least partly, responsible for benefits on cardiovascular health (Hodgson and Croft, 2010). In this regard, there is a shift in polyphenol-related research from testing their antioxidant activities to deeper understanding their molecular mechanisms of action including cell signalling and gene expression (Table 1.5).

1.5 Pro-oxidant properties of polyphenols

Chemical structure of various polyphenols indicates that they cannot only be considered purely as antioxidants, because under certain reaction conditions, they can also display pro-oxidant activity. The pro-oxidant properties of dietary polyphenols may result from several possible mechanisms such as:

- chemical instability;
- depletion of cellular glutathione;
- mobilisation of cellular copper ions (Hu, 2011).

Table 1.5. Paradigm shift in flavonoid research (adapted from Surai, 2014).

Concept	Current view	Traditional view
Flavonoids as radical scavengers	Minor, if at all relevant *in vivo*	Major action
Flavonoids as antioxidants	Yes, but in an indirect sense (inhibition of prooxidant enzymes such as NADPH oxidases, lipoxygenases and MPO)	Major action
Flavonoids as enzyme inhibitors	Few key enzymes, particularly NADPH oxidases and angiotensin-converting enzyme	Many enzymes
Target in cell metabolism	NO* metabolism	Lipid peroxidation
Target in NO metabolism	NO* loss ↓	NOS activity ↑
Role of flavonoid glucuronides	Transport metabolites in blood plasma to target cells	Urinary excretion products
Role of flavonoids in Nrf2 and NF-κB regulation	Main mechanism of protective action	Participates in transcription factor regulation

One common feature shared by several polyphenolic compounds is their sensitivity to auto-oxidation *in vitro* (Halliwell, 2007). The ability of dietary polyphenols to act as antioxidants or pro-oxidants under *in vitro* and *in vivo* conditions is dependent on a number of factors such as concentration, structure and the test system used.

It is well known that both Fe^{2+} and Cu^{+} perform Fenton-like reactions with H_2O_2, and polyphenol compounds containing metal binding catechol and gallol groups have very different activities, depending on the metal ion. Antioxidant activity is commonly observed for polyphenols in Fe^{2+}/H_2O_2 systems, while when testing polyphenols in $Cu+/H_2O_2$ systems, pro-oxidant activity is often observed from the interactions between polyphenols and copper (Perron and Brumaghim, 2009). For example, ferulic and caffeic acids are hydroxycinnamic acid derivatives widely distributed in plant-derived food products, and in Fenton reaction, they behave as pro-oxidants and the possible mechanisms responsible for their pro-oxidant properties may be related to their ferric reducing ability (Maurya and Devasagayam, 2010). Furthermore, any oxidised phenols (such as quinones and semiquinones) formed from phenolics during such redox reactions could also possibly be deleterious. In addition, some polyphenols are likely to act as pro-oxidants by forming quinones that participate in redox cycling (Bors *et al.*, 2000).

It has been shown that several polyphenols are able to bind both DNA and Cu^{2+} forming a ternary complex (Hadi *et al.*, 2007). A redox reaction of the polyphenols and Cu^{2+} in the ternary complex may occur leading to the reduction of Cu^{2+} to Cu^{+}, whose re-oxidation generates a variety of ROS. It was further confirmed that the polyphenol-Cu^{2+} system is capable of causing DNA degradation in cells such as lymphocytes, and polyphenols alone (in the absence of added copper) are also capable of causing DNA breakage in cells. It is worth mentioning that some polyphenol compounds may follow both a redox-cycling pathway and a radical-scavenging pathway, depending on polyphenol concentration (Perron *et al.*, 2011).

There is striking evidence for *in vivo* ROS formation in human lung cancer xenograft tissues after epigallocatechin-3-gallate treatment in mice (Li *et al.*, 2010). It is proven that pro-oxidant activities of various polyphenols in cancer cells are an important feature providing their anticancer effects. An important mechanism for flavonoid pro-oxidant toxicity involves the numerous peroxidases that catalyse the oxidation of polyphenols. For example, the oxidation of phenols by polyphenol oxidase produces extremely reactive free radical intermediates, and this may be associated with the pro-oxidant activity of polyphenols as a result of their tendency to auto-oxidation accompanied by the formation of ROS and H_2O_2 (Rodrigo *et al.*, 2011). In general, it was found that the effectiveness of flavonoids for catalysing the co-oxidation of ascorbate, NADH or GSH increased as their redox potential decreased (Galati *et al.*, 2002). Thus, the more readily oxidisable flavonoids were the most effective. In particular, it was shown that pro-oxidant properties of the flavonoids apigenin, naringenin and naringin related to the fact that their phenoxyl radicals rapidly co-oxidise glutathione or nicotinamide adenine dinucleotide, resulting in extensive oxygen uptake and superoxide radical formation (Galati *et al.*, 1999).

A substantial body of evidence on the pro-oxidant activity of polyphenol compounds has been accumulated. The pro-oxidant characteristic of polyphenols, related to their abilities to generate ROS, has been shown both in cell-free systems and in *in vitro* studies with cells. Reactive oxygen species have been detected in cell culture media and in phosphate buffers amended with polyphenols. For example, time-dependent generation and concentration-dependent generation of H_2O_2 were noted in Dulbecco's modified Eagle's medium amended with green tea, red wine, green tea polyphenol extract, black tea polyphenol extract, Ginkgo biloba extract, pomegranate extract, apple extract, epigallocatechin, epicatechin gallate, catechin gallate, theaflavin, theaflavin-3-monogallate, theaflavin-3-monogallate, theaflavin-3,3-digallate, chrysin, gallic acid and quercetin (Babich *et al.*, 2011; Schweigert *et al.*, 2001).

Pro-oxidant properties of polyphenols could be associated with cell signalling by which flavonoids contribute to the co-ordination of cell functions (Babich *et al.*, 2011). Depending on the scale, pro-oxidant effects can be beneficial; as by imposing a mild degree of oxidative stress, the levels of antioxidant defences and biotransformation enzymes might be raised, leading to overall cytoprotection (Halliwell, 2008). It has been suggested that a potential health benefit for the consumption of polyphenols at dietary levels is associated with boosting antioxidant defence systems by generating low levels of ROS and inducing mild oxidative stress causing an adaptive cellular response (Lambert *et al.*, 2010; Moskaug *et al.*, 2005). At the other end of the scale is a toxic effect of polyphenols in humans (Mazzanti *et al.*, 2009) and animals (Lambert *et al.*, 2010) as a result of their pro-oxidant properties.

1.6 Polyphenol effects in poultry and farm animals

Protective effects in growing chickens of grape and grape seed extracts, by-products of juice and wine production, have been studied by a group of researchers in Spain, and the results have been published in a series of papers from the same department. Firstly, an experiment was conducted to investigate the effect of inclusion of grape pomace (GP) at levels of 5, 15 and 30 g/kg and α-tocopheryl acetate (200 mg/kg) in a corn-soybean basal diet on chicken growth performance, feed digestibility and some antioxidant-related parameters in the body (Goni *et al.*, 2007). It has been shown that growth performance and protein and amino acid digestibility were not affected among the different treatments. Results also showed a linear reduction of lipid oxidation in breast and thigh meats at 4 and 7 days with increasing content of GP in the diet. This research was extended, and higher (60 g/kg) dose of GP was also tested (Brenes *et al.*, 2008). The authors concentrated on protective effects of grape concentrate on the lipid peroxidation in the chicken meat during storage and showed some benefits. Furthermore, in the paper data on total antioxidant activity of the diet and excreta were presented. For example, excreta total antioxidant activity increased from 74.7 μmol/g (control) up to 107.2 μmol/g (experimental group). However, they do not have any physiological significance, as to provide antioxidant protection in the body, an antioxidant component has to be located in a right place (e.g. in biological membranes, where peroxidation has a detrimental effect), in right concentration and in right time. Furthermore, it is surprising that the authors found increased antioxidant activity of the diet due to vitamin E supplementation [(6.29 vs 1.87 and 11.96 vs 8.63, Goni *et al.*, 2007) and (7.9 vs 4.0 and 4.0 vs 3.3, Brenes *et al.*, 2008)]. In the form of tocopherol acetate, vitamin E does not possess any antioxidant activity (Surai, 2002), this puts some doubts on validity of techniques used for the assessment of antioxidant activity in the studies.

Extracts obtained from grape seeds and pomace are complex in composition and contain monomeric phenolic compounds such as (+)-catechins, (-)-epicatechin and (-)-epicatechin-3-O-gallate, and dimeric, trimeric, and tetrameric proanthocyanidins (Saito *et al.*, 1998). It is obvious that the biological activity of these polyphenols depends on their bioavailability (Hervert-Hernandez *et al.*, 2009). It is generally accepted that the availability of phenolic compounds for human and animals is rather low. It is well known that antioxidant absorption, transport, metabolism and tissue distribution are of great importance for its protective effect (Surai, 2002). In this term, a conclusion from the paper of Brenes *et al.* (2008) that 'Grape pomace concentrate supplementation was as equal in antioxidant potential as vitamin E' sounds like a premature one. Similarly, a conclusion from the research conducted in the same lab that 'Grape pomace could be considered as a good alternative to α-tocopheryl acetate supplementation of feeds and to improve vitamin E status' (Goni *et al.*, 2007) is based just on meat stability during storage and some sparing effect of polyphenols on vitamin E level in the chicken liver is not scientifically sound for the same reason.

It is well known that vitamin E possesses membrane-stabilising effects (Surai, 1999; 2002; Surai *et al.*, 2019b) responsible for decreasing lipid peroxidation in the meat during storage. In aforementioned papers, polyphenols were not detected in tissues, and there was little research done to understand a mode of action of the grape extract at the cellular level. It is well known that lipid peroxidation in muscle depends on a range of factors, including amount and composition of lipids, composition and concentration of various natural antioxidants, activities of antioxidant enzymes and other enzymatic factors, concentration and distribution of iron and copper possessing pro-oxidant properties, etc. (Surai, 2018). None of those were studied in aforementioned papers where only final product of lipid peroxidation (MDA) and vitamin E concentration were determined. In another publication from the same lab, it was shown that GP inclusion into the chicken diet at 30 or 60 mg/kg was associated with decreased MDA accumulation in the raw and cooked meat during storage (Sayago-Ayerdi *et al.*, 2009).

It is important to note that in fresh meat or in the meat after 3- or 6-day storage, there was no effect of the dietary GP on lipid peroxidation. Only during longer meat storage (13 or 20 days), protective effect of dietary GB was observed. The authors suggested that polyphenols could be accumulated in tissues and provide antioxidant protection similar to vitamin E. It seems a very speculative suggestion as there are no data on polyphenol content of the meat and, generally speaking, polyphenols are not well absorbed and even if found in muscles, the active concentrations would be much lower than those providing antioxidant protection. It could well be that chelating properties of polyphenols would be responsible for changes in Fe and Cu content of the muscles leading to decrease MDA production. Therefore, mechanisms of protective effects of GP against MDA accumulation in muscles could be completely different from those described for vitamin E. It should be also mentioned that changes in total antioxidant potential of the meat extract due to dietary GP supplementation probably reflect many different changes in meat composition and without additional analysis, it is impossible to explain molecular mechanisms of protective effects of dietary polyphenols.

Relationship between polyphenols and vitamin E is not straightforward and it could well be that phenolics affect vitamin redistribution between tissues and plasma. For example, it has been shown that while mouse groups receiving grape extract, either isolated or in association with α-tocopherol, presented higher vitamin E serum levels, and their hepatic content of this vitamin was significantly lower in relation to control group (Peluzio Mdo *et al.*, 2011). To develop this point further, it would be interesting to analyse some results on effects of polyphenolic extracts in animals. For example, it has been shown that the grape extract treatment of mice did not alter the serum and liver levels of polyphenols (Peluzio Mdo *et al.*, 2011). It has also been shown that inclusion of Camelina meal at 2.5%, 5% and 10% increased phenolic compounds in the diet by 28.4, 31.7 and 46.4% (Aziza *et al.*, 2010a,b). However, those phenolics most likely were not transferred to the muscles because total phenolic compounds concentrations in breast and thigh muscles did not change and total flavonoid concentrations significantly decreased.

Therefore, protective effects of the experimental diets against lipid peroxidation in the stored breast and thigh muscles are probably polyphenol-independent. It seems likely that Camelina meal, similar to other plant extracts, at high levels of inclusion possesses some toxic effects. For example, for the first 21 days, FCR in birds significantly improved (from 1.83 in the control birds down to 1.71; 1.62 and 1.53, respectively, for 2.5; 5% and 10% Camelina meal consumption) (Aziza *et al.*, 2010a). However, during 22-42 days of age, FCR dramatically increased due to Camelina meal consumption (from 1.67 in the control group up to 1.95; 1.91 and 2.0 respectively). Impaired feed conversion and decreased feed intake during the starter phase in birds fed Camelina cake or Camelina meal have been reported by Ryhanen *et al.* (2007) and Pekel *et al.* (2009).

Additional findings suggest that the grape pomace extract does not behave the same way *in vitro* and *in vivo* (Veskoukis *et al.*, 2012). The tested grape extract exhibited potent *in vitro* antioxidant properties because it scavenged the DPPH(•) and ABTS(•+) radicals and inhibited DNA damage induced by peroxyl and hydroxyl radicals. However, administration of the extract in rats generally had a detrimental effect inducing oxidative stress at rest and after exercise, whereas exercise performance was not affected. Similarly, consuming artichoke leaf extract, a natural vegetable preparation of high antioxidant potential, resulted in higher plasma total antioxidant potential than placebo but did not limit oxidative damage to erythrocytes in competitive rowers subjected to strenuous training (Skarpanska-Stejnborn *et al.*, 2008). In addition, supplementation with Rhodiola rosea extract increased total antioxidant potential in the plasma of professional rowers but had no effect on oxidative damage induced by exhaustive exercise (Skarpanska-Stejnborn *et al.*, 2009).

Despite the high antioxidant capacity of individual apple polyphenols and apple extracts and the significant antioxidant effects of apple extract added to human plasma *in vitro*, ingestion of large amounts of apples by humans does not appear to result in equivalent *in vivo* antioxidant effects of apple polyphenols (Lotito and Frei, 2004). Irrespective to antioxidant efficacy *in vitro*, black tea does not protect plasma from lipid peroxidation *in vivo* (Cherubini *et al.*, 1999). Dietary supplementation of growing pigs with green tea polyphenols did not affect serum, liver, lung and muscle vitamin E concentrations, plasma antioxidant capacity or parameters of meat quality including meat temperature, pH, conductivity, colour and drip loss (Augustin *et al.*, 2008). It was concluded that supplementation of pig diets with green tea catechins was not associated with improved antioxidant status and meat quality under commercial conditions.

The striking discrepancy between the *in vitro* and *ex vivo* data is most likely explained by the insufficient bioavailability of polyphenols in humans and animals. Grape extracts are not always effective in decreasing lipid peroxidation in tissues. For example, grape seed extract (GSE) supplementation has limited protective effect in liver tissue of diabetic rats (Belviranli *et al.*, 2012). MDA levels decreased with GSE supplementation in control rats but increased in acute and chronic exercise groups compared with their non-supplemented control. Therefore, GSE has a limited antioxidant effect on exercise-induced oxidative stress in liver tissue. Dietary GSE did not improve oxidative stress in mice as determined by plasma antioxidant potential, glutathione peroxidase and liver lipid peroxidation (Hogan *et al.*, 2010). Natural tocopherols, rosemary, green tea, grape seed and tomato extracts were supplemented singly and in combinations at total concentrations of 100 and 200 mg/kg of feed in a 4% linseed oil-containing diet to investigate the oxidative stability of broiler breast muscle (Smet *et al.*, 2008).

Grape seed extract supplemented at 100 mg/kg showed worse results in comparison with other treatments. Unfortunately, the author did not use any control samples without inclusion of specific antioxidants into the diet, and it is impossible to judge whether there were any protective effects of extracts at the dosage of 100 mg/kg, while lipid peroxidation in the meat was lower in samples obtained from animals fed on 200 mg/kg plant extracts. However, it is not clear from the study whether the protective effect of the plant extracts was directly related to their antioxidant properties or mediated via other mechanisms of action. It is interesting to note that in a later paper by the same group of authors (Vossen *et al.*, 2011), there was no effect of plant extracts on lipid peroxidation index (TBARS) in broiler plasma. These data support the idea that protective effect of dietary plant extract on meat oxidation was an indirect one.

In general, stabilising effect of plant extracts or individual polyphenols is not consistent. For example, the effects of dietary tea catechins (TC) supplementation at levels of 50, 100, 200 and 300 mg/kg feed on susceptibility of chicken breast meat, thigh meat, liver and heart to iron-induced lipid oxidation were investigated (Tang *et al.*, 2000). Tea catechins supplementation at all levels exerted antioxidative effects for all tissues with the exception of 50 mg/kg feed for breast meat, where pro-oxidant action of TC was observed. Similarly, dietary oregano essential oil supplementation also exerted antioxidative effects, the supplementation being most effective in retarding lipid oxidation in stored raw and cooked chicken meat at the 100 mg oregano essential oil/kg feed (Botsoglou *et al.*, 2002).

There were some protective effects of dietary TC against lipid peroxidation in pig meat (Mason *et al.*, 2005). However, dietary rosemary extract failed to show an antioxidative protective effect in pork (Haak *et al.*, 2008). An attempt to increase oxidative stability of beef by dietary supplementation of TC or rosemary extract was not successful (O'Grady *et al.*, 2006). In contrast, adding various extracts to the ground meat *in vitro* is proven to be more effective. For example, the control samples showed significantly higher TBARS and hexanal content over beef storage. Butylated hydroxyanisole (BHA)/butylated hydroxytoluene (BHT), grape seed extract, pine bark extract and oleoresin rosemary retarded the formation of TBARS by 75%, 92%, 94% and 92%, respectively, after 9 days, and significantly lowered the hexanal content throughout the storage period (Ahn *et al.*, 2007).

Recently several review papers devoted to effects of polyphenols on poultry have been published. In particular, Akbarian *et al.* (2016) summarised data (16 papers) on the effects of dietary polyphenols on antioxidant systems of poultry under heat stress conditions. Positive effects of epigallocatechin-3-gallate, genistein, resveratrol, Curcuma xanthorrhiza essential oil, ginger essential oil, Oreganum compactum essential oil, grape seed extract, lemon peel extract, orange peel extract, extract from dried fruits of Forsythia suspensa, Brahma Rasayana extract, ethanol extract of propolis, polyphenols extracted from Tamarindus indica seed coat, Berberis vulgaris root extract, cashew nut shell liquid, Ayurvedic polyherbal preparation, Schisandra chinensis and Ligustrum lucidum, dry powdered leaves of Mentha longifolia, polyherbal mix Stresroak (fruits and leaves from different herbs) and ginger root powder were shown. The aforementioned polyphenol sources in the diets of heat-stressed broiler chickens, laying hens and quails demonstrated ameliorating/protective effects on enzymatic AO (SOD, GPx, CAT, GR), non-enzymatic AO (GSH, vitamin E and ascorbic acid) and decreased lipid peroxidation (MDA) in various tissues (Akbarian *et al.*, 2016).

Polyphenols as potential attenuators of heat stress in poultry production were summarised by Hu *et al.* (2019) demonstrating protective effects of resveratrol, curcumin and epigallocatechin gallate on only on antioxidant defence system but also partly preventing deteriorating effects of heat stress on chicken performance, including growth rate and FCR. Furthermore, immunomodulating effects of various polyphenols in poultry have been reviewed by Lee *et al.* (2019) with a specific emphasis on effects of polyphenols on Nrf2 and NF-κB and showing some positive, but not conclusive, results. Furthermore, another recent review presented an analysis of data related to a range of flavonoids (kaempferol, hesperidin, genistein, naringin, curcumin, baicalein, soybean isoflavone, mix of flavonoids containing quercetin &catechin, citrus flavonoids with 50:50 of quercetin: rutin, alfalfa flavonoids, hawthorn flavonoid and bamboo leaf extract) in relation to poultry nutrition published in 15 papers (Rafiei and Khajali, 2021).

Again, mostly biochemical changes associated with the antioxidant defence network were shown with only few parameters relative to poultry production (reduced incidence of chicken muscular dystrophy and reduced incidence of chicken pulmonary hypertension syndrome) were improved by flavonoid dietary supplementation. Finally, recent review summarising the role of polyphenols (curcumin, nano-curcumin, resveratrol, quercetin, epigallocatechin gallate, turmeric rhizome extract, polyphenol extract from *Terminalia chebula Retz. and Punica granatum L*), in poultry (broiler chickens, laying hens and quails) nutrition was based on analysis of 12 papers (Abdel-Moneim *et al.*, 2020). The authors pointed out that beyond their beneficial effects, polyphenols could also have detrimental impacts on gut health, nutrient digestibility, and absorption of some vitamins and minerals and further research is required to shed light on their molecular mechanisms of action.

A recent review devoted to polyphenols in layer nutrition also indicated that supplementing polyphenols in optimal doses to a layer diet can improve egg production as well as external and internal egg quality (Abd El-Hack *et al.*, 2023). The authors underlined that, excessive dietary polyphenol levels could have detrimental effects on birds leading to compromised egg production and decrease egg quality. In spite of a great progress in studies devoted to polyphenols in poultry/animal nutrition, the connection between health-promoting effects of polyphenols in *in vitro* models and protective effects of these phytochemicals in poultry/animal health are unclear, and somehow understudied in poultry and other farm animals compared to lab animals and humans (Scott *et al.*, 2022).

1.7 Polyphenols vs vitamin E

The main reason for vitamin E dietary supplementation for poultry and farm animals is to maintain their optimal health and high productive and reproductive performances. It includes positive effects of vitamin E on male (Surai, 1999; Surai *et al.*, 2019b) and female (Surai, 2002; Surai *et al.*, 2019b) reproduction, immunocompetence (Surai, 2002), effective growth and development (McIlroy *et al.*, 1993), high quality of eggs and meat (Surai and Fisinin, 2010; Surai and Sparks, 2001), decreased negative consequences of various stresses (Surai and Fisinin, 2012), etc. Extensive research and wide commercial application for a number of years clearly showed essentiality of vitamin E in animal/poultry nutrition.

When the idea of replacement of vitamin E by various other products, including polyphenols, is considered, it is necessary to take into account a range of physiological and biochemical functions played by these compounds. A comparison of vitamin E and polyphenol activities in animals/poultry is shown in Table 1.6.

From the analysis presented above, it is clear that these two groups of biologically active compounds are quite different in their efficacy and mode of action. There is no sufficient evidence to indicate that polyphenols can replace vitamin E in its main biological functions.

For example, some data indicating positive effects of grape extracts on meat quality are not comprehensive enough to justify such a replacement, as meat quality is only one from many important vitamin E-related issues in poultry production.

The concept of the total antioxidant system of the body (Surai, 2002; 2006; 2020a,b; 2022; Surai and Earle-Payne, 2022; Surai *et al.*, 2019a; 2021a,b) combines all the antioxidant compounds of the cell/tissue in such a way that they are effectively interacting with each other, providing an effective antioxidant defence. In this system,

Table 1.6. Comparison of the mode of action of vitamin E and polyphenols (adapted from Surai, 2014).

Action	Vitamin E	Plant extracts (Polyphenols)
Composition	4 tocopherols and 4 tocotrienols, tocopherol-acetate is a supplemental form	Thousands of various compounds with variation in composition
Absorption	Well defined absorption in the small intestine	Poorly absorbed
Metabolic transformation within tissues	Alpha-tocopherol is an active form of vitamin E after dietary supplementation	Quickly transformed to various metabolites
Delivery to target tissues	Effectively delivered to the target tissues	Tissue concentrations are negligible
Effect on nutrient digestion	Improves digestion of many nutrients	Decrease digestion of many nutrients including protein and lipids
Specific effects on sperm function	Positive effect on male reproduction	There are no proven effects on male reproduction
Specific effects on egg/ova and female reproduction	Positive effect on female reproduction	There are no proven effects on female reproduction
Specific effects on immunity	Positive (protective) effects on the immunocompetence	Effects on the immunocompetence is not consistent
Antioxidant properties	Main chain-breaking biological antioxidant	Depending on conditions can be antioxidant or prooxidant
Toxicity	Low toxicity when consumed in excess	Could be toxic at high consumption

vitamin E has a special role being located in the biological membranes, a place where lipid peroxidation takes place. Other compounds of the antioxidant system, including polyphenols, can help vitamin E be effective by its recycling or decreasing free radical load. It seems likely that the gut is the major place of antioxidant action of polyphenols (Surai and Fisinin, 2015; Surai *et al.*, 2004; 2018).

Generally, reduction of oxidative damage, modulation of colonic flora and variation in gene expression are involved in the modulation of intestinal function by polyphenols. For example, to study the molecular effects of wine polyphenols at the gene level, the microarray technology was used: rats were treated with 50 mg/kg wine polyphenols for 14 days, mixed in the diet. Global expression analysis of 5,707 genes revealed an extensive downregulation of genes involved in a wide range of physiological functions, such as metabolism, transport, signal transduction and intercellular signalling (Dolara *et al.*, 2005). It was shown that two major regulatory pathways were downregulated in the colon mucosa of polyphenol-treated rats: inflammatory response and steroid metabolism. Polyphenols target multiple inflammatory components and reinforce anti-inflammatory mechanisms leading to NF-κB, AP-1, HIF, and STAT suppression with reduced proinflammatory mediator generation (Chu, 2014).

It seems likely that non-antioxidant functions of vitamin E are also of great importance for maintaining physiological and biochemical homoeostasis in the cell (Azzi, 2007; 2018; 2021; Han *et al.*, 2010; Miyazawa *et al.*, 2019; Muyrers *et al.*, 2010; Pedeboscq *et al.*, 2012; Ungurianu *et al.*, 2021; Vieira-Filho *et al.*, 2011; Zingg *et al.*, 2010; 2012) and they cannot be performed by other compounds, including polyphenols. After 100 years of extensive research in the field of vitamin E, we greatly appreciate its unique role in biological systems, in maintaining growth, development and general health of human and animals. Therefore, a conclusion from a recent paper 'Plant feed additives (PFA) as natural alternatives to the use of synthetic antioxidant vitamins on yield, quality, and oxidative status of poultry products: A review of the literature of the last 20 years' by Pitino *et al.* (2021) indicated that 'the PFA effects were, in general, less pronounced than the vitamin E ones in poultry products' confirmed the aforementioned suggestions.

In the last decade, studies have attempted to understand the molecular mechanism involved in polyphenol/flavonoids action. Besides scavenging free radicals, many phenolics also exhibit multiple biological properties, for example, anti-inflammatory, anticancer, antiviral, antimicrobial, vasorelaxant and anticlotting activities (Rahman *et al.*, 2007), hepatoprotective activities, prevention of cardiovascular diseases and antitumoral effect (Sies, 2010), as well as anti-protozoans, antiulcer and gastroprotective actions, neuroprotective and antidiabetic properties (Tripoli *et al.*, 2007). Therefore, polyphenols might exert several other specific biological effects beyond their direct antioxidant-pro-oxidant activities. This includes:

- the inhibition of activities of different enzymes, among which telomerase, cyclooxygenase, lipoxygenase; and

- the interaction with signal transduction pathways and cell receptors, affecting caspase-dependent pathways, cell cycle regulation and platelet functions (D'Archivio *et al.*, 2007; Visioli *et al.*, 2011).

Many natural polyphenols affect transcription factor expression/activities, including Nrf2 and NF-κB (Chauhan *et al.*, 2022; Hussain *et al.*, 2022; Yu *et al.*, 2022; Zhou *et al.*, 2019) by:

- regulating the production of ROS;
- affecting Nrf2/NF-κB nuclear translocation;
- affecting DNA binding ability;
- interfering with Keap1-Nrf2 or IκB/NF-κB interaction;
- promoting Keap1 ubiquitination.

In general, major mechanisms of polyphenol protective action against oxidative stress can be summarised as follows (Figure 1.2):

Polyphenols can activate the Nrf2, SIRT1 and inhibit NF-κB, RONS-producing enzymes and RONS production in the mitochondria, thereby enhancing cellular antioxidant defence system First of all, polyphenols can upregulate Nrf2 (Hussain *et al.*, 2017; Nabavi *et al.*, 2016; Pawlowska *et al.*, 2019; Truong *et al.*, 2018; Xing *et al.*, 2020; Zhang *et al.*, 2018; Zhou *et al.*, 2019). This upregulation leads to activation of various protective genes and synthesis of more than 200 antioxidant-related

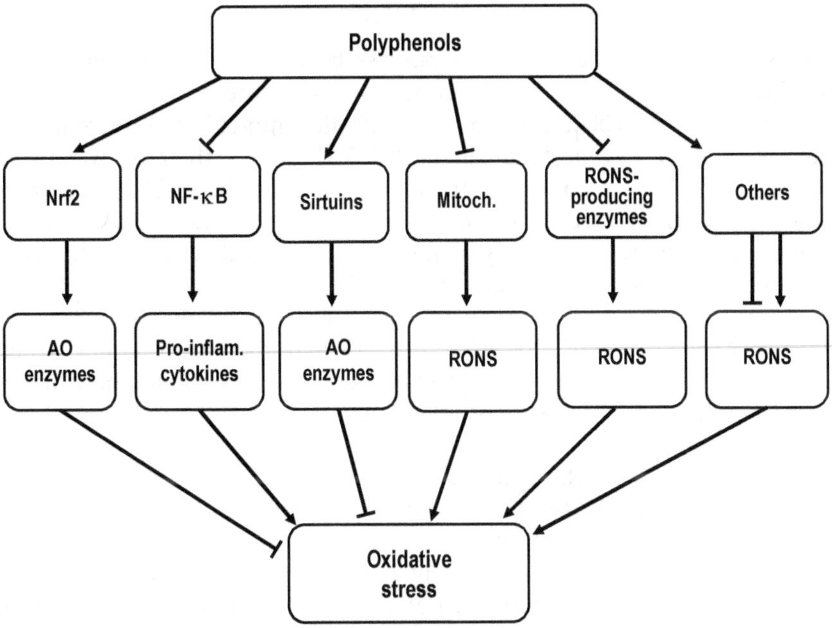

Figure 1.2. Possible protective effects of polyphenols against oxidative stress in animals/poultry. Mitoch = mitochondria; pro-inflam = pro-inflammatory.

compounds which can help decreasing oxidative stress. Secondly, polyphenols can downregulate NF-κB (da Cunha *et al.*, 2019; Liu *et al.*, 2016; Rahman *et al.*, 2018; Serra *et al.*, 2018; Xing *et al.*, 2020; Zhang *et al.*, 2014).

Decreased NF-κB expression and activity are responsible for reduced production of pro-inflammatory cytokines and decreased oxidative stress. It is known that resveratrol is an important activator of SIRT1 (Dai *et al.*, 2018). Furthermore, other polyphenolic compounds, including flavonoids are also considered to have SIRT-activating properties (Sarubbo *et al.*, 2018). Taking into account an important role of SIRTs in regulation of antioxidant enzymes, transcription factors and other elements of the antioxidant defence network (Surai *et al.*, 2021a), SIRT-activating properties of polyphenols is of great importance in oxidative stress prevention and management. Polyphenols are shown to inhibit mitochondrial generation of ROS (Lagoa *et al.*, 2022) and to improve mitochondrial biogenesis (Zielinska-Blizniewska *et al.*, 2019) substantially contributing to decreased RONS production and reduced oxidative stress. Interestingly, polyphenols can inhibit specific enzymes producing RONS, including NADPH oxidase, xanthine oxidase, nitric oxide synthase and p450 cytochromes (Fraga *et al.*, 2018; Mu *et al.*, 2019; Yahfoufi *et al.*, 2018). This could be a vital part of protection against RONS overproduction and oxidative stress. There are also various additional mechanisms of decreasing oxidative stress by polyphenols, including metal (Fe and Cu) chelating and preventing their catalytic role in the RONS formation (Mu *et al.*, 2019; Zielinska-Blizniewska *et al.*, 2019), direct scavenging free radicals in the gut (Surai *et al.*, 2004) and regulation of other stress factors (HSF1) and vitagenes (Surai, 2020b).

Flavonoids are generally accepted to possess potent antioxidant and antiradical activities. This is proven under *in vitro* conditions when these compounds are used in concentrations over 10-100 μM. However, *in vivo* flavonoid plasma concentrations are much lower and only in some cases can reach 1-5 μM, due to their low water solubility and bioavailability (Kren, 2021) and metabolic changes (Surai, 2014). Furthermore, it should be taken into account that measures *in vitro* antioxidant capacity of phytochemicals is an index reflecting their sensitivity to oxidation rather than an index of AO activity. However, there is a range of biological effects of flavonoids observed *in vivo* (Kren, 2021; Surai, 2014). This paradox could be explained by the concept of para-hormesis (Forman *et al.*, 2014; Kren, 2021), hypothesising that phytochemicals could act as weak pro-oxidants to activate Nrf2, responsible for synthesis of an array of protective molecules possessing AO activities.

Therefore, it seems likely that phytochemicals including silymarin do not act *in vivo* as direct antioxidants, but they improve AO defences indirectly, via affecting transcription factors including activation of Nrf2 (Surai *et al.*, 2019a) and suppression of NF-κB (Surai *et al.*, 2021b). In a recent review summarising beneficial effects of polyphenols in health and diseases (Yu *et al.*, 2022) it was clearly showed that the intestinal anti-inflammatory properties of more than 20 polyphenols were associated with modulation/inhibition of the Toll-like receptor (TLR4)/NF-κB-mediated signalling pathway.

1.8 Detrimental effects of polyphenols

Irrespective of a great deal of information claiming health-promoting properties of various polyphenols, it should be mentioned that not all flavonoids are necessarily beneficial, and their physiological effects depend on a range factors including type, concentration, absorption and metabolic transformation, etc. Indeed, the dual role of these substances by producing either toxic or beneficial effects seems also to depend on doses and/or the experimental cell type (Hodek *et al.*, 2002). It should be mentioned that in some aforementioned studies, the authors did not pay much attention to the detrimental consequences of grape extract feeding. In particular, decrease chicken weight gain (by 68 g) and increase FCR (1.79 vs 1.74), while vitamin E supplementation improved FCR (1.69 vs1.74). Furthermore, inclusion GPC into the chicken diet decreased fat digestibility (P<0.05, at 60 g/kg), while vitamin E supplementation improved fat digestibility (86.2 vs 84.53, P<0.05) (Brenes *et al.*, 2008).

In other studies, it has been observed that condensed tannins could bind biliary salts, a limiting factor for efficient fat digestion in poultry (Krogdahl, 1985), with a concomitant reduction in their absorption and an increase in the faecal excretion in mice (Roy and Schneeman, 1981). Another mechanism whereby nutrients are rendered less digestible by polyphenols is through the inactivation of digestive enzymes. For example, proanthocyanidin extracts from bean greatly inhibited digestive enzymes (trypsin, α-amylase and lipase) in young chicks (Longstaff and McNab, 1991). Moreno *et al.* (2003) also demonstrated *in vitro* the inhibitory effects of grape seed extract on fat-metabolizing enzymes and lipoprotein lipase. There is some evidence to show that polyphenols can inhibit a range of enzymes including α-glucosidase and pancreatic lipase (You *et al.*, 2011), α-amylase and α-glucosidase activity (McDougall *et al.*, 2005; Yilmazer-Musa *et al.*, 2012). The inhibition of digestive enzymes may be explained with the ability of condensed tannins to form insoluble complexes with proteins in the gastrointestinal tract (Griffiths, 1986; Horigome *et al.*, 1988). Binding of polyphenolic compounds to both dietary and endogenous protein, such as digestive enzymes and proteins located at the luminal side of the intestinal tract, could be a reason of the reduced apparent digestibility of protein in polyphenol-containing diets. Polyphenols can form complexes with protein due to the interaction of their reactive hydroxyl groups with the carbonyl group of protein. As a consequence of this complexation, protein and amino acid digestibility were reduced by the inclusion in chicken and pig diets of sorghum and faba bean polyphenols (Jansman *et al.*, 1993; Ortiz *et al.*, 1993). Some polyphenolic compounds can also reduce the absorption of iron, and possibly other trace metals, when included in a diet. For example, grape seed extract inhibited Zn absorption (Kim *et al.*, 2011) or haeme iron absorption in a dose-dependent manner (Ma *et al.*, 2010; 2011), altered microbial protein fermentation and/or amino acid metabolism in human (Jacobs *et al.*, 2012), glucose uptake by intestinal cells (Johnston *et al.*, 2005) or folic acid absorption (Lemos *et al.*, 2007).

In general, effect of polyphenol compounds on absorption and assimilation of different nutrients depends on many different factors including type of compounds, its dosage, combination with other compounds, etc. (Martel *et al.*, 2010). The pronounced and significant growth depression was observed with the use of a grape seed extract reported by Hughes *et al.* (2005) and Lau and King (2003). In general, relatively high dietary concentrations of polyphenols in various diets reduced performance in chickens as well as other livestock (Jansman *et al.*, 1993; Nyachotti *et al.*, 1997). While most flavonoids/phenolics at food/feed derived levels are considered safe, inclusion into the diet flavonoid/phenolics-based additives needs to be carefully assessed as there have been reports of toxic flavonoid-drug interactions, liver failure, contact dermatitis, haemolytic anaemia and oestrogenic-related concerns such as male reproductive health and breast cancer associated with dietary flavonoid/phenolic consumption or exposures (Galati and O'Brien, 2004; Mennen *et al.*, 2005).

Hazards, risks and safety of high consumption of polyphenols should always be seriously considered. In particular, Ebrahimi and Schluesener (2012) presented a range of references to the toxic effects of high doses of polyphenols, which showed that quercetin consumption is associated with chronic nephropathy in rats and reduced mice life expectancy, while green tea polyphenols disrupted kidney function in mice and enhanced tumour development in the colon of male rats. Similarly, caffeic acid induced gastrointestinal and kidney tumours in rats and mice. Other side effects of high consumption of polyphenols include thyroid toxicity, malnutrition, oestrogenic activity and compromised infertility. Furthermore, flavonoids could inhibit the absorption of some nutrients, interact with certain drug pharmacokinetics and affect neurobehavioral development (Surai, 2014). However, to date the *in vivo* safety of high doses polyphenols to much extent remains unknown (Cladis *et al.*, 2022).

The intake of polyphenolic (phytoestrogens) that can mimic estrogen function can induce various pathological conditions in the cow female reproductive tract, including ovarian, fallopian, and uterine dysfunction. Furthermore, the metabolism of genistein and daidzein is shown to yield the metabolites equol and p-phenyl-phenol which can compromise cow fertilisation (Bešlo *et al.*, 2022). Similarly, from the summary of recent *in vivo* studies on the effects of polyphenols on the reproductive performance of males and females of farm animals it is clear that animals (rabbits, lambs, goat bucks, boar) consuming diets based on seeds and/or forage with polyphenolic compounds (isoflavones and lignans) were characterised by substantial reproductive disturbances in sexual activity, hormonal balance and gonads function (Hashem *et al.*, 2020).

Grape seed extract (GSE; 7.2 g/kg) in the broiler diets was shown to decrease villi height: crypt depth ratio and significantly decreased weight gain (Viveros *et al.*, 2011). Similarly, GSE (5 g/kg) was reported to compromise weight gain and feed conversion, apparent ileal digestibility of protein with a significant decrease in the concentrations of plasma copper, iron and zinc (Chamorro *et al.*, 2013). Maternal GSE supplementation in breeder hens was found to affect the fertility of the offspring in a sex-specific manner in subsequent generations indicative by decreased semen quality in males of the F1 generation Furthermore, F1-GSE was characterised by a delay in puberty onset and, the number of yellow follicles measurable at 26 weeks of age was markedly lower in F1-GSE than in controls. In addition, offspring (F2) of the

GSE group (F1) were shown to be smaller than control (F2) offspring, reflecting a transgenerational effect (Grandhaye *et al.*, 2021).

Dietary supplementation of grape proanthocyanidins (30 mg/kg) was shown to detrimentally affect the blood biochemical biomarkers in broiler chicks, as evidenced by increased alkaline phosphatase and creatinine content by day 21 and increased alanine aminotransferase by day 42 in plasma (Yang *et al.*, 2017). Similarly, chicken growth performance was indicated to be depressed due to inclusion into the diet of fermented and unfermented grape skin at 30 g/kg and 60 g/kg (Nardoia *et al.*, 2020). It was also suggested that excessive polyphenol levels in the layer diet could have negative impact on gastrointestinal tract health, digestive enzyme activity, nutrient digestion, vitamin and mineral absorption leading to decreased laying hens performance and egg quality (Abd El-Hack *et al.*, 2023).

Clearly, taking into account possible detrimental effects of polyphenols and their unpredicted behaviour in the body depending on the conditions (antioxidant vs pro-oxidant, mutagen vs antimutagen, etc.), a caution should be given for their inclusion into the diet, before more detailed information is available on their absorption and assimilation, pharmacokinetics and metabolic fate in the body and molecular mechanisms of their action. Therefore, there is a need for further research in this exciting area.

1.9 Conclusions

In a search for an ideal human diet, it was identified that vegetables and fruit contain high concentrations of polyphenolic compounds, which could be responsible for their health-promoting properties. Therefore, for the last 30 years polyphenols, including various flavonoids were in a centre of research work of many labs worldwide. Analysis of resent publications in this area indicates that:

1. Antioxidant properties of polyphenols/flavonoids observed in *in vitro* model systems are convincing and, in some cases, polyphenols could be even more effective than traditional biological antioxidants, including vitamins E and C.
2. Antioxidant activities of polyphenols/flavonoids in *in vivo* biological systems are not straightforward and depend on a variety factors including:
   - efficiency of absorption, which is generally low;
   - active concentrations in the target tissues, which are extremely low;
   - metabolic transformation after absorption which could diminish their antioxidant properties and clearly needs more research;
   - surrounding environments that determine whether polyphenols show antioxidant or prooxidant properties;
   - effect on various signalling mechanisms, including vita-gene expression.
3. Non-antioxidant activities of polyphenols/flavonoids seem to be more important and biologically relevant than their antioxidant activities but need more research.
4. Attempts to replace vitamin E in the animal diet with various plant extracts are premature and have no scientific base to fully substantiate the claims.

5. Effects of polyphenols/flavonoids on the gut antioxidant-pro-oxidant balance and gut health in general need further research.
6. Detrimental effects of polyphenols/flavonoids, including inhibitory effects on various enzymes, interference with absorption of some minerals (Zn, Cu. Fe) and vitamins need more attention and additional research.
7. Polyphenols/flavonoids research is an exciting area promising many discoveries in future.

It seems likely that polyphenols can be considered as natural enhancers of the antioxidant defence systems in human and animals/poultry. Their protective effect against oxidative stress is most likely indirect and mediated by various mechanisms where they show mild pro-oxidant, rather than antioxidant effects. The only place where polyphenols can show direct RONS scavenging is gut, but there is a need for more research in this area. It seems likely that polyphenols can alert the antioxidant defence network by imposing mild oxidative stress. In such conditions activation of stress response pathways, transcription factors and vitagenes could improve adaptive ability of human/animals to various stresses. This hormetic actions of polyphenolics are condition-dependent and could have protective or detrimental effects and the exciting area of polyphenolics awaits further research.

There is abundant data obtained from laboratory and farm animal models related to the biological and pharmacological effects of various plant extracts containing high concentrations of polyphenols (Olivares-Vicente *et al.*, 2018). However, there are several important points which to some extent restrict wide usage of polyphenol-rich plant extracts in medical practise and animal/poultry nutrition:

1. It is impossible to guarantee the composition of the extract. Flavonoid/polyphenol concentration and composition would depend on many factors including conditions of plant growth (soil composition, fertilisation, temperature, humidity, etc.), extraction procedure, extract storage conditions, etc.
2. Main polyphenols in plant extracts are characterised, but there could be many other undetected and uncharacterised compounds possessing biological activities.
3. Low bioavailability of most polyphenols makes it difficult to explain molecular mechanisms of their biological activity.
4. Most *in vitro* research showing various benefits of polyphenolic compounds used their concentrations which much higher those achievable in biological tissues.
5. Polyphenol interactions with other nutrients and drugs are not fully addressed at the moment and need more attention.
6. Clearly there is a need for further research in this exciting area.

In the next chapters of this book information will be provided to prove the point that standardised plant extract called silymarin (SM) containing a range of polyphenols could be one of the best examples of polyphenol application in medicine and veterinary medicine.

References

Abd El-Hack, M.E., Salem, H.M., Khafaga, A.F., Soliman, S.M. and El-Saadony, M.T., 2023. Impacts of polyphenols on laying hens' productivity and egg quality: a review. Journal of Animal Physiology and Animal Nutrition 107: 928-947. https://doi.org/10.1111/jpn.13758.

Abdel-Moneim, A.E., Shehata, A.M., Alzahrani, S.O., Shafi, M.E., Mesalam, N.M., Taha, A.E., Swelum, A.A., Arif, M., Fayyaz, M. and Abd El-Hack, M.E., 2020. The role of polyphenols in poultry nutrition. Journal of Animal Physiology and Animal Nutrition 104: 1851-1866.

Ahn, J., Grün, I.U. and Mustapha, A., 2007. Effects of plant extracts on microbial growth, color change, and lipid oxidation in cooked beef. Food Microbiology 24: 7-14.

Akbarian, A., Michiels, J., Degroote, J., Majdeddin, M., Golian, A. and De Smet, S., 2016. Association between heat stress and oxidative stress in poultry; mitochondrial dysfunction and dietary interventions with phytochemicals. Journal of Animal Science and Biotechnology 7: 37.

Andriantsitohaina, R., Auger, C., Chataigneau, T., Étienne-Selloum, N., Li, H., Martínez, M.C., Schini-Kerth, V.B. and Laher, I., 2012. Molecular mechanisms of the cardiovascular protective effects of polyphenols. British Journal of Nutrition 108: 1532-1549.

Ashkar, F., Bhullar, K.S. and Wu, J., 2022. The effect of polyphenols on kidney disease: targeting mitochondria. Nutrients 14: 3115.

Augustin, K., Blank, R., Boesch-Saadatmandi, C., Frank, J., Wolffram, S. and Rimbach, G., 2008. Dietary green tea polyphenols do not affect vitamin E status, antioxidant capacity and meat quality of growing pigs. Journal of Animal Physiology and Animal Nutrition 92: 705-711.

Aziza, A.E., Quezada, N. and Cherian, G., 2010a. Feeding Camelina sativa meal to meat-type chickens: effect on production performance and tissue fatty acid composition. The Journal of Applied Poultry Research 19: 157-168.

Aziza, A.E., Quezada, N. and Cherian, G., 2010b. Antioxidative effect of dietary Camelina meal in fresh, stored, or cooked broiler chicken meat. Poultry Science 89: 2711-2718.

Azzi, A., 2007. Molecular mechanism of alpha-tocopherol action. Free Radical Biology & Medicine 43: 16-21.

Azzi, A., 2018. Many tocopherols, one vitamin E. Molecular Aspects of Medicine 61: 92-103.

Azzi, A., 2021. Reflections on a century of vitamin E research: looking at the past with an eye on the future. Free Radical Biology & Medicine 175: 155-160.

Babich, H., Schuck, A.G., Weisburg, J.H. and Zuckerbraun, H.L., 2011. Research strategies in the study of the pro-oxidant nature of polyphenol nutraceuticals. Journal of Toxicology 2011: 467305.

Bachheti, R.K., Worku, L.A., Gonfa, Y.H., Zebeaman, M., Deepti Pandey, D.P. and Bachheti, A., 2022. Prevention and treatment of cardiovascular diseases with plant phytochemicals: a review. Evidence-Based Complementary and Alternative Medicine eCAM 2022: 5741198.

Belviranli, M., Gökbel, H., Okudan, N. and Büyükbaş, S., 2012. Oxidative stress and anti-oxidant status in diabetic rat liver: effect of plant polyphenols. Archives of Physiology and Biochemistry 118: 237-243.

Bešlo, D., Došlić, G., Agić, D., Rastija, V., Šperanda, M., Gantner, V. and Lučić, B., 2022. Polyphenols in ruminant nutrition and their effects on reproduction. Antioxidants 11: 970.

Bianchi, F., Cappella, A., Gagliano, N., Sfondrini, L. and Stacchiotti, A., 2022. Polyphenols-gut-heart: an impactful relationship to improve cardiovascular diseases. Antioxidants 11: 1700.

Bisht, K., Wagner, K.H. and Bulmer, A.C., 2010. Curcumin, resveratrol and flavonoids as anti-inflammatory, cyto- and DNA-protective dietary compounds. Toxicology 278: 88-100.

Bors, W., Michel, C. and Stettmaier, K., 2000. Electron paramagnetic resonance studies of radical species of proanthocyanidins and gallate esters. Archives of Biochemistry and Biophysics 374: 347-355.

Botsoglou, N.A., Christaki, E., Fletouris, D.J., Florou-Paneri, P. and Spais, A.B., 2002. The effect of dietary oregano essential oil on lipid oxidation in raw and cooked chicken during refrigerated storage. Meat Science 62: 259-265.

Brenes, A., Viveros, A., Goñi, I., Centeno, C., Sayago-Ayerdi, S.G., Arija, I. and Saura-Calixto, F., 2008. Effect of grape pomace concentrate and vitamin E on digestibility of polyphenols and antioxidant activity in chickens. Poultry Science 87: 307-316.

Calatayud-Sáez, F.M., Calatayud, B. and Calatayud, A., 2022. Effects of the Mediterranean diet on morbidity from inflammatory and recurrent diseases with special reference to childhood asthma. Nutrients 14: 936.

Cena, H. and Calder, P.C., 2020. Defining a healthy diet: evidence for the role of contemporary dietary patterns in health and disease. Nutrients 12: 334.

Chamorro, S., Viveros, A., Centeno, C., Romero, C., Arija, I. and Brenes, A., 2013. Effects of dietary grape seed extract on growth performance, amino acid digestibility and plasma lipids and mineral content in broiler chicks. Animal 7: 555-561.

Cherubini, A., Beal, M.F. and Frei, B., 1999. Black tea increases the resistance of human plasma to lipid peroxidation *in vitro*, but not *ex vivo*. Free Radical Biology & Medicine 27: 381-387.

Chauhan, A., Islam, A.U., Prakash, H. and Singh, S., 2022. Phytochemicals targeting NF-κB signaling: potential anti-cancer interventions. Journal of Pharmaceutical Analysis 12: 394-405.

Chen, L., Pu, Y., Xu, Y., He, X., Cao, J., Ma, Y. and Jiang, W., 2022. Anti-diabetic and anti-obesity: efficacy evaluation and exploitation of polyphenols in fruits and vegetables. Food Research International 157: 111202.

Cheng, X., Chen, Q. and Sun, P., 2022. Natural phytochemicals that affect autophagy in the treatment of oral diseases and infections: a review. Frontiers in Pharmacology 13: 970596.

Chu, A.J., 2014. Antagonism by bioactive polyphenols against inflammation: a systematic view. Inflammation & Allergy Drug Targets 13: 34-64.

Cladis, D.P., Weaver, C.M. and Ferruzzi, M.G., 2022. (Poly)phenol toxicity *in vivo* following oral administration: a targeted narrative review of (poly)phenols from green tea, grape, and anthocyanin-rich extracts. Phytotherapy Research 36: 323-335.

da Cunha, L.R., Muniz-Junqueira, M.I. and Dos Santos Borges, T.K., 2019. Impact of polyphenols in phagocyte functions. Journal of Inflammation Research 12: 205-217.

Dai, H., Sinclair, D.A., Ellis, J.L. and Steegborn, C., 2018. Sirtuin activators and inhibitors: promises, achievements, and challenges. Pharmacology & Therapeutics 188: 140-154.

D'Archivio, M., Filesi, C., Di Benedetto, R., Gargiulo, R., Giovannini, C., Masella, R., 2007. Polyphenols, dietary sources and bioavailability. Annali Dell'Istituto Superiore di Sanità 43: 348-361.

De la O, V., Zazpe, I., Goni, L., Santiago, S., Martín-Calvo, N., Bes-Rastrollo, M., Martínez, J.A., Martínez-González, M.Á. and Ruiz-Canela, M., 2022. A score appraising Paleolithic diet and the risk of cardiovascular disease in a Mediterranean prospective cohort. European Journal of Nutrition 61: 957-971.

De la O, V., Zazpe, I., Martínez, J.A., Santiago, S., Carlos, S., Zulet, M.Á. and Ruiz-Canela, M., 2021. Scoping review of Paleolithic dietary patterns: a definition proposal. Nutrition Research Reviews 34: 78-106.

Dolara, P., Luceri, C., De Filippo, C., Femia, A.P., Giovannelli, L., Caderni, G., Cecchini, C., Silvi, S., Orpianesi, C. and Cresci, A., 2005. Red wine polyphenols influence carcinogenesis, intestinal microflora, oxidative damage and gene expression profiles of colonic mucosa in F344 rats. Mutation Research 591: 237-246.

Duthie, G. and Morrice, P., 2012. Antioxidant capacity of flavonoids in hepatic microsomes is not reflected by antioxidant effects *in vivo*. Oxidative Medicine and Cellular Longevity 2012: 165127.

Ebrahimi, A. and Schluesener, H., 2012. Natural polyphenols against neurodegenerative disorders: potentials and pitfalls. Ageing Research Reviews 11: 329-345.

Egert, S. and Rimbach, G., 2011. Which sources of flavonoids: complex diets or dietary supplements? Advances in Nutrition 2: 8-14.

Forman, H.J., Davies, K.J.A. and Ursini, F., 2014. How do nutritional antioxidants really work: Nucleophilic tone and para-hormesis versus free radical scavenging *in vivo*. Free Radical Biology & Medicine 66: 24-35.

Fraga, C.G., Oteiza, P.I. and Galleano, M., 2018. Plant bioactives and redox signaling: (-)-Epicatechin as a paradigm. Molecular Aspects of Medicine 61: 31-40.

Freitas, P.L., Miranda, J., França, L.M. and Paes, A., 2022. Plant-derived (poly)phenols and their metabolic outcomes: The pursuit of a role for the gut microbiota. Nutrients 14: 3510.

Galati, G., Chan, T., Wu, B. and O'Brien, P.J., 1999. Glutathione-dependent generation of reactive oxygen species by the peroxidase-catalyzed redox cycling of flavonoids. Chemical Research in Toxicology 12: 521-525.

Galati, G. and O'Brien, P.J., 2004. Potential toxicity of flavonoids and other dietary phenolics: significance for their chemopreventive and anticancer properties. Free Radical Biology & Medicine 37: 287-303.

Galati, G., Sabzevari, O., Wilson, J.X. and O'Brien, P.J., 2002. Prooxidant activity and cellular effects of the phenoxyl radicals of dietary flavonoids and other polyphenolics. Toxicology 177: 91-104.

Ghaedi, E., Mohammadi, M., Mohammadi, H., Ramezani-Jolfaie, N., Malekzadeh, J., Hosseinzadeh, M. and Salehi-Abargouei, A., 2019. Effects of a Paleolithic diet on cardiovascular disease risk factors: A systematic review and meta-analysis of randomized controlled trials. Advances in Nutrition 10: 634-646.

Goñi, I., Brenes, A., Centeno, C., Viveros, A., Saura-Calixto, F., Rebolé, A., Arija, I. and Estevez, R., 2007. Effect of dietary grape pomace and vitamin E on growth performance, nutrient digest digestibility, and susceptibility to meat lipid oxidation in chickens. Poultry Science 86: 508-516.

Grandhaye, J., Lecompte, F., Chartrin, P., Leconte, M., Riva, A., Barbe, A., JeanPierre, É., Caldas-Silveira, E., Ganier, P., Chahnamian, M., Ramé, C., Dupont, J. and Froment, P., 2021. Maternal dietary supplementation with grape seed extract in reproductive hens increases fertility in females but decreases semen quality in males of the F1 generation. PloS One 16: e0246750.

Griffiths, D.W., 1986. The inhibition of digestive enzymes by polyphenolic compounds. Advances in Experimental Medicine and Biology 199: 509-516.

Haak, L., Raes, K., Van Dyck, S. and De Smet, S., 2008. Effect of dietary rosemary and α-tocopheryl acetate on the oxidative stability of raw and cooked pork following oxidized linseed oil administration. Meat Science 78: 239-247.

Hadi, S.M., Bhat, S.H., Azmi, A.S., Hanif, S., Shamim, U. and Ullah, M.F., 2007. Oxidative breakage of cellular DNA by plant polyphenols: a putative mechanism for anticancer properties. Seminars in Cancer Biology 17: 370-376.

Halliwell, B., 2007. Dietary polyphenols: good, bad, or indifferent for your health? Cardiovascular Research 73: 341-347.

Halliwell, B., 2008. Are polyphenols antioxidants or pro-oxidants? What do we learn from cell culture and *in vivo* studies? Archives of Biochemistry and Biophysics 476: 107-112.

Halliwell, B., 2014. Cell culture, oxidative stress, and antioxidants: avoiding pitfalls. Biomedical Journal 37: 99-105.

Halliwell, B., 2018. Artefacts with ascorbate and other redox-active compounds in cell culture: epigenetic modifications, and cell killing due to hydrogen peroxide generation in cell culture media. Free Radical Research 52: 907-909.

Halliwell, B., Rafter, J. and Jenner, A., 2005. Health promotion by flavonoids, tocopherols, tocotrienols, and other phenols: direct or indirect effects? Antioxidant or not? American Journal of Clinical Nutrition 81: 268S-276S.

Han, S.N., Pang, E., Zingg, J.M., Meydani, S.N., Meydani, M. and Azzi, A., 2010. Differential effects of natural and synthetic vitamin E on gene transcription in murine T lymphocytes. Archives of Biochemistry and Biophysics 495: 49-55.

Hao, Q., Wu, Y., Vadgama, J.V. and Wang, P., 2022. Phytochemicals in inhibition of prostate cancer: Evidence from molecular mechanisms studies. Biomolecules 12: 1306.

Hashem, N.M., Gonzalez-Bulnes, A. and Simal-Gandara, J., 2020. Polyphenols in farm animals: Source of reproductive gain or waste? Antioxidants 9: 1023.

Hervert-Hernández, D., Pintado, C., Rotger, R. and Goñi, I., 2009. Stimulatory effect of grape pomace polyphenols on Lactobacillus acidophilus growth. International Journal of Food Microbiology 136: 119-122.

Hodek, P., Trefil, P. and Stiborová, M., 2002. Flavonoids-potent and versatile biologically active compounds interacting with cytochromes P450. Chemico-Biological Interactions 139: 1-21.

Hodgson, J.M., 2008. Tea flavonoids and cardiovascular disease. Asia Pacific Journal of Clinical Nutrition 17: 288-290.

Hodgson, J.M. and Croft, K.D., 2010. Tea flavonoids and cardiovascular health. Molecular Aspects of Medicine 31: 495-502.

Hogan, S., Canning, C., Sun, S., Sun, X. and Zhou, K., 2010. Effects of grape pomace antioxidant extract on oxidative stress and inflammation in diet induced obese mice. Journal of Agricultural and Food Chemistry 58: 11250-11256.

Horigome, T., Kumar, R., and Okamoto, K., 1988. Effects of condensed tannins prepared from leaves of fodder plants on digestive enzymes *in vitro* and in the intestine of rats. British Journal of Nutrition 60: 275-278.

Howard, A.N. and Constamble, B.J., 1958. The metabolism of adrenocorticotrophic hormone and ascorbic acid in the chick. Biochemical Journal 69: 501-505.

Hu, M-L., 2011. Dietary polyphenols as antioxidants and anticancer agents: More questions than answers. Chang Gung Medical Journal 34: 449-460.

Hu, R., He, Y., Arowolo, M.A., Wu, S. and He, J., 2019. Polyphenols as potential attenuators of heat stress in poultry production. Antioxidants 8: 67.

Hughes, R.J., Brooker, J.D. and Smyl, C., 2005. Growth rate of broiler chickens given condensed tannins extracted from grape seed. Proceedings of Australian Poultry Science Symposium 17: 65-68.

Hussain, T., Tan, B., Liu, G., Murtaza, G., Rahu, N., Saleem, M. and Yin, Y., 2017. Modulatory mechanism of polyphenols and Nrf2 signaling pathway in LPS challenged pregnancy disorders. Oxidative Medicine and Cellular Longevity 2017: 8254289.

Hussain, Y., Khan, H., Alsharif, K.F., Hayat Khan, A., Aschner, M. and Saso, L., 2022. The therapeutic potential of kaemferol and other naturally occurring polyphenols might be modulated by Nrf2-ARE signaling pathway: Current status and future direction. Molecules 27: 4145.

Jacobs, D.M., Fuhrmann, J.C., van Dorsten, F.A., Rein, D., Peters, S., van Velzen, E.J., Hollebrands, B., Draijer, R., van Duynhoven, J. and Garczarek, U., 2012. Impact of short-term intake of red wine and grape polyphenol extract on the human metabolome. Journal of Agricultural and Food Chemistry 60: 3078-3085.

Jansman, A.J.M., Huisman, J. and Van der Poel, A.F.B., 1993. Ileal and faecal digestibility in piglets of field beans (*Vicia faba* L.) varying in tannin content. Animal Feed Science and Technology 42: 83-96.

Jin, H., Leng, Q. and Li, C., 2012. Dietary flavonoid for preventing colorectal neoplasms. Cochrane Database of Systematic Reviews 8: CD009350.

Johnston, K., Sharp, P., Clifford, M. and Morgan, L. 2005. Dietary polyphenols decrease glucose uptake by human intestinal Caco-2 cells. FEBS Letters 579: 1653-1657.

Kim, E.Y., Pai, T.K. and Han, O., 2011. Effect of bioactive dietary polyphenols on zinc transport across the intestinal Caco-2 cell monolayers. Journal of Agricultural and Food Chemistry 59: 3606-3612.

Klimova, B., Dziuba, S. and Cierniak-Emerych, A., 2020. The effect of healthy diet on cognitive performance among healthy seniors – A mini review. Frontiers in Human Neuroscience 14: 325.

Krebs-Smith, S.M., Pannucci, T.E., Subar, A.F., Kirkpatrick, S.I., Lerman, J.L., Tooze, J.A., Wilson, M.M. and Reedy, J., 2018. Update of the healthy eating index: HEI-2015. Journal of the Academy of Nutrition and Dietetics 118: 1591-1602.

Křen, V., 2021. Chirality matters: Biological activity of optically pure silybin and its congeners. International Journal of Molecular Sciences 22: 7885.

Krogdahl, A., 1985. Digestion and absorption of lipids in poultry. Journal of Nutrition 115: 675-685.

Lagoa, R., Marques-da-Silva, D., Diniz, M., Daglia, M. and Bishayee, A., 2022. Molecular mechanisms linking environmental toxicants to cancer development: Significance for protective interventions with polyphenols. Seminars in Cancer Biology 80: 118-144.

Lambert, J.D., Kennett, M.J., Sang, S., Reuhl, K.R., Ju, J. and Yang, C.S., 2010. Hepatotoxicity of high oral dose (-)-epigallocatechin-3-gallate in mice. Food and Chemical Toxicology 48: 409-416.

Lampignano, L., Donghia, R., Sila, A., Bortone, I., Tatoli, R., De Nucci, S., Castellana, F., Zupo, R., Tirelli, S., Giannoccaro, V., Guerra, V., Panza, F., Lozupone, M., Mastronardi, M., De Pergola, G., Giannelli, G. and Sardone, R., 2022. Mediterranean diet and fatty liver risk in a population of overweight older Italians: A propensity score-matched case-cohort study. Nutrients 14: 258.

Lau, D.W. and King, A.J., 2003. Pre- and post-mortem use of grape seed extract in dark poultry meat to inhibit development of thiobarbituric acid reactive substances. Journal of Agricultural and Food Chemistry 51: 1602-1607.

Lee, M.T., Lin, W.C. and Lee, T.T., 2019. Potential crosstalk of oxidative stress and immune response in poultry through phytochemicals – A review. Asian-Australasian Journal of Animal Sciences 32: 309-319.

Lee, J.H., Park, J. and Shin, D.W., 2022. The molecular mechanism of polyphenols with anti-aging activity in aged human dermal fibroblasts. Molecules 27: 4351.

Lemos, C., Peters, G.J., Jansen, G., Martel, F. and Calhau, C., 2007. Modulation of folate uptake in cultured human colon adenocarcinoma Caco-2 cells by dietary compounds. European Journal of Nutrition 46: 329-336.

Li, G.X., Chen, Y.K., Hou, Z., Xiao, H., Jin, H., Lu, G., Lee, M.J., Liu, B., Guan, F., Yang, Z., Yu, A. and Yang, C.S., 2010. Pro-oxidative activities and dose-response relationship of (–)-epigallocatechin-3-gallate in the inhibition of lung cancer cell growth: a comparative study *in vivo* and *in vitro*. Carcinogenesis 31: 902-910.

Li, J., Zhong, X., Zhao, Y., Shen, J., Pilapong, C. and Xiao, Z., 2022. Polyphenols as lung cancer chemopreventive agents by targeting microRNAs. Molecules 27: 5903.

Liu, L., Fu, C., Yan, M., Xie, H., Li, S., Yu, Q., He, S. and He, J., 2016. Resveratrol modulates intestinal morphology and HSP70/90, NF-κB and EGF expression in the jejunal mucosa of black-boned chickens on exposure to circular heat stress. Food & Function 7: 1329-1338.

Liu, S., Lin, F., Wang, J., Pan, X., Sun, L. and Wu, W., 2022. Polyphenols for the treatment of ischemic stroke: New applications and insights. Molecules 27: 4181.

Lobczowska, K., Banik, A., Brukalo, K., Forberger, S., Kubiak, T., Romaniuk, P., Scheidmeir, M., Scheller, D.A., Steinacker, J.M., Wendt, J., Wieczorowska-Tobis, K., Bekker, M., Zeeb, H. and Luszczynska, A., 2022. Meta-review of implementation determinants for policies promoting healthy diet and physically active lifestyle: application of the Consolidated Framework for Implementation Research. Implementation Science 17: 2.

Longstaff, M. and McNab, J.M., 1991. The inhibitory effects of hull polysaccharides and tannins of field beans (Vicia faba L) on the digestion of amino acids, starch and lipid and on digestive enzyme activities in young chicks. British Journal of Nutrition 65: 199-216.

Lotfi, K., Saneei, P., Hajhashemy, Z. and Esmaillzadeh, A., 2022. Adherence to the Mediterranean diet, five-year weight change, and risk of overweight and obesity: A systematic review and dose-response meta-analysis of prospective cohort studies. Advances in Nutrition 13: 152-166.

Lotito, S.B. and Frei, B., 2004. Relevance of apple polyphenols as antioxidants in human plasma: contrasting *in vitro* and *in vivo* effects. Free Radical Biology & Medicine 36: 201-211.

Ma, Q., Kim, E.Y. and Han, O., 2010. Bioactive dietary polyphenols decrease heme iron absorption by decreasing basolateral iron release in human intestinal Caco-2 cells. Journal of Nutrition 140: 1117-1121.

Ma, Q., Kim, E.Y., Lindsay, E.A. and Han, O., 2011. Bioactive dietary polyphenols inhibit heme iron absorption in a dose-dependent manner in human intestinal Caco-2 cells. Journal of Food Science 76: H143-H150.

Manach, C., Scalbert, A., Morand, C., Rémésy, C. and Jiménez, L., 2004. Polyphenols: food sources and bioavailability. The American Journal of Clinical Nutrition 79: 727-747.

Martel, F., Monteiro, R. and Calhau, C., 2010. Effect of polyphenols on the intestinal and placental transport of some bioactive compounds. Nutrition Research Reviews 23: 47-64.

Mason, L.M., Hogan, S.A., Lynch, A., O'Sullivan, K., Lawlor, P.G. and Kerry, J.P., 2005. Effect of restricted feeding and antioxidant supplementation on pig performance and quality characteristics of longissimus dorsi from Landrace and Duroc pigs. Meat Science 70: 307-317.

Maurya, D.K. and Devasagayam, T.P., 2010. Antioxidant and prooxidant nature of hydroxycinnamic acid derivatives ferulic and caffeic acids. Food and Chemical Toxicology 48: 3369-3373.

Mazzanti, G., Menniti-Ippolito, F., Moro, P.A., Cassetti, F., Raschetti, R., Santuccio, C. and Mastrangelo, S., 2009. Hepatotoxicity from green tea: a review of the literature and two unpublished cases. European Journal of Clinical Pharmacology 65: 331-341.

McCullough, M.L., Peterson, J.J., Patel, R., Jacques, P.F., Shah, R. and Dwyer, J.T., 2012. Flavonoid intake and cardiovascular disease mortality in a prospective cohort of US adults. American Journal of Clinical Nutrition 95: 454-464.

McDougall, G.J., Shpiro, F., Dobson, P., Smith, P., Blake, A. and Stewart, D., 2005. Different polyphenolic components of soft fruits inhibit alpha-amylase and alpha-glucosidase. Journal of Agricultural and Food Chemistry 53: 2760-2766.

McIlroy, S.G., Goodall, E.A., Rice, D.A., McNulty, M.S. and Kennedy, D.G., 1993. Improved performance in commercial broiler flocks with subclinical infectious bursal disease when fed diets containing increased concentrations of vitamin E. Avian Pathology 22: 81-94.

McKee, J.S., Harrison, P.C. and Riskowski, G.L., 1997. Effects of supplemental ascorbic acid on the energy conversion of broiler chicks during heat stress and feed withdrawal. Poultry Science 76: 1278-1286.

Menezes, R., Matafome, P., Freitas, M. and García-Conesa, M.T., 2022. Updated information of the effects of (poly)phenols against type-2 diabetes mellitus in humans: Reinforcing the recommendations for future research. Nutrients 14: 3563.

Mennen, L.I., Walker, R., Bennetau-Pelissero, C. and Scalbert, A., 2005. Risks and safety of polyphenol consumption. American Journal of Clinical Nutrition 81: 326S-329S.

Miller, V., Webb, P., Micha, R., Mozaffarian, D. and Global Dietary Database, 2020. Defining diet quality: a synthesis of dietary quality metrics and their validity for the double burden of malnutrition. The Lancet. Planetary Health 4: e352-e370.

Miyazawa, T., Burdeos, G.C., Itaya, M., Nakagawa, K. and Miyazawa T., 2019. Vitamin E: Regulatory redox interactions. IUBMB Life 71: 430-441.

Moreno, D.A., Ilic, N., Poulev, A., Brasaemle, D.L., Fried, S.K. and Raskin, I., 2003. Inhibitory effects of grape seed extract on lipases. Nutrition 19: 876-879.

Moskaug, J.O., Carlsen, H. and Myhrstad, M.C.W., 2005. Polyphenols and glutathione synthesis regulation. American Journal of Clinical Nutrition 81: 277S-283S.

Mori, M., Sagara, M., Mori, H. and Yamori, Y., 2022. Grading of Japanese diet intakes by 24-hour urine analysis of taurine and soy isoflavones in relation to cardiovascular risks. Advances in Experimental Medicine and Biology 1370: 173-184.

Moustafa, B., Trifan, G., Isasi, C.R., Lipton, R.B., Sotres-Alvarez, D., Cai, J., Tarraf, W., Stickel, A., Mattei, J., Talavera, G.A., Daviglus, M.L., González, H.M. and Testai, F.D., 2022. Association of Mediterranean diet with cognitive decline among diverse Hispanic or Latino adults from the Hispanic community health study/Study of Latinos. JAMA Network Open 5: e2221982.

Mu, K., Wang, D. and Kitts, D.D., 2019. Molecular mechanisms that define redox balance function in pathogen-host interactions – Is there a role for dietary bioactive polyphenols?. International Journal of Molecular Sciences 20: 6222.

Muyrers, J., Klingenstein, R., Stitz, L. and Korth, C., 2010. Structure-activity relationship of tocopherol derivatives suggesting a novel non-antioxidant mechanism in antiprion potency. Neuroscience Letters 469: 122-126.

Nabavi, S.F., Barber, A.J., Spagnuolo, C., Russo, G.L., Daglia, M., Nabavi, S.M. and Sobarzo-Sánchez, E., 2016. Nrf2 as molecular target for polyphenols: A novel therapeutic strategy in diabetic retinopathy. Critical Reviews in Clinical Laboratory Sciences 53: 293-312.

Nardoia, M., Romero, C., Brenes, A., Arija, I., Viveros, A., Ruiz-Capillas, C. and Chamorro, S., 2020. Addition of fermented and unfermented grape skin in broilers' diets: effect on digestion, growth performance, intestinal microbiota and oxidative stability of meat. Animal 14: 1371-1381.

Natella, F., Nardini, M., Giannetti, I., Dattilo, C. and Scaccini, C., 2002. Coffee drinking influences plasma antioxidant capacity in humans. Journal of Agricultural and Food Chemistry 50: 6211-6216.

Nyachotti, C.M., Atkinson, J.L. and Leeson, S., 1997. Sorghum tannins a review. World's Poultry Science Journal 53: 5-21.

O'Grady, M.N., Maher, V., Troy, D.J., Moloney, A.P. and Kerry, J.P., 2006. An assessment of dietary supplementation with tea catechins and rosemary extract on the quality of fresh beef. Meat Science 73: 132-146.

Olivares-Vicente, M., Barrajon-Catalan, E., Herranz-Lopez, M., Segura-Carretero, A., Joven, J., Encinar, J.A. and Micol, V., 2018. Plant-derived polyphenols in human health: Biological activity, metabolites and putative molecular targets. Current Drug Metabolism 19: 351-369.

Ortiz, L.T., Centeno, C. and Trevino, J., 1993. Tannin in faba bean seeds: Effects on the digestion of protein and amino acids in growing chicks. Animal Feed Science and Technology 41: 271-278.

Pawlowska, E., Szczepanska, J., Koskela, A., Kaarniranta, K. and Blasiak, J., 2019. Dietary polyphenols in age-related macular degeneration: Protection against oxidative stress and beyond. Oxidative Medicine and Cellular Longevity 2019: 9682318.

Pedeboscq, S., Rey, C., Muriel Petit, M., Harpey, C., De Giorgi, F., Francois Ichas, F. and Lartigue, L., 2012. Non-antioxidant properties of α-tocopherol reduce the anticancer activity of several protein kinase inhibitors *in vitro*. PLoS ONE 7: e36811.

Pekel, Y., Patterson, H.P., Hulet, R.M., Acar, N., Cravener, T.L., Dowler, D.B. and Hunter, J.M., 2009. Dietary Camelina meal versus flaxseed with and without supplemental copper for broiler chickens: Live performance and processing yield. Poultry Science 88: 2392-2398.

Peluzio Mdo, C., Teixeira, T.F., Oliveira, V.P., Sabarense, C.M., Dias, C.M., Abranches, M.V. and Maldonado, I.R., 2011. Grape extract and α-tocopherol effect in cardiovascular disease model of Apo E -/- mice. Acta Cirurgica Brasileira 26: 253-260.

Perron, N.R. and Brumaghim, J.L. 2009. A review of the antioxidant mechanisms of polyphenol compounds related to iron binding. Cell Biochemistry and Biophysics 53: 75-100.

Perron, N.R., García, C.R., Pinzón, J.R., Chaur, M.N. and Brumaghim, J.L., 2011. Antioxidant and prooxidant effects of polyphenol compounds on copper-mediated DNA damage. Journal of Inorganic Biochemistry 105: 745-753.

Pitino, R., De Marchi, M., Manuelian, C.L., Johnson, M., Simoni, M., Righi, F. and Tsiplakou, E., 2021. Plant feed additives as natural alternatives to the use of synthetic antioxidant vitamins on yield, quality, and oxidative status of poultry products: A Review of the literature of the last 20 years. Antioxidants 10: 757.

Procházková, D., Boušová, I. and Wilhelmová, N., 2011. Antioxidant and prooxidant properties of flavonoids. Fitoterapia 82: 513-523.

Quetglas-Llabrés, M.M., Monserrat-Mesquida, M., Bouzas, C., Gómez, C., Mateos, D., Ripoll-Vera, T., Tur, J.A. and Sureda, A., 2022. Inflammatory and oxidative stress markers related to adherence to the Mediterranean diet in patients with metabolic syndrome. Antioxidants 11: 901.

Rafiei, F. and Khajali, F., 2021. Flavonoid antioxidants in chicken meat production: Potential application and future trends. World's Poultry Science Journal 77: 347-361.

Rahman, S.U., Li, Y., Huang, Y., Zhu, L., Feng, S., Wu, J. and Wang, X., 2018. Treatment of inflammatory bowel disease via green tea polyphenols: possible application and protective approaches. Inflammopharmacology 26: 319-330.

Rahman, M., Riaz, M. and Desai, U.R., 2007. Synthesis of biologically relevant biflavanoids – A review. Chemistry and Biodiversity 4: 2495-2527.

Rana, A., Samtiya, M., Dhewa, T., Mishra, V. and Aluko, R.E., 2022. Health benefits of polyphenols: A concise review. Journal of Food Biochemistry 46: e14264.

Robbins, R.J., 2003. Phenolic acids in foods: an overview of analytical methodology. Journal of Agricultural and Food Chemistry 51: 2866-2887.

Rodrigo, R., Miranda, A. and Vergara, L., 2011. Modulation of endogenous antioxidant system by wine polyphenols in human disease. Clinica Chimica Acta 412: 410-424.

Romero-Robles, M.A., Ccami-Bernal, F., Ortiz-Benique, Z.N., Pinto-Ruiz, D.F., Benites-Zapata, V.A. and Casas Patiño, D., 2022. Adherence to Mediterranean diet associated with health-related quality of life in children and adolescents: A systematic review. BMC Nutrition 8: 1-17.

Roy, D.M. and Schneeman, B.O., 1981. Effect of soy protein, casein and trypsin inhibitor on cholesterol, bile acids and pancreatic enzymes in mice. Journal of Nutrition 111: 878-885.

Ryhanen, E.L., Perttila, S., Tupasela, T., Valaja, J., Eriksson, C. and Larkka, K., 2007. Effect of Camelina sativa expeller cake on performance and meat quality of broilers. Journal of the Science of Food and Agriculture 87: 1489-1494.

Sahebnasagh, A., Eghbali, S., Saghafi, F., Sureda, A. and Avan, R., 2022. Neurohormetic phytochemicals in the pathogenesis of neurodegenerative diseases. Immunity & Ageing 19: 36.

Saito, M., Hosoyama, H., Ariga, T., Kataoka, S. and Yamaji, N., 1998. Antiulcer activity of grape seed extract and procyanidins. Journal of Agricultural and Food Chemistry 46: 1460-1464.

Saji, N., Tsuduki, T., Murotani, K., Hisada, T., Sugimoto, T., Kimura, A., Niida, S., Toba, K. and Sakurai, T., 2022. Relationship between the Japanese-style diet, gut microbiota, and dementia: A cross-sectional study. Nutrition 94: 111524.

Santhiravel, S., Bekhit, A., Mendis, E., Jacobs, J.L., Dunshea, F.R., Rajapakse, N. and Ponnampalam, E.N., 2022. The impact of plant phytochemicals on the gut microbiota of humans for a balanced life. International Journal of Molecular Sciences 23: 8124.

Sarubbo, F., Esteban, S., Miralles, A. and Moranta, D., 2018. Effects of resveratrol and other polyphenols on Sirt1: Relevance to brain function during aging. Current Neuropharmacology 16: 126-136.

Sáyago-Ayerdi, S.G., Brenes, A., Viveros, A. and Goñi, I., 2009. Antioxidative effect of dietary grape pomace concentrate on lipid oxidation of chilled and long-term frozen stored chicken patties. Meat Science 83: 528-533.

Scalbert, A. and Williamson, G., 2000. Dietary intake and bioavailability of polyphenols. The Journal of Nutrition 130: 2073S-2085S.

Schewe, T., Steffen, Y. and Sies, H., 2008. How do dietary flavanols improve vascular function? A position paper. Archives of Biochemistry and Biophysics 476: 102-106.

Schweigert, N., Zehnder, A.J. and Eggen, R.I., 2001. Chemical properties of catechols and their molecular modes of toxic action in cells, from microorganisms to mammals. Environmental Microbiology 3: 81-91.

Scott, M.B., Styring, A.K. and McCullagh, J., 2022. Polyphenols: bioavailability, microbiome interactions and cellular effects on health in humans and animals. Pathogens 11: 770.

Serra, G., Incani, A., Serreli, G., Porru, L., Melis, M.P., Tuberoso, C., Rossin, D., Biasi, F. and Deiana, M., 2018. Olive oil polyphenols reduce oxysterols-induced redox imbalance and pro-inflammatory response in intestinal cells. Redox Biology 17: 348-354.

Sharifi-Rad, J., Rapposelli, S., Sestito, S., Herrera-Bravo, J., Arancibia-Diaz, A., Salazar, L.A., Yeskaliyeva, B., Beyatli, A., Leyva-Gómez, G., González-Contreras, C., Gürer, E.S., Martorell, M. and Calina, D., 2022. Multi-target mechanisms of phytochemicals in Alzheimer's disease: Effects on oxidative stress, neuroinflammation and protein aggregation. Journal of Personalized Medicine 12: 1515.

Shirota, M., Watanabe, N., Suzuki, M. and Kobori, M., 2022. Japanese-style diet and cardiovascular disease mortality: A systematic review and meta-analysis of prospective cohort studies. Nutrients 14: 2008.

Si, W., Zhang, Y., Li, X., Du, Y. and Xu, Q., 2021. Understanding the functional activity of polyphenols using omics-based approaches. Nutrients 13: 3953.

Sies, H., 2010. Polyphenols and health: update and perspectives. Archives of Biochemistry and Biophysics 501: 2-5.

Skarpanska-Stejnborn, A., Pilaczynska-Szczesniak, L., Basta, P. and Deskur-Smielecka, E., 2009. The influence of supplementation with Rhodiola rosea L. extract on selected redox parameters in professional rowers. International Journal of Sport Nutrition and Exercise Metabolism 19: 186-199.

Skarpanska-Stejnborn, A., Pilaczynska-Szczesniak, L., Basta, P., Deskur-Smielcka, E. and Horoszkiewicz-Hassan, M., 2008. The influence of supplementation with artichoke (Cynara scolymus L.) extract on selected redox parameters in rowers. International Journal of Sport Nutrition and Exercise Metabolism 18: 313-327.

Skibola, C.F. and Smith, M.T., 2000. Potential health impacts of excessive flavonoid intake. Free Radical Biology & Medicine 29: 375-383.

Smet, K., Raes, K., Huyghebaert, G., Haak, L., Arnouts, S. and De Smet, S., 2008. Lipid and protein oxidation of broiler meat as influenced by dietary natural antioxidant supplementation. Poultry Science 87: 1682-1688.

Sohouli, M.H., Fatahi, S., Lari, A., Lotfi, M., Seifishahpar, M., Găman, M.A., Rahideh, S.T., AlBatati, S.K., Al Hossan, A.M., Alkhalifa, S.A., Alomar, S.A. and Abu-Zaid, A., 2022. The effect of Paleolithic diet on glucose metabolism and lipid profile among patients with metabolic disorders: a systematic review and meta-analysis of randomized controlled trials. Critical Reviews in Food Science and Nutrition 62: 4551-4562.

Stagos, D., Amoutzias, G.D., Matakos, A., Spyrou, A., Tsatsakis, A.M. and Kouretas, D., 2012. Chemoprevention of liver cancer by plant polyphenols. Food and Chemical Toxicology 50: 2155-2170.

Surai, K.P., Surai, P.F., Speake, B.K. and Sparks, N.H.C., 2004. Antioxidant-prooxidant balance in the intestine: Food for thought. 2. Antioxidants. Current Topics in Nutraceutical Research 2: 27-46.

Surai, P.F., 1999. Vitamin E in avian reproduction. Poultry and Avian Biology Reviews 10: 1-60.

Surai, P.F., 2002. Natural antioxidants in avian nutrition and reproduction. Nottingham University Press, Nottingham, UK.

Surai, P.F., 2006. Selenium in nutrition and health. Nottingham University Press, Nottingham, UK.

Surai, P.F., 2014. Polyphenol compounds in the chicken/animal diet: from the past to the future. Journal of Animal Physiology and Animal Nutrition 9: 19-31.

Surai, P.F., 2018. Selenium in poultry nutrition and health. Wageningen Academic Publishers, Wageningen, The Netherlands.

Surai, P.F., 2020a. Antioxidants in poultry nutrition and reproduction: An update. Antioxidants 9: 105.

Surai, P.F., 2020b. Vitagenes in avian biology and poultry health. Wageningen Academic Publishers, Wageningen, The Netherlands.

Surai, P.F., 2022. Silymarin as a vitagene modulator: effects on mitochondria integrity in stress conditions. In: Ostojik, S.M. (ed) Molecular nutrition and mitochondria. Elsevier, Academic Press, London, UK, pp. 535-559.

Surai, P.F. and Earle-Payne, K., 2022. Antioxidant defences and redox homeostasis in animals. Antioxidants 11: 1012.

Surai, P.F. and Fisinin, V.I., 2010. Ill health effects of food lipids: Consequences of inadequate food processing, storage and cooking. In: De Meester, F., Zibadi, S. and Ross, R.R. (eds) Modern dietary fat intakes in disease promotion. Humana Press, Springer, New York, USA, pp. 251-274.

Surai, P.F. and Fisinin, V.I., 2012. Feeding breeders to avoid oxidative stress in embryos. Proceedings of the XXIV World's Poultry Science Congress, Salvador, Brazil, World's Poultry Science Journal. 68: 1-12.

Surai, P.F. and Fisinin, V.I., 2015. Antioxidant-prooxidant balance in the intestine: Applications in chick placement and pig weaning. Journal of Veterinary Science & Medicine 3: 1-16.

Surai, P.F., Kochish, I.I., Fisinin, V.I. and Kidd, M.T., 2019a. Antioxidant defence systems and oxidative stress in poultry biology: An update. Antioxidants 8: 235.

Surai, P.F., Kochish, I.I., Romanov, M.N. and Griffin, D.K., 2019b. Nutritional modulation of the antioxidant capacities in poultry: the case of vitamin E. Poultry Science, 98: 4030-4041.

Surai, P.F., Kochish, I.I. and Fisinin, V.I., 2021a. Vitagenes in avian biology: protective functions of sirtuins. In: Maise, K. (ed) Sirtuin biology in medicine. Academic Press, UK, USA, pp. 353-372.

Surai, P.F., Kochish, I.I. and Kidd, M.T., 2021b. Redox homeostasis in poultry: Regulatory roles of NF-κB. Antioxidants 10: 186.

Surai, P.F., Kochish, I.I., Fisinin, V.I., Grozina, A.A. and Shatskikh E.V., 2018. Molecular mechanisms of chicken gut health maintenance: role of microbiota. Agricultural Technologies, Moscow, Russia.

Surai, P.F. and Sparks, N.H.C., 2001. Designer eggs: from improvement of egg composition to functional food. Trends in Food Science and Technology 12: 7-16.

Suzuki, N., Goto, Y., Ota, H., Kito, K., Mano, F., Joo, E., Ikeda, K., Inagaki, N. and Nakayama, T., 2018. Characteristics of the Japanese diet described in epidemiologic publications: A qualitative systematic review. Journal of Nutritional Science and Vitaminology 64: 129-137.

Szliszka, E. and Krol, W., 2011. The role of dietary polyphenols in tumor necrosis factor-related apoptosis inducing ligand (TRAIL)-induced apoptosis for cancer chemoprevention. European Journal of Cancer Prevention 20: 63-69.

Tang, S.Z., Kerry, J.P., Sheehan, D., Buckley, D.J. and Morrissey, P.A., 2000. Dietary tea catechins and iron-induced lipid oxidation in chicken meat, liver and heart. Meat Science 56: 285-290.

Theodoratou, E., Kyle, J., Cetnarskyj, R., Farrington, S.M., Tenesa, A., Barnetson, R., Porteous, M., Dunlop, M. and Campbell1, H., 2007. Dietary flavonoids and the risk of colorectal cancer. Cancer Epidemiology, Biomarkers & Prevention 16: 684-693.

Tripoli, E., La Guardia, M., Giammanco, S., Di Majo, D. and Giammanco M., 2007. Citrus flavonoids: Molecular structure, biological activity and nutritional properties: A Review. Food Chemistry 104: 466-479.

Truong, V.L., Jun, M. and Jeong, W.S., 2018. Role of resveratrol in regulation of cellular defense systems against oxidative stress. Biofactors 44: 36-49.

Ungurianu, A., Zanfirescu, A., Niţulescu, G. and Margină, D., 2021. Vitamin E beyond Its antioxidant label. Antioxidants 10: 634.

Vauzour, D., 2012. Dietary polyphenols as modulators of brain functions: biological actions and molecular mechanisms underpinning their beneficial effects. Oxidative Medicine and Cellular Longevity 2012: 914273.

Veskoukis, A.S., Kyparos, A., Nikolaidis, M.G., Stagos, D., Aligiannis, N., Halabalaki, M., Chronis, K., Goutzourelas, N., Skaltsounis, L. and Kouretas, D., 2012. The antioxidant effects of a polyphenol-rich grape pomace extract *in vitro* do not correspond in vivo using exercise as an oxidant stimulus. Oxidative Medicine and Cellular Longevity 2012: 185867.

Vieira-Filho, L.D., Lara, L.S., Silva, P.A., Santos, F.T.J., Luzardo, R., Fabiana S.T., Oliveira, F.S.T., Paixão, A.D.O. and Vieyra, A., 2011. Placental malnutrition changes the regulatory network of renal Na-ATPase in adult rat progeny: Reprogramming by maternal a-tocopherol during lactation. Archives of Biochemistry and Biophysics 505: 91-97.

Visioli, F., De La Lastra, C.A., Andres-Lacueva, C., Aviram, M., Calhau, C., Cassano, A., D'Archivio, M., Faria, A., Favé, G., Fogliano, V., Llorach, R., Vitaglione, P., Zoratti, M. and Edeas, M., 2011. Polyphenols and human health: a prospectus. Critical Reviews in Food Science and Nutrition 51: 524-546.

Viveros, A., Chamorro, S., Pizarro, M., Arija, I., Centeno, C. and Brenes, A., 2011. Effects of dietary polyphenol-rich grape products on intestinal microflora and gut morphology in broiler chicks. Poultry Science 90: 566-578.

Vladu, A.F., Ficai, D., Ene, A.G. and Ficai, A., 2022. Combination therapy using polyphenols: An efficient way to improve antitumoral activity and reduce resistance. International Journal of Molecular Sciences 23: 10244.

Vossen, E., Ntawubizi, M., Raes, K., Smet, K., Huyghebaert, G., Arnouts, S. and De Smet, S., 2011. Effect of dietary antioxidant supplementation on the oxidative status of plasma in broilers. Journal of Animal Physiology and Animal Nutrition 95: 198-205.

Wang, S., Du, Q., Meng, X. and Zhang, Y., 2022. Natural polyphenols: a potential prevention and treatment strategy for metabolic syndrome. Food & Function 13: 9734-9753.

Willemsen, H., Swennen, Q., Everaert, N., Geraert, P.A., Mercier, Y., Stinckens, A., Decuypere, E. and Buyse, J., 2011. Effects of dietary supplementation of methionine and its hydroxy analog DL-2-hydroxy-4-methylthiobutanoic acid on growth performance, plasma hormone levels, and the redox status of broiler chickens exposed to high temperatures. Poultry Science 90: 2311-2320.

Xing, C., Wang, Y., Dai, X., Yang, F., Luo, J., Liu, P., Zhang, C., Cao, H. and Hu, G., 2020. The protective effects of resveratrol on antioxidant function and the mRNA expression of inflammatory cytokines in the ovaries of hens with fatty liver hemorrhagic syndrome. Poultry Science 99: 1019-1027.

Yahfoufi, N., Alsadi, N., Jambi, M. and Matar, C., 2018. The Immunomodulatory and anti-inflammatory role of polyphenols. Nutrients 10: 1618.

Yang, J.Y., Zhang, H.J., Wang, J., Wu, S.G., Yue, H.Y., Jiang, X.R. and Qi, G.H., 2017. Effects of dietary grape proanthocyanidins on the growth performance, jejunum morphology and plasma biochemical indices of broiler chicks. Animal 11: 762-770.

Yeung, S.S.Y., Kwan, M. and Woo, J., 2021. Healthy diet for healthy aging. Nutrients 13: 4310.

Yilmazer-Musa, M., Griffith, A.M., Michels, A.J., Schneider, E. and Frei, B., 2012. Grape seed and tea extracts and catechin 3-gallates are potent inhibitors of a-amylase and a-glucosidase activity. Journal of Agricultural and Food Chemistry 60: 8924-8929.

You, Q., Chen, F., Wang, X., Luo, P.G. and Jiang, Y., 2011. Inhibitory effects of muscadine anthocyanins on a-glucosidase and pancreatic lipase activities. Journal of Agricultural and Food Chemistry 59: 9506-9511.

Yu, C., Wang, D., Yang, Z. and Wang, T., 2022. Pharmacological effects of polyphenol phytochemicals on the intestinal inflammation via targeting TLR4/NF-κB signaling pathway. International Journal of Molecular Sciences 23: 6939.

Zhang, Y., Xia, M., Weng, S., Wang, C., Yuan, P. and Tang, S., 2022. Effect of Mediterranean diet for pregnant women: a meta-analysis of randomized controlled trials. The Journal of Maternal-Fetal & Neonatal Medicine 35: 4824-4829.

Zhang, C., Chen, K., Zhao, X. and Geng, Z., 2018. Protective effects of resveratrol against high ambient temperature-induced spleen dysplasia in broilers through modulating splenic redox status and apoptosis. Journal of the Science of Food and Agriculture, 98: 5409-5417.

Zhang, C., Tian, Y., Yan, F., Kang, X., Han, R., Sun, G. and Zhang, H., 2014. Modulation of growth and immunity by dietary supplementation with resveratrol in young chickens receiving conventional vaccinations. American Journal of Veterinary Research 75: 752-759.

Zheng, Z., Zhang, L. and Hou, X., 2022. Potential roles and molecular mechanisms of phytochemicals against cancer. Food & Function 13: 9208-9225.

Zhou, Y., Jiang, Z., Lu, H., Xu, Z., Tong, R., Shi, J. and Jia, G., 2019. Recent advances of natural polyphenols activators for Keap1-Nrf2 signaling pathway. Chemistry & Biodiversity 16: e1900400.

Zielinska-Blizniewska, H., Sitarek, P., Merecz-Sadowska, A., Malinowska, K., Zajdel, K., Jablonska, M., Sliwinski, T. and Zajdel, R., 2019. Plant extracts and reactive oxygen species as two counteracting agents with anti- and pro-obesity properties. International Journal of Molecular Sciences 20: 4556.

Zingg, J.M., Meydani, M. and Azzi, A., 2010. alpha-Tocopheryl phosphate – an active lipid mediator? Molecular Nutrition & Food Research 54: 679-692.

Zingg, J.M., Meydani, M. and Azzi, A., 2012. a-Tocopheryl phosphate – an activated form of vitamin E important for angiogenesis and vasculogenesis? BioFactors 38: 24-33.

Chapter 2
From milk thistle to silymarin: chemical and pharmacological properties

A stich in time saves nine

Peter F. Surai[1-6] and Anton Surai[7]*
[1]Vitagene and Health Research Centre, Bristol, UK; [2]Department of Microbiology and Biochemistry, Faculty of Veterinary Medicine, Trakia University, Stara Zagora, Bulgaria; [3]Department of Animal Nutrition, Faculty of Agricultural and Environmental Sciences, Szent Istvan University, Hungary; [4]Saint-Petersburg State Academy of Veterinary Medicine, St. Petersburg, Russia; [5]Sumy National Agrarian University, Sumy, Ukraine; [6]Odessa National Academy of Food Technologies, Odessa, Ukraine; [7]Healthy Food Services, Bristol, UK
psurai@feedfood.co.uk

Abstract

Milk thistle is an important source of polyphenolics, including mixture of flavonolignans, mainly silibinin (also known as silybin), as well as silycristine, silydianin, quercetin and taxifolin. The aforementioned phytochemicals comprise a major part of the standardised formulation prepared from the extract from the fruits of milk thistle, namely silymarin (SM). From the data presented in this chapter it is clear that SM is non-toxic, commonly used supplement, which in some countries considered as a drug. Low bioavailability of SM compounds, similar to other polyphenolics, is an important limitation in SM efficacy in many studies and the development of new formulations with increased SM solubility and availability is an important topic of current research. Some of publications are dealing with SM, others describe effects of its major constituents, including silibinin/silybin (SB). It is noteworthy that SB is used mainly in *in vitro* studies as well as in research devoted to elucidation of pharmacology and pharmacodynamics of the active ingredients of the SM preparations. At the same time, clinical applications and veterinary/animal nutrition studies are mainly based on SM and milk thistle usage. In this chapter major milestones in thistle/SM investigation are described, chemical composition and structure of silymarin, as well as its pharmacokinetics, toxicity and practical applications are presented. In the scientific literature the potential therapeutic role of SM in various diseases have been described including liver diseases, cancer, diabetes, neurodegenerative disorders, β-thalassemia. Furthermore, SM has been investigated for its anti-inflammatory and anti-toxic effects in allergic rhinitis, asthma, cancer treatment-related adverse effects, rheumatoid arthritis, drug-induced hepatotoxicity, drug-induced nephrotoxicity, dyslipidaemia, etc. Therefore, in the literature there is a great deal of information about SM protective actions in various *in vitro* and *in vivo* model systems, however, clinical trials supporting these uses are limited. In the next chapters of the book more detailed information related to SM biological activity, molecular mechanisms of its action and benefits of its clinical usage will be presented.

Peter F. Surai and Anton Surai **Silymarin puzzle**
DOI:10.3920/978-90-8686-944-2_002, © Wageningen Academic Publishers, 2023

Keywords: silymarin, silibinin/silybin, composition, structure, pharmacokinetics, toxicity

2.1 Introduction

Milk thistle (MT) is an important source of polyphenolics, including mixture of flavonolignans, mainly silybin A and silybin B (also used under common name silybin or silibinin, SB), as well as silycristine, silydianin, quercetin, taxifolin and some others. The aforementioned phytochemicals comprise a major part of the standardised formulation prepared from the extract from the fruits of milk thistle, namely silymarin (SM). This preparation has received tremendous attention for the last 50 years being used as a food supplement and sometimes as a prescribed drug to deal with various health-related problems in human and to support productive and reproductive performance of farm animals and poultry under various commercially-relevant stress conditions. In the chapter history of MT usage, chemical composition and structure of its major active constituents, their pharmacokinetic and possible toxicity will be addressed.

2.2 History of milk thistle/SM investigation

Silybum marianum (L.) *Gaertn.*, also known as milk thistle (MT), is an annual or biannual species belonging to the Asteraceae family and is native to Southern Europe, Asia Minor and Northern Africa and it is also naturalised in North and South America, Australia and New Zealand (Martinelli *et al.*, 2017). The name 'milk thistle' is believed to come from the story of the Virgin Mary who was sheltering under the thorny leaves of the milk thistle while nursing baby Jesus. According to this story, a drop of Mary's milk fell, causing the distinctive white veins on the leaves of milk thistle. Milk thistle is the English common name for this species and there is a range of other names including Mary thistle, Holy thistle, St. Mary's thistle, Lady's thistle, Marian thistle, Christ's crown, Venus thistle, Variegated thistle, Heal thistle, Pig leaves, Royal thistle, Snake milk, Sow thistle and Wild artichoke (Qavami *et al.*, 2013).

This medicinal plant has been known for over 2,000 years and ever since ancient times, *S. marianum* has been cultivated for its wide pharmacological properties and the plant history can be summaries as follows (Abenavoli *et al.*, 2010; 2018; Bijak, 2017; Devi, 2019; Ross, 2008; Schuppan *et al.*, 1999):

- The first record is in the Bible under its older Latin name *Lebanon cardus* (the Old Testament; Genesis 3:18).
- Theophrastus, the successor to Aristotle in the Peripatetic school (371-287 BC), mentioned that MT was used as a general medicinal herb. Therefore, MT has been used medicinally since the fourth century BC.
- Dioscorides, a Greek physician, pharmacologist, and botanist (40-90 AD) was the first to describe the healing properties of TM.
- Pliny the Elder, a Roman author, naturalist and natural philosopher (AD 23-79) reported that the plant's juice had the ability to remove/carry off bile.

- The ancient Greeks and Romans are believed to use MT for snake bites treatment.
- Hildegard von Bingen, a German Benedictine abbess, in 1152, described milk thistle usage.
- John Gerard, an English herbalist, in 1597 indicated that milk thistle is 'the best remedy against melancholy diseases'.
- Even Nicolas Culpeper, an English botanist, herbalist, physician and astrologer (1616-1654) mentioned usage of the plant to prevent/treat liver/spleen disorders/obstructions.
- Albrecht von Haller, a Swiss anatomist, physiologist and naturalist (1708-1777) mentioned the efficacy of the plant in preventing liver disease and liver pain.
- Johannes Gottfried Rademacher, a German physician (1772-1850), recommended it to treat liver ailments.
- For several centuries MT has been used by Indian and Chinese medicines in clinical practice for liver and gallbladder problems.
- In the USA, MT was a part of the naturopathic medical tradition of the native Americans.
- A renewal interest to MT was created in central Europe, especially in Germany, in the late 1960s, when research studies refocused attention on milk thistle and its constituents as natural hepatoprotective compounds.
- In 1968-1974 active compounds of MT were characterised and in 1971 first animal experimental studies on liver protection by MT were conducted.
- During the 1970s and 1980s, German scientists validated the potential value of milk thistle as a liver herb.
- SM, an extract of milk thistle fruits, in the 1970s was classified as an official medicine with hepatoprotective properties by the WHO.
- Elucidation of molecular mechanisms of silibinin (SB) was conducted in 1976-1988 and in 1980s first controlled clinical studies of protective effect of MT in acute viral hepatitis and alcoholic cirrhosis were performed.
- SM is included in the pharmacopoeia of many countries under various trademarks.
- At present, *S. marianum* (MT) is grown as a medicinal plant in Europe and Asia and SM, SB, and milk thistle extract currently rank among the top-selling botanical supplements or phytomedicines/herbal dietary supplements in the US, Italy and in other countries (Martinelli *et al.*, 2017; Xie *et al.*, 2019);
- The USA is expected to account for 26% of global milk thistle supplement revenue, while India is expected to be the major market for milk thistle supplements, accounting for 1/3 of global sales, while UK is expected to hold a market share of 28% during the forecast period, 2022-2032 (Cision PR Newswire, 2022a).
- According to Fact. MR (2022), the global milk thistle supplements market size was valued at over US$ 90-94 million in 2019 and is projected to grow at an impressive CAGR of ~7.4% in the forecast period (2020-2030) and is expected to reach a valuation of US$ 120.7 million by 2025 and more than US$ 178 million by 2030.
- In accordance with the Fact.MR's latest report (Cision PR Newswire, 2022b). the milk thistle supplements global market is expected to reach US$ 103.14 million by 2022 with a forecast to double for the next 10 years and reaching US$204 million in 2031.

- Canada has approved around 70 different products containing this herb (Sornsuvit *et al.*, 2018) and SM is especially popular in Germany (Dixit *et al.*, 2007).
- MT products are sold in the form of soft gel, capsules, liquids, tablets, powder and granules and sales channels include drug stores, health & beauty stores, supermarkets, direct selling, third party online channels, company online channels, etc.
- Top manufactures of milk thistle extract include Nourished, Bio-Botanica, Euromed, BI Nutraceuticals, Blackmores, Maypro, Naturex, Indena, etc.
- Milk thistle (*Silybum marianum*) is known to contain a mixture of flavonolignans, mainly silibinin (also known as silybin), as well as silycristine, silydianin, quercetin and taxifolin Main constituents of milk thistle fruits are shown in Table 2.1.
- SM is a standardised formulation prepared from the extract from the fruits (seeds) of milk thistle.
- SM has long been approved in Europe, where it is the drug of choice for amatoxin poisoning (Mullins *et al.*, 2015).
- While the market for SB in the United States is too small to justify efforts by the manufacturer to pursue US Food and Drug Administration approval, the drug is essentially available for compassionate use under the National Institutes of Health-registered study protocol referenced in the original case report (NIHCC, 2014).

There is a great number of brand names for SM produced all over the world (Table 2.2).

Table 2.1. Main constituents of milk thistle fruits (adapted from Abenavoli *et al.*, 2010).

Silybin	Dihydrokaempferol
Silychristin	Kaempferol
Silydianin	Apigenin
3-Deoxyderivatives of silychristin and silydianin (silymonin)	Naringin
Neosilyhermin A	Eriodyctiol
Neosilyhermin B	Chrysoerinol
2,3-Dehydrosilybin	5,7-Dihydroxy chromone
Taxifolin	Dehydroconiferyl alcohol
Quercetin	Silyhermin
15-30% lipids (~60% linoleic acid; ~30% oleic acid; ~9% palmitic acid)	
~0.038% tocopherol	
~0.63% sterols (cholesterol, campesterol, sigmasterol and sitosterol)	
~25-30% protein	
Carbohydrates (arabinose, rhamnose, xylose, glucose)	
Other compounds	

Table 2.2. Silymarin Brand Names (adapted from Drugs.com, 2022a).

Country	*Brand Names*/producer
Argentina	*Laragon 150*, Roemmers
Austria	*Legalon 140 mg*, Meda Pharm; *Legalon 70 mg*, Meda Pharm; *Legalon SIL*, Meda Pharm
Bahrain	*Legalon*, Maskati
Belgium	*Legalon SIL*, Meda Pharma
Bosnia & Herzegowina	*Silymarin Forte*, Belupo
Bulgaria	Carsil 110 mg, Carsil 22.5 mg, Carsil 90 mg, Sopharma; Legalon, Madaus
Chile	*Legalon*, Bayer; *Legalon Forte*, Bayer
China	*Ci Ning*, Shanxi C&Y Pharmaceutical Co., *Legalon*, Madaus GmbH; *Shui Lin Jia*, Tasly Group
Colombia	*Apotox*, Incobra; *Hepabiol*, Gruinfacol; *Hepabionta*, Asher Pharma; *Silimarina*, Bawiss
Costa Rica	*Silimarina Genfar*, Genfar S.A.
Croatia	*Silymarin*, Belupo
Czech Republic	*Flavobion*, Takeda, *Lagosa*, Wörwag Pharma; *Legalon*, Meda Pharma; *Silymarin AL*, Aliud
Egypt	*Hepaguard [+ Acetylcysteine]*, Eva; *Hepamarin*, Uni Pharma; *Hepaticum*, MUP; *Legalex*, Alexandria Co.; *Legalon*, Madaus; *Livamarin*, Eep co; *Livoprotec*, Pharaonia; *Mariagon*, Acapi; *Mepasil*, Mepaco; *Seralon E [+ Tocopherol, α-]*, Tiba; *Silymarin Sedico*, Sedico; *Silymarin Zinc Health Line [+ Zinc]*, Health Line; *Urso Plus [+ Ursodeoxycholic Acid]*, Minapharm
Ecuador	*Kufer Q Forte [+ Ubidecarenone]*, BioGenet; *Kufer Q Recargado [+ Ubidecarenone]*, BioGenet; *Kufer Q-C [+ Ubidecarenone]*, BioGenet; *Lipositol Q10 Forte [+ Ubidecarenon]*, Kronos; *Silimarina*, Genfar; *Silime*, ECU
El Salvador	*Silimarina Genfar*, Genfar S.A
Estonia	*Ardeyhepan*, Ardeypharm; *Carsil*, Sopharma
Georgia	*Carsil*, Sopharma; *Carsil Forte*, Sopharma; *Legalon*, Madaus; *Silarsil*, Uni Pharma
Germany	*Legalon*, Meda Pharma; *Legalon Forte*, Rottapharm/Madaus; *Silicur*, DR. KADE Pharmazeutische Fabrik; *Legalon SIL*, Meda Pharma
Guatemala	*Silimarina Genfar*, Genfar S.A.
Hong Kong	*Silymarin*, Quality Pharm
Hungary	*Hegrimarin*, Strathmann; *Legalon 140 mg*, Meda; *Legalon 70 mg*, Meda; *Legalon SIL 10 mg/ml*, Meda; *Silygamma 86.5 mg*, Wörwag Pharma
India	*Actimarin Forte [+ Ursodeoxycholic Acid]*, Alb. David; *Arosi [+ Ornithine]*, Arvincare; *Hepagreen Plus [+ Aspartic Acid, L-]*, Santiago; *Limarin*, Serum Intl.; *Liverubin*, Alchem; *Livosil Forte*, Centaur; *Livosil-B [+ Thiamine, + Riboflavin, + Pyridoxine], Centaur; Nitlor Plus [+ Ornithine]*, BMW; *Prohep Forte*, Lupin; *Similar*, Zydus; *Silybon*, Micro Labs; *Silyrin*, Talent; *Sivylar Daiichi*, Ranbaxy; *Tyrin*, TNT; *Tyrin-Forte [+ Ursodeoxycholic Acid]*, TNT; *Urdohep-SL [+ Ursodeoxycholic Acid], Macleods; Ursolic Plus [+ Ursodeoxycholic Acid]*, Stadmed
Indonesia	*Liparin*, Guardian Pharmatama
Italy	*Legalon*, Rottapharm; *Silimarin*, Germed Pharma; *Silmar*, BioHealth Pharmaceuticals
Kuwait	*Legalon*, Madaus
Latvia	*BioSilymarin*, Irel, *Carsil*, Sopharma; *Lagosa*, Woerwag Pharma
Lithuania	*Carsil*, Alvogen; *Carsil*, Lex ano; *Carsil*, Sopharma; *Helar*, Aconitum; *Livosil*, Aconitum; *Silymarin Siromed*, IBE Pharma

Table 2.2. Silymarin Brand Names (adapted from Drugs.com, 2022a).

Country	***Brand Names*/producer**
Luxembourg	*Legalon 140 mg*, Madaus; *Legalon SIL*, Meda
Macedonia	*Carsil*, Sopharma; *Silymarin Belupo*, Belupo
Malaysia	*Cefasily*, Cefak/Bio-Pharmaceuticals
Malta	*Legalon*, Rottapharm
Mexico	*Legalon*, Takeda México; *Neo-Cholal [+ Inositol, + Magnesium]*, Italmex
Nicaragua	*Silimarina Genfar*, Genfar S.A.
Oman	*Legalon*, Madaus GmbH; *Silymarin*, Sedico Pharma
Pakistan	*Equadin*, Wilson; *Hepamyrin*, Qintar Pharma; *Hepar*, Fynk; *Hepasil*, Helicon; *Heptosil*, Medisearch; *Liprotec*, Olive Labs
Paraguay	*Silimarina Pharma Arte*, Pharma Arte
Peru	*Hepactor B*, Pharma-C; *Hepalab-B*, Drog. Infarval; *Hepalivio*, Naturgen; *Higalab B*, Keyfarm; *Higanatur*, Sherfarma; *Lagosa*, Wörwag Pharma; *Silimarina-Genfar*, Genfar
Philippines	*Hepavit*, Littman; *Legalon*, Madaus; *Liver Plus*, XL Lab
Poland	*Lagosa*, Wörwag Pharma; *Legalon*, Madaus; *Silimax*, Filofarm
Portugal	*Legalon*, Neo-Farmacêutica
Romania	*Lagosa*, Wörwag Pharma; *Legalon 140*, Rottapharm-Madaus; *Legalon 70*, Rottapharm-Madaus; *Silibina Arena*, Arena; *Silimarinã Biofarm*, Biofarm
Slovakia	*Flavobion*, Takeda; *Lagosa*, Wörwag, *Legalon*, Madaus
South Africa	*Legalon*, Nycomed
Spain	*Legalon*, Meda Pharma Sau; *Silarine*, Vir
Switzerland	*Allsan*, Mariendistel Biomed, *Legalon 140 mg*, MEDA Pharma; *Legalon 70 mg*, MEDA Pharma; *Phytopharma Leber Galle*, Phytopharma; *Legalon SIL*, Meda Pharma
Taiwan	*Bao-Gan*, Chen Ta; *Dilacan Silymarin*, CanCap; *Durasilymarin*, Wyeth; *Econlin*, Health Chemical; *Eliamine*, Panion & BF; *Elianine*, Panion & BF; *Enpex*, Yuan Chou; *Forliver*, Root; *Gen Bo*, Chen Ho; *Hepanat*, Yung Shin; *Hepa-V*, UBI; *Hepawell*, Quest Vitamins; *Heprin*, Dong Kook; *Kenbo*, Yung Chang; *Lemarin*, Hans-E Lembecke; *Livercon*, Sheng Chung Tang; *Liveron*, Hua Shin; *Livorin*, Weidar; *Lolian*, Hwang's; *Poken*, Meider; *Pougenin*, Hua Shin; *Poulican-U*, Sinphar; *Procam*, Everest; *Sican*, Astar; *Silibin*, Hwang's; *Siligen*, Synmosa; *Silima*, Souriree; *Silimin*, Kojar; *Silin*, Shun Sheng; *Silirin*, Chin Teng Pharmaceutical Industrial; *Silliver*, Chung Mei; *Siluma*, Ming Ta; *Silycon*, AND; *Silygen*, Siu Guan; *Silygen-F*, Hor Chen; *Silygen-H*, Hor Chen; *Silyhep*, Kojar; *Silyma*, Ming Ta; *Silymarin*, Pei Li; Shou Chan; Tai Yu; *Silyme-V*, Oriental; *Silymin*, Swiss Pharm; *Sucan*, Yu Sheng; *Suganlin*, Fisherman; *Sulican*, Yu Sheng; *Symatone*, Patron; *Winmarin*, Winston
Thailand	*Legalon*, Madaus; *Leveron*, Vesco Pharma; *Livotone*, Mega Lifesciences; *Sivylar*, Daiichi; *Pharmarin*, Pharmaland; *Samarin*, Berlin
Uruguay	*Silimarina Disfarm*, Bernard; *Tendencil*, Szabó
Venezuela	*Legalon*, Zuoz
Vietnam	*Liverstad*, Stada-VN JV; *Silygamma 150 mg*, Woerwag Pharma

Among major manufacturers of the milk thistle supplements are 21st Century Healthcare Inc., Amway, Bio-Botanica Inc., Blackmores Ltd., Divine Bounty, Doctor's Best, Euromed S.A., Halal-Pharma International Ltd., Indena SPA, Inner Mongolia Ever Brilliance Biotechnology Co. Ltd., Integra Nutrition Inc., Jarrow Formulas Inc., Maypro Industries, Natural Field Enterprise Limited, Nature's Best, Nature's Bounty Co., Naturex, Nested Naturals Inc., North Folk Nutra, Now Foods, Otsuka Pharmaceutical Co. Ltd., Sunergetic, Swanson Health Products, The Bioforce Group and many others.

2.3 Chemical composition and structure

The active ingredient in milk thistle is silymarin (SM). It is obtained from the fruits, which are reported to be pressed to remove most of the fats and further defatted with solvent (petroleum ether). The resulting cake is further extracted with other solvents (acetone or ethyl acetate), and the remaining fat is separated after dilution with water (Kren, 2021). In fact, SM, a standardised extract from the milk thistle *Silybum marianum* contains as its main constituents (65-80%) a complex of flavonolignans: silybin A, silybin B, isosilybin A, isosilybin B, silychristin, isosilychristin, silydianin, and the flavonoids taxifolin, quercetin, and kaempferol (Table 2.3). The remainder is reported to consist of fatty acids, betaine, apigenin, silybonol, proteins, fixed oil, various polyphenols including a mixture of undefined polyphenolic compounds (about 30%), often referred to as 'polymeric fraction' (Bijak, 2017; Křen and Valentová, 2022) composed mostly of oligomers and polymers of flavonolignans (Tvrdy *et al.*, 2021). To obtain flavonolignans, the seed meal is usually subjected to successive washes with petroleum ether to remove lipids, and flavonolignans are then extracted with ethanol (Wang *et al.*, 2020).

Table 2.3. Composition of commercially available silymarin and its constituents (adapted from Viktorova *et al.*, 2019).

Compound	Summary formula	MW, g/mol	Concentration, mg/g
Silybin B	$C_{25}H_{22}O_{10}$	482.44	133
Silybin A	$C_{25}H_{22}O_{10}$	482.44	113
Silychristin[1]	$C_{25}H_{22}O_{10}$	482.44	110
Isosilybin A	$C_{25}H_{22}O_{10}$	482.44	67.4
Isosilybin B	$C_{25}H_{22}O_{10}$	482.44	26.1
Silydianin	$C_{25}H_{22}O_{10}$	482.44	32.0
Taxifolin	$C_{15}H_{12}O_7$	304.25	25.3
2,3-Dehydrosilybin	$C_{25}H_{22}O_{10}$	480.43	5.0
SILYMARIN (sum of constituents			511.8
Silymarin content in commercial preparation (%)			51.2±2.8

[1] In some publications its spelling is silycristine, silychristine, or silycristin.

SM is reported to contain about 30% silybin A and B, about 5% isosilybin A and B, 7-10% silychristin A, 10% silydianin, a smaller amount of taxifolin (2-5%), and ≤3% 2,3-dehydroflavonolignans (Křen and Valentová, 2022). It should be mentioned that the composition of SM varies greatly between the variety of *S. marianum* (Aziz *et al.*, 2020) and the conditions under which it is grown (Martinelli *et al.*, 2021) including soil composition, climatic conditions as well as techniques of plant processing (Abenavali *et al.*, 2018; Devi, 2019; Křen and Valentová, 2022). For example, a positive correlations of SM content in milk thistle seeds with average rainfall and soil organic matter were established. At the same time negative correlation between temperature, humidity, soil pH and SM production by milk thistle was shown (Javeria and Hussain, 2022). Therefore, since SM is a crude extract of plant material, it has a high degree of compositional variability (Kren, 2021) which could be responsible for experimental results variability.

The chemical structure of silybin was established in 1968 (Pelter and Hänsel, 1968) and the absolute configuration of the compound at the C-2 and C-3 positions was revealed 7 years later by the same authors (Pelter and Hänsel, 1975). Silybin (also known as flavobin, silibinin, silliver, silymarin I) was reported to have a molecular weight of 482.441, a molecular formula of $C_{25}H_{22}O_{10}$, and a CAS Number of 22888-70-6 (PubChem, Fallah *et al.*, 2021). In scientific literature terms silybin and silibinin are used as synonyms (Kren, 2021). There are two domains, connected by a 1, 4-dioxane ring, in the molecular structure of silybin: the first one is related to the flavononol group, found in flavonoids such as taxifolin (dihydroquercetin), and the second domain is the phenylpropanoid group, found in coniferyl alcohol. Silybin molecule has five hydroxyl groups serving as the main targets for derivatisation (Fallah *et al.*, 2021). Silybin A and B diastereoisomers comprising up to 70% of the SM extract, are believed to be the most biologically active components. Therefore, natural silybin is a mixture of silybin A and B, with a ratio of these two stereoisomers to be about 3:7 (Křen and Valentová, 2022). In older literature this ratio was reported to be 1:1 (Kim *et al.*, 2003). Indeed, this ratio is variable depending on the source and processing conditions of SM (Kren, 2021). SB has a low solubility in water and it is practically insoluble in polar solvents. It is quite resistant to reduction but easily oxidises to 2,3-dehydrosilybin, being stable under acidic conditions and unstable in the presence of Lewis acids or in basic conditions (Abenavali *et al.*, 2018).

2.4 Pharmacokinetics

There are over 200 papers dealing with various pharmacological aspects of SM including its absorption, distribution, metabolism, and excretion and results were well reviewed by Abenavoli *et al.*, (2010), Kren (2013, 2021), Theodosiou *et al.* (2014), Tvrdý *et al.* (2021), Křen and Valentová (2022) and can be summarised as follows:

- Orally administered SM is rapidly taken up by gastrointestinal tract cells in all parts of the intestine with the highest uptake to be found in the duodenum followed by the jejunum, ileum, and colon. After entering the intestinal cells, SM flavonolignans undergo rapid conjugation, primary glucuronidation and the process continues in the liver. In human plasma, near the plasma peak times (1-3 h), the average portions of free, sulphated, and glucuronidated total SM flavonolignans are approximately 17%, 28%, and 55%, respectively (Tvrdý *et al.*, 2021).

- In rats, SB is believed to be mainly bound to plasma triglyceride-rich lipoproteins, while in human plasma, it is associated with a specific site on serum albumin (Tvrdý *et al.*, 2021).
- After single oral administration of a standardised dose of SB 100 to 360 mg to male volunteers, plasma SB C_{max} was reached after approximately 2 h and it was mainly present (75%) in the conjugated form (Abenavoli *et al.*, 2010).
- The plasma half-life ($t_{1/2}$) of free silybin after a single intravenous dose in rabbits, mice, rats and humans were reported to be 60-72, 72-96, 15-48 and 60-240 minutes, respectively (Křen and Valentová, 2022).
- Intravenously administered SB is found in different organs including the heart, liver, spleen, lung, and kidney with the heart having the highest concentration in comparison to other mentioned organs (Tvrdý *et al.*, 2021).
- Tissue distribution of SB in mice (6 to 7 weeks old) after oral administration of 50 mg/kg is shown in Table 2.4. Peak concentrations of free SB were observed after 30 minutes in the liver, lungs, stomach and pancreas, while in the skin and prostate, peak concentrations of SB were reached 60 minutes after administration (Zhao and Agarwal, 1999). Similarly, conjugated SB (sulphate conjugates and β-glucuronides) in the liver, skin, prostate and pancreas exhibited peak tissue concentrations after 1 hour, while the lungs and stomach showed peak SB values after 30 minutes. The concentrations of free and conjugated SB diminished exponentially (Zhao and Agarwal, 1999).
- SB concentrations in bile was reported to be approximately 100-fold higher than those found in serum with peak concentrations reached within 2-9 h (Abenavoli *et al.*, 2010).
- Bile SB levels greatly exceed serum levels, showing that substantial levels are achieved in the liver (14.5 μg/g corresponding to about 30 μM) and may remain high due to enterohepatic recirculation. Therefore, the liver would greatly benefit from exposure to the SM flavonolignans (Zhao and Agarwal, 1999; Filburn *et al.*, 2007).

Table 2.4. Tissue distribution of silibinin (SB; 50 mg/kg) orally administered to mice (adapted from Zhao and Agarwal, 1999).

Tissue	Maximum SB concentration, μg/g		Elimination half-life, min	
	Free SB	Conjugated SB	Free SB	Conjugated SB
Liver	8.8	5.7	57	71
Lung	4.3	2.8	95	94
Stomach	123	270	127	70
Skin	1.4	4.3	105	74
Prostate	2.5	6.1	107	67
Pancreas	5.8	10.6		45

- After i.p. administration of tritium-labelled SB to rats, its concentration in membranes was slowly rising and reached 77% of total liver content after 6 h, while little SB was found in the nucleus (Tvrdý *et al.*, 2021).
- For total SB, an elimination half-life of approximately 6 h was estimated and SM bioavailability (the portion of the administered compound reaching the systemic circulation) is relatively low comprising less than 1% for SB (Tvrdý *et al.*, 2021).
- SB and other components of SM are reported to rapidly conjugate with sulphate and glucuronic acid in the liver. The conjugates pass into the plasma and into the bile, where they are found in amounts corresponding to 80% of the total dose administered, while a small portion is eliminated in the urine. These findings indicate the existence of enterohepatic circulation (intestinal absorption, conjugation in the liver, excretion in the bile, hydrolysis by the intestinal flora, and reuptake in the intestine), making the study of the intestinal absorption of SM very difficult (Zhao and Agarwal, 1999).
- In the rat, intestinal absorption of labelled SB (a dose of 20 mg/kg) amounts to about 35% with peak radioactivity was demonstrated in the plasma 30 minutes after ingestion (Zhao and Agarwal, 1999).
- SB is characterised by rapid metabolism, comparatively low bioavailability, and its plasma concentration is commonly within the nanomolar range limits (Fallah *et al.*, 2021).
- The bioavailability of SM flavonolignans in rats and humans has been reported to be very low (in a range of 0.45-5%; Křen and Valentová, 2022).
- Many factors contribute to a low oral bioavailability of SM including (Tvrdý *et al.* (2021)):
  - *Drug solubility*. In accordance with the biopharmaceutics classification system defined by the Food and Drug Administration (FDA) guideline, SB belongs to class IV, being a compound with a low aqueous solubility and low absorption from the gut.
  - *Dissolution of formulation*. There is a range of patented techniques to improve SM water solubility and bioavailability.
  - *Stability in gastrointestinal fluids.*
  - *Permeability across the intestinal barrier*. Relatively good lipidic solubility helps SM penetrating into gut cells.
  - *First-pass metabolism both in the intestine and the liver*. SM compounds are quickly metabolised by various pathways including conjugation.
  - *Efflux transporters*. Flavonolignans from SM are known to be substrates of efflux transporters limiting the net permeability.
- After oral administration, flavonolignans undergo both phase I and phase II biotransformation, with increased glutathione *S*-transferase and quinone reductase activity observed in the liver, stomach, lungs, small bowel, and skin, in a time- and dose-dependent manner (Zhao and Agarwal, 1999).
- The phase I biotransformation (functionalisation) of flavonolignans by cytochromes P-450 was found to account for about 1-2% of the total parent substance (Kren, 2021).
- Conjugation reactions of phase II were reported to be the main biotransformation pathway of flavonolignans and methylations, glucuronidations, sulfations, and

glutathione conjugation occur in intestinal cells and in the liver (Kren, 2021; Křen and Valentová, 2022). Among them, glucuronylation is considered to be the major conjugation pathway of SM flavonolignans. After oral consumption of SM in healthy volunteers plasma silybin was found mainly (83-90%) in the conjugated form (Fallah *et al.*, 2021). The rapid and extensive phase II metabolism of SB has been considered as the major factor responsible for its low bioavailability (Xie *et al.*, 2019).

- Silybin B is shown to be metabolised to a much larger extent and significantly faster than silybin A (Kren, 2021).
- Thirty-one metabolites were identified in human urine after SM consumption. Monoglucuronides were shown to be the most common excreted form, followed by sulphate-glucuronides and diglucuronides, respectively (Rickling, *et al.*, 1995).
- After oral administration of silibinin capsules to rat and human 18 metabolites were identified in urine samples. Interestingly, 27.6% and 23.3% of silibinin were excreted in urine in the form of metabolites over a 72-h period. Five major metabolites were as follows: silibinin A-7-O-β-glucuronide, silibinin B-7-O-β-glucuronide, silibinin A-5-O-β-glucuronide, silibinin B-5-O-β-glucuronide and silibinin A-20-O-glucuronide (Xu *et al.*, 2022a).
- The excretion of monoglucuronides was reported to peak 2 h after SM consumption, whereas sulphate-glucuronide and diglucuronide excretion peaked at 8 h (Calani *et al.*, 2012).
- Both free and conjugated SB are reported to be rapidly eliminated *in vivo*. However, the renal excretion of SB is low (1-2% of an original oral dose over 24 h) and it is believed that 20-40% of bile SB is recovered by enterohepatic circulation, and the remaining part is excreted via faeces (Tvrdý *et al.*, 2021).
- Excretion of total flavonolignans including their conjugates in urine was shown to be only 0.45%, while excretion of parent SB and its conjugates varied in a range of 1% to 5% (Tvrdý *et al.*, 2021).
- The microbial degradation of flavonolignans is not well characterised, but they appear to be relatively resistant to the gut microbiota (Křen and Valentová, 2022). At the same time dietary SM supplementation in sows was reported to reduce the gut bacterial community and its richness. Furthermore, SM was able to increase the relative abundance of *Fibrobacteres and Actinobacteria* at the phylum level (Xu *et al.*, 2022b).
- SB concentration achievable in human plasma is about 1 μM (Filburn, 2007) and varies depending on SM dosage: 0.37-1.3 μM (Lorenz *et al.*, 1984), 0.7-2.9 μM (Saller *et al.*, 2001) or 0.54-3.13 μM (Sornsuvit *et al.*, 2018). In general, the maximum achievable plasma concentration of silybin is approximately 10 μM (Křen and Valentová, 2022).
- Various approaches have been tested to enhance water solubility and bioavailability of SM, including complexing with N-methylglucamine, succinate, β-cyclodextrin and phosphatidylcholine (Filburn *et al.*, 2007). In fact, when dogs were dosed with equal amount of SB in a silybin-phosphatidylcholine complex (SPC) and SM extract, the mean C_{max} plasma levels of SB increased by 2.7-fold in comparison to SM extract (Filburn *et al.*, 2007).

- To improve SM bioavailability, self-microemulsifying drug delivery system, sugar coated tablets, floating effervescent tablets, dripping pills, microspheres, proliposomes and β-cyclodextrin molecular inclusion complexes have been widely used (Eita, 2022).
- Pharmacokinetic parameters of SB following oral administration of four different commercial SM products in rats indicates that SB concentrations (C_{max}) were 0.52; 0.94; 1.54; and 6.49 μM and T_{max} were 30, 10, 10 and 20 min respectively (Ha *et al.*, 2019).
- In spite of a great body of *in vitro* data showing interactions of SM or individual flavonolignans with a range of enzymes and transporters, the clinical relevance of these interactions is not clear, and they have not been confirmed in human trials, but the risk of potential pharmacokinetic interaction in humans cannot be fully excluded (Tvrdý *et al.*, 2021).
- The recommended dosage for active disease is 140 mg of SM (200 mg of extract) three times daily. If the silymarin-phosphatidylcholine is used, 100 mg three times daily is considered to be the appropriate dosage (Fraschini *et al.*, 2002).

2.5 Silymarin toxicity

The acute toxicity of SM has been studied in mice, rats, rabbits and dogs after intravenous infusion. The LD50 values for the acute SM toxicity after intravenous infusion was reported to be approximately 400 mg/kg BW in mice, 385 mg/kg BW in rats and 140 mg/kg BW in rabbits and dogs. After oral SM administration, LD50 is much higher with values ranging over 10 g/kg BW. The mean lethal dose for rabbits and the maximum tolerated dose in dogs were calculated to be about 300 mg/kg (Lecomte, 1975). In the cases of acute intoxication, the main cause of death was associated with cardiovascular failure (Radko, and Cybulski, 2007). Indeed, the acute, subacute and chronic toxicity of SM were reported to be very low without embryotoxic potential.

SM was shown to be safe at therapeutic doses in human, well tolerated even at a high dose of 700 mg three times a day for 24 weeks, and only transient side effects like gastrointestinal upsets and mild allergic reactions, urticaria, nausea, headache, joint pain, itching, and mild laxative symptoms have been detected in some studies. Total percentage of adverse events observed in a meta-analysis of clinical trials was reported to be 2.36% with SB versus 5.05% with placebo and no deaths or life-threatening adverse events have been reported (Saller *et al.*, 2008). In animals, SM was reported to be non-toxic and symptom free with the maximum oral doses of 2,500 and 5,000 mg/kg but had mutagenic activity in *Salmonella typhimurium* strains in the presence of metabolic enzymes. Furthermore, major active compounds of SM, namely silybin, silydianin, and silychristin, were not cytotoxic and genotoxic at concentration of 100 μM (Soleimani *et al.*, 2019).

Current findings on drug-drug interactions of SM, including results from clinical trials, concluded that SM does not pose a clinically relevant risk of drug-drug interaction (Xie *et al.*, 2019). However, pharmacokinetic studies carried out in healthy volunteers indicated that SM pretreatment increased the exposure of talinolol and domperidone, decreased the AUC of indinavir and metronidazole, reduced losartan biotransformation into its active form and affected the pharmacokinetics of pyrazinamide (Xie *et al.*, 2019). It is demonstrated that SM is an inhibitor of CYP2C9 enzyme and could displace the site I ligand warfarin from human serum albumin (Poór *et al.*, 2018). SB is also shown to affect the pharmacokinetics of methadone in rats (Pan *et al.*, 2018). Therefore, SM may interfere with the pharmacokinetics of several drugs and drug-drug interactions in relation to SM warrant more research.

2.6 Silymarin applications

The potential therapeutic role of SM in various diseases have been described including

- liver diseases (Abenavoli *et al.*, 2010; 2011; 2013; 2018);
- cancer (Polachi *et al.*, 2016; Zhu *et al.*, 2016);
- diabetes (Stolf *et al.*, 2017);
- neurodegenerative disorders (Devi *et al.*, 2017);
- or β-thalassemia (Moayedi Esfahani *et al.*, 2015).

Furthermore, SM has been investigated for its anti-inflammatory and CNS effects in allergic rhinitis, asthma, cancer treatment-related adverse effects, rheumatoid arthritis, drug-induced hepatotoxicity, drug-induced nephrotoxicity, dyslipidemia, etc. However clinical trials supporting these uses are limited. In the next chapters of the book more detailed information related to SM biological activity, molecular mechanisms of its action and benefits of its clinical usage will be presented.

2.7 Conclusions

Milk thistle is an important source of polyphenolics, including mixture of flavonolignans, mainly silibinin (also known as silybin), as well as silycristine, silydianin, quercetin and taxifolin. The aforementioned phytochemicals comprise a major part of the standardised formulation prepared from the extract from the fruits of milk thistle, namely silymarin. From the data presented above it is clear that SM is non-toxic, commonly used supplement, which in some countries considered as a drug. Low bioavailability of SM compounds, similar to other polyphenolics, is an important limitation in SM efficacy in many studies and the development of new formulations with increased SM solubility and availability is an important topic of current research.

In the literature there is a great deal information about SM protective actions in various *in vitro* and *in vivo* model systems and clinical trials and it will be considered in detail in the next chapters of this book. Some of publications are dealing with SM, others describe effects of its major constituents, including SB. Therefore, a specific emphasis will be given to that and in many cases when talking about molecular mechanisms of SM action we will be using SM/SB abbreviation meaning that we combine information related to SM and its main constituent, namely silybin/silibinin, to make some conclusions. It is noteworthy that SB is used mainly in *in vitro* studies as well as in research devoted to elucidation of pharmacology and pharmacodynamics of the active ingredients of the SM preparations. At the same time, clinical applications and veterinary/animal nutrition studies are mainly based on SM and milk thistle usage.

References

Abenavoli, L. and Bellentani, S., 2013. Milk thistle to treat non-alcoholic fatty liver disease: Dream or reality? Expert Review of Gastroenterology & Hepatology 7: 677-679.

Abenavoli, L., Aviello, G., Capasso, R., Milic, N. and Capasso, F., 2011. Milk thistle for non-alcoholic fatty liver disease treatment. Hepatitis Monthly 11: 173-177.

Abenavoli, L., Capasso, R., Milic, N. and Capasso, F., 2010. Milk thistle in liver diseases: past, present, future. Phytotherapy Research 24:1423-1432.

Abenavoli, L., Izzo, A.A., Milić, N., Cicala, C., Santini, A. and Capasso, R., 2018. Milk thistle (*Silybum marianum*): A concise overview on its chemistry, pharmacological, and nutraceutical uses in liver diseases. Phytotherapy Research 32: 2202-2213.

Aziz, M., Saeed, F., Ahmad, N., Ahmad, A., Afzaal, M., Hussain, S., Mohamed, A.A., Alamri, M.S. and Anjum, F.M., 2020. Biochemical profile of milk thistle (*Silybum marianum* L.) with special reference to silymarin content. Food Science & Nutrition 9: 244-250.

Bijak, M., 2017. Silybin, a major bioactive component of milk thistle (*Silybum marianum* L. Gaernt.) – Chemistry, bioavailability, and metabolism. Molecules 22: 1942.

Calani, L., Brighenti, F., Bruni, R. and Del Rio, D., 2012. Absorption and metabolism of milk thistle flavanolignans in humans. Phytomedicine 20: 40-46.

A Cision Company (Cision PR Newswire), 2022a. Powder dietary supplements market to surpass US$ 75.2 billion by 2032 amidst growing focus on preventive healthcare. A Cision Company, Pundong Shanghai, China. Available at: https:// tinyurl.com/2p82p3yh.

A Cision Company (Cision PR Newswire), 2022b. Milk thistle supplements market to garner US$ 204 Mn by 2032: Exclusive Fact.MR study. A Cision Company, Pundong Shanghai, China. Available at: https://www.tinyurl.com/2tur8yzn.

Devi, K.P., Malar, D.S., Braidy, N., Nabavi, S.M. and Nabavi, S.F., 2017. A mini review on the chemistry and neuroprotective effects of silymarin. Current Drug Targets 18: 1529-1536.

Devi, K.P., 2019. Milk thistle (*Silybum marianum*). In: Seyed, N. and Silva, A. (eds) Nonvitamin and nonmineral nutritional supplements. Elsevier, Academic Press, London, UK, pp. 321-325.

Dixit, N., Baboota, S., Kohli, K., Ahmad, S. and Ali, J., 2007. Silymarin: A review of pharmacological aspects and bioavailability enhancement approaches. Indian Journal of Pharmacology 39: 172-179.

Drugsite Trust (Drugs.com), 2022a. Silibinin. Drugsite Trust, Auckland, New Zealand Available at: https://tinyurl.com/4kfvrxtb.

Drugsite Trust (Drugs.com), 2022b. Milk thistle. Drugsite Trust, Auckland, New Zealand. Available at https://tinyurl.com/ycyxyw5f.

Eita, A.A.B., 2022. Milk thistle (*Silybum marianum* (L.)Gaertn.): An overview about its pharmacology and medicinal uses with an emphasis on oral diseases. Journal of Oral Biosciences 64: 71-76.

Fact. MR, 2022. Milk thistle supplements demand outlook (2022-2032). Fact MR, Rockville, MD, USA. Available at: https://www.tinyurl.com/4mupetcr.

Fallah, M., Davoodvandi, A., Nikmanzar, S., Aghili, S., Mirazimi, S., Aschner, M., Rashidian, A., Hamblin, M.R., Chamanara, M., Naghsh, N. and Mirzaei, H., 2021. Silymarin (milk thistle extract) as a therapeutic agent in gastrointestinal cancer. Biomedicine & Pharmacotherapy 142: 112024.

Filburn, C.R., Kettenacker, R. and Griffin, D.W., 2007. Bioavailability of a silybin-phosphatidylcholine complex in dogs. Journal of Veterinary Pharmacology and Therapeutics 30: 132-138.

Fraschini, F., Demartini, G. and Esposti, D., 2002. Pharmacology of silymarin. Clinical Drug Investigation 22: 51-65.

Ha, E.S., Han, D.G., Seo, S.W., Kim, J.M., Lee, S.K., Sim, W.Y., Yoon, I.S. and Kim, M.S., 2019. A simple HPLC method for the quantitative determination of silybin in rat plasma: Application to a comparative pharmacokinetic study on commercial silymarin products. Molecules 24: 2180.

Javeria, M. and Hussain, K., 2022. Relationship between different agro-climatic conditions and silymarin production in wild milk thistle (*Silybum marianum* l. gaert.) in pakistan. Pakistan Journal of Botany 54: 179-185.

Kim, N.C., Graf, T.N., Sparacino, C.M., Wani, M.C. and Wall, M.E., 2003. Complete isolation and characterization of silybins and isosilybins from milk thistle (*Silybum marianum*). Organic & Biomolecular Chemistry 1: 1684-1689.

Křen, V., 2021. Chirality matters: Biological activity of optically pure silybin and Its congeners. International Journal of Molecular Sciences 22: 7885.

Křen, V., Marhol, P., Purchartová, K., Gabrielová, E. and Modrianský, M., 2013. Biotransformation of silybin and its congeners. Current Drug Metabolism 14: 1009-1021.

Křen, V. and Valentová, K., 2022. Silybin and its congeners: from traditional medicine to molecular effects. Natural Product Reports 39: 1264-1281.

Lecomte, J., 1975. Les propriétés pharmacologiques de la silybine et de la silymarine [Pharmacologic properties of silybin and silymarin]. Revue Medicale de Liege 30: 110-114.

Lorenz, D., Lücker, P.W., Mennicke, W.H. and Wetzelsberger, N., 1984. Pharmacokinetic studies with silymarin in human serum and bile. Methods and Findings in Experimental and Clinical Pharmacology 6: 655-661.

Martinelli, T., Whittaker, A., Benedettelli, S., Carboni, A. and Andrzejewska, J., 2017. The study of flavonolignan association patterns in fruits of diverging *Silybum marianum* (L.) Gaertn. chemotypes provides new insights into the silymarin biosynthetic pathway. Phytochemistry 144: 9-18.

Martinelli, T., Fulvio, F., Pietrella, M., Focacci, M., Lauria, M. and Paris, R., 2021. In *Silybum marianum* Italian wild populations the variability of silymarin profiles results from the combination of only two stable chemotypes. Fitoterapia 148: 104797.

Moayedi Esfahani, B.A., Reisi, N. and Mirmoghtadaei, M., 2015. Evaluating the safety and efficacy of silymarin in β-thalassemia patients: A review. Hemoglobin 39: 75-80.

Mullins, M.E., Schwarz, E.S., Dribben, W.H., Halcomb, S.E. and Arroyo-Plasencia, A.M., 2015. Silibinin: where is the ethical conundrum? Chest 147: e105.

National Institutes of Health Clinical Center (NIHCC), 2014. Intravenous milk thistle (silibinin-legalon) for hepatic failure induced by amatoxin/ amanita mushroom poisoning. National Institutes of Health; Bethesda, MD, USA. Available at: https://www.tinyurl.com/mrxwu79m.

Pan, P.P., Wang, J., Luo, J., Wang, S.H., Zhou, Y.F., Chen, S.Z. and Du, Z., 2018. Silibinin affects the pharmacokinetics of methadone in rats. Drug Testing and Analysis 10: 557-561.

Pelter, A. and Hänsel, R., 1968. The structure of silybin (silybum substance E6), the first flavonolignan. Tetrahedron Letters 9: 2911-2916.

Pelter, A. and Hansel, R., 1975. Structure of silybin. 1. Degradative experiments. Chemische Berichte 108: 790-802.

Polachi, N., Bai, G., Li, T., Chu, Y., Wang, X., Li, S., Gu, N., Wu, J., Li, W., Zhang, Y., Zhou, S., Sun, H. and Liu, C., 2016. Modulatory effects of silibinin in various cell signaling pathways against liver disorders and cancer – A comprehensive review. European Journal of Medicinal Chemistry 123: 577-595.

Poór, M., Boda, G., Mohos, V., Kuzma, M., Bálint, M., Hetényi, C. and Bencsik, T., 2018. Pharmacokinetic interaction of diosmetin and silibinin with other drugs: Inhibition of CYP2C9-mediated biotransformation and displacement. Biomedicine & Pharmacotherapie 102: 912-921.

Qavami, N., Naghi, B.H., Labbafi, M.R. and Mehrafarin, A., 2013. A review on pharmacological, cultivation and biotechnology aspects of milk thistle (*Silybum marianum* (L.) Gaertn.). Journal of Medicinal Plants 12: 19-37.

Radko, L. and Cybulski, W., 2007. Application of silymarin in human and animal medicine. Journal of Pre-Clinical and Clinical Research 1: 22-26.

Rickling, B., Hans, B., Kramarczyk, R., Krumbiegel, G. and Weyhenmeyer, R., 1995. Two high-performance liquid chromatographic assays for the determination of free and total silibinin diastereomers in plasma using column switching with electrochemical detection and reversed-phase chromatography with ultraviolet detection. Journal of Chromatography. B, Biomedical Applications 670: 267-277.

Ross, S.M., 2008. Milk thistle (*Silybum marianum*): an ancient botanical medicine for modern times. Holistic Nursing Practice 22: 299-300.

Saller, R., Brignoli, R., Melzer, J. and Meier, R., 2008. An updated systematic review with meta-analysis for the clinical evidence of silymarin. Forschende Komplementarmedizin 15: 9-20.

Saller, R., Meier, R. and Brignoli, R., 2001. The use of silymarin in the treatment of liver diseases. Drugs 61: 2035-2063.

Schuppan, D., Jia, J.D., Brinkhaus, B. and Hahn, E.G. 1999. Herbal products for liver diseases: a therapeutic challenge for the new millennium. Hepatology 30: 1099-1104.

Soleimani, V., Delghandi, P.S., Moallem, S.A. and Karimi, G., 2019. Safety and toxicity of silymarin, the major constituent of milk thistle extract: An updated review. Phytotherapy Research 33: 1627-1638.

Sornsuvit, C., Hongwiset, D., Yotsawimonwat, S., Toonkum, M., Thongsawat, S. and Taesotikul, W., 2018. The bioavailability and pharmacokinetics of silymarin SMEDDS formulation study in healthy Thai volunteers. Evidence-Based Complementary and Alternative Medicine 2018: 1507834.

Stolf, A.M., Cardoso, C.C. and Acco, A., 2017. Effects of silymarin on diabetes mellitus complications: A review. Phytotherapy Research 31: 366-374.

Theodosiou, E., Purchartová, K., Stamatis, H., Kolisis, F. and Křen, V., 2014. Bioavailability of silymarin flavonolignans: drug formulations and biotransformation. Phytochemistry Reviews 13: 1-18.

Tvrdý, V., Pourová, J., Jirkovský, E., Křen, V., Valentová, K. and Mladěnka, P., 2021. Systematic review of pharmacokinetics and potential pharmacokinetic interactions of flavonolignans from silymarin. Medicinal Research Reviews 41: 2195-2246.

Viktorova, J., Stranska-Zachariasova, M., Fenclova, M., Vitek, L., Hajslova, J., Kren, V. and Ruml, T., 2019. Complex evaluation of antioxidant capacity of milk thistle dietary supplements. Antioxidants 8: 317.

Wang, X., Zhang, Z. and Wu, S.C., 2020. Health benefits of *Silybum marianum*: Phytochemistry, pharmacology, and applications. Journal of Agricultural and Food Chemistry 68: 11644-11664.

Xie, Y., Zhang, D., Zhang, J. and Yuan, J., 2019. Metabolism, transport and drug-drug interactions of silymarin. Molecules 24: 3693.

Xu, C., Yuan, Y., Pang, P., Yang, H., Zhang, Q., Yuan, D. and Qi, W., 2022a. Urinary excretion of silibinin diastereoisomers and their conjugated metabolites in rat and human at different dosages. Biomedical Chromatography 36: e5480.

Xu, S., Jiang, X., Jia, X., Jiang, X., Che, L., Lin, Y., Zhuo, Y., Feng, B., Fang, Z., Li, J., Wang, J., Ren, Z. and Wu, D., 2022b. Silymarin modulates microbiota in the gut to improve the health of sow from late gestation to lactation. Animals 12: 2202.

Zhao, J. and Agarwal, R., 1999. Tissue distribution of silibinin, the major active constituent of silymarin, in mice and its association with enhancement of phase II enzymes: implications in cancer chemoprevention. Carcinogenesis 20: 2101-2108.

Zhu, X.X., Ding, Y.H., Wu, Y., Qian, L.Y., Zou, H. and He, Q., 2016. Silibinin: A potential old drug for cancer therapy. Expert Review of Clinical Pharmacology 9: 1323-1330.

Chapter 3
Antioxidant defence systems in health and diseases

The first blow is half the battle

Peter F. Surai[1-6] and Anton Surai[7]*
[1]Vitagene and Health Research Centre, Bristol, UK; [2]Department of Microbiology and Biochemistry, Faculty of Veterinary Medicine, Trakia University, Stara Zagora, Bulgaria; [3]Department of Animal Nutrition, Faculty of Agricultural and Environmental Sciences, Szent Istvan University, Hungary; [4]Saint-Petersburg State Academy of Veterinary Medicine, St. Petersburg, Russia; [5]Sumy National Agrarian University, Sumy, Ukraine; [6]Odessa National Academy of Food Technologies, Odessa, Ukraine; [7]Healthy Food Services, Bristol, UK
psurai@feedfood.co.uk

Abstract

Redox (antioxidant-prooxidant) balance in the body/tissues/cells is an important determinant of various physiological functions. Indeed, oxidative stress occurs when this balance is disturbed due to overproduction of free radicals or compromised antioxidant defences. Free radical overproduction and oxidative stress are considered as a pathobiochemical mechanism involved in the initiation or progression phase of various diseases in human and farm animals. The antioxidant defence includes several options, including decrease localised oxygen concentration, decrease activity of pro-oxidant enzymes, improve efficiency of electron chain in the mitochondria and decreasing electron leakage leading to superoxide production, induction of various transcription factors (e.g. Nrf2, NF-κB and others) and ARE-related synthesis of AO enzymes (SOD, GPx, CAT, GR, GST, etc.). Furthermore, it includes binding metal ions (metal-binding proteins) and metal chelating, decomposition of peroxides by converting them to non-radical, nontoxic products, chain breaking by scavenging intermediate radicals such as peroxyl and alkoxyl radicals, repair and removal of damaged molecules (methionine sulfoxide reductase, DNA-repair enzymes, HSPs and other chaperons, etc.). In addition, redox-signalling and vitagene activation with synthesis and increased expression of protective molecules (GSH, thioredoxins, SOD, HSPs, sirtuins, etc.), antioxidant recycling mechanisms, including vitamin E recycling, protein glutathionylation is a way to prevent its irreversible oxidation, apoptosis activation and removal of terminally damaged cells and restriction of mutagenesis are also important parts of the AO defence strategy. All antioxidants in the body are working as a 'team' responsible for antioxidant defence and we call this team the antioxidant system. In this team one member helps another one working efficiently. The regulation of gene expression by oxidants, antioxidants, and redox state has emerged as a novel subdiscipline in molecular biology that has promising implications for medical practises as well as for animal production. However, there are still many gaps in our knowledge of the basic molecular mechanisms of oxidative damage and antioxidant defences. It seems likely that in future more attention will be paid to various approaches to regulate redox homeostasis

DOI:10.3920/978-90-8686-944-2_003,

in human and animals, including vitagene activation, and antioxidant-regulating properties of SM/SB would be of great importance and they will be considered in detail in the next chapters of the book.

Keywords: antioxidants, redox balance, Nrf2, NF-κB, vitagenes, oxidative stress, silymarin

3.1 Introduction

It is well known that oxygen is an essential element for eukaryotes, and they rely on oxygen for the efficient production of energy. However, energy production in mitochondria is not 100% efficient and some electrons can escape from the electron transport chain (ETC) forming free radicals. For the last three decades free radical research has generated valuable information for deeper understanding not only detrimental, but also beneficial role of free radicals in cell signalling, stress adaptation and other physiological processes. The benefit or harm of free radicals ultimately depend on the level of their production and efficiency of antioxidant defence. In fact, disturbances of redox balance and oxidative stress are responsible for the development of a range human diseases (Table 3.1).

3.2 Free radicals and reactive oxygen and nitrogen species

Free radicals are atoms or molecules containing one or more unpaired electrons. Free radicals are highly unstable and reactive and are capable of damaging biologically relevant molecules such as DNA, proteins, lipids or carbohydrates.

The animal body is under constant attack from free radicals, formed as a natural consequence of the body's normal metabolic activity and as part of the immune system's strategy for destroying invading microorganisms. The internal and external sources of free radicals are shown in Table 3.2. Collective terms reactive oxygen species (ROS) and reactive nitrogen species (RNS) have been introduced (Halliwell and Gutteridge, 2015) and combined by a term RONS, including not only the oxygen or nitrogen radicals, but also some non-radical reactive derivatives of oxygen and nitrogen (Table 3.3).

Therefore, RONS (Table 3.3) are constantly produced *in vivo* in the course of the physiological metabolism in tissues. It is generally accepted that the electron-transport chain in the mitochondria is responsible for major part of superoxide production in the body. Mitochondrial electron transport system consumes more than 85% of all oxygen used by the cell and, because the efficiency of electron transport is not 100%, about 1-3% of electrons escape from the chain and the univalent reduction of molecular oxygen results in superoxide anion formation. About 10^{12} O_2 molecules processed by each rat cell daily and if the leakage of partially reduced oxygen molecules is about 2%, this will yield about 2 x10^{10} molecules of ROS per cell per day (for a review see Surai, 2020). An interesting calculation has been made by Halliwell (1994), showing

Table 3.1. Free radical involvement in the development of human diseases (adapted from Surai and Sparks, 2001).

Liver	**Eye**
Reperfusion	Retinopathy of prematurity
Toxic effects of chemicals: halogenated hydrocarbons, quinones, iron, ethanol acetaminophen	Photic retinopathy
Endotoxin	Macular degeneration
	Ocular hemorrhages
	Cataracts
Kidney	**Muscle**
Autoimmune nephrosis: inflammation	Muscular dystrophy
Toxic effects of chemicals: aminoglycosides, heavy metals	Multiple sclerosis
	Exercise
Lung	**Skin**
Normobaric hyperoxic injury	Radiation (UV or ionizing)
Bronchopulmonary dysplasia	Thermal injury
Toxic effects of chemicals: paraquat, bleomycin	Toxic effects of chemicals: tetracyclines
Emphysema	Porphyria
Asbestosis	Contact dermatitis
Idiopathic pulmonary fibrosis	
Heart and cardiovascular system	**Brain and nervous system**
Atherosclerosis	Parkinson's disease
Hemochromatosis	Alzheimer's disease
Ischemia/reperfusion	Tardive dyskinesia
Myocardial infarction	Neuronal ceroid lipofuscinosis
Selenium deficiency (Keishan disease)	Neurotoxins
Toxic effects of chemicals: ethanol, doxorubicin	Hypertensive cerebrovascular injury
	Allergic encephalomyelitis
Gastrointestinal tract	**Inflammatory-immune system**
Reperfusion	Glomerulonephritis
Toxic effects of chemicals: nonsteroidal and anti-inflammatory agents, alloxan, iron	Vasculitis
Pancreatitis	Autoimmune disease
Colitis	Rheumatoid arthritis
Blood	**Miscellaneous/general**
Malaria	Aging
Various anaemias	AIDS
Protoporphyrin photooxidation	Cancer
Fanconi's anemia	Diabetes
Favism	Inflammation
Toxic effects of chemicals: phenylhydrazine, primaquine and related drugs, sulphonamides, lead, etc.	Trauma
	Rheumatoid arthritis and lupus
	Acute pancreatitis

Table 3.2. Internal and external sources of free radicals (adapted from Surai, 2020).

Internally generated	Factors promoting ROS formation
Mitochondria (ETC)	Cigarette smoke
Phagocytes (NADPH-Oxidase)	Radiation
Xanthine oxidase	UV light
Reactions with Fe^{2+} or Cu^{+}	Pollution
Arachidonate pathways	Certain drugs
Peroxisomes	Chemical reagents
Inflammation	Industrial solvents
Biomolecule oxidation (adrenaline, dopamine, tetrahydrofolates, etc.)	High level of ammonia
	Mycotoxins

Table 3.3. Reactive oxygen and nitrogen species (adapted from Surai, 2020).

Radicals	Non-radicals
Alkoxyl, RO*	Hydrogen peroxide, H_2O_2
Hydroperoxyl, HOO*	Hypochlorous acid, HOCl
Hydroxyl, *OH	Ozone, O_3
Peroxyl, ROO*	Singlet oxygen, $^1O_2$
Superoxide, O_2*	Peroxynitrite, $ONOO^-$
Nitric oxide, NO*	Nitroxyl anion, NO^-
Nitrogen dioxide, NO_2*	Nitrous acid, HNO_2

that in the human body about 1.72 kg/year of superoxide radical is produced. In stress condition it would be substantially increased. Clearly, these calculations showed that free radical production in the body is substantial and many thousand biological molecules can be easily damaged if are not protected. The activation of phagocytes in stress conditions is another important source of free radical generation. Immune cells produce RONS and use them as an important weapon to destroy pathogens.

Free radicals are implicated in the initiation or progression phase of various human diseases, including cardiovascular disease, some forms of cancer, cataracts, age-related macular degeneration, rheumatoid arthritis and a variety of neuro-degenerative diseases (Table 3.1). In animal/poultry production, overproduction of free radicals and oxidative stress are considered to be related to various type of stresses, including, nutritional, technological, environmental and internal stresses. In general, it is widely believed that most human and animal/poultry diseases at different stages of their development are associated with free radical production and metabolism (Surai, 2020). Normally, there is a delicate balance between the amount of free radicals generated in the body and the antioxidants to protect against them. For the majority of organisms on Earth, life without oxygen is impossible, animals, plants and many micro-organisms relying on oxygen for the efficient production of energy. However, they pay a high price for pleasure of living in an oxygenated atmosphere since high oxygen concentration in the atmosphere is potentially toxic for living organisms.

3.3 Three levels of antioxidant defence

During evolution living organisms have developed specific antioxidant protective mechanisms to deal with RONS. Therefore, it is only the presence of natural antioxidants in living organisms which enable them to survive in an oxygen-rich environment. These mechanisms are described by the general term 'antioxidant system'. It is diverse and responsible for the protection of cells from the actions of free radicals. This system includes:

- natural fat-soluble antioxidants (vitamin E, carotenoids, ubiquinones, etc.);
- water-soluble antioxidants (ascorbic acid, uric acid, carnitine, taurine (TAU), etc.);
- antioxidant enzymes: glutathione peroxidase (GPx), catalase (CAT) and superoxide dismutase, including cytosolic Cu/ZnSOD called SOD1, mitochondrial MnSOD called SOD2 and extracellular SOD called SOD3);
- thiol redox system consisting of the glutathione system (glutathione/glutathione reductase/glutaredoxin/glutathione peroxidase and a thioredoxin system (thioredoxin/thioredoxin peroxidase/thioredoxin reductase).

The antioxidant capacity of a compound is determined by multiple factors in addition to the reactivity toward free radicals, including the chemical reactivity toward free radicals; fate of antioxidant-derived radicals; interaction with other antioxidants; concentration, distribution, mobility, and metabolism at the micro-environment. The protective antioxidant compounds are located in organelles, subcellular compartments or the extracellular space enabling maximum cellular protection to occur. Thus, the antioxidant system of the living cell includes three major levels of defence (Surai, 2020):

The first level of defence is responsible for prevention of free radical formation by removing precursors of free radicals or by inactivating catalysts and consists of three antioxidant enzymes namely SOD, GPx and CAT plus metal-binding proteins (Figure 3.1).

Since the superoxide radical is the main free radical produced in physiological conditions in the cell (Halliwell, 1994) superoxide dismutase (EC 1.15.1.1) is considered to be the main element of the first level of antioxidant defence in the cell. This enzyme dismutates the superoxide radical in the following reaction:

$$\mathbf{2O_2^{*} + 2H+ \xrightarrow{SOD} H_2O_2 + O_2}$$

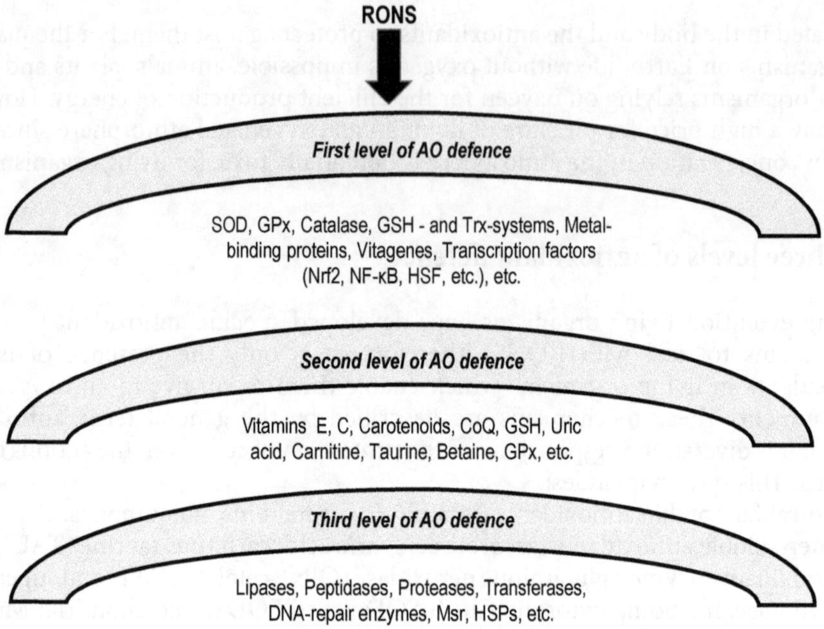

Figure 3.1. Three lines of antioxidant defence in animal cells (adapted from Surai, 2020).

The hydrogen peroxide formed by SOD action can be detoxified by GPx or CAT which reduce it to water as follows:

$$H_2O_2 + 2GSH \xrightarrow{GPx} GSSG + 2H_2O$$

$$2H_2O_2 \xrightarrow{CAT} 2H_2O + O_2$$

Catalase (EC 1.11.1.6) is a tetrameric enzyme consisting of four identical subunits of 60 kDa containing a single ferriprotoporphyrin group per subunit. It plays an important role in the acquisition of tolerance to oxidative stress in the adaptive response of cells. In mammalian cells, NADPH is bound to CAT protecting it from inactivation by H_2O_2. Since GPx has a much higher affinity for H_2O_2 than CAT and wider distribution in the cell (CAT is located mainly in peroxisomes), the H_2O_2 removal from the cell is very much dependent on GPx.

Recently it has been shown that thioredoxin peroxidases are also capable of directly reducing hydrogen peroxide. It is interesting that the levels of antioxidant enzymes are regulated by gene expression as well as by post-translational modifications (Surai, 2020).

Hydrogen peroxide can also be detoxified by peroxiredoxins (Prx):

$$\textbf{Prx (reduced)} + H_2O_2 \longrightarrow \textbf{Prx (oxidised)} + 2H_2O$$

The oxidised form of Prx is inactive, requiring the donation of electrons from reduced thioredoxin (Trx) to restore its catalytic activity:

$$\textbf{Prx (oxidised) + Trx (reduced)} \longrightarrow \textbf{Prx (reduced) + Trx (oxidised)}$$

Furthermore, Se-dependent enzyme TR reduce oxidised Trx to its reduced active form:

$$\textbf{Trx (oxidised)} \xrightarrow{\text{TR}} \textbf{Trx (reduced)}$$

Mammalian cells express 6 Prx isoforms, including Prx3 and Prx5 in the mitochondria. Prxs function by undergoing oxidation by H_2O_2 at an active site cysteine and then subsequent reduction by thioredoxin, thioredoxin reductase, and NADPH. There are eight GPXs, which are oxidised by H_2O_2 and reduced by glutathione (GSH), and CAT is found in peroxisomes (Surai, 2020). Therefore, GSH- and Trx-systems, as well as vitagenes and some transcription factors (e.g. Nrf2, NF-κB, HSF, etc.) also belong to the first level of the antioxidant defence. Transition metal ions also accelerate the decomposition of lipid hydroperoxides into cytotoxic products such as aldehydes, alkoxyl radicals and peroxyl radicals:

$$\textbf{LOOH} + Fe^{2}+ \longrightarrow \textbf{LO*} + Fe^{3}+ + OH^{-}$$

$$\textbf{LOOH} + Fe^{3}+ \longrightarrow \textbf{LOO*} + Fe^{2}+ + H+$$

Thus, metal-binding proteins (transferrin, lactoferrin, haptoglobin, hemopexin, metallothionenin, ceruloplasmin, ferritin, albumin, myoglobin, etc.) also belong to the first level of defence. It is necessary to take into account that iron and copper are powerful promoters of free radical reactions and therefore their availability in 'catalytic' forms is carefully regulated *in vivo* (Surai, 2020). Therefore, organisms have evolved to keep transition metal ions safely sequestered in storage or transport proteins.

Unfortunately, this first level of antioxidant defence in the cell is not sufficient to completely prevent free radical formation and some radicals do escape through the preventive first level of antioxidant safety screen initiating lipid peroxidation and causing damage to DNA and proteins. Therefore, the second level of defence consists of chain-breaking antioxidants – vitamin E, ubiquinol, carotenoids, vitamin A, ascorbic acid, TAU, carnitine, uric acid and some other antioxidants. Glutathione and thioredoxin systems also have a substantial role to play in the second level of antioxidant defence. Chain-breaking antioxidants inhibit peroxidation by keeping the chain length of the propagation reaction as small as possible. Therefore, they prevent the propagation step of lipid peroxidation by scavenging peroxyl radical intermediates in the chain reaction:

$$\text{LOO*} + \text{Toc} \longrightarrow \text{Toc*} + \text{LOOH}$$

Where LOO* is lipid peroxyl radical; Toc is tocopherol, Toc* = tocopheroxyl radical and LOOH = lipid hydroperoxide.

Some specific enzymes which hydrolyse oxidised bases preventing their incorporation into DNA can also be considered as a part of the second level of antioxidant defence. However, even the second level of antioxidant defence in the cell is not able to prevent damaging effects of ROS and RNS on lipids, proteins and DNA. In this case, the third level of defence is based on systems that eliminate damaged molecules or repair them. This level of antioxidant defence includes lipolytic (lipases), proteolytic (peptidases or proteases) and other enzymes (Msr, DNA repair enzymes, ligases, nucleases, polymerases, proteinases, phospholipases, various transferases, etc.) as well as protein chaperones, including HSPs. All the antioxidants are operating in the body in association with each other forming integrated antioxidant system. The co-operative interactions between antioxidants in the cell are vital for maximum protection from the deleterious effects of free radicals and toxic products of their metabolism.

3.4 Antioxidant defence network

Living cells permanently balance the process of formation and inactivation of RONS and as a result RONS level remains low but still above zero. Adverse environmental conditions initiate attempts of organisms to resist the environment that became more aggressive (Skulachev, 1998). Cells can usually tolerate mild oxidative stress by additional synthesis of various antioxidants (GSH, antioxidant enzymes, etc.) in an attempt to restore antioxidant/oxidant balance. At the same time, energy expenditures increased, and respiration activated leading to the increased yield of RONS. However, these adaptive mechanisms have limited ability. Once the free radical production exceeds the ability of antioxidant systems to neutralise them, lipid peroxidation develops and causes damage to unsaturated lipids in cell membranes, amino acids in proteins and nucleotides in DNA and as a result, membrane and cell integrity is disrupted. Membrane damage is associated with a decreased efficiency of absorption of different nutrients and leads to an imbalance of vitamins, amino acids, inorganic elements and other nutrients in the organism. All these events result in health-related problems in human and lead to decreased productive and reproductive performances of farm animals/poultry. Immunity incompetence and unfavourable changes in the cardio-vascular system, brain and neurones and muscle system due to increased lipid peroxidation and protein oxidation make the situation even worse.

Therefore, the antioxidant defence includes several options (Figure 3.2; Surai, 2020):

- decrease localised oxygen concentration;
- decrease activity of pro-oxidant enzymes;

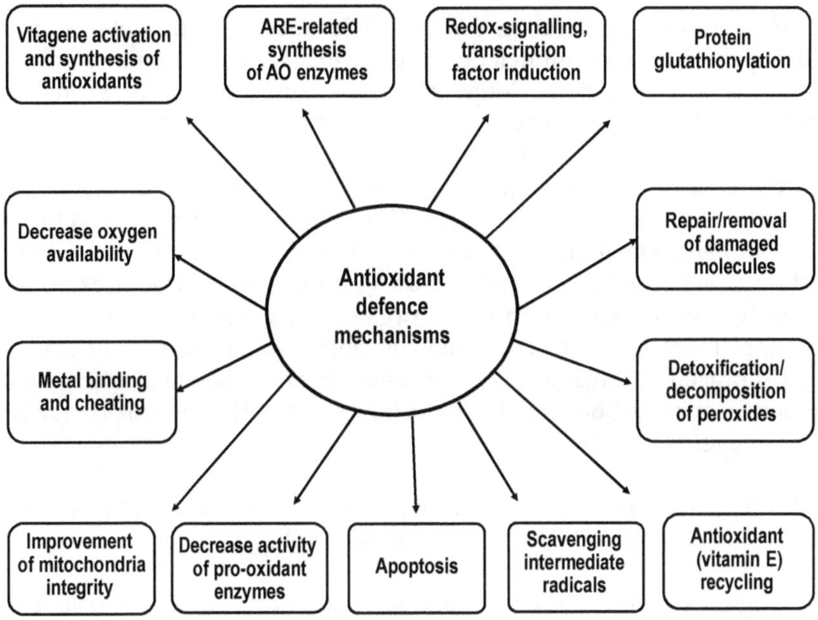

Figure 3.2. Antioxidant defence mechanisms (adapted from Surai, 2020).

- improve efficiency of electron chain in the mitochondria and decreasing electron leakage leading to superoxide production;
- induction of various transcription factors (e.g. NF-E2-related factor 2 [Nrf2], nuclear factor-κB [NF-κB] and others) and ARE-related synthesis of AO enzymes (SOD, GPx, CAT, glutathione reductase [GR], glutathione S-transferase [GST], etc.);
- binding metal ions (metal-binding proteins) and metal chelating;
- decomposition of peroxides by converting them to non-radical, nontoxic products;
- chain breaking by scavenging intermediate radicals such as peroxyl and alkoxyl radicals;
- repair and removal of damaged molecules (methionine sulfoxide reductase, DNA-repair enzymes, HSPs and other chaperons, etc.);
- redox-signalling and vitagene activation with synthesis and increased expression of protective molecules (GSH, thioredoxins, SOD, HSPs, sirtuins, etc.);
- antioxidant recycling mechanisms, including vitamin E recycling;
- protein glutathionylation is a way to prevent its irreversible oxidation;
- apoptosis activation and removal terminally damaged cells and restriction of mutagenesis.

As it was shown above all antioxidants in the body are working as a 'team' responsible for antioxidant defence and we call this team the antioxidant system. In this team one member helps another one working efficiently. In general vitamin E and coenzyme Q are considered to be a 'head-quarter' of the antioxidant defences, while Se is a 'chief executive' of antioxidant defence, since from 25 known selenoproteins, more than half participate in antioxidant defences (Surai, 2020). Furthermore, a central role in antioxidant system regulation belongs to vitagene expression and additional synthesis of protective molecules in stress conditions ('ministry of defence') to improve adaptive ability to stress. Therefore, if relationships in this team are effective, which happens only in the case of balanced diet and sufficient provision of dietary antioxidant nutrients, then even low doses of such antioxidants as vitamin E could be effective. On the other hand, when this team is subjected to high stress conditions, free radical production is increased dramatically. During these times, without external help it is difficult to prevent damage to major organs and systems. This 'external help' is dietary supplementation with increased concentrations of natural antioxidants. For nutritionist or feed formulator it is a great challenge to understand when the internal antioxidant team in the body requires help, how much of this help to provide and what the economic return will be.

It is well accepted that in the body a delicate critical balance exists between antioxidant defence, repair systems and free radical generation (Figure 3.3).

In physiological conditions the right and left parts of the so-called 'balances' are in equilibrium i.e. free radical generation is neutralised by the antioxidant system to maintain the redox homeostasis. Exogenous factors are among the most important elements, which increase an efficiency of the antioxidant system of the body. Natural

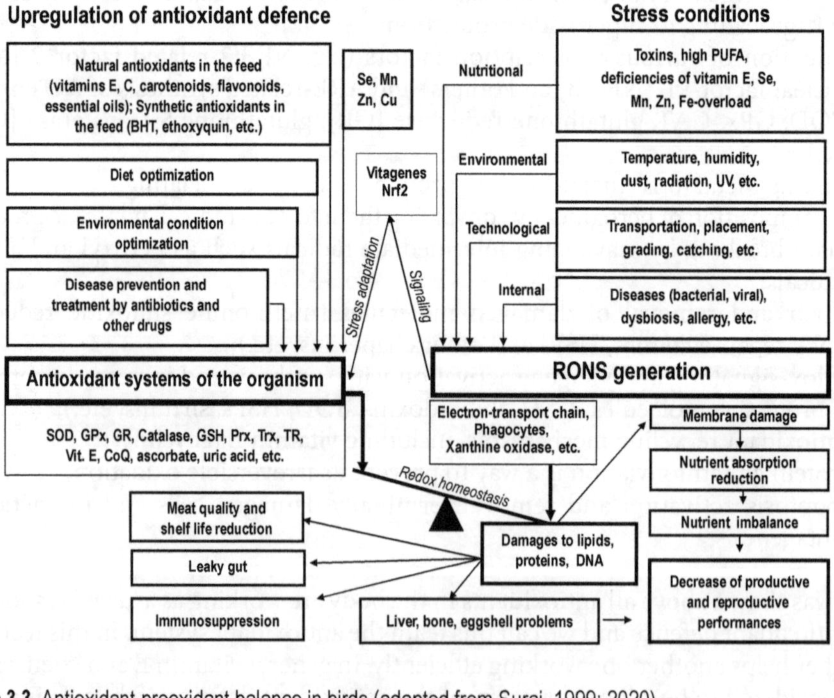

Figure 3.3. Antioxidant-prooxidant balance in birds (adapted from Surai, 1999; 2020).

and synthetic antioxidants in the feed as well as optimal levels of Mn, Cu, Zn and Se help maintain the efficient levels of endogenous antioxidants in the tissues. Optimal diet composition allows the antioxidants of the feed to be efficiently absorbed and metabolised. Optimal temperature, humidity and other environmental conditions are also required for the effective protection against RONS production. The prevention of different diseases is an integral part of the efficient antioxidant defence as well. Different stress conditions are associated with overproduction of RONS and cause oxidative stress i.e. a disturbance in the redox balance leading to potential tissue damage (Surai, 2020). It is generally accepted that RONS also have beneficial effects by participating in redox signalling and stress adaptation via regulating various transcription factors and vitagenes.

3.5 Oxidative stress and redox biology

The concept of oxidative stress as an imbalance between oxidants and antioxidants and oxidative stress responses was formulated by Sies in 1985 (Sies and Jones, 2020) and later it was updated (Surai, 2020) to include current development and understanding of the topic. To deal with the oxidative challenge and to maintain redox homeostasis a stress response is initiated including the activation of gene expression of defence systems. There are two major 'master regulators' of the stress response, including the Nrf2/Keap1 and the NF-κB/IκB systems. Booth transcription factors are translocated to the nucleus and create protective, but in many cases opposite responses. While Nrf2 activates genes responsible for synthesis of an array of protective antioxidant molecules, NF-κB activates the expression of genes involved in inflammatory, immune, and acute phase responses. The stress response also includes other important factors such as the hypoxia induced response, the heat shock response, the unfolded protein response, and various repair programs as well as removal programs including autophagy, mitophagy, apoptosis, necroptosis, ferroptosis, etc. (Surai, 2020). Oxidative stress and its relationship to redox signalling is shown in Figure 3.4. Redox signalling is shown to be integrated with main homeostatic mechanisms at the molecular, organellar, cellular, tissue and organismic levels (Sies and Jones, 2020) and associated with the vitagene network and various transcription factors (Surai, 2020).

3.6 Stress-response pathways

Animals and human manage stress via adopting various mechanisms generally called 'stress response' (SR) associated with induction of various genes responsible for synthesis of various cyto-protective molecules. Depending on conditions, SR can be immediate, lasting from a few seconds to several hours and associated with receptor-mediated intracellular signalling or SR may be delayed with involvement of various modulators and downstream effectors (Bhattacharya and Rattan, 2019). There are at least 8 stress-response pathways responsible for stress sensing and development of the adequate response (Figure 3.5).

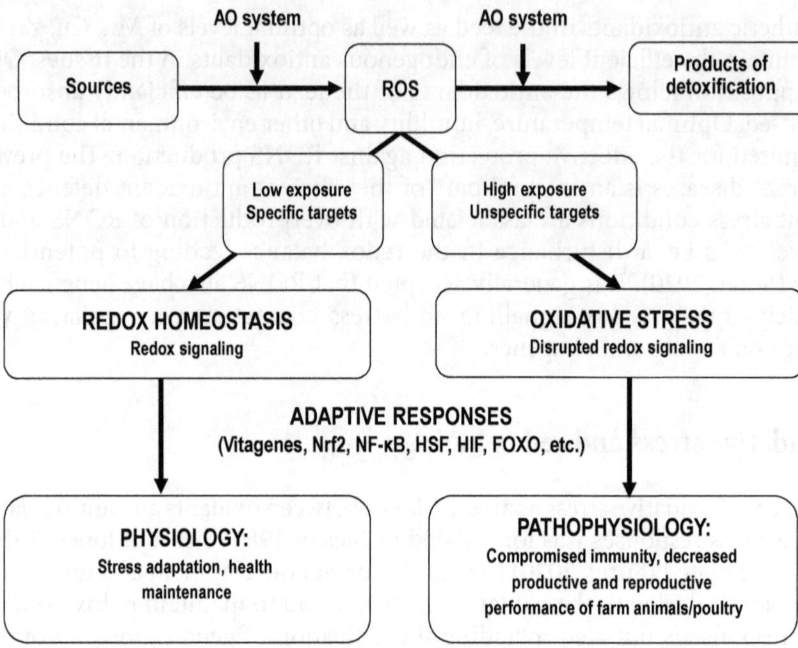

Figure 3.4. Oxidative stress and its relationship to redox signalling (adapted from Surai, 2020).

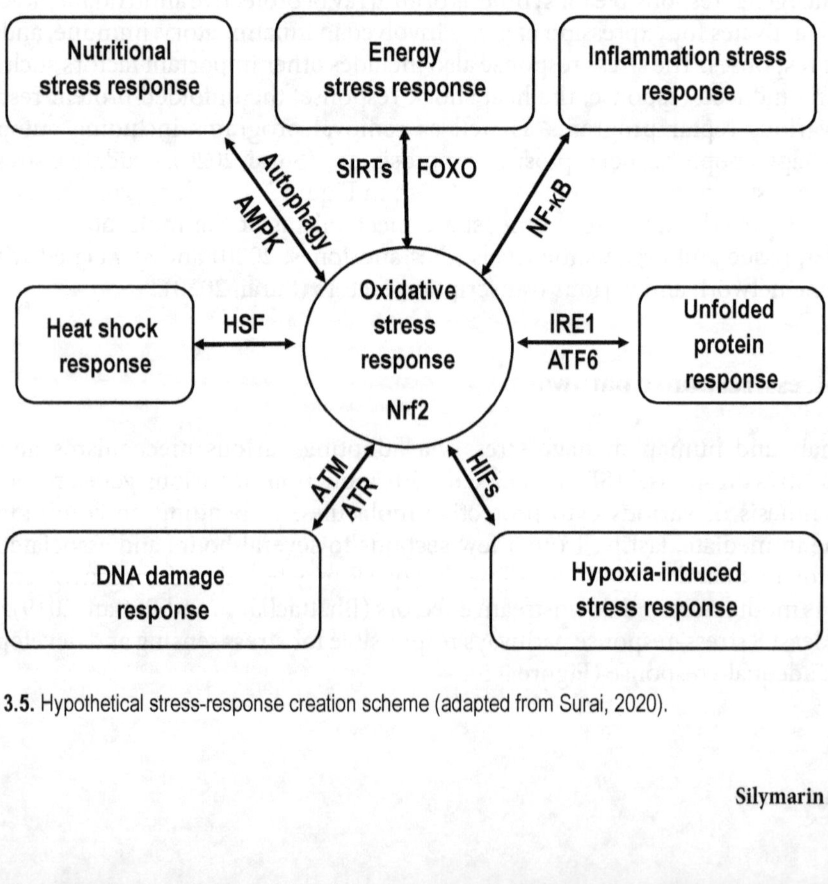

Figure 3.5. Hypothetical stress-response creation scheme (adapted from Surai, 2020).

AMPK: AMP-activated protein kinase; ATF6: activating transcription factor 6; ATM: Ataxia-telangiectasia-mutated; ATR: Ataxia-telangiectasia and Rad 3-related; FOXO: forkhead box protein; HIF: hypoxia inducible factor; HSF: heat shock factor; IRE1: inositol-requiring enzyme 1; NF-κβ: nuclear factor kappa-light-chain-enhancer of activated B cells; Nrf2: nuclear factor erythroid-2 related factor 2; SIRTs-sirtuins.

For example, various stresses in animal/poultry production caused by increased/reduced temperature, dust in air, mycotoxins, etc. can activation of HSF1 with following HSP activation (Surai, 2020). Oxidative stress can cause an accumulation of unfolded proteins in the ER lumen triggering an SR called the unfolded protein response (UPR) or ER stress response. Low oxygen levels, some metals and various chemicals can activate hypoxia-induced stress response (HISR) associated with activation of HIF inducible genes responsible for synthesis of protective molecules, including erythropoietin, HO-1, etc. helping deal with homeostasis disturbance. Radiation, various pro-oxidants (pesticides, mycotoxins, etc.), as well as RONS can cause DNA damage and activate DNA damage response (DDR) associated with activation of a key serine/threonine protein signalling kinase (ATM) and Rad3-related (ATR). In the next step, ATM and ATR are recruited to double-strand and single strand breaks with following activation of DNA repair enzymes to repair damaged DNA or remove it (Surai, 2020).

Various pathogens, damaged macromolecules, allergens and various chemicals can activate inflammatory stress response (ISR) associated with activation/translocation to nucleus of NF-κB and synthesis of various pro-inflammatory cytokines (Surai *et al.*, 2021a). Low ATP/AMP or NAD+/NADH ratio due to lack of energy could cause energy stress response (ESR) mediated mainly via sirtuin system activation, AMPK activation and deacetylation of PGC-1α, FOXO and other important molecules. Nutritional disbalance/inadequacy, hypoxia and damaged cellular organelles can lead to nutritional stress response (NSR) associated with AMPK activation and autophagosome formation with following lysosomal digestion of damaged mitochondria. Finally, oxidative stress response is related to Nrf2 activation and synthesis of a range protective molecules (Surai, 2020). Interestingly, all 8 stress-responses are interrelated, and oxidative stress response can be placed into the centre of stress-response creation (Figure 3.5).

An interconnected core of reactions and components mediating cross talk between essential bioenergetic processes and signalling pathways is called a redox hub (Foyer and Noctor, 2011). Major redox hubs in mammalian cells include Nrf2, NF-κB, HIF, FOXO, p53, oestrogen-related receptor (ERR), peroxisome proliferator-activated receptor-γ co-activator 1α (PGC1α), 5′-adenosine monophosphate-activated protein kinase (AMPK), uncoupling proteins (UCP) and glyceraldehyde 3-phosphate dehydrogenase (GAPDH; Sies and Jones, 2020; Sies and Ursini, 2022; Sies *et al.*, 2022; Figure 3.6).

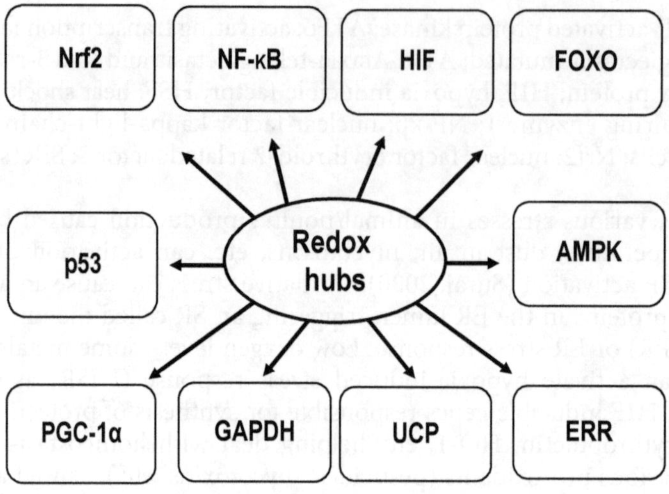

Figure 3.6. Redox hubs in mammals (adapted from Sies and Jones, 2020; Sies and Ursini, 2022; Sies *et al.*, 2022). AMPK = AMP-activated protein kinase; ERR = oestrogen-related receptor; GAPDH = glyceraldehyde 3-phosphate dehydrogenase; FOXO = forkhead box protein; HIF = hypoxia inducible factor; NF-κβ = nuclear factor kappa-light-chain-enhancer of activated B cells; Nrf2 = nuclear factor erythroid-2 related factor 2; PGC1α = peroxisome proliferator-activated receptor-γ co-activator 1α; p53 = tumour protein P53, UCP = uncoupling proteins.

Furthermore, 2-cys peroxiredoxins are considered to be emerging hubs determining redox dependency of mammalian signalling networks (Park *et al.*, 2014) and sirtuins roles in redox regulation is of paramount importance (Surai *et al.*, 2021b).

Therefore, the aforementioned redox hubs can buffer the production of oxidants and reductants and are responsible for sensing changes in redox state and integration of information from the environment and metabolism leading to adaptation via gene expression and synthesis of protective molecules, repairing or removing damages molecules and re-establishing adaptive homeostasis.

While oxidative stress pathways are now well studied, little is known about how cells initially sense the accumulation of ROS (Heo *et al.*, 2021). There is a range of redox sensors responsible for oxidative stress/redox disbalance detection and transmission oxidative stress signals to chaperones and inducing various protective mechanisms. The redox-dependent signalling pathways in biological systems are highly conserved and based on the oxidation and reduction of cysteine residues in proteins. It was demonstrated that in mitochondrial proteins >90% of the Cys residues were conserved among vertebrates, whereas only about 70% of other amino acids in the same proteins were conserved and therefore the thiol of Cys is believed to serve as a versatile sulphur switch to link redox chemistry with structure and function (Go and Jones, 2013). Importantly, the human Cys proteome was reported to include 214,000 Cys residues encoded in the genome (Go and Jones, 2013). It seems likely that methionine and selenocysteine (Sec) residues can also be post-translationally modified by ROS and the human genome was reported to encode 174,000 Met residues (Go and Jones, 2013). Furthermore, Sec is found only in 25 selenoproteins, but such selenoproteins as TR, GPx and MsrB1 are most important enzymes in the redox status homeostasis maintenance (Surai, 2018).

Therefore, the redox sensing and signalling are known to control cell functions by modifying the activity of transcription factors and metabolic enzymes as well as regulating gene expression and controlling epigenetic modifications (Lennicke and Cochemé, 2021). The regulatory actions include sulfhydryl groups forming a reversible disulphide bridges in various proteins, including transcription factors and their inhibitors (e.g. Nrf2-Keap1; Surai *et al.*, 2019; NF-κB-IκB; Surai *et al.*, 2021a) as well as antioxidant enzymes (e.g. GPx7; Surai, 2020) and antioxidant-relating proteins (e.g. Sestrins, Ro *et al.*, 2020; HSP70, Surai and Kochish, 2017); Trx in the Trx redox system and GSH in the GSH redox system, misfolded proteins, oxidised proteins and lipids, etc. Endoplasmic reticulum (ER) stress-sensing proteins include PKR-like ER kinase (PERK), inositol-requiring enzyme 1 (IRE1) and activating transcription factor 6 (ATF6; Huang *et al.*, 2019). Recently it has been reported that the Cys/N-degron pathway can function as a sensor of ROS/oxidative stress under various physiological conditions (Heo *et al.*, 2021). Furthermore, stress-responsive mitogen-activated protein (MAP) three kinase 1 (MTK1) has been recently identified to serve as a cellular redox sensor detecting changes in the intracellular redox state and transducing them into the stress-activated p38 and JNK MAPK (SAPK) signalling involved in cell fate decision making, including oxidative stress-induced cell death, and cytokine production (Matsushita *et al.*, 2020).

3.7 Conclusions

Redox (antioxidant-prooxidant) balance in the cell is an important determinant of various physiological functions. There is a large body of data indicating that oxidative stress occurs when this balance is disturbed due to overproduction of free radicals or compromised antioxidant defences. Free radical overproduction and oxidative stress are considered as a pathobiochemical mechanism involved in the initiation or progression phase of various diseases. In human free radial overproduction, lipid peroxidation and protein oxidation are responsible for the development of various diseases while in animal/poultry production they cause decrease of productive and reproductive performance as well as decreased product quality. Dietary antioxidants are important players in protecting against the development of the oxidative stress in stress conditions of human life and commercial egg and meat production. However, recent evidence suggests that oxidative stress can induce changes in gene expression. Some ROS, such as H_2O_2, are now considered to be signal molecules taking part in signal transduction in the cell, affecting redox homeostasis and stress adaptation. There is a range of redox-sensitive transcription factors, including Nrf2, NF-κB, FOXO, p53, PGC-1α, HIF-1 and HSF1 (Figure 3.7), which participate in regulation of various cellular processes including adaptation to stress.

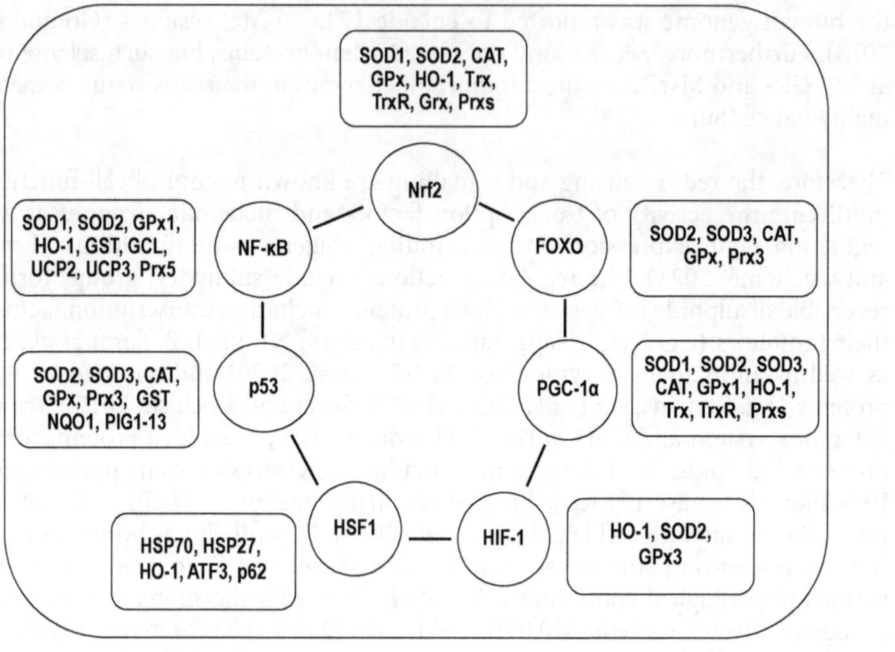

Figure 3.7. Transcription factors and their clients involved in redox status regulation (adapted from Surai, 2020).

The regulation of gene expression by oxidants, antioxidants, and redox state has emerged as a novel subdiscipline in molecular biology that has promising implications for human health and farm animal and poultry production. Thus, the redox state/homeostasis of the cell, which reflects antioxidant/prooxidant balance, can be considered as an important element of gene regulation.

Therefore, the effect of antioxidants on human and animal health is much deeper than one could expect several years ago. The mechanisms by which natural antioxidants act at the molecular and cellular level include their roles in gene expression and regulation, apoptosis, and signal transduction. Antioxidants are involved in fundamental metabolic and homeostatic processes. However, there are still many gaps in our knowledge of the basic molecular mechanisms of oxidative damage and antioxidant defences.

Therefore, once redox disbalance is detected there is an activation of protective intracellular signalling pathways, including vitagenes, leading to re-establishment of the adaptive redox homeostasis by additional synthesis of antioxidant molecules as well as repairing damaged molecules and removal of those molecules which are not repairable. These elements of the antioxidant defence network are dealing mainly with proteostasis (Surai, 2020). There is also an effective system to deal with lipid peroxides. This includes such enzymes as GPx4 and vitamin E. It is generally accepted that vitamin E is main chain-breaking antioxidant in biological membranes responsible for prevention of lipid peroxidation and for membrane integrity maintenance. As mentioned above, vitamin E recycling is of paramount importance for its protective effects in biological systems. It seems likely that CoQ is also important antioxidant helping in prevention of lipid peroxidation.

More detailed description of two major transcription factors in redox homeostasis maintenance, namely Nrf2 and NF-κB, and effect of SM on these transcription factors will be presented in the next chapters of the book. The transcription factors interact with each other and with other important signalling pathways including the vitagene network, which will be in detail considered in the next chapters of the book. This interaction occurs in a cooperative and interactive way to stimulate additional synthesis of various antioxidants to deal with oxidative stress and to re-establish adaptive homeostasis under various stress conditions. Molecular mechanisms of interactions between antioxidants, transcription factors and vitagenes and their participation in stress adaptation and establishment of adaptive homeostasis will be considered in the next chapters of this book.

Taking into account inability of human and animals to synthesise vitamin E it should be provided with the diet. At the same time Se, as an integral part of 25 selenoproteins, participating in the antioxidant defence network should also be provided in optimal form and effective dosage with food/feed as well as Cu, Zn and Mn as essential parts of SOD and Fe as an integral part of CAT. Generally speaking, it seems likely that in future more attention will be paid to various approaches to regulate redox homeostasis in human and animals, including vitagene activation, and antioxidant-regulating properties of SM/SB would be of great importance and they will be considered in detail in the next chapters of the book.

References

Bhattacharya, S. and Rattan, S.I., 2019. Primary stress response pathways for preconditioning and physiological hormesis. In: Rattan, S.I.S. and Kyriazis, M. (eds) The science of hormesis in health and longevity. Academic Press, London, UK, pp. 35-51.

Go, Y.M. and Jones, D.P., 2013. The redox proteome. The Journal of Biological Chemistry 288: 26512-26520.

Foyer, C.H. and Noctor, G., 2011. Ascorbate and glutathione: the heart of the redox hub. Plant Physiology 155: 2-18.

Halliwell, B., 1994. Free radicals and antioxidants: A personal view. Nutrition Reviews 52: 253-265.

Halliwell, B. and Gutteridge, J.M.C., 2015. Free radicals in biology and medicine. Oxford University Press, Oxford, UK.

Heo, A.J., Kim, S.B., Ji, C.H., Han, D., Lee, S.J., Lee, S.H., Lee, M.J., Lee, J.S., Ciechanover, A., Kim, B.Y. and Kwon, Y.T., 2021. The N-terminal cysteine is a dual sensor of oxygen and oxidative stress. Proceedings of the National Academy of Sciences of the United States of America 118: e2107993118.

Huang, S., Xing, Y. and Liu, Y., 2019. Emerging roles for the ER stress sensor IRE1α in metabolic regulation and disease. The Journal of Biological Chemistry 294: 18726-18741.

Lennicke, C. and Cochemé, H.M., 2021. Redox metabolism: ROS as specific molecular regulators of cell signaling and function. Molecular Cell 81: 3691-3707.

Matsushita, M., Nakamura, T., Moriizumi, H., Miki, H. and Takekawa, M., 2020. Stress-responsive MTK1 SAPKKK serves as a redox sensor that mediates delayed and sustained activation of SAPKs by oxidative stress. Science Advances 6: eaay9778.

Park, J., Lee, S., Lee, S. and Kang, S.W., 2014. 2-cys peroxiredoxins: emerging hubs determining redox dependency of Mammalian signaling networks. International Journal of Cell Biology 2014: 715867.

Ro, S.H., Fay, J., Cyuzuzo, C.I., Jang, Y., Lee, N., Song, H.S. and Harris, E.N., 2020. SESTRINs: Emerging dynamic stress-sensors in metabolic and environmental health. Frontiers in Cell and Developmental Biology 8: 603421.

Sies, H. and Jones, D.P., 2020. Reactive oxygen species (ROS) as pleiotropic physiological signalling agents. Nature Reviews. Molecular Cell Biology 21: 363-383.

Sies, H., Belousov, V.V., Chandel, N.S., Davies, M.J., Jones, D.P., Mann, G.E., Murphy, M.P., Yamamoto, M. and Winterbourn, C., 2022. Defining roles of specific reactive oxygen species (ROS) in cell biology and physiology. Nature Reviews. Molecular Cell Biology 23: 499-515.

Sies, H. and Ursini, F., 2022. Homeostatic control of redox status and health. IUBMB Life 74: 24-28.

Skulachev, V.P., 1998. Biochemical mechanisms of evolution and the role of oxygen. Biochemistry (Moscow) 63: 1335-1343.

Surai, P.F., 1999. Vitamin E in avian reproduction. Poultry and Avian Biology Reviews 10: 1-60.

Surai, P.F., 2018. Selenium in poultry nutrition and health. Wageningen Academic Publishers, Wageningen, The Netherlands.

Surai, P.F., 2020. Vitagene in avian biology and poultry health. Wageningen Academic Publishers, Wageningen, The Netherlands.

Surai, P.F. and Kochish, I.I., 2017. Antioxidant systems and vitagenes in poultry biology: heat shock proteins. In: Asea, A.A.A. and Kaur, P. (eds) Heat shock proteins in veterinary. Springer, Switzerland, pp. 123-177.

Surai, P.F., Kochish, I.I., Fisinin, V.I. and Kidd, M.T., 2019. Antioxidant defence systems and oxidative stress in poultry biology: An update. Antioxidants 8; 235.

Surai, P.F., Kochish, I.I. and Kidd, M.T., 2021a. Redox homeostasis in poultry: Regulatory roles of NF-κB. Antioxidants 10: 186.

Surai, P.F., Kochish, I.I. and Fisinin, V.I., 2021b. Vitagenes in avian biology: protective functions of sirtuins. In: Maiese, K. (ed) Sirtuin biology in medicine. Academic Press, London, UK, pp. 353-372.

Surai, P.F. and Sparks, N.H.C., 2001. Designer eggs: from improvement of egg composition to functional food. Trends in Food Science & Technology 12: 7-16.

Part II.
Molecular mechanisms of silymarin action

Live and learn

Chapter 4
Antioxidant properties of silymarin

A chain is no stronger than its weakest link

Peter F. Surai[1-6] and Anton Surai[7]*
[1]Vitagene and Health Research Centre, Bristol, UK; [2]Department of Microbiology and Biochemistry, Faculty of Veterinary Medicine, Trakia University, Stara Zagora, Bulgaria; [3]Department of Animal Nutrition, Faculty of Agricultural and Environmental Sciences, Szent Istvan University, Hungary [4]Saint-Petersburg State Academy of Veterinary Medicine, St. Petersburg, Russia; [5]Sumy National Agrarian University, Sumy, Ukraine; [6]Odessa National Academy of Food Technologies, Odessa, Ukraine; [7]Healthy Food Services, Bristol, UK
psurai@feedfood.co.uk

Abstract

The data presented in this chapter indicate that direct AO action of silymarin (SM) is only relevant to the gut, while other antioxidant-related activities are of great importance. In fact, protective effects of SM on mitochondria shown in various *in vitro* and *in vivo* model systems in many cases are a driving force of protective effects of SM under various stress conditions. SM is responsible for maintaining an optimal redox balance in the cell by activating a range of antioxidant enzymes and non-enzymatic antioxidants, mainly via Nrf2 induction. Decreasing inflammatory responses in the gut and other tissues by inhibiting NF-κB pathways is an emerging mechanism of SM protective effect in liver toxicity and diseases. Activating vitagenes, responsible for synthesis of protective molecules, including HSP, Trx, sirtuins, etc., and providing additional protection in stress conditions deserves more attention in future research. Various effects on the microenvironment of the gut, including SM-bacteria interactions, await future investigation. Various phytochemicals, including flavonoids, are an essential part of our diet responsible for turning on and maintaining an optimal status of our antioxidant defences. Since flavonoids are not well absorbed in the gut, their active concentration in the plasma and target tissues are comparatively low, but probably sufficient for Nrf2 activation and NF-κB suppression as well as vitagene activation. Therefore, consumption of phytochemicals, including SM, could have a pre-conditioning effect on the antioxidant system of the body. This could explain the beneficial health-promoting effects of a diet rich in fruits and vegetables as important sources of the aforementioned chemicals (polyphenols and other phytochemicals) maintaining the body's ability to be highly adaptive to various stresses. SM and its main component SB are responsible for regulation of the antioxidant defences in the gut and in the whole body.

Keywords: antioxidants, mitochondria, oxidative stress, silymarin, silibinin

DOI:10.3920/978-90-8686-944-2_004,

4.1 Introduction

- Silymarin can contribute to the antioxidant defences in different ways (Surai, 2015; 2020):
- Firstly, by direct free radical scavenging.
- Secondly, by preventing free radical formation as a result of inhibition of specific enzymes responsible for free radical production.
- Thirdly, by maintaining the integrity of mitochondria including ETC under various stress conditions.
- Fourthly, by participating in the maintenance of optimal redox status of the cell/tissue by activating a range of antioxidant enzymes and non-enzymatic antioxidants, mainly via transcription factors, including Nrf2 and NF-κB.
- Finally, by activating an array of vitagenes, responsible for the synthesis of protective molecules, including SOD, HSPs, elements of Trx- and GSH systems, sirtuins and providing additional protection in stress conditions.

It seems likely that direct free radical scavenging and inhibiting specific enzymes responsible for free radical production by SM play only minor role in antioxidant protective activity of SM (Surai, 2015; 2020). In this chapter first three options of AO properties of SM will be considered while effects of SM on transcription factors, on vitagenes and anti-toxic effects of SM (because of substantial amount of information) will be considered in the separate chapters.

4.2 Direct free radical scavenging

The effects of SB on the formation of ROS and eicosanoids by human platelets, white blood and endothelial cells were investigated (Dehmlow *et al.*, 1996a). SB is shown to be a strong scavenger of HOCI at 50% inhibitory concentration (IC_{50}) to be 7 μM, but not of O_2- (IC_{50}>200 μM) produced by human granulocytes. Similarly, production of O_2- and NO in isolated rat Kupffer cells were suppressed by SB in a dose-dependent manner, with IC_{50} 80 μM (Dehmlow *et al.*, 1996b). In addition, SB had no superoxide anion scavenging capability but was able to significantly decrease (at 20 μM) hem-mediated LDL oxidation and showed slight inhibition of hydroxyl radical formation (Varga *et al.*, 2006). The rate constants of SB with OH radical (1.8×10^{10} dm/mol/s) is diffusion controlled, suggesting that SB is a potent free radical scavenger (Fu *et al.*, 2009). SB (2.5 μM) was illustrated to significantly decrease the concentration of H_2O_2 in Ab_{1-42}-stressed neurons and prevented oxidative-related injuries (Yin *et al.*, 2011). Furthermore, SB (10 μM and higher) is shown to have protective activity in ameliorating DNA damage in a model system (Fu *et al.*, 2009). Treatment *in vitro* of monocytes from pre-eclamptic women with SB significantly inhibited spontaneous O_2- and H_2O_2 release and tumour necrosis factor alpha (TNF-α) production. The main effect of SB was obtained at 50 μM concentration (Cristofalo *et al.*, 2013). Thus, SB exerts antioxidant and anti-inflammatory effects on monocytes from preeclamptic pregnant women by inhibiting the *in vitro* endogenous release of ROS and TNF-α production.

Antioxidant action of SM (equal to 62 μM of SB) has been shown in various model systems. For example, IC_{50} for H_2O_2 was 38 μM, while IC_{50} for NO was 266 μM (Domitrovic *et al.*, 2013). It was shown that SM inhibited 82.7% lipid peroxidation of linoleic acid emulsion; while BHA, BHT, alpha-tocopherol and Trolox indicated inhibition of 83.3, 82.1, 68.1 and 81.3% on peroxidation of linoleic acid emulsion at the same concentration, respectively (Köksal *et al.*, 2009). In another *in vitro* study free radical scavenging activity and antioxidant properties of SM (>200 μM) were showed by four different assays (Asghar and Masood, 2008). It is important to mention that the free radical scavenging activity of pure individual compounds of the SM is reported to vary considerably, with silydianin and silychristin being 2-10-fold more active than the SB and on a mass basis, SM is shown to be about 8-fold more potent than SB as a free radical scavenger (Dvorak *et al.*, 2003). Indeed, SM and SB are not the same compounds and their AO activities could differ substantially depending on their concentrations in the target tissues. Therefore, in the following sections a distinction will be made between AO activities of SM and its active constituent silybin (SB), containing two major diastereomers, silybins A and B.

4.3 Inhibition of free-radical producing enzymes by silybin

4.3.1 Xanthine oxidase

Xanthine oxidase (XO) catalyses the terminal two steps of purine degradation, converting hypoxanthine to uric acid and considered to be a critical source of both O_2^- and H_2O_2 in inflammatory diseases (Doehner and Landmesser, 2011). In particular, XO in its oxidase form is considered to be a main source of oxidative stress and destructive free radicals in ischemia reperfusion injury associated with heart attacks and stroke, spinal cord injury, as well as being a destructive force in myocardial or renal hypoxia and infarctions (Pauff and Hille, 2009). It seems likely that SB can affect XO activity and inhibition of XO by SB in the steady-state appeared to be independent of the SB concentration. Furthermore, in the presence of 50 μM SB, the production of superoxide by XO was decreased by approximately 20% relative to the control at 100 μM xanthine (Pauff and Hille, 2009). When O_2^- production was induced in xanthine/xanthine oxidase system, SB inhibited uric acid formation with an IC_{50} of 32.2 μM (Varga *et al.*, 2004). Interestingly, inhibition in uric acid formation occurred parallel with inhibition of cytochrome C reduction (e.g. with O_2^- formation) suggesting that the observed effects are due to the inhibition of xanthine oxidase activity rather than the scavenging of O_2^- radicals.

4.3.2 NADPH oxidase

ROS generation by NADPH oxidase enzyme complex plays a critical role in several physiological processes including host defence, posttranslational modification of proteins, cell differentiation and regulation of gene expression (Bedard and Krause, 2007). SB and its derivatives inhibited the NADPH oxidase activity in PMA-stimulated cell lysate in a concentration dependent manner. The most distinct inhibition was observed when cell lysate was preincubated with 5,7,4″-trimethylsilybin possessing high lipid solubility. Indeed, 50% inhibition of NADPH oxidase activity was achieved when using 5 μM of 5,7,4″-trimethylsilybin and 10 μM of SB at final concentrations (Varga *et al.*, 2004). As-intoxicated rats showed a significant up-regulation of myocardial NADPH (NOX) oxidase subunits such as NOX2 and NOX4 as well as Keap1 and down-regulation of Nrf2 and HO-1 protein expressions. Pre-administration of SB (75 mg/kg BW) remarkably recovered all these altered parameters to near normalcy in As-induced cardiotoxic rat (Muthumani and Prabu, 2014). Co-administration of SB (75 mg/kg day) along with As resulted in a reversal of As-induced biochemical changes in kidney accompanied by a significant decrease in lipid peroxidation and an increase in the level of renal antioxidant defence system (Prabu and Muthumani, 2012) and decreased the NADPH oxidase, inducible nitric oxide synthase (iNOS) and NF-κB over expression by As and upregulated the Nrf2 expression in the renal tissue.

The effect of SB in cultures of mouse podocytes and in the OVE26 mouse, a model of type 1 diabetes mellitus and diabetic nephropathy was investigated. Exposure of podocytes to high glucose (HG) increased 60% the intracellular superoxide production, 90% the NADPH oxidase activity, 100% the Nox4 expression, and 150% the number of apoptotic cells, effects that were completely blocked by 10 μM SB. These *in vitro* observations were confirmed by similar *in vivo* findings. The kidney cortex of vehicle-treated control OVE26 mice displayed greater Nox4 expression and twice as much superoxide production than cortex of SB-treated mice (Khazim *et al.*, 2013). Therefore, the *in vitro* data demonstrated that SB decreased superoxide generation in cultured podocytes and the *in vivo* study showed a similar effect in the kidney cortex. This is not surprising considering that oxidative stress and enhanced generation of ROS is the underlying mechanism of injury to multiple cell types. It is tempting to speculate that inhibition of Nox4 function may be the common protective mechanism of SB in all these cell types, since it is also known that Nox4-derived ROS play a key role in glucose-mediated mesangial cell injury.

4.4 Protective effects of silybin on mitochondria, a main source of free radical production in the cell

4.4.1. Mitochondria as an important source of ROS

It is generally accepted that the ETC in the mitochondria is responsible for major part of superoxide production in the body (Halliwell and Gutteridge, 2015). Mitochondria are shown to contain up to 12 sites for ROS production associated with nutrient oxidation and respiration. Mitochondria are the primary cellular consumers of oxygen and contain numerous redox enzymes capable of transferring single electrons to oxygen, generating the ROS superoxide (O_2^-). It is well appreciated that mitochondria are the main cellular consumers of oxygen and primary source of free radicals in the cell. It is proven that mitochondrial enzymes producing ROS include (Lin and Beal, 2006):

- aconitase and α-ketoglutarate dehydrogenase, important the tricarboxylic acid cycle enzymes;
- complexes I, II and III of the ETC;
- glycerol-3-phosphate dehydrogenase and pyruvate dehydrogenase;
- dihydroorotate dehydrogenase;
- the monoamine oxidases A and B;
- cytochrome b5 reductase.

Although energy generation in the mitochondrion is an essential and extremely important process for cell survival, excessive mitochondrial ROS production also has detrimental consequences for the cell and the whole body. In general, ubiquinone reduction site of complex I, the outer quinone-binding site of the Q-cycle in complex III and glycerol 3-phosphate dehydrogenase are considered as major contributors to ROS production (Brand, 2010). Evidence has been increasingly emerged that there are at least 12 sites of ROS (superoxide and/or hydrogen peroxide) formation in mammalian mitochondria. Mitochondria exhibit a highly dynamic and complicated ROS release profile that varies depending on physiological conditions and carbon source, type, and availability and cell type. However, it seems likely that complex III has consistently the highest capacity of ROS production in all tissue and cell types examined so far (Young *et al.*, 2019). Mitochondrial ETC consumes more than 85% of all oxygen used by the cell and, because the efficiency of electron transport is not 100%, about 1-3% of electrons could escape from the chain and the univalent reduction of molecular oxygen results in superoxide anion formation.

Recently, it has been calculated that less than 0.1% of the electrons passing through the respiratory chain could leak on to O_2 to form superoxide in normal physiological conditions of electron transfer (Larosa and Remacle, 2018). Even in such conditions about 10^9 molecules of ROS per cell per day could be produced. Generally, this number would depend on many factors including animal species, age, sex, tissue, etc. An interesting calculation has been made by Halliwell (1994), showing that in the human body about 1.72 kg/year of superoxide radical is produced. In stress condition it would be substantially increased. Clearly, these calculations showed that free radical production in the body is substantial and many thousand biological molecules can be easily damaged if are not protected. Furthermore, mitochondrial insults, including oxidative damage itself, can cause an imbalance between ROS production and removal, resulting in net ROS production. For example, ROS, which is an inevitable by-product of oxidative phosphorylation, induce protein modifications, lipid peroxidation and mitochondrial DNA damage, which ultimately results in mitochondrial dysfunction (Sekine and Ichijo, 2015).

For many years the detrimental effects of ROS have been a focus of research, but it is now clear that mitochondrially generated ROS have a light side being involved in regulation of intracellular signal transduction pathways (Forrester *et al.*, 2018; Larosa and Remacle, 2018), leading to cell adaptation to stress (Calabrese *et al.*, 2010; Surai, 2020). Mitochondrially generated ROS are involved in regulating intracellular signal transduction pathways that result in cell adaptation to stress (Surai *et al.*, 2019).

The crosstalk of the mitochondria with various transcription factors, including Nrf2 (Tsushima *et al.*, 2020), FOXO (Fasano *et al.*, 2019), NK-κB (Surai *et al.*, 2021) has primary importance, since the mitochondria are considered to be signalling hubs for stress adaptation (Surai, 2020) as well as for regulated cell death, immunity and other important physiological functions (Tsushima *et al.*, 2020). Therefore, polyphenolic compounds potentially could affect mitochondria functions via regulation of various transcription factors and one of the mechanisms responsible for the decrease in oxidative stress is the protective effect of SM/SB on mitochondrial structure and function.

4.4.2 Protective effects of SM/SB on mitochondria

4.4.2.1 *In vitro* evidence

Protective effects of SM on mitochondria *in vitro* were initially shown in 1970's. In fact, swelling effects produced *in vitro* by inorganic phosphate and lysolecithin on liver mitochondria was partly counteracted by SM (1 mM) added into the medium (Boccini *et al.*, 1973). Furthermore, SM was shown to protect both liver mitochondria and microsomes from lipid peroxide formation induced by various agents and protective AO effect of SM in the model systems used was about 10-fold higher than that for α-tocopherol (Bindoli *et al.*, 1977). However, those SM concentrations used in the aforementioned studies are not achievable in biological systems and it seems likely that direct AO activity of SM is of great importance only in the gut (Surai, 2015; 2020). It seems likely that regulatory effects of SM on AO enzyme expression and activity, especially in mitochondria, could substantially contribute to AO activity and protective effects of SM. It was reported that SM addition (250 μM) *in vitro* was associated with increased SOD activity and upregulated mitochondrial membrane potential leading to prevention of mitochondrial dysfunction and cell injury (Rolo *et al.*, 2003). Therefore, SM demonstrated a reduction of the main parameters of mitochondrial dysfunction induced by ischemia/reperfusion (I/R) including alterations in mitochondrial respiration, reduction in membrane potential and increased susceptibility to MPT induction.

SB, at a concentration as low as 10 μM, was found to fully mitigate the rise in metabolic flow-driven ROS formation in perfused rat hepatocytes. In addition, studies on isolated liver mitochondria showed that this low dose of SB depressed ROS production linked to the electron transfer chain activity (Detaille *et al.*, 2008). It has been reported that cold preservation and warm reperfusion of the rat liver were associated with increased lipid peroxidation and superoxide anion generation, as well as with decreased GSH, mitochondrial ATP content and respiratory control ratio (RCR). However, preservation conducted in presence of SB (100 μM) improved parameters affected by preservation and reperfusion. SB promoted an increase of ATP and RCR by 39 and 16% respectively and decreased oxidative stress to values observed in livers never preserved nor perfused (Ligeret *et al.*, 2008). It has been suggested that the uncoupler-like activity of dehydrosilybin could be the background of its ROS modulation effect in various experimental systems. In reality, dehydrosilybin uncoupled the respiration of isolated rat heart mitochondria with a very high potency in suppressing ROS production in isolated rat heart mitochondria with IC_{50}=0.15 μM (Gabrielová *et al.*, 2010). It is worth noting that SB in mitochondria was far more effective than in other model systems based on generating superoxide or in cells cultures, where the IC_{50} for dehydrosilybin exceeds 50 μM.

It is important to mention that 50-300 μM of SB exerted pronounced effects on liver carbohydrate metabolism (Colturato *et al.*, 2012). The authors suggested four different sites of metabolic action of SB, including:

- glucose 6-phosphatase activity;
- pyruvate carrier (monocarboxylate carrier, which operates in the plasma and mitochondrial membranes);
- mitochondrial respiratory chain at complex I;
- deviation of NADH supply for gluconeogenesis and mitochondria.

Furthermore, the authors showed that SB at tested concentrations acted as uncoupler of oxidative phosphorylation and inhibitor of the respiratory chain and ATPase activity in mitochondria, being responsible for an impairment of the mitochondrial energy transduction (Colturato *et al.*, 2012). SB (10 μM) was found to protect primary cultured neurons against 1-methyl-4-phenylpyridine-induced cell death and mitochondrial membrane disruption (Lee *et al.*, 2015). In an *in vitro* model of non-alcoholic fatty liver disease progression based on sequential exposure of hepatocytes to high concentrations of fatty acids (FA) and TNF-α it was suggested that SB (50 μM) was able to counteract the FA-induced mitochondrial damage by acting on the following pathways (Vecchione *et al.*, 2017):

- increased the mitochondrial size and improved the mitochondrial cristae organisation;
- stimulated mitochondrial FA oxidation;
- reduced basal and maximal respiration and ATP production in SH cells;
- stimulated ATP production in SS cells;
- rescued the FA-induced apoptotic signals and oxidative stress in SH cells.

It was demonstrated that mitochondrial abnormalities contributed to advanced glycation end products (AGE)-induced apoptosis of osteoblastic cells associated with enhanced mitochondrial oxidative stress, reduction in mitochondrial membrane potential and ATP production, abnormal mitochondrial morphology, and altered mitochondrial dynamics. The aforementioned AGE-induced mitochondrial abnormalities were indicated to be mediated by the receptor of AGEs (RAGE). In such conditions SB (100 μM) was able to downregulate the expression of RAGE and ameliorate RAGE-mediated mitochondrial pathways (Mao *et al.*, 2018). In an *in vitro* model based on cultured hepatocytes exposed to excess fructose and fatty acids mimicking a severe non-alcoholic fatty liver disease (NAFLD), SB (50 μM) was shown to exert beneficial action by inhibiting mitochondrial respiration, which is stimulated in steatosis progression (Grasselli *et al.*, 2019). SB (10 μM) was reported to ameliorate palmitic acid-induced mitochondrial dysfunction in pancreatic β-cells (INS-1 cells; Sun *et al.*, 2019). The expression of cytosolic cytochrome C, mitochondrial mass and mitochondrial membrane potential (ΔΨm) were markedly affected after palmitic acid treatment, but these changed were partly reversed by SB treatment and the authors speculated that protective roles of SB are mediated by ERα (Sun *et al.*, 2019).

It was found that effects of silibinin A (Sil A) on mitochondria are condition-dependent, including its concentration, level of stress and cell type. For example, incubation of liver HepG2 cells with 25 μM and 50 μM SIL A for 24 hours showed a significant improvement on the basal ATP level, while 150 μM did not show any effect on ATP levels, and 500 μM significantly reduced ATP levels being toxic. However, SIL A can protect against sodium nitroprusside (SNP)-induced nitrosative stress at the level of mitochondria. Obviously, under conditions of nitrosative stress, a concentration of 150 μM SIL A was shown to protect HepG2 cells from the SNP-induced drop in ATP levels, while lower concentrations, did not demonstrate any protective effects (Esselun *et al.*, 2019). Interestingly, in PC12 cells (a neuronal model), SIL A did not affect basal ATP levels. Furthermore, in comparison to HepG2 cells, PC12 cells were more vulnerable to SIL A, since incubation with 150 μM SIL A significantly reduced basal ATP levels. PC12 cells were also more vulnerable to nitrosative stress and their incubation with 25 μM, 50 μM, 100 μM, and 150 μM SIL A prior to SNP treatment showed a concentration-dependent, protective effect in PC12 cells (Esselun *et al.*, 2019). The authors showed that protective effect of SIL A was also observed at the level of mitochondrial membrane potential maintenance in stress conditions.

Interestingly, that SM effect of mitochondria *in vitro* is concentration and condition dependent. For example, SM at 100 μM was reported to impair the mitochondrial activity in human primary chondrocytes (Wu *et al.*, 2021). Bovine insulin amyloid fibrils were shown to cause SH-SY5Y cell death by inducing necrosis/apoptosis and affected membrane permeability. Adding SB (250 μM or 500 μM) to the medium was reported to attenuate insulin fibrillation, neuronal toxicity, and mitochondria membrane damage (Katebi *et al.*, 2018). H_2O_2 administration was shown to induce apoptosis in HTR-8/SVneo trophoblast cells associated with decline of mitochondrial membrane potential and release of cytochrome C from mitochondria to cytoplasm. H_2O_2 also imposed oxidative stress evidenced by increased ROS production, elevated levels of MDA, and reduced activity of SOD and GPx. SB (250 and 500 μM) was able to ameliorate H_2O_2-induced cell apoptosis and oxidative stress by activating Nrf2 signalling in trophoblast cells (Guo *et al.*, 2020).

In various *in vitro* model systems SM was also shown to inhibit pro-oxidant enzymes. It was demonstrated that SB inhibited the activity of ROS-generating monoamine oxidase (MAO) that catalyses the oxidative deamination of monoamines (Mazzio *et al.*, 1998). The formation of leukotrienes via the 5-lipoxygenase pathway was indicated to be strongly inhibited by SB. In particular, in human granulocytes IC_{50}-values of 15 μM and 14.5 μM SB were detected for LTB4 and LTC4/D4/E4/F4 formation respectively. However, much higher SB concentrations (45-69 μM) were necessary to inhibit the cyclooxygenase pathway (Dehmlow *et al.*, 1996a).

It seems likely that SM effects on normal and cancer cells differ. For-example, SB (150 μM) was shown to induce mitochondrial NOX4-mediated endoplasmic reticulum stress response and its subsequent apoptosis in human prostate cell lines, PC-3 (Kim *et al.*, 2016). Therefore, NOX4-driven mitochondrial ROS production was considered to be a potential target for development of the cancer therapy and management. SB (100 μM) was found to induce autophagic cell death through ROS-dependent mitochondrial dysfunction and ATP depletion involving BNIP3 in human MCF7 breast cancer cells (Jiang *et al.*, 2015). SB at higher concentrations (150-250 μM) was indicated to enhance fission of mitochondria, leading to apoptosis of MCF-7 and MDA-MB-231 cells (Si *et al.*, 2019). It is important to note that SB at lower concentrations (30-90 μM) was reported to enhance fusion of mitochondria, inhibiting migration and invasion capacity of the MDA-MB-231 cells (Si *et al.*, 2020). SB was found to induce apoptosis of human epidermal cancer A431 cells by activating the AMPK-endothelial nitric oxide synthase (eNOS) pathway, leading to mitochondrial dysfunction and apoptosis (Yu *et al.*, 2019).

SB (150, 300 and 450 μM) was also shown to induce G2/M cell cycle arrest by activating Drp1-dpendent mitochondrial fission dysfunction in cervical cancer cells (You *et al.*, 2020b). It seems likely that autophagy activated by SB could contribute to glioma cell death via induction of oxidative stress-mediated BNIP3-dependent nuclear translocation of apoptosis inducing factor (Wang *et al.*, 2020). In a doxorubicin-induced injury model SB was demonstrated to protect cardiomyocytes by eliminating mitochondrial ROS and restoring autophagy through IL6ST/JAK2/STAT3 signalling pathway (Li *et al.*, 2022).

SM and its active derivatives are shown to induce apoptosis, enhance expression of several tumour suppressors and cell cycle inhibitors, inhibit the growth and transcription factors, and mediators of cell proliferation showing strong anti-cancer effects (Boojar *et al.*, 2020). In great contrast to cancer cells, SB can regulate mitochondrial fission in normal cells providing increased stress resistance. In particular, it was shown (You *et al.*, 2020a) that in normal cells SB (12.5- 50 μM):
- markedly promoted cell proliferation by facilitating G1/S transition via activating dynamin-related protein 1 (Drp1), which is responsible for mitochondrial fission in normal cells;
- dose-dependently increased the mitochondrial mass, mtDNA copy number, cellular ATP production and mitochondrial membrane potential;
- dose-dependently increased the expression of Drp1.

Importantly, protective effects of SB against ethanol- or acetaldehyde-caused damage in liver cell lines was illustrated to involve the repression of mitochondrial fission (Song *et al.*, 2022).

The aforementioned data obtained in various *in vitro* systems can be summarised as follows:
- SM/SB has regulatory effects on AO enzyme expression and activity in mitochondria;
- SB demonstrate a reduction of the main parameters of mitochondrial dysfunction induced by I/R;

- at a concentration as low as 10 μM (achievable in the liver *in vivo*), SB was found to depress ROS production linked to the electron transfer chain activity;
- at 10 μM SB was effective in protection of primary cultured neurons against toxicant-induced cell death and mitochondrial membrane disruption;
- at 10 μM SB ameliorated palmitic acid-induced mitochondrial dysfunction in pancreatic β-cells;
- at 12.5-5- μM SB can regulate mitochondrial fission in normal cells providing increased stress resistance;
- effects of SB on mitochondria are condition-dependent, including its concentration, level of stress and cell type.

4.4.2.2 *In vivo* evidence

In rats hepatic accumulation of MDA-protein adducts and formation of mitochondrial MDA after iron overload were significantly decreased by treatment with SB (100 mg/kg BW/day for 4 months): mitochondrial energy wasting and tissue ATP depletion induced by iron overload were successfully counteracted by SB (Pietrangelo *et al.*, 1995). An iron chelating ability of SB was, at least partly, responsible for its protective effects. In a later study it was confirmed that the protective action of SB against iron-induced oxidative injury strictly depended on its capability to counteract the rise of mitochondrial chelatable iron level (Masini *et al.*, 2000). By using in situ detection of oxidative stress gene response, membrane oxidation by-products and electron microscopy, it was clearly demonstrated that, in acutely iron-dosed gerbil, iron-induced oxidant stress was accompanied by irreversible mitochondrial dysfunctions. *In vivo* administration of SB (100 mg/kg BW/day for 8 weeks) was shown to be able to prevent oxidative stress and mitochondrial defects (Pietrangelo *et al.*, 2002).

SB (0.4 g/kg) in complex with phospholipid (SILIPHOS) was effective in decreasing severe oxidative stress and preserving hepatic mitochondrial bioenergetics and mitochondrial proton leak and ATP reduction in nonalcoholic steatohepatitis induced by the methionine- and choline-deficient diet (Serviddio *et al.*, 2010). In a rat model of non-alcoholic steatohepatitis a control group of animals was fed a standard liquid diet for 12 weeks, while the experimental groups were fed a high-fat liquid diet for 12 weeks without (NASH) or with simultaneous daily supplement with silibinin-phosphatidylcholine complex (200 mg/kg) for the last 5 weeks. Treatment with SB was demonstrated to improve liver steatosis and inflammation and decreased NASH-induced lipid peroxidation, plasma insulin and TNF-α and returned GSH concentration back to normal. However, SB was not able to correct cellular energetic imbalance indicative by a significant decrease in hepatic mitochondrial ATP production (Haddad *et al.*, 2011).

In a fatty liver model based on feeding a high-fat diet to rats for 6 weeks SB treatment (26 mg/kg/day, was shown to significantly protect against fatty liver by stabilising mitochondrial membrane fluidity (Yao *et al.*, 2011). In a model of nonalcoholic steatohepatitis a four-week daily dose of SB (20 mg/kg i.p.) was administrated to db/db mice fed a methionine-choline deficient diet. SB was found to decrease levels of isoprostanes, 8-deoxyguanosine and nitrites/nitrates and restored GSH levels in the liver and in the heart of the experimental animals. Furthermore, liver mitochondrial respiratory chain activity was reported to be dramatically impaired in untreated mice, while it was completely restored in SB-treated animals (Salamore *et al.*, 2012). Changes in mitochondrial respiratory complexes in fatty hepatocytes were attenuated by SB-vitamin E complex (15 mg vitamin E and 47 mg SB) fed to rats with a major protective effect on Complex II subunit CII-30 (Grattagliano *et al.*, 2013).

It was shown that chronic cholestasis was associated with cardiolipin oxidation leading to impairment of mitochondrial function and increased ROS production. Interestingly, SB (0.4 g/kg diet) was found to limit mitochondrial failure. For example, cirrhosis was illustrated to induce a significant reduction in $\Delta\Psi$ from complex I that was completely prevented by treatment with SB. In addition, SB was reported to positively affect complex V activity, strongly reduced in cirrhotic liver, and also limited proton leak, ameliorated the decrease in ATP synthesis. Furthermore, SB restored the normal expression of PGC-1α (a key transcription regulator of cellular energy metabolism and mitochondrial biogenesis) and mtDNA copy number in cirrhotic liver (Serviddio, *et al.*, 2014). Silymarin oil (10 ml/kg/BW) significantly increased levels of membrane fluidity and membrane potential of liver mitochondria (Zhu *et al.*, 2014). It has been suggested that protective mechanism of action of SB (50-200 μM) in intrastriatal MPP+-injected rats was associated with maintenance of mitochondrial bioenergetics and integrity (Geed *et al.*, 2014). Rats exposed to a carcinogen (1,2-di-methylhydrazine; DMH) showed increased activities of phase I enzymes (cytochrome b5, cytochrome b5 reductase, cytochromeP450, cytochromeP450 reductase, cytochromP4502E1) in the liver and colonic mucosa as compared to control rats. SB supplementation (50 mg/kg/BW) modulates the xenobiotic metabolising enzymes including decreasing activity of ROS-producing cytochrome b5 reductase (Sangeetha *et al.*, 2012).

SM was shown to protect mitochondria from pathological events by triggering pro-survival cell signalling. For example, SB supplementation is reported to optimise electron-transport chain, decreasing electron leakage and ROS formation and directly reducing activities of ROS-producing enzymes in the mitochondria. The administration of SM (30 mg/kg body weight/d for 4 weeks) was reported to significantly ameliorate high fat diet (HFD)- induced glucose metabolic disorders, oxidative stress, mitochondrial biogenesis and pathological alterations in the kidney. SM (12.5-100 μM) also significantly mitigated renal mitochondrial biogenesis and partly restored mitochondrial membrane potential in palmitic acid-treated HK2 cells (Feng *et al.*, 2017). Activation of SIRT1 by SB was illustrated to improve mitochondrial health and to alleviate the oxidative damage in experimental diabetic neuropathy and high glucose-mediated neurotoxicity models (Khan *et al.*, 2022).

In a model system based on streptozotocin (STZ)-induced diabetes in mice, SM (104 mg/kg) was found to increase/restore oxygen flux through NADH oxidase and succinate oxidase in the liver mitochondria that were compromised in the diabetic group (Stolf *et al.*, 2018). The authors showed that SM not only restored oxidase activity, but also significantly increased it in comparison to a control non-diabetic animals, reflecting an improvement in AO defences in general. In a stress model of rat cardiac hypertrophy induced by partial abdominal aortic constriction (PAAC) a significant reduction in cardiac mtDNA concentration as compared to normal control rats was observed. Treatment with SM (100 mg/kg/day, p.o.) was shown to significantly prevent oxidative stress (restoration of SOD activity and GSH concentration) and partly restored mtDNA concentration in PAAC-treated rats (Sharma *et al.*, 2019). In the mice model of myocardial I/R SB was indicated to reduce cardiomyocytes apoptosis, attenuated mitochondrial impairment and endoplasmic reticulum (ER) stress, alleviated ROS generation, neutrophil infiltration and cytokines release (Chen *et al.*, 2020). Clinical applications of SM and its constituents are quite diverse. In particular, SB was demonstrated to be effective in the control of neuropathy, retinopathy, impaired healing, hepatopathy, cardiomyopathy, and osteoporosis in diabetic patients by regulating insulin sensitivity, oxidative stress, inflammation, apoptosis, proliferation, differentiation, and ECM remodelling (Chu *et al.*, 2018).

Therefore, in a variety of *in vivo* studies, a range of stress-related model systems were used including iron overload, non-alcoholic steatohepatitis induced by the methionine- and choline-deficient diet or by a high-fat liquid diet, chronic cholestasis and cirrhosis, exposure to carcinogens, HFD-induced metabolic disorders, STZ-induced diabetes, cardiac hypertrophy induced by partial abdominal aortic constriction, myocardial I/R and others. SM supplementation was associated with:

- prevention of oxidative stress and mitochondrial defects;
- preservation of hepatic mitochondrial bioenergetics, proton leak and ATP content;
- stabilising mitochondrial integrity, membrane fluidity and membrane potential;
- restoring mitochondrial respiratory chain activity, cellular energy metabolism and mitochondrial biogenesis;
- triggering pro-survival cell signalling;
- inhibiting cardiomyocytes apoptosis.

There are many possible mechanisms by which SM can improve the antioxidant defence network efficacy in the body. They include direct and indirect SM actions. First of all, a direct scavenging free radicals and chelating free Fe and Cu are mainly effective in the gut. Secondly, preventing free radical formation by inhibiting specific ROS-producing enzymes, or improving the integrity of electron-transport chain of mitochondria in stress conditions as a result of SM consumption, is of great importance. Thirdly, maintaining an optimal redox balance in the cell by activating a range of antioxidant enzymes and non-enzymatic antioxidants, mainly via Nrf2 induction, is probably the main driving force of AO action of SM. Fourthly, decreasing inflammatory responses in the gut and other tissues by inhibiting NF-κB pathways is an emerging mechanism of SM protective effect in liver toxicity and diseases. Fifthly, activating vitagenes, responsible for synthesis of protective molecules, including HSP, Trx, sirtuins, etc., and providing additional protection in stress conditions deserves more attention in future research. Finally, various effects on the microenvironment of the gut, including SM-bacteria interactions, await future investigation. The last four points will be addressed in detail in the next chapters.

4.5 Is effective silybin concentration *in vitro* achievable *in vivo*?

As mentioned above, because of their poor absorption and rapid elimination, plasma values of SB will rarely exceed micromolar concentrations. Therefore, the SM concentration used in the most aforementioned studies are not achievable in the *in vivo* target tissues, where the SB concentration usually at least 10-100-fold lower. The available evidence indicates that the active free SB concentration in plasma after oral consumption of SM depending on dose of supplementation could be in a range 0.2-2.0 μM. In healthy volunteers, after an oral administration of SM (equivalent to 120 mg SB), total (unconjugated + conjugated) SB concentration in plasma was 1.1-1.3 μg/ml (Kim *et al.*, 2003). Lower bioavailability of SB was shown in another study with higher dose of SM consumption (equivalent to 240 mg SB), where maximum SB concentration was about 0.7 μM (Lorenz *et al.*, 1984). A comparable SB concentrations (0.3-1.9 μM) were reported in healthy volunteers receiving about 240 mg SB (Hoh *et al.*, 2006).

More recently, silybin A maximal concentration in human plasma was observed to be 0.2-0.6 μM and Silybin B concentrations comprised about 30% of those shown for silybin A (Zhu *et al.*, 2013). The concentrations of free and conjugated SB in the target tissues of mice have been shown to reach their maximum levels within 1 h after 50 mg/kg SB administration. The C_{max} of free/conjugated SB in the tissues were 18.3/11.8; 8.9/5.8; 255/560; 2.9/8.9; 5.3/12.6; 12.0/21.9 μM for liver, lung, stomach, skin, prostate and pancreas, respectively (Zhao and Agarwal, 1999).

The average concentration of most plant polyphenols in plasma rarely exceeds 1-2 μM in healthy subjects (Bell *et al.*, 2000; Lapidot *et al.*, 1998). Furthermore, the effect of SM in physiologically relevant concentrations would be relatively limited when taking into account concentrations of other antioxidants in plasma. For example, vitamin C (26.1 to 84.6 μM), vitamin E (20-30 μM), urate (150-200 μM), and albumin (several hundred μM) are found in plasma (Holman, 2014; Hu, 2011) and polyphenol contribution to plasma TAC will certainly be less than 2% (Hollman, 2014). Similar situation could be found in animals (chickens) where antioxidant concentrations in plasma are in the same range (vitamin C: 61-66 μM, Howard and Constamble, 1958; McKee *et al.*, 1997; vitamin E: 13-15 μM, Surai, 2002; and total antioxidant value in plasma could vary from 336.9 μM, Brenes *et al.*, 2008; up to 740-830 μM, Willemsen *et al.*, 2011). The general concentration of antioxidants in human plasma to be about 1,000 μM (Benzie *et al.*, 1999), therefore 20-50 μM additional antioxidant from dietary sources would be required to make a significant contribution to systemic antioxidant capacity (Halliwell *et al.*, 2005). While SM displays potent antioxidant activity *in vitro*, the bioactive forms of flavonoids *in vivo* are not those forms found in plants (e.g. flavonoid glycosides) due to their extensive biotransformation in the intestine and hepatic metabolism upon absorption. Therefore, metabolic modifications occurring *in vivo* may substantially influence the antioxidant activity of dietary flavonoids. SB, similar to other flavonoids, is considered by the body as foreign matter and quickly metabolised via phase II enzymes.

4.6 Oxidability and pro-oxidant properties of silymarin

It has been sown that the oxidation of Keap1 cysteine thiols can be mediated by some polyphenols. It is an interesting fact that among flavonoids, the higher their intrinsic potential to generate oxidative stress and redox cycling, the stronger their potency as inducers of ARE-mediated gene expression (Lee-Hilz *et al.*, 2006). It was hypothesised that low concentrations of polyphenols could generate H_2O_2, at very low concentration and by diffusion it activates Nrf2 signalling, inducing cell adaptation to oxidative stress (Erlank *et al.*, 2011). Thus, polyphenols act as nutritional 'medicinals,' which might have a preventative nature, rather than functioning as therapeutic agents. Therefore, the activation of Nrf2-ARE signalling by antioxidant polyphenols to induce various AO molecules is probably attributable to their prooxidant activity (Surh *et al.*, 2008a,b). It seems likely that the same can be applied for SB. If fact, pure SB was found to be unstable whilst silybin in SM was stable in buffers from pH 1.0 to 7.8. The metabolism of SB was more severe when in its pure form as compared to silybin as a part of SM, as tested in a range of biological fluids including plasma, intestinal fluid and liver homogenates. It would appear that components in SM have a stabilisation effect on its main component SB (Tang *et al.*, 2009).

Therefore, it could well be that in some *in vitro* experiments with cell cultures SB could be oxidised and its affect would be a reflection of the oxidised form of the flavonoid or ROS generated during SB oxidation. For example, SB and 2,3-dehydrosilybin were shown to chelate transition metals, especially Cu^{2+} and pro-oxidant properties of such a complex *in vitro* have been shown (Zatloukalová *et al.*, 2011). Similarly, SB can cause pro-oxidant effect via iron-catalysed oxidation with the subsequent generation of ROS (Gharagozloo *et al.*, 2008). SB has been shown to be a strong pro-oxidative agent, i.e. it was able to oxidise NADH *in vitro* in the presence of peroxidase and H_2O_2 (Colturato *et al.*, 2012). This pro-oxidative action results from the production of free-radical derivatives and subsequent NADH oxidation (Awad *et al.*, 2001; 2002). Treatment with SM (50, 100, or 200 μM) for 24 h affected the cellular redox status and induced a dose-dependent increase in ROS generation in HepG2 cells. There was also a dose-dependent decrease in intracellular GSH level and decreased total AO potential in HepG2 cells (Zhang *et al.*, 2013). SB induced cell death in human breast cancer cell lines MCF7 and MDA-MB-231 and it was attenuated by antioxidants, suggesting that the effect of SB was dependent on ROS generation (Kim *et al.*, 2014). Similarly, treatment of HT29 cells with SB increased the intracellular ROS level (Woo *et al.*, 2014). It has been suggested that SM at 100 mg/kg without stressors might exert pro-oxidant effect in animals. In fact, the levels of NO and MDA increased in CCl_4 and SM (100 mg/kg)-treated groups, while SM at lower doses (25 and 50 mg/kg) did not alter the NO and MDA content in the rat hippocampus. The concentration of total thiol molecules increased in the SM50 group and showed a remarkable decrease in

CCl_4 and SM100 groups (Malekinejad *et al.*, 2012). From the aforementioned results we can suggest that SB can affect Nrf2 activity via its oxidation-reduction potential.

4.7 Conclusions

The data presented in this chapter indicate that direct AO action of SM is only relevant to the gut, while other antioxidant-related activities are of great importance (Figure 4.1) and they will be considered in detail in the next chapters. Various phytochemicals, including flavonoids, are an essential part of our diet, which are responsible for turning on and maintaining an optimal status of our antioxidant defences. Since flavonoids are not well absorbed in the gut, their active concentration in the plasma and target tissues are comparatively low, but probably sufficient for Nrf2 activation and NF-κB suppression as well as vitagene activation (for more details see next chapters of the book).

Therefore, consumption of phytochemicals, including SM, could have a pre-conditioning effect on the antioxidant system of the body. This could explain the beneficial health-promoting effects of a diet rich in fruits and vegetables as important sources of the aforementioned chemicals (polyphenols and other phytochemicals) maintaining the body's ability to be highly adaptive to various stresses. SM and its main component SB are responsible for regulation of the antioxidant defences in the gut and in the whole body.

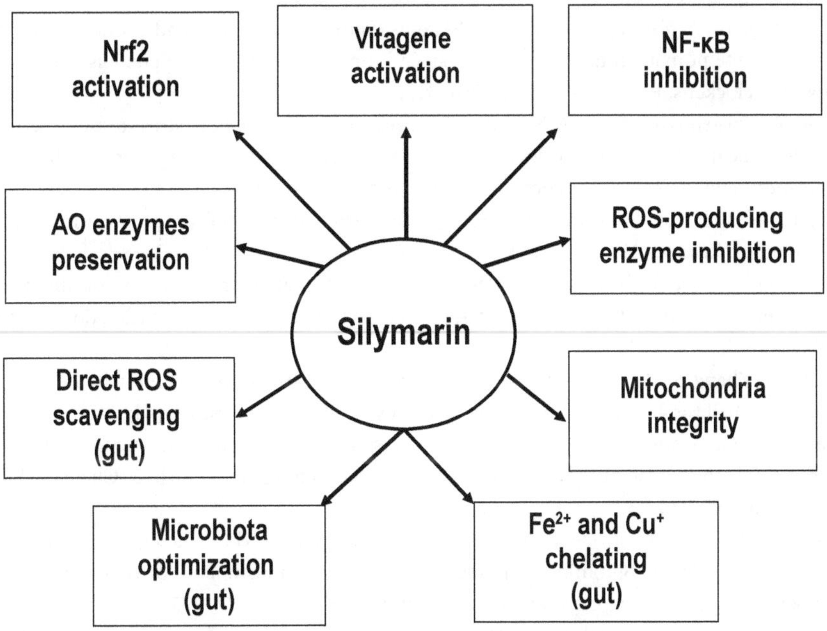

Figure 4.1. Antioxidant effects of SM/SB.

References

Asghar, Z. and Masood, Z., 2008. Evaluation of antioxidant properties of silymarin and its potential to inhibit peroxyl radicals *in vitro*. Pakistan Journal of Pharmaceutical Sciences 21: 249-254.

Awad, H.M., Boersma, M.G., Boeren, S., van Bladeren, P.J., Vervoort, J. and Rietjens, I.M., 2001. Structure-activity study on the quinone/quinone methide chemistry of flavonoids. Chemical Research in Toxicology 14: 398-408.

Awad, H.M., Boersma, M.G., Boeren, S., van Bladeren, P.J., Vervoort, J. and Rietjens, I.M., 2002. The regioselectivity of glutathione adduct formation with flavonoid quinone/quinone methides is pH-dependent. Chemical Research in Toxicology 15: 343-351.

Bedard, K. and Krause, K.H., 2007. The NOX family of ROS-generating NADPH oxidases: physiology and pathophysiology. Physiological Reviews 87: 245-313.

Bell, J.R., Donovan, J.L., Wong, R., Waterhouse, A.L., German, J.B., Walzem, R.L. and Kasim-Karakas, S.E., 2000. (+)-Catechin in human plasma after ingestion of a single serving of reconstituted red wine. The American Journal of Clinical Nutrition 71: 103-108.

Benzie, I.F., Szeto, Y.T., Strain, J.J. and Tomlinson, B., 1999. Consumption of green tea causes rapid increase in plasma antioxidant power in humans. Nutrition and Cancer 34: 83-87.

Bindoli, A., Cavallini, L. and Siliprandi, N., 1977. Inhibitory action of silymarin of lipid peroxide formation in rat liver mitochondria and microsomes. Biochemical Pharmacology 26: 2405-2409.

Bocchini, B., Cordani, A.M., Brunetti, M. and Porcellati, G., 1973. The activity of silymarin on mitochondrial swelling in the rat. Pharmacological Research Communications 5: 231-238.

Boojar, M.M.A., Boojar, M.M.A. and Golmohammad, S., 2020. Overview of silibinin anti-tumor effects. Journal of Herbal Medicine 23: 100375.

Brand, M.D., 2010. The sites and topology of mitochondrial superoxide production. Experimental Gerontology 45: 466-472.

Brenes, A., Viveros, A., Goñi, I., Centeno, C., Sáyago-Ayerdy, S.G., Arija, I. and Saura-Calixto, F., 2008. Effect of grape pomace concentrate and vitamin E on digestibility of polyphenols and antioxidant activity in chickens. Poultry Science 87: 307-316.

Calabrese, V., Cornelius, C., Stella, A.M.G. and Calabrese, E.J., 2010. Cellular stress responses, mitostress and carnitine insufficiencies as critical determinants in aging and neurodegenerative disorders: role of hormesis and vitagenes. Neurochemical Research, 35: 1880-1915.

Chance, B., Sies, H. and Boveris, A., 1979. Hydroperoxide metabolism in mammalian organs. Physiological Reviews 59: 527-605.

Chen, Y.H., Lin, H., Wang, Q., Hou, J.W., Mao, Z.J. and Li, Y.G., 2020. Protective role of silibinin against myocardial ischemia/reperfusion injury-induced cardiac dysfunction. International Journal of Biological Sciences 16: 1972-1988.

Chu, C., Li, D., Zhang, S., Ikejima, T., Jia, Y., Wang, D. and Xu, F., 2018. Role of silibinin in the management of diabetes mellitus and its complications. Archives of Pharmacal Research 41: 785-796.

Colturato, C.P., Constantin, R.P., Maeda Jr, A.S., Constantin, R.P., Yamamoto, N.S., Bracht, A., Ishii-Iwamoto, E.L. and Constantin, J., 2012. Metabolic effects of silibinin in the rat liver. Chemico-Biological Interactions 195: 119-132.

Cristofalo, R., Bannwart-Castro, C.F., Magalhaes, C.G., Borges, V.T.M., Peraçoli, J.C., Witkin, S.S. and Peracoli, M.T., 2013. Silibinin attenuates oxidative metabolism and cytokine production by monocytes from preeclamptic women. Free Radical Research 47: 268-275.

Dehmlow, C., Murawski, N. and de Groot, H., 1996a. Scavenging of reactive oxygen species and inhibition of arachidonic acid metabolism by silibinin in human cells. Life Sciences 58: 1591-1600.

Dehmlow, C., Erhard, J. and de Groot, H., 1996b. Inhibition of Kupffer cell functions as an explanation for the hepatoprotective properties of silibinin. Hepatology 23: 749-754.

Detaille, D., Sanchez, C., Sanz, N., Lopez-Novoa, J.M., Leverve, X. and El-Mir, M.Y., 2008. Interrelation between the inhibition of glycolytic flux by silibinin and the lowering of mitochondrial ROS production in perfused rat hepatocytes. Life Sciences 82: 1070-1076.

Doehner, W. and Landmesser, U., 2011. Xanthine oxidase and uric acid in cardiovascular disease: clinical impact and therapeutic options. Seminars in Nephrology 31: 433-440.

Domitrović, R., Jakovac, H., Marchesi, V.V. and Blažeković, B., 2013. Resolution of liver fibrosis by isoquinoline alkaloid berberine in CCl4-intoxicated mice is mediated by suppression of oxidative stress and upregulation of MMP-2 expression. Journal of Medicinal Food 16: 518-528.

Dvořák, Z., Kosina, P., Walterová, D., Šimánek, V., Bachleda, P. and Ulrichová, J., 2003. Primary cultures of human hepatocytes as a tool in cytotoxicity studies: cell protection against model toxins by flavonolignans obtained from *Silybum marianum*. Toxicology Letters 137: 201-212.

Erlank, H., Elmann, A., Kohen, R., and Kanner, J., 2011. Polyphenols activate Nrf2 in astrocytes via H2O2, semiquinones, and quinones. Free Radical Biology & Medicine 51: 2319-2327.

Esselun, C., Bruns, B., Hagl, S., Grewal, R. and Eckert, G.P., 2019. Differential effects of silibinin A on mitochondrial function in neuronal PC12 and HepG2 liver cells. Oxidative Medicine and Cellular Longevity 2019: 1652609.

Fasano, C., Disciglio, V., Bertora, S., Lepore Signorile, M. and Simone, C., 2019. FOXO3a from the nucleus to the mitochondria: A round trip in cellular stress response. Cells 8: 1110.

Feng, B., Meng, R., Huang, B., Bi, Y., Shen, S. and Zhu, D., 2017. Silymarin protects against renal injury through normalization of lipid metabolism and mitochondrial biogenesis in high fat-fed mice. Free Radical Biology & Medicine 110: 240-249.

Forrester, S.J., Kikuchi, D.S., Hernandes, M.S., Xu, Q. and Griendling, K.K., 2018. Reactive oxygen species in metabolic and inflammatory signaling. Circulation Research 122: 877-902.

Fu, H., Lin, M., Muroya, Y., Hata, K., Katsumura, Y., Yokoya, A., Shikazono, N. and Hatano, Y., 2009. Free radical scavenging reactions and antioxidant activities of silybin: mechanistic aspects and pulse radiolytic studies. Free Radical Research 43: 887-897.

Gabrielová, E., Jabůrek, M., Gažák, R., Vostálová, J., Ježek, J., Křen, V. and Modrianský, M., 2010. Dehydrosilybin attenuates the production of ROS in rat cardiomyocyte mitochondria with an uncoupler-like mechanism. Journal of Bioenergetics and Biomembranes 42: 499-509.

Geed, M., Garabadu, D., Ahmad, A. and Krishnamurthy, S., 2014. Silibinin pretreatment attenuates biochemical and behavioral changes induced by intrastriatal MPP+ injection in rats. Pharmacology Biochemistry and Behavior 117: 92-103.

Gharagozloo, M., Khoshdel, Z. and Amirghofran, Z., 2008. The effect of an iron (III) chelator, silybin, on the proliferation and cell cycle of Jurkat cells: a comparison with desferrioxamine. European Journal of Pharmacology 589: 1-7.

Grasselli, E., Baldini, F., Vecchione, G., Oliveira, P.J., Sardão, V.A., Voci, A., Portincasa, P. and Vergani, L., 2019. Excess fructose and fatty acids trigger a model of non-alcoholic fatty liver disease progression *in vitro*: Protective effect of the flavonoid silybin. International Journal of Molecular Medicine 44: 705-712.

Grattagliano, I., Diogo, C.V., Mastrodonato, M., de Bari, O., Persichella, M., Wang, D.Q., Liquori, A., Ferri, D., Carratù, M.R., Oliveira, P.J. and Portincasa, P., 2013. A silybin-phospholipids complex counteracts rat fatty liver degeneration and mitochondrial oxidative changes. World Journal of Gastroenterology 19: 3007-3017.

Guo, H., Wang, Y. and Liu, D., 2020. Silibinin ameliorates H_2O_2-induced cell apoptosis and oxidative stress response by activating Nrf2 signaling in trophoblast cells. Acta Histochemica 122: 151620.

Haddad, Y., Vallerand, D., Brault, A. and Haddad, P.S., 2011. Antioxidant and hepatoprotective effects of silibinin in a rat model of nonalcoholic steatohepatitis. Evidence-based Complementary and Alternative Medicine 2011: nep164.

Halliwell, B., 1994. Free radicals and antioxidants: A personal view. Nutrition Reviews 52: 253-265.

Halliwell, B. and Gutteridge, J.M.C., 2015. Free radicals in biology and medicine. Oxford University Press, USA.

Halliwell, B., Rafter, J. and Jenner, A., 2005. Health promotion by flavonoids, tocopherols, tocotrienols, and other phenols: direct or indirect effects? Antioxidant or not?. The American Journal of Clinical Nutrition 81: 268S-276S.

Hoh, C., Boocock, D., Marczylo, T., Singh, R., Berry, D.P., Dennison, A.R., Hemingway, D., Miller, A., West, K., Euden, S. and Garcea, G., 2006. Pilot study of oral silibinin, a putative chemopreventive agent, in colorectal cancer patients: silibinin levels in plasma, colorectum, and liver and their pharmacodynamic consequences. Clinical Cancer Research 12: 2944-2950.

Hollman, P.C., 2014. Unravelling of the health effects of polyphenols is a complex puzzle complicated by metabolism. Archives of Biochemistry and Biophysics 559: 100-105.

Howard, A.N. and Constamble, B.J., 1958. The metabolism of adrenocorticotrophic hormone and ascorbic acid in the chick. The Biochemical Journal 69: 501-505.

Hu, M.L., 2011. Dietary polyphenols as antioxidants and anticancer agents: more questions than answers. Chang Gung Medical Journal 34: 449-460.

Jiang, K., Wang, W., Jin, X., Wang, Z., Ji, Z. and Meng, G., 2015. Silibinin, a natural flavonoid, induces autophagy via ROS-dependent mitochondrial dysfunction and loss of ATP involving BNIP3 in human MCF7 breast cancer cells. Oncology Reports 33: 2711-2718.

Katebi, B., Mahdavimehr, M., Meratan, A.A., Ghasemi, A. and Nemat-Gorgani, M., 2018. Protective effects of silibinin on insulin amyloid fibrillation, cytotoxicity and mitochondrial membrane damage. Archives of Biochemistry and Biophysics 659: 22-32.

Khan, I., Preeti, K., Kumar, R., Khatri, D.K. and Singh, S.B., 2022. Activation of SIRT1 by silibinin improved mitochondrial health and alleviated the oxidative damage in experimental diabetic neuropathy and high glucose-mediated neurotoxicity. Archives of Physiology and Biochemistry. https://doi.org/10.1080/13813455.2022.2108454.

Khazim, K., Gorin, Y., Cavaglieri, R.C., Abboud, H.E. and Fanti, P., 2013. The antioxidant silybin prevents high glucose-induced oxidative stress and podocyte injury *in vitro* and *in vivo*. American Journal of Physiology-Renal Physiology 305: F691-F700.

Kim, N.C., Graf, T.N., Sparacino, C.M., Wani, M.C. and Wall, M.E., 2003. Complete isolation and characterization of silybins and isosilybins from milk thistle (*Silybum marianum*). Organic & Biomolecular Chemistry 1: 1684-1689.

Kim, S.H., Kim, K.Y., Yu, S.N., Seo, Y.K., Chun, S.S., Yu, H.S. and Ahn, S.C., 2016. Silibinin induces mitochondrial NOX4-mediated endoplasmic reticulum stress response and its subsequent apoptosis. BMC Cancer 16: 1-10.

Kim, T.H., Woo, J.S., Kim, Y.K. and Kim, K.H., 2014. Silibinin induces cell death through reactive oxygen species-dependent downregulation of notch-1/ERK/Akt signaling in human breast cancer cells. The Journal of Pharmacology and Experimental Therapeutics 349: 268-278.

Köksal, E., Gülçin, İ., Beyza, S., Sarikaya, O. and Bursal, E., 2009. *In vitro* antioxidant activity of silymarin. Journal of Enzyme Inhibition and Medicinal Chemistry 24: 395-405.

Lapidot, T., Harel, S., Granit, R. and Kanner, J., 1998. Bioavailability of red wine anthocyanins as detected in human urine. Journal of Agricultural and Food Chemistry 46: 4297-4302.

Larosa, V. and Remacle, C., 2018. Insights into the respiratory chain and oxidative stress. Bioscience Reports 38: BSR20171492.

Lee, Y., Park, H.R., Chun, H.J. and Lee, J., 2015. Silibinin prevents dopaminergic neuronal loss in a mouse model of Parkinson's disease via mitochondrial stabilization. Journal of Neuroscience Research 93: 755-765.

Lee-Hilz, Y.Y., Boerboom, A.M., Westphal, A.H., Berkel, W.J., Aarts, J.M. and Rietjens, I.M., 2006. Pro-oxidant activity of flavonoids induces EpRE-mediated gene expression. Chemical Research in Toxicology 19: 1499-1505.

Ligeret, H., Brault, A., Vallerand, D., Haddad, Y. and Haddad, P.S., 2008. Antioxidant and mitochondrial protective effects of silibinin in cold preservation-warm reperfusion liver injury. Journal of Ethnopharmacology 115: 507-514.

Li, W., Qu, X., Kang, X., Zhang, H., Zhang, X., Hu, H., Yao, L., Zhang, L., Zheng, J., Zheng, Y., Zhang, J. and Xu, Y., 2022. Silibinin eliminates mitochondrial ROS and restores autophagy through IL6ST/JAK2/STAT3 signaling pathway to protect cardiomyocytes from doxorubicin-induced injury. European Journal of Pharmacology 929: 175153.

Lin, M.T. and Beal, M.F., 2006. Mitochondrial dysfunction and oxidative stress in neurodegenerative diseases. Nature 443: 787-795.

Lorenz, D., Lücker, P.W., Mennicke, W.H. and Wetzelsberger, N., 1984. Pharmacokinetic studies with silymarin in human serum and bile. Methods and Findings in Experimental and Clinical Pharmacology 6: 655-661.

Malekinejad, H., Janbaz-Acyabar, H., Razi, M. and Varasteh, S., 2012. Preventive and protective effects of silymarin on doxorubicin-induced testicular damages correlate with changes in c-myc gene expression. Phytomedicine 19: 1077-1084.

Mao, Y.X., Cai, W.J., Sun, X.Y., Dai, P.P., Li, X.M., Wang, Q., Huang, X.L., He, B., Wang, P.P., Wu, G., Ma, J.F. and Huang, S.B., 2018. RAGE-dependent mitochondria pathway: a novel target of silibinin against apoptosis of osteoblastic cells induced by advanced glycation end products. Cell Death & Disease 9: 674.

Masini, A., Ceccarelli, D., Giovannini, F., Montosi, G., Garuti, C. and Pietrangelo, A., 2000. Iron-induced oxidant stress leads to irreversible mitochondrial dysfunctions and fibrosis in the liver of chronic iron-dosed gerbils. The effect of silybin. Journal of Bioenergetics and Biomembranes 32: 175-182.

Mazzio, E.A., Harris, N. and Soliman, K.F., 1998. Food constituents attenuate monoamine oxidase activity and peroxide levels in C6 astrocyte cells. Planta Medica 64: 603-606.

McKee, J.S., Harrison, P.C. and Riskowski, G.L., 1997. Effects of supplemental ascorbic acid on the energy conversion of broiler chicks during heat stress and feed withdrawal. Poultry Science 76: 1278-1286.

Muthumani, M. and Prabu, S.M., 2014. Silibinin potentially attenuates arsenic-induced oxidative stress mediated cardiotoxicity and dyslipidemia in rats. Cardiovascular Toxicology 14: 83-97.

Pauff, J.M. and Hille, R., 2009. Inhibition studies of bovine xanthine oxidase by luteolin, silibinin, quercetin, and curcumin. Journal of Natural Products 72:725-731.

Pietrangelo, A., Borella, F., Casalgrandi, G., Montosi, G., Ceccarelli, D., Gallesi, D., Giovannini, F., Gasparetto, A. and Masini, A., 1995. Antioxidant activity of silybin *in vivo* during long-term iron overload in rats. Gastroenterology 109: 1941-1949.

Pietrangelo, A., Montosi, G., Garuti, C., Contri, M., Giovannini, F., Ceccarelli, D. and Masini, A., 2002. Iron-induced oxidant stress in nonparenchymal liver cells: mitochondrial derangement and fibrosis in acutely iron-dosed gerbils and its prevention by silybin. Journal of Bioenergetics and Biomembranes 34: 67-79.

Prabu, S.M. and Muthumani, M., 2012. Silibinin ameliorates arsenic induced nephrotoxicity by abrogation of oxidative stress, inflammation and apoptosis in rats. Molecular Biology Reports 39: 11201-11216.

Rolo, A.P., Oliveira, P.J., Moreno, A.J. and Palmeira, C.M., 2003. Protection against post-ischemic mitochondrial injury in rat liver by silymarin or TUDC. Hepatology Research 26: 217-224.

Salamone, F., Galvano, F., Marino, A., Paternostro, C., Tibullo, D., Bucchieri, F., Mangiameli, A., Parola, M., Bugianesi, E. and Volti, G.L., 2012. Silibinin improves hepatic and myocardial injury in mice with nonalcoholic steatohepatitis. Digestive and Liver Disease 44: 334-342.

Sangeetha, N., Viswanathan, P., Balasubramanian, T. and Nalini, N., 2012. Colon cancer chemopreventive efficacy of silibinin through perturbation of xenobiotic metabolizing enzymes in experimental rats. European Journal of Pharmacology 674: 430-438.

Sekine, S. and Ichijo, H., 2015. Mitochondrial proteolysis: its emerging roles in stress responses. Biochimica et Biophysica Acta (BBA)-General Subjects 1850: 274-280.

Serviddio, G., Bellanti, F., Giudetti, A.M., Gnoni, G.V., Petrella, A., Tamborra, R., Romano, A.D., Rollo, T., Vendemiale, G. and Altomare, E., 2010. A silybin-phospholipid complex prevents mitochondrial dysfunction in a rodent model of nonalcoholic steatohepatitis. Journal of Pharmacology and Experimental Therapeutics 332: 922-932.

Serviddio, G., Bellanti, F., Stanca, E., Lunetti, P., Blonda, M., Tamborra, R., Siculella, L., Vendemiale, G., Capobianco, L. and Giudetti, A.M., 2014. Silybin exerts antioxidant effects and induces mitochondrial biogenesis in liver of rat with secondary biliary cirrhosis. Free Radical Biology & Medicine 73: 117-126.

Sharma, B., Chaube, U. and Patel, B.M., 2019. Beneficial effect of silymarin in pressure overload induced experimental cardiac hypertrophy. Cardiovascular Toxicology 19: 23-35.

Si, L., Fu, J., Liu, W., Hayashi, T., Nie, Y., Mizuno, K., Hattori, S., Fujisaki, H., Onodera, S. and Ikejima, T., 2020. Silibinin inhibits migration and invasion of breast cancer MDA-MB-231 cells through induction of mitochondrial fusion. Molecular and Cellular Biochemistry 463: 189-201.

Si, L., Liu, W., Hayashi, T., Ji, Y., Fu, J., Nie, Y., Mizuno, K., Hattori, S., Onodera, S. and Ikejima, T., 2019. Silibinin-induced apoptosis of breast cancer cells involves mitochondrial impairment. Archives of Biochemistry and Biophysics 671: 42-51.

Song, X.Y., Liu, P.C., Liu, W.W., Hayashi, T., Mizuno, K., Hattori, S., Fujisaki, H. and Ikejima, T., 2022. Protective effects of silibinin against ethanol- or acetaldehyde-caused damage in liver cell lines involve the repression of mitochondrial fission. Toxicology In Vitro 80: 105330.

Stolf, A.M., Campos Cardoso, C., Morais, H., Alves de Souza, C.E., Lomba, L.A., Brandt, A.P., Agnes, J.P., Collere, F.C., Galindo, C.M., Corso, C.R., Spercoski, K.M., Locatelli Dittrich, R., Zampronio, A.R., Cadena, S. and Acco, A., 2018. Effects of silymarin on angiogenesis and oxidative stress in streptozotocin-induced diabetes in mice. Biomedicine & Pharmacotherapy 108: 232-243.

Sun, Y., Yang, J., Liu, W., Yao, G., Xu, F., Hayashi, T., Onodera, S. and Ikejima, T., 2019. Attenuating effect of silibinin on palmitic acid-induced apoptosis and mitochondrial dysfunction in pancreatic β-cells is mediated by estrogen receptor alpha. Molecular and Cellular Biochemistry 460: 81-92.

Surai, P.F., 2002. Natural antioxidants in avian nutrition and reproduction. Nottingham University Press, Nottingham, UK.

Surai, P.F., 2015. Silymarin as a natural antioxidant: an overview of the current evidence and perspectives. Antioxidants 4: 204-247.

Surai, P.F., 2020. Vitagene in avian biology and poultry health. Wageningen Academic Publishers, Wageningen, The Netherlands.

Surai, P.F., Kochish, I.I., Fisinin, V.I. and Kidd, M.T., 2019. Antioxidant defence systems and oxidative stress in poultry biology: An update. Antioxidants 8: 235.

Surai, P.F., Kochish, I.I. and Kidd, M.T., 2021. Redox homeostasis in poultry: Regulatory roles of NF-κB. Antioxidants 10, 186.

Surh, Y.J., 2008. NF-kappa B and Nrf2 as potential chemopreventive targets of some anti-inflammatory and antioxidative phytonutrients with anti-inflammatory and antioxidative activities. Asia Pacific Journal of Clinical Nutrition, 17: 269-272.

Surh, Y.J., Kundu, J.K. and Na, H.K., 2008. Nrf2 as a master redox switch in turning on the cellular signaling involved in the induction of cytoprotective genes by some chemopreventive phytochemicals. Planta Medica 74: 1526-1539.

Tang, N., Wu, D., Lu, Y., Chen, J., Zhang, B. and Wu, W., 2009. A comparative study on the stability of silybin and that in silymarin in buffers and biological fluids. Drug Metabolism Letters 3: 115-119.

Tsushima, M., Liu, J., Hirao, W., Yamazaki, H., Tomita, H. and Itoh, K., 2020. Emerging evidence for crosstalk between Nrf2 and mitochondria in physiological homeostasis and in heart disease. Archives of Pharmacal Research 43: 286-296.

Varga, Z., Seres, I., Nagy, E., Ujhelyi, L., Balla, G., Balla, J. and Antus, S., 2006. Structure prerequisite for antioxidant activity of silybin in different biochemical systems *in vitro*. Phytomedicine 13: 85-93.

Varga, Z., Ujhelyi, L., Kiss, A., Balla, J., Czompa, A. and Antus, S., 2004. Effect of silybin on phorbol myristate acetate-induced protein kinase C translocation, NADPH oxidase activity and apoptosis in human neutrophils. Phytomedicine 11: 206-212.

Vecchione, G., Grasselli, E., Cioffi, F., Baldini, F., Oliveira, P.J., Sardão, V.A., Cortese, K., Lanni, A., Voci, A., Portincasa, P. and Vergani, L., 2017. The nutraceutic silybin counteracts excess lipid accumulation and ongoing oxidative stress in an *in vitro* model of non-alcoholic fatty liver disease progression. Frontiers in Nutrition 4: 42.

Wang, C., He, C., Lu, S., Wang, X., Wang, L., Liang, S., Wang, X., Piao, M., Cui, J., Chi, G. and Ge, P., 2020. Autophagy activated by silibinin contributes to glioma cell death via induction of oxidative stress-mediated BNIP3-dependent nuclear translocation of AIF. Cell Death & Disease 11: 630.

Willemsen, H., Swennen, Q., Everaert, N., Geraert, P.A., Mercier, Y., Stinckens, A., Decuypere, E. and Buyse, J., 2011. Effects of dietary supplementation of methionine and its hydroxy analog DL-2-hydroxy-4-methylthiobutanoic acid on growth performance, plasma hormone levels, and the redox status of broiler chickens exposed to high temperatures. Poultry Science 90: 2311-2320.

Woo, S.M., Min, K.J., Kim, S., Park, J.W., Kim, D.E., Chun, K.S., Kim, Y.H., Lee, T.J., Kim, S.H., Choi, Y.H., Chang, J.S. and Kwon, T.K., 2014. Silibinin induces apoptosis of HT29 colon carcinoma cells through early growth response-1 (EGR-1)-mediated non-steroidal anti-inflammatory drug-activated gene-1 (NAG-1) up-regulation. Chemico-Biological Interactions 211: 36-43.

Wu, W.T., Chen, Y.R., Lu, D.H., Senatov, F.S., Yang, K.C. and Wang, C.C., 2021. Silymarin modulates catabolic cytokine expression through Sirt1 and SOX9 in human articular chondrocytes. Journal of Orthopaedic Surgery and Research 16: 147.

Yao, J., Zhi, M. and Minhu, C., 2011. Effect of silybin on high-fat-induced fatty liver in rats. Brazilian Journal of Medical and Biological Research 44: 652-659.

Yin, F., Liu, J., Ji, X., Wang, Y., Zidichouski, J. and Zhang, J., 2011. Silibinin: A novel inhibitor of Aβ aggregation. Neurochemistry International 58: 399-403.

You, Y., Chen, L., Wu, Y., Wang, M., Lu, H., Zhou, X., Liu, H., Fu, Z., He, Q., Ou, J., Fu, X., Liu, Y., Kwan, H., Liang, D., Zhao, X. and Dai, J., 2020a. Silibinin promotes cell proliferation through facilitating G1/S transitions by activating Drp1-mediated mitochondrial fission in cells. Cell Transplantation 29: 963689720950213.

You, Y., He, Q., Lu, H., Zhou, X., Chen, L., Liu, H., Lu, Z., Liu, D., Liu, Y., Zuo, D., Fu, X., Kwan, H. and Zhao, X., 2020b. Silibinin induces G2/M cell cycle arrest by activating Drp1-dependent mitochondrial fission in cervical cancer. Frontiers in Pharmacology 11: 271.

Young, A., Gill, R. and Mailloux, R.J., 2019. Protein S-glutathionylation: The linchpin for the transmission of regulatory information on redox buffering capacity in mitochondria. Chemico-Biological Interactions 299: 151-162.

Yu, Y., Li, L.F., Tao, J., Zhou, X.M. and Xu, C., 2019. Silibinin induced apoptosis of human epidermal cancer A431 cells by promoting mitochondrial NOS. Free Radical Research 53: 714-726.

Zatloukalová, M., Křen, V., Gažák, R., Kubala, M., Trouillas, P., Ulrichová, J. and Vacek, J., 2011. Electrochemical investigation of flavonolignans and study of their interactions with DNA in the presence of Cu(II). Bioelectrochemistry 82: 117-124.

Zhang, S., Yang, Y., Liang, Z., Duan, W., Yang, J., Yan, J., Wang, N., Feng, W., Ding, M., Nie, Y. and Jin, Z., 2013. Silybin-mediated inhibition of Notch signaling exerts antitumor activity in human hepatocellular carcinoma cells. PloS One 8: e83699.

Zhao, J. and Agarwal, R., 1999. Tissue distribution of silibinin, the major active constituent of silymarin, in mice and its association with enhancement of phase II enzymes: implications in cancer chemoprevention. Carcinogenesis 20: 2101-2108.

Zhu, H.J., Brinda, B.J., Chavin, K.D., Bernstein, H.J., Patrick, K.S. and Markowitz, J.S., 2013. An assessment of pharmacokinetics and antioxidant activity of free silymarin flavonolignans in healthy volunteers: a dose escalation study. Drug Metabolism and Disposition 41: 1679-1685.

Zhu, S.Y., Dong, Y., Tu, J., Zhou, Y., Zhou, X.H. and Xu, B., 2014. *Silybum marianum* oil attenuates oxidative stress and ameliorates mitochondrial dysfunction in mice treated with D-galactose. Pharmacognosy Magazine 10: S92-S99.

Chapter 5
Silymarin and Nrf2

You never know what you can do till you try

Peter F. Surai[1-6] and Anton Surai[7]*
[1]Vitagene and Health Research Centre, Bristol, UK; [2]Department of Microbiology and Biochemistry, Faculty of Veterinary Medicine, Trakia University, Stara Zagora, Bulgaria; [3]Department of Animal Nutrition, Faculty of Agricultural and Environmental Sciences, Szent Istvan University, Hungary; [4]Saint-Petersburg State Academy of Veterinary Medicine, St. Petersburg, Russia; [5]Sumy National Agrarian University, Sumy, Ukraine; [6]Odessa National Academy of Food Technologies, Odessa, Ukraine; [7]Healthy Food Services, Bristol, UK
psurai@feedfood.co.uk

Abstract

The data presented in this chapter clearly showed that Nrf2 activation is an important adaptive mechanism to deal with various stresses in human and animals. A great deal of accumulating evidence indicates that Nrf2 is responsible for metabolic control of the cellular redox homeostasis as a result of regulation of the key antioxidants (SOD, GPx, GSH, Trx, peroxiredoxin), detoxification enzymes and various proteins possessing anti-inflammatory properties. Indeed, by improving ROS scavenging and restoring redox homeostasis under stress condition, Nrf2 can prevent/decrease stress-related detrimental changes in human and farm animals/poultry and plays a crucial role in antistress strategy development. However, in the case of excessive stress, decreased Nrf2 expression and oxidative stress can occur leading to detrimental consequences in terms of human health and productive and reproductive performance of farm animals/poultry. There is a range of nutrients, including various phytochemicals (e.g. silymarin) able to prevent detrimental effects of stressors on Nrf2 expression. Transcription factors, including Nrf2, NF-κB, HSF1 and others are working in concert and are responsible for adaptive response of the eukaryotic cell under various forms of oxidative, electrophilic, thermal, inflammatory and other stresses by orchestrating effective transcriptional programs. In general, induction of these programs is associated with upregulation of various protective mechanisms including molecular chaperones, responsible for proteostasis, antioxidant and drug-metabolising enzymes, dealing with various RONS, as well as specific proteins responsible for the repair and clearance of damaged macromolecules as well as for the maintenance of cell structure, redox homeostasis, and intermediary metabolism. It sems likely that regulatory effects of silymarin/silibinin on Nrf2 are among major molecular mechanisms of protective effects of the phytochemicals in humans and farm animals/poultry.

Keywords: antioxidants, Nrf2, oxidative stress, adaptation, redox homeostasis, silymarin, silibinin

5.1 Introduction

Accumulating evidence indicates that ROS are no longer viewed as just toxic by-products of mitochondrial respiration but are now appreciated for their role in regulating a myriad of cellular signalling pathways (Reczek and Chandel, 2015). It has been suggested that the signalling ROS are produced in a subtly regulated manner, while many deleterious ROS are produced and react randomly (Niki, 2014). Therefore, it is unlikely that nutritional antioxidants affect detrimentally physiologically important signalling, since the antioxidants do not scavenge signalling ROS/RNS nor do they inhibit the formation of signalling molecules (Niki, 2012; 2016).

Oxidation-reduction (redox) based regulation of gene expression is a fundamental regulatory mechanism in cell biology acting at the cell-signalling level. The field of redox signalling that is the overlap of signal transduction with redox biology was established. It is commonly acknowledged that redox signalling is essential in physiological homeostasis and alterations in redox signalling are observed in stress conditions and aging and sustained deviation from redox homeostasis results in disease (Forman, 2016) and decreased productive and reproductive performance of fam animals/poultry (Surai, 2020). Since ROS are damaging to many biological molecules, the antioxidant systems are responsible for prevention of the damages. However, a basal level of oxidative stress is essential for cell adaptation and survival, since a moderate level of oxidative stress can create adaptive responses and improve adaptive ability to stressful challenges/conditions (Yan, 2014). There is strong evidence that, in human and animals, redox-signalling pathways use ROS as signalling molecules to activate genes responsible for regulation of various functions including growth, differentiation, proliferation and apoptosis (Surai, 2020).

It is well appreciated that the antioxidant defence systems are also under regulation by various transcription factors (Ma and He, 2012; Kweider *et al.*, 2014; Majzunova *et al.*, 2013; Song and Zou, 2014). Redox balance is controlled by a battery of transcriptional factors, including Nrf2, NF-κB, PPARs, PGC-1α, p53, FOXO, AP-1, etc. (Lushckak, 2011, Wang and Hai, 2016). They regulate redox status through modulating ROS-generating enzymes and antioxidant enzymes in a cooperative and interactive way being critically important for animal adaptation to various stresses. In recent years great attention has been paid to a basic leucine zipper transcription factor, Nuclear factor-erythroid-2- (NF-E2-) related factor 2 (Nrf2) and, therefore, we consider briefly its important roles in stress adaptation and its regulation by various factors, including dietary SM/SB.

5.2 Transcription factor Nrf2

It is well appreciated that the antioxidant defence systems are under regulation by various transcription factors (Ma and He, 2012; Kweider *et al.*, 2014; Majzunova *et al.*, 2013; Song and Zou, 2014). Oxidative stress is believed to activate a range of transcription factors/pathways including Nrf2, NF-κB, AP-1, TP53, HIF-1α,

HSF1, PPAR-γ, MAPK, FOXO, NOTCH, CREB, β-catenin/Wnt, etc. (Lushckak, 2011; Marinho *et al.*, 2014; Tu *et al.*, 2019; Wang and Hai, 2016). Activation of these transcription factors is associated with the expression of over 500 different genes (Tu *et al.*, 2019). They regulate redox status through modulating ROS-generating enzymes and antioxidant enzymes in a cooperative and interactive way being critically important for human/animal adaptation to various stresses.

Nrf2 was discovered (as a member of the human CNC-bZIP transcription factor family) and isolated in the year 1994 from the human erythroleukemia cell line K562 during a research related to β-globin gene regulation (Moi *et al.*, 1994). It is known that Nrf2 is the redox-sensitive master regulator of oxidative stress signalling and oxidative stress responses being critical for cell adaptation and survival in stressful conditions (Itoh *et al.*, 2010). Clearly, Nrf2 has a vital role in adaptive responses to oxidative stress via induction of the expression of various protective molecules (Howden, 2013; Keum and Choi, 2014; Tang *et al.*, 2014; Vriend and Reiter, 2015). Nrf2 is thought to be expressed in all cell types and its basal protein levels necessary for housekeeping functions are usually low in physiological/unstressed conditions mainly due to its KEAP1 mediated proteasomal degradation (He *et al.*, 2020b). It is worth mentioning that Nrf2-associated response to stresses takes place withing few minutes. For example, oxidative stress in cultured cardiomyocytes or mild ischemic reperfusion in mice were shown to be associated with rapid (about 10 min) onset of Nrf2 protein translation to limit tissue injury (Chen, 2021).

The existing evidence suggests that under normal physiological conditions, Nrf2, a 605-amino acid transcription factor composed of seven functional domains (Neh1-7) regulating its stability or/and its transcriptional activity (transactivation) is located in the cytoplasm. Nrf2 exists as an inactive complex with the negative regulator called Kelch-like-ECH-associated protein 1 (Keap1), a 624-amino acid, cysteine-rich, homodimeric zinc-finger protein, identified as a negative regulator of Nrf2 in 1999 (Itoch *et al.*, 1999). Keap1 is known to be responsible for forwarding Nrf2 to a Cul3-based E3 ligase with the following rapid 26S proteasomal degradation with a half-life under physiological conditions of 15-20 min (Choi *et al.*, 2014; Helou *et al.*, 2019). The intracellular concentration of Nrf2 is believed to be determined by a complex equilibrium between its synthesis and its proteasomal degradation. Nrf2 abundance within the cell is thought to be tightly regulated and controlled by four E3 ubiquitin ligase complexes-mediated ubiquitylation and proteasomal degradation (He *et al.*, 2020b).

The cysteine residues of Keap1 have been shown to be susceptible to covalent modification by a range of electrophilic species (Madden and Itzhaki, 2020). Keap1 was found to contain more than 27 cysteine residues possessing different reactivity and having various functional impact on Nrf2. Cys151, located within the BTB homodimerization domain, was shown to be responsible for Nfr2 activation, while Cys273, 288, and 297, located in the intervening region, were indicated to inhibit Nrf2 activity facilitating its interaction with Keap1. Furthermore, highly conserved and redox-sensitive cysteines (Cys119, 235, 311, 316, 414, and 516) have been also identified in Nrf2 and their oxidative modification could prevent Keap1 recognition and binding (Panieri and Saso, 2019). Therefore, Keap1 serves as a sensitive cellular redox sensor and main intracellular regulator of Nrf2 (Bellezza *et al.*, 2018). It is generally believed that oxidative or electrophilic stress, causing increased ROS production can modify/oxidise critical cysteine thiols of Keap1 leading to the Keap1-Nrf2 complex dissociation and prevention of Nrf2 degradation in proteosome. For example, alkylation or oxidation of cysteine residues was indicated to disable Keap1 from recruiting the E3 ligase for Nrf2 ubiquitination leading to an extension of the Nrf2 half-life to nearly 60 mins (Chen, 2021).

Therefore, Nrf2 translocates to the nucleus, heterodimerises with one of the small Maf (musculoaponeurotic fibrosarcoma oncogene homolog) proteins and binds to antioxidant/electrophile-response elements (ARE) in the upstream promoter region of genes encoding various antioxidant molecules to activate their transcription (Bellezza *et al.*, 2018; Figure 5.1). Many antioxidant and detoxification genes are shown to contain such elements in their promoters. Computational analyses predicted 10 068 human genes containing AREs (Wang *et al.*, 2007) participating in creating cellular responses to various stress conditions. Particularly, *NFE2L2* gene (coding Nrf2) is shown to contain ARE within its promoter region that renders Nrf2 the ability to directly activate its own transcription, providing a positive feedback mechanism to amplify Nrf2 effects (He *et al.*, 2020b). Interestingly, *NFE2L2* promoter is reported to contain an NF-κB binding site and could potentially be regulated by NF-κB (Rushworth *et al.*, 2012). There is growing evidence that Nrf2 activity is

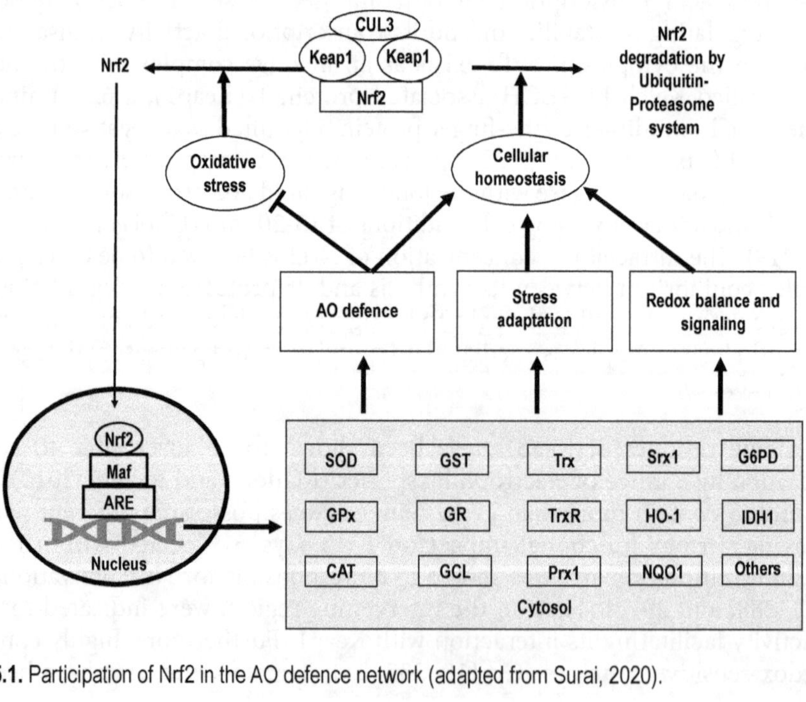

Figure 5.1. Participation of Nrf2 in the AO defence network (adapted from Surai, 2020).

tightly regulated. Nrf2-activated genes were shown to require the recruitment of both Nrf2 and Nrf2-binding partners including transcription factors, cofactors, and mediators for a complete activation (He *et al.*, 2020b). Recently a mutant mouse helped to demonstrate that Cys151/Cys273/Cys288 play a vital role in the sensing of electrophilic Nrf2-inducing chemicals (Saito *et al.*, 2015).

In cells under physiological homeostatic conditions, cytosolic transcription factor Nrf2 is kept at low levels being bound to Keap1 by the ubiquitin ligase complex Cullin (Cul)3-RING-box protein (Rbx)1 (Cul3). This complex ubiquitinates Nrf2, triggering its constant proteasomal degradation. Under oxidative stress, ROS modify/oxidise SH-groups within Keap1 leading to conformational changes inducing the Nrf2 release from Keap1. This prevents Nrf2 proteasomal degradation and Nrf2 translocates to the nucleus. In the nucleus, Nfr2 binds to the ARE and initiates the transcription of an array of direct or indirect antioxidant enzymes including SOD, GPx, CAT, GST, GR, GCL, Trx, TrxR, Prx1, Srx1, HO-1, NQO1, G6PD, IDH2, etc. These enzymes contribute to the improvement of the antioxidant defence network and reduce the cellular oxidative stress. The Nrf2 induced synthesis of AO enzymes also participates in regulation of stress adaptation and redox signalling. The restoration of cellular homeostasis leads to Nrf2-Keap1 complex formation and activation of Nrf2 degradation by ubiquitin-proteosome system and decreases the Nrf2 mediated synthesis of AO enzymes.

By binding to antioxidant/electrophile-response elements (ARE) in the upstream promoter region of genes encoding various antioxidant molecules, Nrf2 regulates the expression of an array of protective molecules. They are responsible for multiple pathways, including provision of direct antioxidants or enzymes that directly inactivate oxidants, increasing levels of GSH, Trx and NADPH synthesis, enhancing toxin export via the multidrug response transporters, inhibiting cytokine mediated inflammation, enhancing recognition, repair, and removal of damaged proteins, increasing chaperones and regulating posttranslational modifications (Loboda *et al.*, 2016; Sussan and Biswal, 2014; Table 5.1). Nrf2 initiates synthesis of enzymes of the first line of the antioxidant defence, namely SOD, GPx and CAT, detoxification enzymes (HO-1, NQO1, and GST), enzymes catalysing GSH synthesis (GCL) and NADPH-synthesising enzymes, as well as others stress-response proteins responsible for protection against oxidative and inflammatory damages (Cuadrado *et al.*, 2019; Gureev *et al.*, 2019; Helou *et al.*, 2019; Zhou *et al.*, 2014).

Accumulating evidence clearly shows that Nrf2 can also regulate many important biological processes (for review and references see Chen, 2021; Panieri and Saso, 2019), including

- cell signalling;
- cell proliferation and differentiation;
- detoxification;
- transcription;
- inflammation;

Table 5.1. Principal functions of enzymes encoded by Nrf2 target genes and involved in the antioxidant defence (Cuadrado *et al.*, 2019; Gureev *et al.*, 2019; Helou *et al.*, 2019; Loboda, 2016; Tu *et al.*, 2019).

Gene name	Abbreviation	Enzyme principal functions
Superoxide dismutase	SOD	Dismutation of superoxide radicals to molecular oxygen and hydrogen peroxide
Glutathione peroxidase	GPx	Detoxification of hydrogen peroxide, organic hydroperoxides and lipid peroxides
Glutamate cysteine ligase	GCL	Synthesis of GSH (rate-limiting step)
Glutathione reductase	GR	Conversion of glutathione disulphide into the reduced glutathione
Glutathione S-transferase	GST	Detoxification of xenobiotics and electrophiles by conjugation with GSH
Sulfiredoxin	Srx	Reduction of cysteine sulfinic acid formed in peroxiredoxins
Catalase	CAT	Transformation of H_2O_2 into water and oxygen
Thioredoxin 1	Trx	Reduction of other proteins by cysteine thiol-disulphide exchange
Thioredoxin reductase	TrxR	AO defence and maintaining redox balance
Thioredoxin peroxidase (peroxiredoxins)	Prx	Reduction of hydrogen peroxide and alkyl hydroperoxides
Heme oxygenase 1	HO-1	Heme degradation to carbon monoxide
Glucose 6-phosphate dehydrogenase	G6PD	Generation of NADPH, the critical cofactor fuelling antioxidant reaction
6-phosphogluconate dehydrogenase	6PGDH	
Malic enzyme 1	ME1	
Isocitrate dehydrogenase 1	IDH1	
NAD(P)H quinone oxidoreductase-1	NQO1	Reduction of quinones to hydroquinones

- autophagy;
- apoptosis;
- mitochondrial function or biogenesis; as well as
- several metabolic pathways involved in iron/heme, glucose, glutamine, lipid, NADPH and pentose phosphate metabolism.

It is widely believed that Nrf2 is involved in regulation of the expression of about 250 genes (Cuadrado *et al.*, 2019) and gene products (proteins) support the maintenance and responsiveness of the cellular antioxidant systems. In accordance with earlier study, Nrf2 has been found to directly or indirectly alter the expression of approximately 15,000 genes, and the number of directly inducible genes has been estimated at 654. Interestingly, the inducible targets of Nrf2 are primarily categorised as antioxidative genes (Sussan and Biswal, 2014). Therefore, a well-orchestrated adaptive change in gene expression in response to stress via Nrf2 and the ARE is a key mechanism of effective protection against oxidative stress (Figure 5.2; Cuadrado *et al.*, 2019; Gureev *et al.*, 2019).

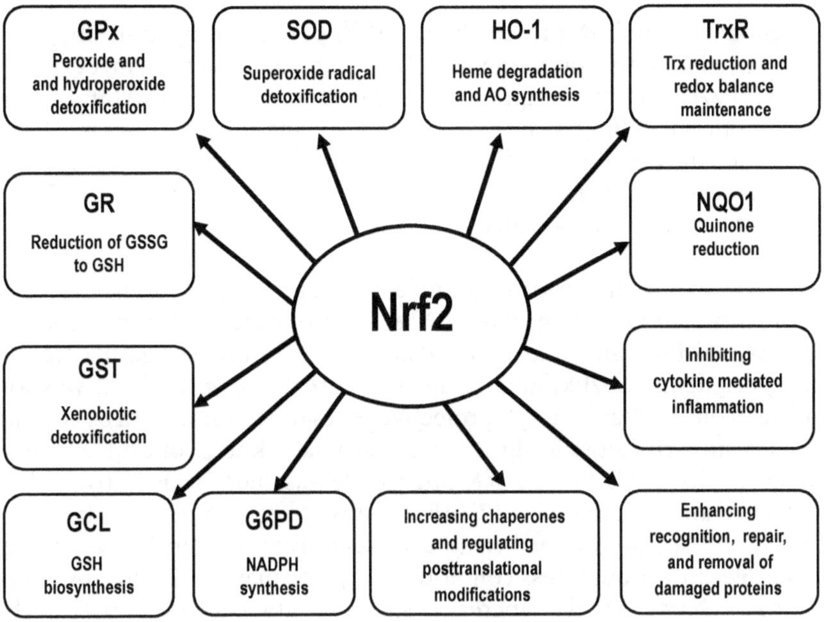

Figure 5.2. Cytoprotective genes and processes regulated by Nrf2 transcription factor (adapted from Loboda *et al.*, 2016; Surai, 2020; Sussan and Biswal, 2014). GPx = glutathione peroxidase; SOD = superoxide dismutase; HO-1 = heme oxigenase-1; TR = thioredoxin reductase; GR = glutathione reductase; GST = glutathione S-transferase; GCL = γ-glutamylcysteine ligase; G6PD = glucose-6-phosphate dehydrogenase; NQO1 = NAD(P)H:quinone dehydrogenase 1.

It has become increasingly apparent that Nrf2 expression and location is controlled through a complex transcriptional/epigenetic and post-translational network activation of Nrf2 in response to various stimulus (Bellezza *et al.*, 2018; Hayes and Dinkova-Kostova, 2014), including:

- redox disturbances;
- endoplasmic reticulum stress;
- autophagy impairment;
- inflammation;
- growth factor stimulation; and
- nutrient/energy fluxes orchestrating adaptive responses to diverse forms of stress.

Furthermore, it is proven that effects of Nrf2 on the adaptive ability of cells is quite broad and in addition to activation of synthesis of antioxidant molecules, Nrf2 also upregulate the repair and degradation of damaged macromolecules and directs metabolic reprogramming during stress by modulating intermediary metabolism (Zhou *et al.*, 2014). Nrf2 is involved in protein quality control by induction of proteasome subunits associated with a decrease in unfolded proteins and restoring the physiological protein turnover (Bellezza *et al.*, 2018). Furthermore, Nrf2 was reported to upregulate various transcription factors, including heat shock factor 1 (HSF1),

CCAAT-enhancer-binding protein beta (c/EBPβ), activating transcription factor (ATF)3, ATF4, nuclear factor interleukin (IL)-3 regulated (NFIL3), myocyte enhancer factor 2 (MEF2A), and transcription factor MafG to orchestrate cytoprotection and tissue repair or remodelling (Chen, 2021). Thus, elucidating molecular mechanisms of the cooperation or competition of Nrf2 with other transcription factors and co-factors at the ARE and ARE-like sites is a key for complete understanding of Nrf2-mediated gene transactivation (He *et al.*, 2020b).

Keap1 is shown to be the critical negative regulator of Nrf2 *in vivo*, as confirmed by experiments using mouse genetics. Direct Keap1 knock-out mice (*Keap1*$^{-/-}$) died around the time of weaning due to hyperkeratosis of the upper digestive tract leading to feeding problems (Suzuki and Yamamoto, 2017). However, Nrf2 was found to accumulate in the nucleus, and cytoprotective genes were indicated to be constitutively up-regulated in various tissues in these global Keap1 knock-out mice. The authors showed that the lethal phenotype of *Keap1*$^{-/-}$ mice was due to constitutive stabilisation of Nrf2 (Suzuki and Yamamoto, 2017). The adverse effects of Nrf2 activation/activators need further investigations. Furthermore, it was proven that Nrf2 plays an important protective roles in various stress conditions. In particular, Nrf2 knockout mice were reported to be characterised by increased susceptibility to a wide variety of chemical insults, including lung injury in response to BHT, carcinogenesis in response to benzopyrene, liver toxicity in response to acetaminophen (APAP), and DNA damage in response to diesel exhaust fumes (Baird and Yamamoto, 2020a,b).

It is important to mention that comprehensive studies of Nrf2 targets using *Nfe2l2*-knockout mice, *Keap1*-knockdown mice and *Keap1*-knockout mice allowed to identify a range of antioxidant response element (ARE) containing genes having important physiological significance beyond the conventional antioxidant stress response (He *et al.*, 2020b), including regulation of:

- aerobic glycolysis and glycogen synthesis and inhibition of gluconeogenesis;
- expression of genes encoding enzymes involved in the pentose phosphate pathway. For example, in mouse hepatocytes Nrf2 regulates the expression of almost all of the enzymes involved in the pentose phosphate pathway (Baird and Yamamoto, M., 2020b);
- de novo purine biosynthesis pathway;
- amino acid metabolism;
- lipid metabolism;
- heme and iron metabolism;
- unfolded protein response and proteostasis;
- autophagy. Deficiency in autophagy leads to competitive interaction with the DLG motif of Nrf2 for the Keap1 binding site with following stabilisation of Nrf2 (Vasileva *et al.*, 2020);
- mitochondrial physiology and biogenesis;
- inflammation and immunity.

5.3 Pharmacological/nutritional Nrf2 activation

There is a range of chemical compounds and conditions which can induce Nrf2 activity, including endogenous signalling compounds/metabolites, oncometabolites, immunometabolites, dietary compounds, pharmaceuticals, microorganisms and extracellular inducers (Figure 5.3).

Based on the chemical structures, at least 10 classes of Nrf2 activators can be established (Sihvola and Levonen, 2017), including

- diphenols;
- Michael reaction acceptors;
- isothiocyanates;
- thiocarbamates;
- trivalent arsenicals;
- 1,2-dithiole-3-thiones;
- Hydroperoxides;
- vicinal dimercaptans;
- heavy metals; and
- polyenes.

Chemical inducers of Nrf2 were categorised into the following five classes (Figure 5.4).

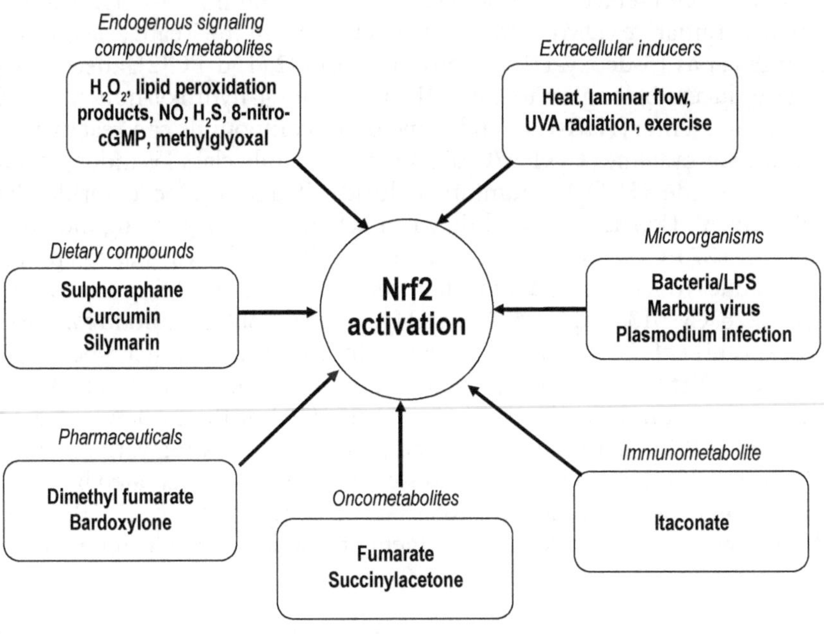

Figure 5.3. Inducers of Nrf2 activity (Adapted from Imai *et al.*, 2021; Baird and Yamamoto, 2020a; Surai, 2020).

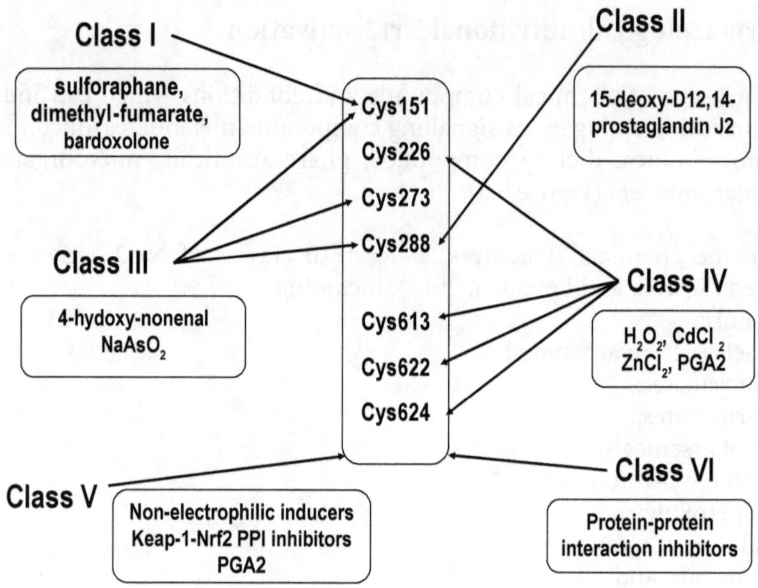

Figure 5.4. Keap1-sensing mechanisms (adapted from Baird and Yamamoto, 2020a; Suzuki *et al.*, 2019).

Class I inducers, represented by sulforaphane (SFN), curcumin, tert-butylhydroquinone, and dimethyl-fumarate (DMF) affect Nrf2 via Cys151 in the Keap1; class II, includes such an inducer as 15-deoxy-D12,14-prostaglandin J2 (15d-PGJ2), affecting Cys288. Chemical inducers belonging to Class III, including 4-hydroxy-nonenal (4-HNE), sodium meta-arsenite ($NaAsO_2$), and some other compounds can react with any of the three sensor cysteines Cys151/Cys273/Cys288, while class IV inducers, includes hydrogen peroxide (H_2O_2), cadmium chloride (CdCl2), zinc chloride (ZnCl2), prostaglandin A2 (PGA2), etc. and they can activate Nrf2 signalling independently of Cys151/Cys273/Cys288. For example, it was clearly shown that Keap1 uses the cysteine residues to set up an elaborate fail-safe mechanism enabling any combination among Cys226, Cys613, and Cys622/Cys624 to form a disulphide bond for the sensing of H_2O_2 (Suzuki *et al.*, 2019). Finally, class V inducers represent other types of inducers such as Keap1-Nrf2 protein-protein interaction inhibitors (Suzuki and Yamamoto, 2017) and function independently of Cys151/273/288 or the oxidative stress sensor Cys226/613/622/624 (Baird and Yamamoto, 2020b). Interestingly, the regulation of the Nrf2 protein level during stress responses is shown to be mediated by the activity but not the composition of the Nrf2-Keap1-Cul3 complex (Iso *et al.*, 2016). A list of some known Nrf2 enhancers for the treatment of oxidative stress-promoted disorders are shown in Table 5.2.

There is also a range of endogenously produced signalling mediators (e.g. H_2O_2, NO, fumarate, products of lipid peroxidation) effectively activating Nrf2 (Sihvola and Levonen, 2017). Currently, a number of natural and synthetic Nrf2-activating compounds have been described, and there is growing body of evidence showing the

Table 5.2. Nrf2 enhancers for the treatment of oxidative stress-promoted disorders (Adapted from Sivandzade *et al.*, 2019; Vasileva, *et al.*, 2020).

NRF2 enhancers	Category	The role in antioxidative systems
Sulforaphane	Organic isothiocyanate	Activates the Nrf2-Keap1 pathway through direct modifications of Keap1 cysteines
		Promotes the ribosomal internalisation of Nrf2 mRNA for protein synthesis
Metformin	Biguanide	Activates AMPK related pathways
		Activates the Nrf2-ARE signalling pathways reducing oxidative stress, inflammation, and loss of blood-brain barrier integrity
		Promotes the neurogenesis and spatial memory formation
		Attenuates blood-brain barrier disruption and reduces post- ischemic brain injury
Astragaloside IV	Bioactive saponin	Inhibits ROS generation and activating the Nrf2-ARE pathway in neuronal cells
		Protects the blood-brain barrier integrity from LPS-induced disruption by activating the Nrf2-ARE pathway
		Anti-inflammatory activities on blood-brain barrier endothelial cells
		Decreases the adhesion of murine dendritic cells JAWS II onto bEnd.3 cells
Curcumin	Polyphenol	Activates the Nrf2-ARE signalling pathways leading to attenuating brain injury in the traumatic brain injury
		Increases the activities of antioxidant enzymes such as SOD and GPx
		Antioxidant, anti-inflammatory and anti-infective properties
Epigallocatechin gallate (EGCG)	Polyphenol	Up-regulates Nrf2/HO-1 via activation of the p38 MAPK and ERK1/2 signalling pathways
		Promotes the dissociation of Nrf2 from Keap1 and its nuclear translocation
Genistein	Isoflavone	Up-regulates Nrf2/HO-1 via Keap1 S-nitrosylation
		Activates the Nrf2-ARE signalling pathway via modulation of PI3K activity in cerebrovascular endothelial cells
Fisetin	Flavonoid	Activates the Nrf2-ARE signalling pathway
		Possesses anti-carcinogenic, anti-inflammatory, anti-viral, and immune-stimulatory activity properties
Melatonin	Hormone	Enhances expression and activity of antioxidant enzymes
		Attenuates brain injury in traumatic brain injury, potentially through activation of the Nrf2-ARE signalling pathway
Bardoxolone methyl (CDDO-Me)	Synthetic cyanoenone triterpenoid	Binds to Cys151 in Keap1 leading to Nrf2 activation
Dimethyl fumarate	Synthetic fumaric acid derivative	Binds to Cys151 in Keap1 leading to Nrf2 activation
Mitoquinone	Synthetic quinone	Activates Nrf2 through induction of Atg7-dependent autophagy, which leads to degradation of Keap1

beneficial effects of Nrf2 activation in various stress conditions (Cuadrado *et al.*, 2019). It is proven that most small-molecule Nrf2 inducers have a common feature: they are electrophiles, which can either oxidise or alkylate Keap1 to release the checkpoint on Nrf2 (Chen, 2021).

In addition, Keap1 dependent but cysteine independent mechanisms were described to stabilise Nrf2 by interfering with formation of the Nrf2-Keap1 complex (He *et al.*, 2020b). There is also a range of other mechanisms activating Nrf2, including its phosphorylation which causes a Nfr2-Keap1 dissociation and Nrf2 translocation to nucleus (Bhakkiyalakshmi *et al.*, 2015). In particular, at least four different mechanisms could lead to dissociation of Keap1 from Nrf2 (Zolnourian *et al.*, 2019):

- oxidation of Cys residues (lower molecular weight reactive oxygen species);
- covalent modification of Cys residues (electrophiles);
- phosphorylation of Nrf2 at Ser40 by protein kinase C and PKR-like ER kinase (PERK);
- protein-protein interaction between p62 and Keap1.

Furthermore, recently it has been shown that post-translational modifications of Keap1 leading to changes in Nrf2 activity are quite diverse (Kopacz *et al.*, 2020). It should also be mentioned that ubiquitination of Nrf2 at the Neh2 is shown to suppress Nrf2 activity, whereas acetylation of Nrf2 at the Neh1 and Neh3 is associated with increased Nrf2 activity. Furthermore, SUMOylation of Nrf2 at the Neh1 andNeh3 could result in either Nrf2 activation or Nrf2 repression (Zang *et al.*, 2020). Phosphorylation of serine 40 of Nrf2 could partially regulate the association of Nrf2 with Keap1, leading to Nrf2 activation (Huang *et al.*, 2000). It is interesting that Nrf2 can also be modulated by metabolites from both the tricarboxylic acid (TCA) cycle (succinate or fumarate) and glycolysis (Baird and Yamamoto, M., 2020b).

AccordingtoZhou*etal.*(2019)themodulationmechanismofKeap1-Nrf2/AREsignalling pathway could be divided into two major categories, including Keap1-dependent and Keap1-independent manners. There are several models for Keap1-dependent regulation mechanisms, including 'hinge and latch model', 'Keap1-CUL3 dissociation model' and 'Keap1 ubiquitination' (Zhou *et al.*, 2019). Furthermore, Nrf2 can be regulated independently of Keap1 (Zhou *et al.*, 2019), including:

- Nrf2 transcriptional regulation and self-regulation;
- posttranscriptional regulation by microRNAs;
- phosphorylation and ubiquitination of various protein kinases;
- binding with other protein molecules, including P21;
- regulation by various transcription factors (CBP, BRG1, c-Jun, p21, p53, p65, ATF1, ATF3, etc.);
- regulation by other modifications, including DNA methylation and histone modification (Figure 5.5).

Although the main form of regulation of the Nrf2 pathway is the aforementioned modification of Keap1 cysteines, disabling its ubiquitination activity (i.e. the 'canonical pathway'), there is a range of other forms of regulation of this pathway, so-called

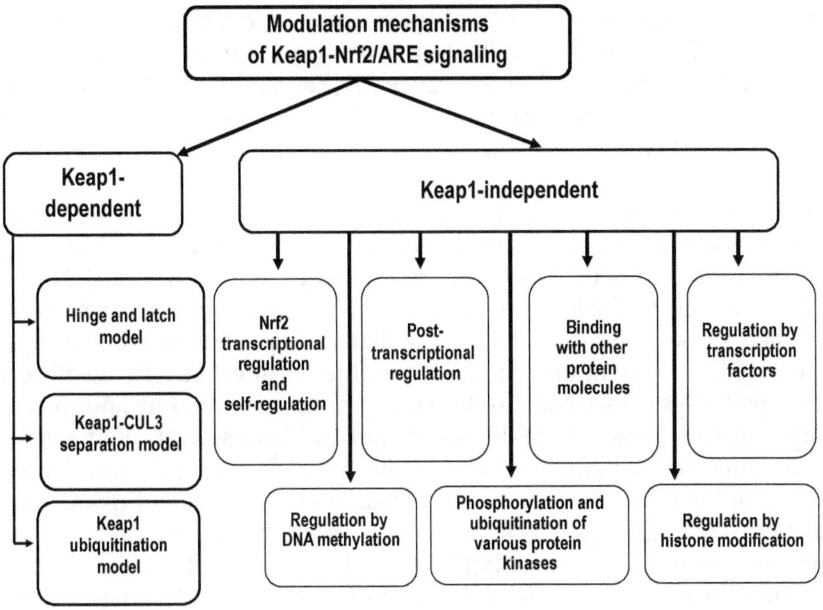

Figure 5.5. Molecular mechanisms of regulation of Keap1-Nrf2/ARE signalling (adapted from Surai, 2020; Zhou *et al.*, 2019).

'noncanonical pathway', at the transcriptional, post-transcriptional, translational and posttranslational level (Guerrero-Hue *et al.*, 2020; Kasai *et al.*, 2020):

- Several transcription factors are known to regulate the expression of the *NFE2L2* gene that encodes Nrf2.
- Besides Keap1, several proteins are involved in Nrf2 degradation. Keap1-independent proteasomal degradation of Nrf2 was shown to involve the β-TrCP-SKP1-CUL1-RBX1, CR6-interacting factor 1 (CRIF1), WDR-23, and HRD1 ubiquitin ligase complexes (He *et al.*, 2020a).
- Translation regulation mechanisms responsible for a low Nrf2 translation efficiency under basal conditions and markedly increased under oxidative stress conditions.
- Post-transcriptional or epigenetic regulation: it seems likely that Keap1/Nrf2 signalling is regulated by epigenetic mechanisms, including DNA methylation, histone modification, chromatin remodelling and microRNAs. Nrf2 synthesis is shown to be downregulated by several miRNAs, including miR27a, miR-28, miR-34a, miR-93, miR-129-5p, miR-142-5p, miR-144, miR-153, miR-155, miR-200c, miR-340-5p, miR-350a, miR-507, and miR-634 at the posttranscriptional level (Zhang *et al.*, 2020).

It seems likely that p62, a multifunctional protein located throughout the cell and a classical receptor of autophagy, is often responsible for activation of Nrf2 in response to various cellular stresses independently of Keap1 modification/oxidation (Kasai *et al.*, 2020). The expression and activity of Nrf2 are tightly regulated at multiple levels. The transcription of Nrf2 is activated by itself and other transcription factors, including the aryl hydrocarbon receptor (AhR), peroxisome proliferator-activated receptor (PPARα or PPARγ), NF-κB, specificity protein 1, p53, myocyte-specific enhancer factor 2 D, c-Jun, c-Myc, and breast cancer 1 (Zang *et al.*, 2020). Nevertheless, it is believed that the Nrf2 protein stability and its transcriptional activity are mainly regulated by Keap1 (Zang *et al.*, 2020).

Molecular mechanisms of regulating roles of transcription factors in cellular adaptation to stress were extensively studied. In particular, it has been suggested that low intensity oxidative stress is predominantly sensed by Keap1/Nrf2 system (Lushchak, 2011) with the following downstream up-regulation of the protective AO genes. It is interesting to note that intermediate oxidative stress could also increase the activity of antioxidant enzymes, but by different mechanisms involved NF-κB and AP-1 pathways (Lushchak, 2011). Furthermore, at both, low and intermediate intensity oxidative stresses, MAP-kinases and other kinases (e.g. protein kinase C and phosphatidylinositol-3-kinase) can participate in signal sensing and cellular response, being an additional adaptive mechanism leading to enhanced antioxidant potential (Zhou *et al.*, 2014). Emerging evidence clearly indicates that Nrf2 can interact with other transcription factors, including heat shock factor (HSF1; Dayalan Naidu *et al.*, 2015) to provide additional options for AO system regulation. Furthermore, the Nrf2 stress pathway intimately communicates with mitochondria to maintain cellular homeostasis during oxidative stress (Itoh *et al.*, 2015). Nrf2 performs its regulatory functions in concert with other transcription factors to further integrate and enhance the effectiveness of adaptive response and to produce acquired resilience.

5.4 Nrf2 and inflammation

It seems likely that Nrf2 may protect against inflammation, beyond its antioxidant activity (Huang *et al.*, 2015). Nrf2 is proven to be responsible for reduction of the expression of pro-inflammatory genes, and enhancing anti-inflammatory signalling (Mohan and Gupta, 2018). For example, Nrf2 activation was shown to reduce lipopolysaccharide (LPS)-induced transcriptional upregulation of pro-inflammatory cytokines (IL-6 and IL-1β) in macrophages by blocking proinflammatory cytokine transcription (Kobayashi, *et al*, 2016). Similar effect of Nrf2 on other pro-inflammatory cytokines (TNF-α, IL-6) and chemokines (CCL2 and CXCL2) was observed in neutrophils (Huang *et al.*, 2015). Since NF-κB is considered to be the major transcription factor responsible for synthesis of pro-inflammatory cytokines (Surai *et al.*, 2021), inhibitory effects of Nrf2 on NF-κB signalling pathway (Ahmed *et al.*, 2017) deserves more attention. For example, Keap1 is reported to promote the ubiquitination and degradation of the upstream kinase IKKβ, leading to the inhibition of NF-κB activation (Lee *et al.*, 2009). Furthermore, reduced oxidative stress was found to further reduce IKKβ activation (Brigelius-Flohé and Flohé, 2011). In addition, Nrf2 is shown to compete with NF-κB for binding to the transcriptional coactivator CBP, leading to reducing the expression of NF-κB-regulated genes (Liu *et al.*, 2008). *In vivo* studies were able to confirm that Nrf2 negatively regulates NF-κB transcriptional activity (Thimmulappa *et al.*, 2006).

5.5 Nrf2 activation as a clinical strategy

Chronic oxidative stress has been associated with the development and exacerbation of various diseases including cancer, diabetes, autoimmune, cutaneous, pulmonary, cardiovascular, neurodegenerative diseases and various inflammatory condition (Dayalan Naidu and Dinkova-Kostova, 2020). Since cytoprotective proteins encoded by NRF2-target genes are essential for protection against a variety of toxic and oxidative insults, protection and treatment of many different oxidative stress-related diseases (e.g. cardiovascular disease, metabolic syndrome, neuronal degeneration, autoimmune disorders, cancer, etc.) can include Nrf2 manipulation by targeted drugs (He *et al.*, 2020b). Nrf2 is shown to be inactivated in certain pathological conditions, such as diabetes, but Keap1 down-regulation or mitochondrial ROS elimination are able to rescue Nrf2 expression and improves the pathology (Kasai *et al.*, 2020). There is a growing body of evidence demonstrating beneficial effects of Nrf2 activation in various pathologies, including renal disease (Guerrero-Hue *et al.*, 2020), fatty liver disease (Kay *et al.*, 2011; Galicia-Moreno *et al.*, 2020), cardiovascular diseases (Vashi and Patel, 2021; Wu *et al.*, 2004), diabetes (Axelsson *et al.*, 2017), neurodegenerative diseases (Kubben, *et al.*, 2016), Alzheimer and Parkinson diseases (Lu *et al.*, 2016) and relapsing multiple sclerosis (Baird and Yamamoto, M., 2020a,b). The pharmacological modulation of Nrf2 by the dimethyl ester of fumaric acid (Tecfidera) was reported to be used in the therapy of psoriasis and multiple sclerosis (Vasileva *et al.*, 2020). There are also ongoing pre-clinical and clinical investigations exploring the potential benefits of Keap1-dependent Nrf2 activation in various pathologies such as T2D, chronic obstructive pulmonary disease, certain types of cancer, kidney and eye diseases (Vasileva *et al.*, 2020). However, overactivation of the Nrf2 pathway could be associated with progressive tissue damage and cancer promotion (Ngo *et al.*, 2017) and development of resistance to multiple therapies in cancer cells (Vasileva *et al.*, 2020). Furthermore, because of complex interactions of Nrf2 with other transcription factors and various pathways, there could be side effects of Nrf2 activation. For example, the phase 3 BEACON clinical trial of the Nrf2 inducer Bardoxolone for the treatment of chronic kidney disease failed due to safety concerns related to an increase in cardiovascular events (Baird and Yamamoto, M., 2020b).

5.6 Silymarin and Nrf2 regulation

An interesting approach to explain health-promoting properties of polyphenols could be to explore the modulation of signalling pathways, e.g. the Nrf2/Keap1/ARE and NF-κB pathways, resulting in increased expression of genes encoding for cytoprotective molecules, including AO enzymes and phase II detoxification enzymes. In addition, decreased expression of NF-κB-regulated genes would reduce production of pro-inflammatory cytokines. It has been shown that some phytochemicals (sulforaphane, curcumin, EGCG, diallyl sulphide, resveratrol, etc.) at concentrations as low as 10 μM can activate Nrf2 signalling by inducing phosphorylation of Nrf2 via activation of upstream protein kinases and/or through direct interaction with Keap1 cysteine thiols (Surh *et al.*, 2008). It is interesting to note that anthocyanins activate the antioxidant transcription factor Nrf2, at a concentration as low as 1 μM (Zhang *et al.*, 2013). Silymarin's ability to upregulate the master antioxidant coordinator Nrf2 has also been investigated in various *in vitro* and *in vivo* model systems. Initially, the SM-containing supplement Protandim (ashwagandha, bacopa extract, green tea extract, SM, and curcumin) was shown to induce HO-1 in a cell culture primarily through Nrf2 activation (Velmurugan *et al.*, 2009). Protandim also induces Nrf2 nuclear localisation and antioxidant enzyme expression (Donovan *et al.*, 2012). However, it is difficult to distinguish the SM effect in the mixture. Furthermore, it was reported that SM (a water-soluble formulation Legalon-SIL containing a succinate-modified active compounds) at 50 and 100 μM significantly upregulated Nrf2 protein levels in CON1 cells after 48 h treatment (Mehrab-Mohseni *et al.*, 2015). SM (104 μM) protected human cells against the damage from the herbicide paraquat (PQ) via triggering anti-oxidant related genes, including Nrf2, NQO1 and HO-1 (Podder *et al.*, 2012). In an *in vitro* experiment with human hepatic HepG2 cells, SM (100 μM) was reported to be protective against 2,2'-Azobis(2-amidinopropane) dihydrochloride (AAPH)-induced oxidative stress and apoptosis and the antioxidant potential of SM was correlated with induction of antioxidant genes including HO-1, NQO-1, γ-GCLC and SOD via transcriptional activation of Nrf2 (Gokila Vani *et al.*, 2013).

In a dietary rat model of non-alcoholic steatohepatitis there was an increase in nuclear translocation of Nrf2 protein in SM-fed animals (Kim *et al.*, 2012) which could enhance its protective effect against oxidative stress. Numerically, there was also a trend in increasing Nrf2 endogenous expression protein in rat liver tissue damaged by CCl_4 by pre-treatment with SM (100 mg/kg/BW; Wu *et al.*, 2013) as well as in an alcohol-pyrazole-fed rat model (50 mg/kg/BW; Choi *et al.*, 2013). It seems likely that the effect of SM on the Nrf2 activation in various oxidative-stress related animal models depends on the dose of SM used. For example, at 10 mg/kg/BW SM showed protective effects against dimerumic acid-induced changes in GSH and HO-1 levels, but did not change Nrf2 levels (Lee *et al.*, 2013). SB-treatment (75 mg/kg/BW) ameliorated arsenic-induced nephrotoxicity by abrogation of oxidative stress, inflammation and apoptosis in rats (Prabu and Muthumani, 2012). It is interesting to note that beyond the preventive action of SB, in rats fed SB alone there was a significant increase in Nrf2 mRNA levels in the kidney. The same SB-treated rats were characterised by increased antioxidant defences as indicated by increased renal SOD and GPx activities, as well as enhanced levels of GSH, vitamins E and C. SM was reported to protect the rats against PQ-induced acute kidney injury including improved renal function, decreased injury score and inhibited apoptosis and oxidative stress through the activating the signalling pathway of Nrf2 (Jia *et al.*, 2022).

SB-induced activation of Nrf2 and HO-1 played a significant role in cellular defence against As-induced oxidative cardiac damage. In a recent study, co-treatment with SM (86 mg/kg/BW) significantly enhanced the antioxidant defence systems of the ethanol-consuming mice via the activation of Nrf2 and HO-1 expression in damaged livers (Cao *et al.*, 2015). Furthermore, SM (200 mg/kg/BW) significantly up-regulated HO-1 and Nrf-2 in the liver of AAPH-treated mice (Gokila Vani *et al.*, 2013). Recently Nrf2-activating effects of SM and its components have been reviewed (Vargas-Mendoza *et al.*, 2020) with a conclusion that further research with in silico, *in vitro*, and *in vivo* models are necessary to elucidate molecular mechanisms of modulating effects of SM and/or its flavolignans on Nrf2.

Therefore, it is clear from the aforementioned data that SM/SB, similar to other polyphenols, acts as an indirect antioxidant through its ability to induce Nrf2 transactivation, which is responsible for the synthesis of an array of antioxidant molecules decreasing oxidative stress and providing effective protection in various stress conditions. Recently the binding properties of SM compounds (silybin A, silybin B, isosilybin A, isosilybin B, silychristin A, silychristin B, silydianin, 2,3-dehydrosilybin, 2,3-dehydrosilychristin, and 2,3-dehydrosilydianin) with Keap1 have been investigated. The study used docking and molecular dynamics simulations combined with the Poisson-Boltzmann and generalised Born and surface area methods and quantum mechanics-molecular mechanics calculations (Bello, 2023). Indeed, in the study silybin A and 2,3-dehydrosilybin demonstrated the ability to bind to the Kelch domain. These SM constituents were found to interact with the same pockets as those observed for the Cpd16 (a novel small molecule Nrf2 activator)-Keap1 complex but with more favourable binding free energies (Bello, 2023). The authors also demonstrated that the Keap1-silybin A and Keap1-2,3-dehydrosilybin complexes are characterised by interactions with Arg415, known to be the critical residue of Keap1-Nrf2 stabilization in humans.

This changes an attitude to SM, a compound that has been assumed to act typically as a free radical scavenger and traditional antioxidant. It is still not clear if physiologically relevant (up to 2 μM) SB concentrations would upregulate Nrf2, but *in vivo* results obtained with various model systems clearly indicated an activation of Nrf2 by SB. In general, most of the experimental studies suggest that dietary SM/SB activates antioxidant pathways such as Nrf2/HO1 and downregulates NF-κB and effect PPAR (Pferschy-Wenzig *et al.*, 2014; Prakash *et al.*, 2014), HIF-1 (Jung *et al.*, 2009; Lin *et al.*, 2013; Wang *et al.*, 2012) and STAT (Agarwal *et al.*, 2007; Hou *et al.*, 2010; Tyagi *et al.*, 2012) pathways.

5.7 Conclusions

The aforementioned data clearly showed that Nrf2 activation is an adaptive mechanism to deal with various stresses in human and animals. The available evidence indicates that Nrf2 is responsible for metabolic control of the cellular redox homeostasis as a result of regulation of the key antioxidants (SOD, GPx, GSH, Trx, peroxiredoxin), detoxification enzymes catalysing phase I, II and III cytoprotective detoxification reactions and proteins possessing anti-inflammatory properties (Dayalan Naidu1 and Dinkova-Kostova, 2020). Indeed, by improving ROS scavenging and restoring redox homeostasis in stress condition, Nrf2 can prevent/decrease stress-related detrimental changes in human and farm animals/poultry and plays a crucial role in antistress strategy development. However, when stress is too high to deal with decreased Nrf2 expression and oxidative stress occur leading to detrimental consequences in terms of human health and productive and reproductive performance of farm animals/poultry. There is a range of nutrients, including various phytochemicals, including SM/SB, as well as carnitine and TAU, able to prevent detrimental effects of stressors on Nrf2 expression (Surai *et al.*, 2019). Furthermore, interest in this transcription factor is beyond stresses. For example, when a comparison between a single male modern broiler line compared to a foundational Barred Plymouth Rock chicken line was conducted, it was shown that Nrf2 expression in breast muscle was much higher in modern broiler compared to the foundational BPR line (Kong *et al.*, 2017) and it was suggested Nrf2-mediated oxidative stress response pathways are involved in breast muscle growth in chickens (Khatri *et al.*, 2018). Transcription factors Nrf2, NF-κB and HSF1 enable the eukaryotic cell to adapt to various forms of oxidative, electrophilic, thermal, inflammatory and other stresses by orchestrating elaborate transcriptional programs termed the Keap1/Nrf2 pathway, NF-κB/IκB pathway and the heat shock response (Dayalan Naidu *et al.*, 2015). In general, induction of these programs is associated with upregulation of various protective mechanisms including molecular chaperones, antioxidant and drug-metabolising enzymes, proteins responsible for the repair and clearance of damaged macromolecules as well as for the maintenance of cell structure, redox, and intermediary metabolism (Dayalan Naidu *et al.*, 2015).

References

Agarwal, C., Tyagi, A., Kaur, M. and Agarwal, R., 2007. Silibinin inhibits constitutive activation of Stat3 and causes caspase activation and apoptotic death of human prostate carcinoma DU145 cells. Carcinogenesis 28: 1463-1470.

Ahmed, S.M., Luo, L., Namani, A., Wang, X.J. and Tang, X., 2017. Nrf2 signaling pathway: Pivotal roles in inflammation. Biochimica et Biophysica Acta. Molecular Basis of Disease 1863: 585-597.

Axelsson, A.S., Tubbs, E., Mecham, B., Chacko, S., Nenonen, H.A., Tang, Y., Fahey, J.W., Derry, J., Wollheim, C.B., Wierup, N., Haymond, M.W., Friend, S.H., Mulder, H. and Rosengren, A.H., 2017. Sulforaphane reduces hepatic glucose production and improves glucose control in patients with type 2 diabetes. Science Translational Medicine 9: eaah4477.

Baird, L. and Yamamoto, M., 2020a. The molecular mechanisms regulating the KEAP1-NRF2 pathway. Molecular and Cellular Biology 40: e00099-20.

Baird, L. and Yamamoto, M., 2020b. The Keap1-Nrf2 pathway: From mechanism to medical applications. In: Sies, H. (ed) Oxidative stress eustress and distress. Academic Press, London, UK, pp. 125-147.

Bellezza, I., Giambanco, I., Minelli, A. and Donato, R., 2018. Nrf2-Keap1 signaling in oxidative and reductive stress. Biochimica et Biophysica Acta. Molecular Cell Research 1865: 721-733.

Bello, M., 2023. Structural basis of Nrf2 activation by flavonolignans from silymarin. Research Square 119: 108393. https://doi.org/10.21203/rs.3.rs-1761632/v1.

Bhakkiyalakshmi, E., Sireesh, D., Rajaguru, P., Paulmurugan, R. and Ramkumar, K.M., 2015. The emerging role of redox-sensitive Nrf2-Keap1 pathway in diabetes. Pharmacological Research 91: 104-114.

Brigelius-Flohé, R. and Flohé, L., 2011. Basic principles and emerging concepts in the redox control of transcription factors. Antioxidants & Redox Signaling 15: 2335-2381.

Cao, Y.W., Jiang, Y., Zhang, D.Y., Wang, M., Chen, W.S., Su, H., Wang, Y.T. and Wan, J.B., 2015. Protective effects of Penthorum chinense Pursh against chronic ethanol-induced liver injury in mice. Journal of Ethnopharmacology 161: 92-98.

Chen, Q.M., 2021. Nrf2 for cardiac protection: pharmacological options against oxidative stress. Trends in Pharmacological Sciences 42: 729-744.

Choi, B.H., Kang, K.S. and Kwak, M.K., 2014. Effect of redox modulating NRF2 activators on chronic kidney disease. Molecules 19: 12727-12759.

Choi, M.K., Han, J.M., Kim, H.G., Lee, J.S., Lee, J.S., Wang, J.H., Son, S.W., Park, H.J. and Son, C.G., 2013. Aqueous extract of Artemisia capillaris exerts hepatoprotective action in alcohol-pyrazole-fed rat model. Journal of Ethnopharmacology 147: 662-670.

Cuadrado, A., Rojo, A.I., Wells, G., Hayes, J.D., Cousin, S.P., Rumsey, W.L., Attucks, O.C., Franklin, S., Levonen, A.L., Kensler, T.W. and Dinkova-Kostova, A.T., 2019. Therapeutic targeting of the NRF2 and KEAP1 partnership in chronic diseases. Nature Reviews. Drug discovery 18: 295-317.

Dayalan Naidu, S. and Dinkova-Kostova, A.T., 2020. KEAP1, a cysteine-based sensor and a drug target for the prevention and treatment of chronic disease. Open Biology 10: 200105.

Dayalan Naidu, S., Kostov, R.V. and Dinkova-Kostova, A.T., 2015. Transcription factors Hsf1 and Nrf2 engage in crosstalk for cytoprotection. Trends in Pharmacological Sciences 36: 6-14.

Donovan, E.L., McCord, J.M., Reuland, D.J., Miller, B.F. and Hamilton, K.L., 2012. Phytochemical activation of Nrf2 protects human coronary artery endothelial cells against an oxidative challenge. Oxidative Medicine and Cellular Longevity 2012: 132931.

Forman, H.J., 2016. Redox signaling: an evolution from free radicals to aging. Free Radical Biology and Medicine 97: 398-407.

Galicia-Moreno, M., Lucano-Landeros, S., Monroy-Ramirez, H.C., Silva-Gomez, J., Gutierrez-Cuevas, J., Santos, A. and Armendariz-Borunda, J., 2020. Roles of Nrf2 in liver diseases: Molecular, pharmacological, and epigenetic aspects. Antioxidants 9: 980.

Gokila Vani, M., Kumar, K.J., Liao, J.W., Chien, S.C., Mau, J.L., Chiang, S.S., Lin, C.C., Kuo, Y.H. and Wang, S.Y., 2013. Antcin C from Antrodia cinnamomea protects liver cells against free radical-induced oxidative stress and apoptosis *in vitro* and *in vivo* through Nrf2-dependent mechanism. Evidence-Based Complementary and Alternative Medicine 2013: 296082.

Guerrero-Hue, M., Rayego-Mateos, S., Vázquez-Carballo, C., Palomino-Antolín, A., García-Caballero, C., Opazo-Rios, L., Morgado-Pascual, J.L., Herencia, C., Mas, S., Ortiz, A., Rubio-Navarro, A., Egea, J., Villalba, J.M., Egido, J. and Moreno, J.A., 2020. Protective role of Nrf2 in renal disease. Antioxidants 10: 39.

Gureev, A.P., Shaforostova, E.A. and Popov, V.N., 2019. Regulation of mitochondrial biogenesis as a way for active longevity: Interaction between the Nrf2 and PGC-1α signaling pathways. Frontiers in Genetics 10: 435.

Hayes, J.D. and Dinkova-Kostova, A.T., 2014. The Nrf2 regulatory network provides an interface between redox and intermediary metabolism. Trends in Biochemical Sciences 39: 199-218.

He, F., Antonucci, L. and Karin, M., 2020a. NRF2 as a regulator of cell metabolism and inflammation in cancer. Carcinogenesis 41: 405-416.

He, F., Ru, X. and Wen, T., 2020b. NRF2, a transcription factor for stress response and beyond. International Journal of Molecular Sciences 21: 4777.

Helou, D.G., Martin, S.F., Pallardy, M., Chollet-Martin, S. and Kerdine-Römer, S., 2019. Nrf2 involvement in chemical-induced skin innate immunity. Frontiers in Immunology 10: 1004.

Hou, Y.C., Liou, K.T., Chern, C.M., Wang, Y.H., Liao, J.F., Chang, S., Chou, Y.H. and Shen, Y.C., 2010. Preventive effect of silymarin in cerebral ischemia-reperfusion-induced brain injury in rats possibly through impairing NF-κB and STAT-1 activation. Phytomedicine 17: 963-973.

Howden, R., 2013. Nrf2 and cardiovascular defense. Oxidative Medicine and Cellular Longevity 2013: 105308.

Huang, H.C., Nguyen, T. and Pickett, C.B., 2000. Regulation of the antioxidant response element by protein kinase C-mediated phosphorylation of NF-E2-related factor 2. Proceedings of the National Academy of Sciences of the United States of America 97: 12475-12480.

Huang, Y., Li, W., Su, Z.Y. and Kong, A.N., 2015. The complexity of the Nrf2 pathway: beyond the antioxidant response. The Journal of Nutritional Biochemistry 26: 1401-1413.

Imai, T., Matsubara, H., & Hara, H., 2021. Potential therapeutic effects of Nrf2 activators on intracranial hemorrhage. Journal of Cerebral Blood Flow and Metabolism 41: 1483-1500.

Iso, T., Suzuki, T., Baird, L. and Yamamoto, M., 2016. Absolute amounts and status of the Nrf2-Keap1-Cul3 complex within cells. Molecular and Cellular Biology 36: 31003112.

Itoh, K., Wakabayashi, N., Katoh, Y., Ishii, T., Igarashi, K., Engel, J.D. and Yamamoto, M., 1999. Keap1 represses nuclear activation of antioxidant responsive elements by Nrf2 through binding to the amino-terminal Neh2 domain. Genes & Development 13: 76-86.

Itoh, K., Ye, P., Matsumiya, T., Tanji, K. and Ozaki, T., 2015. Emerging functional cross-talk between the Keap1-Nrf2 system and mitochondria. Journal of Clinical Biochemistry and Nutrition 56: 91-97.

Itoh, K., Mimura, J. and Yamamoto, M., 2010. Discovery of the negative regulator of Nrf2, Keap1: a historical overview. Antioxidants & Redox Signaling 13: 1665-1678.

Jia, C., Zhang, Z., Wang, J. and Nie, Z., 2022. Silymarin protects the rats against paraquat-induced acute kidney injury via Nrf2. Human & Experimental Toxicology 41: 9603271221074334.

Jung, H.J., Park, J.W., Lee, J.S., Lee, S.R., Jang, B.C., Suh, S.I., Suh, M.H. and Baek, W.K., 2009. Silibinin inhibits expression of HIF-1α through suppression of protein translation in prostate cancer cells. Biochemical and Biophysical Research Communications 390: 71-76.

Kasai, S., Shimizu, S., Tatara, Y., Mimura, J. and Itoh, K., 2020. Regulation of Nrf2 by mitochondrial reactive oxygen species in physiology and pathology. Biomolecules 10: 320.

Kay, H.Y., Kim, W.D., Hwang, S.J., Choi, H.S., Gilroy, R.K., Wan, Y.J. and Kim, S.G., 2011. Nrf2 inhibits LXRα-dependent hepatic lipogenesis by competing with FXR for acetylase binding. Antioxidants & Redox Signaling 15: 2135-2146.

Keum, Y.S. and Choi, B.Y., 2014. Molecular and chemical regulation of the Keap1-Nrf2 signaling pathway. Molecules 19: 10074-10089.

Khatri, B., Seo, D., Shouse, S., Pan, J.H., Hudson, N.J., Kim, J.K., Bottje, W. and Kong, B.C., 2018. MicroRNA profiling associated with muscle growth in modern broilers compared to an unselected chicken breed. BMC Genomics 19: 1-10.

Kim, M., Yang, S.G., Kim, J.M., Lee, J.W., Kim, Y.S. and Lee, J.I., 2012. Silymarin suppresses hepatic stellate cell activation in a dietary rat model of non-alcoholic steatohepatitis: Analysis of isolated hepatic stellate cells. International Journal of Molecular Medicine 30: 473-479.

Kobayashi, E.H., Suzuki, T., Funayama, R., Nagashima, T., Hayashi, M., Sekine, H., Tanaka, N., Moriguchi, T., Motohashi, H., Nakayama, K. and Yamamoto, M., 2016. Nrf2 suppresses macrophage inflammatory response by blocking proinflammatory cytokine transcription. Nature Communications 7: 11624.

Kong, B.W., Hudson, N., Seo, D., Lee, S., Khatri, B., Lassiter, K., Cook, D., Piekarski, A., Dridi, S., Anthony, N. and Bottje, W., 2017. RNA sequencing for global gene expression associated with muscle growth in a single male modern broiler line compared to a foundational Barred Plymouth Rock chicken line. BMC Genomics 18: 82.

Kopacz, A., Kloska, D., Forman, H.J., Jozkowicz, A. and Grochot-Przeczek, A., 2020. Beyond repression of Nrf2: An update on Keap1. Free Radical Biology & Medicine 157: 63-74.

Kubben, N., Zhang, W., Wang, L., Voss, T.C., Yang, J., Qu, J., Liu, G.H. and Misteli, T., 2016. Repression of the antioxidant NRF2 pathway in premature aging. Cell 165: 1361-1374.

Kweider, N., Huppertz, B., Kadyrov, M., Rath, W., Pufe, T. and Wruck, C.J., 2014. A possible protective role of Nrf2 in preeclampsia. Annals of Anatomy 196: 268-277.

Lee, D.F., Kuo, H.P., Liu, M., Chou, C.K., Xia, W., Du, Y., Shen, J., Chen, C.T., Huo, L., Hsu, M.C., Li, C.W., Ding, Q., Liao, T.L., Lai, C.C., Lin, A.C., Chang, Y.H., Tsai, S.F., Li, L.Y. and Hung, M.C., 2009. KEAP1 E3 ligase-mediated downregulation of NF-kappaB signaling by targeting IKKbeta. Molecular Cell 36: 131-140.

Lee, B.H., Hsu, W.H., Hsu, Y.W. and Pan, T.M., 2013. Dimerumic acid attenuates receptor for advanced glycation end products signal to inhibit inflammation and diabetes mediated by Nrf2 activation and promotes methylglyoxal metabolism into d-lactic acid. Free Radical Biology and Medicine 60: 7-16.

Lin, C.H., Li, C.H., Liao, P.L., Tse, L.S., Huang, W.K., Cheng, H.W. and Cheng, Y.W., 2013. Silibinin inhibits VEGF secretion and age-related macular degeneration in a hypoxia-dependent manner through the PI-3 kinase/Akt/mTOR pathway. British Journal of Pharmacology 168: 920-931.

Liu, G.H., Qu, J. and Shen, X., 2008. NF-kappaB/p65 antagonizes Nrf2-ARE pathway by depriving CBP from Nrf2 and facilitating recruitment of HDAC3 to MafK. Biochimica et Biophysica Acta 1783: 713-727.

Loboda, A., Damulewicz, M., Pyza, E., Jozkowicz, A. and Dulak, J., 2016. Role of Nrf2/HO-1 system in development, oxidative stress response and diseases: an evolutionarily conserved mechanism. Cellular and Molecular Life Sciences 73: 3221-3247.

Lu, M.C., Ji, J.A., Jiang, Z.Y. and You, Q.D., 2016. The Keap1-Nrf2-ARE pathway as a potential preventive and therapeutic target: An update. Medicinal Research Reviews 36: 924-963.

Lushchak, V.I., 2011. Adaptive response to oxidative stress: Bacteria, fungi, plants and animals. Comparative Biochemistry and Physiology. Toxicology & Pharmacology 153: 175-190.

Ma, Q. and He, X., 2012. Molecular basis of electrophilic and oxidative defense: promises and perils of Nrf2. Pharmacological Reviews 64: 1055-1081.

Madden, S.K. and Itzhaki, L.S., 2020. Structural and mechanistic insights into the Keap1-Nrf2 system as a route to drug discovery. Biochimica et Biophysica Acta. Proteins and Proteomics 1868: 140405.

Marinho, H.S., Real, C., Cyrne, L., Soares, H. and Antunes, F., 2014. Hydrogen peroxide sensing, signaling and regulation of transcription factors. Redox Biology 2: 535-562.

Majzunova, M., Dovinova, I., Barancik, M. and Chan, J.Y., 2013. Redox signaling in pathophysiology of hypertension. Journal of Biomedical Science 20: 69.

Mehrab-Mohseni, M., Sendi, H., Steuerwald, N., Ghosh, S., Schrum, L.W. and Bonkovsky, H.L., 2011. Legalon-SIL downregulates HCV core and NS5A in human hepatocytes expressing full-length HCV. World Journal of Gastroenterology 17: 1694-1700.

Mohan, S. and Gupta, D., 2018. Crosstalk of toll-like receptors signaling and Nrf2 pathway for regulation of inflammation. Biomedicine & Pharmacotherapy 108: 1866-1878.

Moi, P., Chan, K., Asunis, I., Cao, A. and Kan, Y.W., 1994. Isolation of NF-E2-related factor 2 (Nrf2), a NF-E2-like basic leucine zipper transcriptional activator that binds to the tandem NF-E2/AP1 repeat of the beta-globin locus control region. Proceedings of the National Academy of Sciences of the United States of America 91: 9926-9930.

Ngo, H., Kim, D.H., Cha, Y.N., Na, H.K. and Surh, Y.J., 2017. Nrf2 Mutagenic activation drives hepatocarcinogenesis. Cancer Research 77: 4797-4808.

Niki, E., 2012. Do antioxidants impair signaling by reactive oxygen species and lipid oxidation products? FEBS Letters 586: 3767-3770.

Niki, E., 2014. Antioxidants: basic principles, emerging concepts, and problems. Biomedical Journal 37: 106-111.

Niki, E., 2016. Oxidative stress and antioxidants: distress or eustress? Archives of Biochemistry and Biophysics 595: 19-24.

Panieri, E. and Saso, L., 2019. Potential applications of NRF2 inhibitors in cancer therapy. Oxidative Medicine and Cellular Longevity 2019: 8592348.

Pferschy-Wenzig, E.M., Atanasov, A.G., Malainer, C., Noha, S.M., Kunert, O., Schuster, D., Heiss, E.H., Oberlies, N.H., Wagner, H., Bauer, R. and Dirsch, V.M., 2014. Identification of isosilybin a from milk thistle seeds as an agonist of peroxisome proliferator-activated receptor gamma. Journal of Natural Products 77: 842-847.

Podder, B., Kim, Y.S., Zerin, T. and Song, H.Y., 2012. Antioxidant effect of silymarin on paraquat-induced human lung adenocarcinoma A549 cell line. Food and Chemical Toxicology 50: 3206-3214.

Prabu, S.M. and Muthumani, M., 2012. Silibinin ameliorates arsenic induced nephrotoxicity by abrogation of oxidative stress, inflammation and apoptosis in rats. Molecular Biology Reports 39: 11201-11216.

Prakash, P., Singh, V., Jain, M., Rana, M., Khanna, V., Barthwal, M.K. and Dikshit, M., 2014. Silymarin ameliorates fructose induced insulin resistance syndrome by reducing de novo hepatic lipogenesis in the rat. European Journal of Pharmacology 727: 15-28.

Reczek, C.R. and Chandel, N.S., 2015. ROS-dependent signal transduction. Current Opinion in Cell Biology 33: 8-13.

Rushworth, S.A., Zaitseva, L., Murray, M.Y., Shah, N.M., Bowles, K.M. and MacEwan, D.J., 2012. The high Nrf2 expression in human acute myeloid leukemia is driven by NF-kappaB and underlies its chemo-resistance. Blood 120: 5188-5198.

Saito, R., Suzuki, T., Hiramoto, K., Asami, S., Naganuma, E., Suda, H., Iso, T., Yamamoto, H., Morita, M., Baird, L., Furusawa, Y., Negishi, T., Ichinose, M. and Yamamoto, M., 2015. Characterizations of three major cysteine sensors of Keap1 in stress response. Molecular and Cellular Biology 36: 271-284.

Sihvola, V. and Levonen, A.L., 2017. Keap1 as the redox sensor of the antioxidant response. Archives of Biochemistry and Biophysics 617: 94-100.

Sivandzade, F., Prasad, S., Bhalerao, A. and Cucullo, L., 2019. NRF2 and NF-κB interplay in cerebrovascular and neurodegenerative disorders: Molecular mechanisms and possible therapeutic approaches. Redox Biology 21: 101059.

Song, P. and Zou, M.H., 2014. Redox regulation of endothelial cell fate. Cellular and Molecular Life Sciences 71: 3219-3239.

Surai, P.F., 2020. Vitagene in avian biology and poultry health. Wageningen Academic Publishers, Wageningen, The Netherlands.

Surai, P.F., Kochish, I.I., Fisinin, V.I. and Kidd, M.T., 2019. Antioxidant defence systems and oxidative stress in poultry biology: An update. Antioxidants 8; 235.

Surai, P.F., Kochish, I.I. and Kidd, M.T., 2021. Redox homeostasis in poultry: Regulatory roles of NF-κB. Antioxidants 10, 186.

Surh, Y.J., 2008. NF-kappa B and Nrf2 as potential chemopreventive targets of some anti-inflammatory and antioxidative phytonutrients with anti-inflammatory and antioxidative activities. Asia Pacific Journal of Clinical Nutrition, 17: 269-272.

Sussan, T.E. and Biswal, S. (2014). Oxidative stress and respiratory diseases: the critical role of Nrf2. In: Ganguly, N.K., Jindal, S.K., Biswal, S., Barnes, P.J. and Pawankar, R. (eds) Studies on respiratory disorders. Humana Press, New York, USA, pp. 335-348.

Suzuki, T., Muramatsu, A., Saito, R., Iso, T., Shibata, T., Kuwata, K., Kawaguchi, S.I., Iwawaki, T., Adachi, S., Suda, H., Morita, M., Uchida, K., Baird, L. and Yamamoto, M., 2019. Molecular mechanism of cellular oxidative stress sensing by Keap1. Cell Reports 28: 746-758.

Suzuki, T. and Yamamoto, M., 2017. Stress-sensing mechanisms and the physiological roles of the Keap1-Nrf2 system during cellular stress. The Journal of Biological Chemistry 292: 16817-16824.

Tang, W., Jiang, Y.F., Ponnusamy, M. and Diallo, M., 2014. Role of Nrf2 in chronic liver disease. World Journal of Gastroenterology 20: 13079-13087.

Thimmulappa, R.K., Lee, H., Rangasamy, T., Reddy, S.P., Yamamoto, M., Kensler, T.W. and Biswal, S., 2006. Nrf2 is a critical regulator of the innate immune response and survival during experimental sepsis. The Journal of Clinical Investigation 116: 984-995.

Tyagi, A., Agarwal, C., Dwyer-Nield, L.D., Singh, R.P., Malkinson, A.M. and Agarwal, R., 2012. Silibinin modulates TNF-α and IFN-γ mediated signaling to regulate COX2 and iNOS expression in tumorigenic mouse lung epithelial LM2 cells. Molecular Carcinogenesis 51: 832-842.

Tu, W., Wang, H., Li, S., Liu, Q. and Sha, H., 2019. The anti-inflammatory and anti-oxidant mechanisms of the Keap1/Nrf2/ARE signaling pathway in chronic diseases. Aging and Disease 10: 637-651.

Vargas-Mendoza, N., Morales-González, Á., Morales-Martínez, M., Soriano-Ursúa, M.A., Delgado-Olivares, L., Sandoval-Gallegos, E.M., Madrigal-Bujaidar, E., Álvarez-González, I., Madrigal-Santillán, E. and Morales-Gonzalez, J.A., 2020. Flavolignans from silymarin as Nrf2 bioactivators and their therapeutic applications. Biomedicines 8: E122.

Vashi, R. and Patel, B.M., 2021. NRF2 in cardiovascular diseases: a ray of hope! Journal of Cardiovascular Translational Research 14: 573-586.

Vasileva, L.V., Savova, M.S., Amirova, K.M., Dinkova-Kostova, A.T. and Georgiev, M.I., 2020. Obesity and NRF2-mediated cytoprotection: Where is the missing link?. Pharmacological Research 156: 104760.

Velmurugan, K., Alam, J., McCord, J.M. and Pugazhenthi, S., 2009. Synergistic induction of heme oxygenase-1 by the components of the antioxidant supplement Protandim. Free Radical Biology and Medicine 46: 430-440.

Vriend, J. and Reiter, R.J., 2015. The Keap1-Nrf2-antioxidant response element pathway: a review of its regulation by melatonin and the proteasome. Molecular and Cellular Endocrinology 401: 213-220.

Wang, X., Tomso, D.J., Chorley, B.N., Cho, H.Y., Cheung, V.G., Kleeberger, S.R. and Bell, D.A., 2007. Identification of polymorphic antioxidant response elements in the human genome. Human Molecular Genetics 16: 1188-1200.

Wang, C., Wang, Z., Zhang, X., Zhang, X., Dong, L., Xing, Y., Li, Y., Liu, Z., Chen, L., Qiao, H. and Wang, L., 2012. Protection by silibinin against experimental ischemic stroke: up-regulated pAkt, pmTOR, HIF-1α and Bcl-2, down-regulated Bax, NF-κB expression. Neuroscience Letters 529: 45-50.

Wang, X. and Hai, C., 2016. Novel insights into redox system and the mechanism of redox regulation. Molecular Biology Reports 43: 607-628.

Wu, L., Noyan Ashraf, M.H., Facci, M., Wang, R., Paterson, P.G., Ferrie, A. and Juurlink, B.H., 2004. Dietary approach to attenuate oxidative stress, hypertension, and inflammation in the cardiovascular system. Proceedings of the National Academy of Sciences of the United States of America 101: 7094-7099.

Wu, S., Yue, Y., Tian, H., Li, Z., Li, X., He, W. and Ding, H., 2013. Carthamus red from Carthamus tinctorius L. exerts antioxidant and hepatoprotective effect against CCl4-induced liver damage in rats via the Nrf2 pathway. Journal of Ethnopharmacology 148: 570-578.

Yan, L.J., 2014. Positive oxidative stress in aging and aging-related disease tolerance. Redox Biology 2C: 165-169.

Zang, H., Mathew, R.O. and Cui, T., 2020. The dark side of Nrf2 in the heart. Frontiers in Physiology 11: 722.

Zhang, S., Yang, Y., Liang, Z., Duan, W., Yang, J., Yan, J., Wang, N., Feng, W., Ding, M., Nie, Y. and Jin, Z., 2013. Silybin-mediated inhibition of Notch signaling exerts antitumor activity in human hepatocellular carcinoma cells. PloS One 8: e83699.

Zhou, Y., Jiang, Z., Lu, H., Xu, Z., Tong, R., Shi, J. and Jia, G., 2019. Recent advances of natural polyphenols activators for Keap1-Nrf2 signaling pathway. Chemistry & Biodiversity 16: e1900400.

Zhou, S., Sun, W., Zhang, Z. and Zheng, Y., 2014. The role of Nrf2-mediated pathway in cardiac remodeling and heart failure. Oxidative Medicine and Cellular Longevity 2014: 260429.

Zolnourian, A., Galea, I. and Bulters, D., 2019. Neuroprotective role of the Nrf2 pathway in subarachnoid haemorrhage and its therapeutic potential. Oxidative Medicine and Cellular Longevity 2019: 6218239.

Chapter 6
Silymarin and NF-κB

Do not boast until you see the enemy dead

Peter F. Surai[1-6] and Anton Surai[7]*
[1]Vitagene and Health Research Centre, Bristol, UK; [2]Department of Microbiology and Biochemistry, Faculty of Veterinary Medicine, Trakia University, Stara Zagora, Bulgaria; [3]Department of Animal Nutrition, Faculty of Agricultural and Environmental Sciences, Szent Istvan University, Hungary; [4]Saint-Petersburg State Academy of Veterinary Medicine, St. Petersburg, Russia; [5]Sumy National Agrarian University, Sumy, Ukraine; [6]Odessa National Academy of Food Technologies, Odessa, Ukraine; [7]Healthy Food Services, Bristol, UK
psurai@feedfood.co.uk

Abstract

This chapter is devoted to NF-κB with a special emphasis to the regulatory roles of silymarin (SM). NF-κB is known as a redox-sensitive, inducible nuclear transcription factor that regulates the expression of a number of genes associated with important biological processes, including innate and adaptive immune responses, cell growth, maturation, survival, and adaptive homeostasis establishment via interactions with other transcription factors and vitagenes. NF-κB signalling is an important element in cell adaptation to a diverse array of environmental stimuli, including oxidative stress. These stimuli can be recognised by various receptors, and the subsequent response involves specific adapter proteins. Under normal physiological conditions, the antioxidant defence network and the optimised redox balance in the cell/tissue are responsible for orchestrating important biological processes associated with cell protection, repair, and growth. This includes T-cell maturation, fighting against infections, DNA damage repair, and tissue healing and integrity restoration after injury. However, under various stress conditions, associated with redox disbalance, aberrant NF-κB activation can lead to detrimental changes, including the development of many age-related diseases. A variety of endogenous and exogenous stimuli have been characterised, including danger signals, damage, and survival signals from viral and bacterial components, proinflammatory cytokines, DNA damage, growth factors, and other stressors. Nutritional modulation of NF-κB expression and activity was shown to be achieved by using various antioxidants, including selenium, various polyphenols, taurine, carnitine, retinoic acid, vitamin E, etc. Under various stress conditions, these nutrients can ameliorate (partly or completely) the increased NF-κB expression and activity imposed by stressors. The same nutrients can upregulate Nrf2 and vitagenes. An opportunity to use nutritional/pharmacological means to modulate NF-κB expression and activity should be exploited further and SM is proven to possess NF-κB-modulating properties. In fact, downregulation of NF-κB by silymarin is considered as the main mechanism of anti-inflammatory and other health-related properties of this phytochemical mixture.

DOI:10.3920/978-90-8686-944-2_006,

Keywords: NF-κB, oxidative stress, inflammation, adaptation, redox homeostasis, silymarin

6.1 Introduction

Among various transcription factors NF-κB has a special place being a master regulator of pro-inflammatory cytokines expression and synthesis leading to inflammation progression. Furthermore, NF-κB is also involved in redox balance maintenance and stress adaptation. On the one hand, inflammation is involved in the development of various human diseases. On the other hand, animal and poultry industries suffer from over-inflammation leading to problems with gut integrity and decreased productive and reproductive performance of poultry and pigs. Since SM/SB possesses anti-inflammatory activities it is important to characterise NF-κB and show effects of SM/SB on its expression and activity under various stress conditions. Therefore, this chapter is devoted to NF-κB with a special emphasis to the regulatory roles of SM/SB.

6.2 Transcription factor NF-κB

Nuclear factor kappa B (NF-κB) was discovered in the lab of the Nobel Prize winner, David Baltimore, as an inducible transcription factor in lymphocytes (Sen and Baltimore, 1986). In general, NF-κB structure, functions, and regulation have been extensively characterised in recent comprehensive reviews (Chawla *et al.*, 2020; Lambrou *et al.*, 2020; Yu *et al.*, 2020); however, in this review, the major emphasis is given to oxidative stress and the roles of NF-κB in the regulation of adaptive homeostasis.

The NF-κB family consists of several transcription factors characterised by Rel-homology domains (RHDs) that are able to bind to specific DNA sequences known as κB sites located in the promoter and enhancer regions of various genes (Kopitar-Jerala, 2015). It has been found that NF-κB is conserved across different phyla, and, in mammalian and avian species, it consists of a group of five related proteins (subunits) that are capable of binding to DNA: p50 (a 50 kDa protein also known as NF-κB1), p52 (known as NF-κB2), p65 (also known as RelA), c-Rel, and RelB. In fact, p65, RelB, and c-Rel are characterised by a C-terminal transcription activation domain (TAD) that participates in the positive regulation of gene expression (Sehnert *et al.*, 2020). Interestingly, the other NF-κB family members, NF-κB1 and NF-κB2, were shown to be synthetised as larger precursor proteins (p105 and p100) with subsequent proteolytic processing to p50 and p52 (Lambrou *et al.*, 2020). Transcription factor subunits of NF-κB, for example, p65, can combine to form hetero- and homodimers of different composition, defined as the NF-κB complex. As a result of binding to a variety of DNA sequences called κB sites, NF-κB can effectively regulate different gene targets (Grilli and Memo, 1997).

By using two independent LC-MS/MS experiments, 365 NF-κB/RelA-associated proteins were identified (Li *et al.*, 2014). The functional categories enriched in the newly identified NF-κB/RelA-associated proteins identified by the authors include DNA-binding factors and enzymes, RNA-binding factors and enzymes, nuclear matrix and cytoskeleton components, ribosome biogenesis, protein degradation, and mitochondrial proteins. For the maintenance of redox balance and development of adaptive homeostasis, the last category related to mitochondrial proteins, including antioxidant proteins, namely, peroxiredoxins 3 and 1 (Prx3, and Prx1), is of great importance. Functional analysis of the newly identified RelA-binding proteins conducted by the authors confirmed the complexity of the NF-κB actions and its involvement in the regulation of important biological functions including regulation of protein ubiquitination, chromatin organisation, response to DNA damage stimulus, post-transcriptional regulation of gene expression, cell-cycle progress, and microtubule cytoskeleton translation (Li *et al.*, 2014). Interestingly, an update on NF-κB and proteomics published earlier (Niederberger and Geisslinger, 2013) indicated that stimulation of specific receptors by RNA, DNA, or LPS is associated with the interactions of a number of unique proteins regulating NF-κB expression and activity, which activate a range of genes creating an adaptive response. In this context, it is noteworthy that molecular mechanisms of the maintenance of redox balance and the creation of adaptive homeostasis via modulating transcription factors and vitagenes deserve more attention. Dimerization takes place at a region named the RHD, which is essential for DNA binding, dimerization, and interaction with the inhibitory κB (IκB) proteins (Wu *et al.*, 2018; Thoma and Lightfoot, 2018). The p65/50 dimer is considered to be the most important dimer activating transcription. Hence, RelA-deficient mice are shown to be embryonically lethal as a result of liver apoptosis (McGuire, *et al.*, 2013).

As a result of action of various stimuli, IκB proteins are known to be rapidly phosphorylated by IκB kinase (IKK) on specific serine residues (e.g. Ser-32 and Ser-36 of IκBα; Ser-19 and Ser-23 of IκBβ), followed by ubiquitination (by E2- and E3-ligases), and degradation by the 26S proteasome (Awasthee *et al.*, 2019). To make signalling more effective, on the one hand, NF-κB is shown to encode gene effectors potentiating and amplifying its activation in a feedforward fashion. On the other hand, NF-κB activation is associated with programming default feedback mechanisms responsible for its automatic termination (post mission completion) by regulating the amount/activity/expression of negative effectors including microRNAs (miRNAs), decoy receptors, and anti-inflammatory cytokines, which can lead to the inhibition of the signalling pathways, affecting inhibitory proteins IκBα and IκBε, etc. (Baker *et al.*, 2011; Lingappan, 2018; Zhang *et al.*, 2019a).

There are some similarities in the regulation of Nrf2 and NF-κB in biological systems. For example, in physiological resting conditions, NF-κB is known to be located in the cytoplasm of cells in an inactive state tightly bound to the inhibitory IκB proteins (e.g. IκBα, IκBβ, IκBγ, IκBδ, IκBε, etc.) preventing its binding to target sites. It seems likely that the IκB proteins are responsible for masking the DNA-binding domain of NF-κB/REL proteins, leading to their sequestering in the cytoplasm. Interestingly, IκB proteins are responsible for checking and controlling the pathway due to nuclear export signals and their ability to remove NF-κB proteins from the nucleus (Lingappan, 2018).

It seems likely that key steps in the NF-κB pathway include activation by the IκB kinase (IKK) complex, leading to the phosphorylation-induced proteasomal degradation of IκB proteins, dimer formation, and entering the nucleus, with subsequent binding to κB sites in promotor or enhancer regions of target genes (Patel, *et al.*, 2018); along with other cofactors and histone acetyl transferases (Sivandzade *et al.*, 2019). NF-κB is responsible for the transcription of more than 400 target genes regulating inflammation, immunity, apoptosis, stress adaptation, cell proliferation, and differentiation (Hayden and Ghosh, 2014; Jones and Kounatidis, 2017). Major classes of target genes for NF-κB are shown in Figure 6.1.

As can be seen from the data presented in Figure 6.1, NF-κB target genes can be divided into several groups. The main group includes genes directly related to immunity such as immunoreceptors, proteins involved in antigen presentation, cytokines/chemokines and their modulators, and acute phase proteins. The second group of genes regulated by NF-κB are associated with stress adaptation and homeostasis maintenance under various stress conditions, including transcription factors and regulators, stress response genes, and early response genes. The third group of NF-κB-regulated genes are responsible for the regulation of various cellular function, including regulators of apoptosis, cell-surface receptors, cell adhesion molecules, growth factors, and

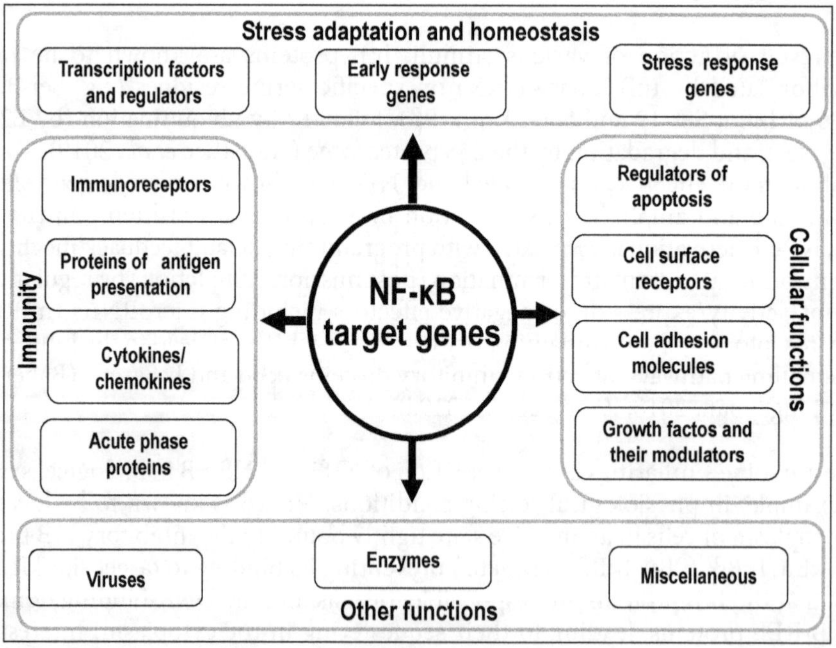

Figure 6.1. NF-κB target genes (adapted from Surai *et al.*, 2021a).

their modulators. There are also NF-κB-regulated genes related to viruses, enzymes, and some other important signalling molecules. Therefore, the great variety of NF-κB-regulated genes explains the pivotal roles of this transcription factor in major physiological and pathophysiological processes in mammalian and avian species.

Generally, the NF-κB system is tightly regulated and can be activated by more than 15 pathways, with the two most common pathways being canonical (classical) and noncanonical (alternative) pathways (Awasthee *et al.*, 2019). The canonical pathway (i.e. the classical pathway) is based primarily on usage of p50 (the product of p105) in conjunction with p65 (p65/p50 nuclear dimer), IKKβ, and NF-κB Essential Modulator, and it can be activated by pro-inflammatory cytokine receptors (e.g. interleukin 1 receptor, IL-1R and tumour necrosis factor receptor, TNFR), by pattern recognition receptors including the TLRs, and by various genotoxic agents. It seems likely that the NF-κB stimulation by various external and internal stressors takes place via the canonical pathway. This includes a response to genotoxic and oxidative stresses, caused by ultraviolet radiation, ionising radiation, ROS, hypoxia, and dysfunctional mitochondria or endoplasmic reticulum by activating NF-κB IKK-dependently, IKK-independently, or both (Scott and Roifman, 2018; Zhang *et al.*, 2019a,b). In particular, NF-κB can be activated by DNA damage via the canonical pathway (Park, 2017).

The noncanonical pathway (known as the alternative pathway) is associated with p52 (the product of p100), RelB, NF-κB-inducing kinase (NIK), and IKKα and it is known to be triggered by a range of stimuli, including lymphotoxin B receptor, B-cell activating factor receptor 3, cluster of differentiation 40 (CD40), and receptor activator of NF-κB ligand. Therefore, ligand-induced activation of the aforementioned receptors leads to the activation of NF-κB-inducing kinase (NIK), which specifically activates IKK1, inducing the phosphorylation and proteolytic processing of p100 to p52, followed by heterodimer formation with RelB to regulate target gene expression (McGuire *et al.*, 2013). It is established that the noncanonical NF-κB pathway is deeply involved in regulation of the immune system, including creation of the adaptive immune response (Sun, 2017). This includes regulation of B-cell development and function, including their differentiation into long-lived antibody-producing plasma cells and memory B cells (for a review, see Giridharan and Srinivasan, 2018; Yu *et al.*, 2020), both being an integral part of the humoral immune response. Since, in comparison to mammals, avian spices are characterised by a different set of immunoglobulin (Ig) classes (IgD and IgE molecules are absent in birds) and a different cytokine repertoire (Kaspers and Göbel, 2016), understanding the molecular mechanisms underlying regulation of the noncanonical NF-κB pathway in birds is a priority for avian scientists. Furthermore, a range of vaccinations used in poultry production are based on humoral response activation and memory B-cell formation (Rabie and Amin Girh, 2020; Schijns *et al.*, 2014), and the noncanonical NF-κB pathway could be a target for improvement of vaccination efficacy. It should be mentioned that the noncanonical NF-κB pathway was also shown to be involved in T-cell development in the thymus, and in orchestrating the formation and maintenance of effector and memory T cells (Sun, 2017). The cell-mediated immunity based on T-cell activity is of paramount importance for poultry, including resistance to viral diseases and vaccination efficacy (Gimeno and Schat, 2018; Kim *et al.*, 2019).

It is important to mention that canonical and noncanonical NF-κB pathways interact with each other. For example, in the classical NF-κB pathway, the first protein transcribed is IκBα. Therefore, it is believed that, in order to inhibit further transcription and restore the original latent state of NF-κB signalling, newly synthesised IκBα can enter the nucleus, remove NF-κB from DNA, and export the complex back to the cytoplasm (Kopitar-Jerala, 2015). Interestingly, the canonical NF-κB pathway is considered to be antiapoptotic, while the noncanonical pathway is proapoptotic (Sehnert *et al.*, 2020).

It well known that NF-κB responds to a large variety of external and internal stress signals/stimuli including oxidative stress (Sivandzade *et al.*, 2019), playing essential roles in the development and maintenance of tissue homeostasis by regulating the transcription of an array of different genes, including proinflammatory cytokines, as well as adhesion molecules, antimicrobial peptides, and acute phase proteins (Buelna-Chontal and Zazueta, 2013; Pedruzzi *et al.*, 2012; Tkach *et al.*, 2014). NF-κB signalling can be considered as an emergency response system, since activation of NF-κB was shown to occur very quickly (within minutes) as a result of release from IκB or as a consequence of cleavage of the inhibitory ankyrin repeat domains of p100 and p105 (Sehnert *et al.*, 2020). Under physiological conditions, the majority of NF-κB-activated genes regulate biological processes associated with cell growth, protection, and repair. They are involved in T-cell maturation, DNA damage repair, tissue healing after injury, and orchestrating the fight against infections (Zhang *et al.*, 2019a,b). It has been proven that activation of NF-κB is an evolutionarily conserved, effective mechanism of host defence against infection and stress (Pal *et al.*, 2014). However, excessive NF-κB activation in commercially relevant stress conditions in poultry and farm animal production systems can lead to detrimental consequences, including chronic inflammation, compromised health status, and decreased productive and reproductive performance. The repertoire of stimuli implicated in the NF-κB activation is very diverse and also includes inhibitory κB kinases, cell-surface receptors, and NF-κB-inducible inhibitor proteins (IB proteins), as well as factors regulating the post-translational modification of the Rel proteins, etc. (Buelna-Chontal and Zazueta, 2013; Hayden and Ghosh, 2014; Jones and Kounatidis, 2017; Pedruzzi *et al.*, 2012; Tkach *et al.*, 2014). Furthermore, p65 and p50 are the targets of many other post-translational modifications such as ubiquitination, acetylation, methylation, phosphorylation, oxidation/reduction, and prolyl-isomerisation, leading to a change in NF-κB transcriptional activity due to affecting the interaction with DNA or as a result of changes in the protein-protein association of NF-κB (Salles *et al.*, 2014).

NF-κB signalling in numerous cell types is involved in the development of various metabolic disorders. In particular, it is thought that resident tissue cells activate NF-κB in response to stress associated with nutrient excesses (Baker *et al.*, 2011). Furthermore, oxidised lipids in the bloodstream can induce NF-κB in vascular endothelia, while, in adipocytes, hepatocytes, and neurons, NF-κB is induced by metabolic or oxidative stress in the ER due to overnutrition. Furthermore, an excess of free fatty acids could also activate NF-κB via TLR4 (Baker *et al.*, 2011). Some examples of activation of NF-κB associated with regulation of downstream transcriptional antioxidant and pro-oxidant targets in the canonical pathway are shown in Figure 6.2.

Depending on physiological context, the activation of NF-κB can have different consequences. Recent findings show that NF-κB does not function alone but is a part of various networks, including crosstalk with other transcription factors (Nrf2, STAT3, FOXO3; etc.), upstream kinases, sirtuins, Wingless-related MMTV integration site 4 (Wnt4), ROS, p53, and miRNAs, which determine the pattern of its effects on the expression of a battery of various genes (Chawla *et al.*, 2020; Zhang *et al.*, 2019a,b). Furthermore, there are regulatory mechanisms coordinating NF-κB association with various important pathways (Sehnert *et al.*, 2020). It has been suggested to consider NF-κB as a stress response factor, since NF-κB signalling is condition-dependent, and NF-κB-dependent cell death or survival would depend on the stimulus and the cell type involved. It seems likely that this complexity is responsible for many apparent contradictions in the literature (Tilborghs *et al.*, 2017). However, most research data indicate that NF-κB signalling pathway enables cells to maintain homeostasis and survive under various stress conditions, including genotoxic stress (Zhang *et al.*, 2019a,b).

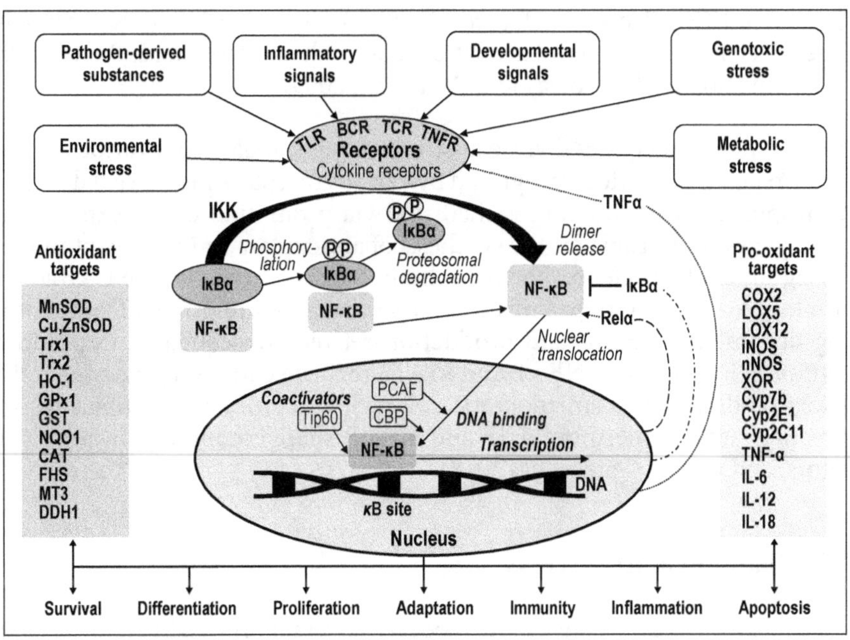

Figure 6.2. Activation of NF-κB and regulation of downstream transcriptional antioxidant and pro-oxidant targets in the canonical pathway (adapted from Surai *et al.*, 2021a).

NF-κB is involved in the modulation of many different molecular events, including inflammation, immune function, cellular growth, and apoptosis (Giridharan and Srinivasan, 2018; Yu *et al.*, 2020). There are a range of NF-κB activators, including pathogen-derived substances (LPS) and inflammatory signals (TNF-α, IL-1), as well as other signals recognised by various receptors, including TNFRs, TLRs, T-cell receptors (TCRs), B-cell receptors (BCRs), and cytokine receptors, which lead to an activation of IκB kinase (IKK) with subsequent phosphorylation of NF-κB inhibitor. This leads to proteasomal degradation of IκB. As a result, the released NF-κB migrates into the nucleus and binds with its corresponding DNA-responsive elements in the presence of coactivators. This results in the transcription of antioxidant (anti-inflammatory) or pro-oxidant (proinflammatory) mediators (Yu *et al.*, 2020; Zhang *et al.*, 2017). It is believed that p65 can induce the expression of both negative regulators (IκBα, IκBε, etc.) and positive regulators (Relα, TNF-α, etc.) participating in tuning the NF-κB pathway (Nelson and Nelson, 2018). It is important to mention that NF-κB can be directly activated or inhibited by ROS in a context-dependent manner, including levels of ROS, exposure, and cell type (Gloire *et al.*, 2006; Lepetsos *et al.*, 2019; Lingappan, 2018). Several findings indicate that ROS-mediated oxidation of redox-sensitive cysteine residues of NF-κB subunits has dual effects (inducing or inhibiting) on the NF-κB signalling depending on the level of ROS, the cell type, and the types of stimuli (Gloire and Piette, 2009; Morgan and Liu, 2011). On the one hand, ROS can activate the NF-κB pathway by imposing disulphide bond formation between Cys54 and Cys347 in IKKγ (Herscovitch *et al.*, 2008). On the other hand, ROS can have an opposite effect: inhibiting NF-κB activation as a result of restricting IκBα degradation, due to inactivation of the proteasome (Wu *et al.*, 2009).

The NF-κB system integrates diverse upstream input signals (from various stresses to pathogen-related molecules) recognised by various receptors into varied downstream output responses. This function is mediated via promotion of the expression of a variety of genes responsible for the synthesis of antioxidant or prooxidant molecules, improving antioxidant defences and redox homeostasis. Alternatively, NF-κB activation can also lead to synthesis of proinflammatory cytokines, imposing inflammation and causing detrimental health- and production-related consequences in poultry and farm animals. In particular, NF-κB and STAT3 regulate common processes and share regulatory binding sites of antiapoptotic, cell cycle and proliferation, tissue resistance, and repair genes. Furthermore, HIF and NF-κB share common activating stimuli, regulators, and targets (Patel *et al.*, 2018).

6.3 NF-κB and oxidative stress

Free-radical production is considered to be an important process in biological systems responsible for the antibacterial action of oxidative burst in phagocytes, cell signalling, and stress adaptation (Sies and Jones, 2020). However, an excess of RONS due to high level of stress or a compromised antioxidant system leads to damages to major biological molecules (proteins, PUFAs, DNA, etc.) associated with immunosuppression, gut health problems, and decreased productive and reproductive performance of poultry

(Surai *et al.*, 2018). Therefore, a variety of protective mechanisms have been developed during evolution to deal with RONS excess, and many transcription factors are involved in this process via regulating vitagenes and a myriad of antioxidant enzymes in stress conditions (Surai, 2020).

There are a range of transcription factors acting cooperatively with NF-κB. For-example, NF-κB and STAT3 are shown to regulate common pathways and share regulatory binding sites of various protective genes, while HIF and NF-κB are reported to share common activating stimuli, regulators, and targets (Patel *et al.*, 2018). The redox balance is believed to be orchestrated by a range of transcription factors, including Nrf2, NF-κB, AP-1, FoxO, PPARs, PGC-1α, p53, and MAPK (Lushchak, 2011; Wang and Hai, 2016). It seems likely that transcription factors and vitagenes are involved in the regulation of redox status by effectively modulating the expression and activity of ROS-generating enzymes and antioxidant enzymes (Dayalan Naidu *et al.*, 2015).

NF-κB has long been considered to be a prototypical proinflammatory signalling pathway stimulating the immune system in response to various stimuli, including physical, physiological, and/or oxidative stress. For example, NF-κB is a key target in receptor-independent hypothalamic microinflammation (Cai and Khor, 2019) associated with intracellular organelle stress, including RNA stress response (Yan *et al.*, 2014), ER stress (Zhang *et al.*, 2008), and defective autophagy (Meng and Cai, 2011). NF-κB is involved in the regulation of many important physiological processes; however, its overactivation has been shown to be associated with increased risk of disease, while NF-κB suppression is associated with risk reduction (Jones and Kounatidis, 2017). Taking the former into account, understanding the role of NF-κB signalling in stress adaptation awaits further investigation. For example, HO-1 can improve cell protection from apoptosis by stimulating free heme catabolism. Interestingly, the HO-1 promoter region contains an NF-κB responsive element and, therefore, HO-1 expression is regulated by NF-κB, as well as by other transcription factors (Kurata *et al.*, 1996). A central role for NF-κB in regulating mitochondrial respiration has been suggested (Tornatore *et al.*, 2012). It seems likely that by controlling the balance between glycolysis and respiration for energy provision, NF-κB is involved in energy homeostasis and metabolic adaptation (Mauro *et al.*, 2011). The authors suggested to consider NF-κB as an important checkpoint connecting cell activation and proliferation with energy sensing and metabolic homeostasis. Since mitochondria are the main ROS source in the cell, it could be that NF-κB signalling is involved in the regulation of ROS formation, detoxification, and the maintenance of redox homeostasis.

6.4 Nutritional modulation of NF-κB

There is a range of nutrients affecting NF-κB expression and activity including amino acids, vitamins and minerals as well as various probiotics (Surai *et al.*, 2021a). In relation to the topic of this book we will consider effects of phytogenic supplements and SM on NF-κB. Recently, various phytogenic supplements received tremendous attention in human and animal/poultry nutrition, and the molecular mechanisms of their protective actions in many cases were related to their antioxidant properties. However, our analysis of the current data in this area showed that polyphenolic compounds are poorly absorbed and their concentrations in target tissues are several orders lower than those used in *in vitro* studies (Surai, 2014). Furthermore, their antioxidant properties are condition-dependent, and, in many cases, polyphenols could show pro-oxidant activities. Therefore, it was suggested that the polyphenolic effects on NF-κB and Nrf2 expression could be a major molecular mechanism of their protective action in various model systems and in poultry nutrition in general (Surai, 2014; 2015d, 2020). Data showing the activation effects of polyphenol compounds on Nrf2 expression and activity with simultaneous suppression of the NF-κB pathway confirmed that idea. There are also a range of publications showing protective effects of phytogenic supplements in animal/poultry nutrition under various stress conditions.

In chickens receiving conventional vaccinations, the NF-κB gene mRNA relative expression in hepatocytes linearly decreased as a result of increasing resveratrol, a plant-derived polyphenolic compound, with a dietary concentration from 200 to 800 mg/kg of diet (Zhang *et al.*, 2014). Similarly, dietary resveratrol (200-600 mg/kg) was shown to reduce the protein expression of NF-κB, HSP70, and HSP90 in the jejunal chicken villi after 15 days of heat stress (Liu *et al.*, 2016). Dietary resveratrol (400 mg/kg) was also indicated to protect quail hepatocytes against heat stress by decreasing the expression of NF-κB, Hsp70, and Hsp90, and increasing the hepatic SOD, CAT, and GPx activities (Sahin *et al.*, 2012). Daidzein (DA), a soy isoflavone, included into the breeder diet at 20 mg/kg was shown to activate the NF-κB, MAPK, and TLR signalling pathways of the offspring broilers. Furthermore, DA promoted lymphocyte development and differentiation and downregulated the expression of genes regulating lymphocyte apoptosis. It also increased the proportion of B cells, leading to promotion of Ig secretion with increased serum IgA and IgG levels and serum ND virus antibody titers (Fan *et al.*, 2018). In healthy Arbor Acre broilers, quercetin supplementation (0.04% and 0.06% for 6 weeks) was found to significantly increase the expression of TNF-α, TNF receptor associated factor-2, TNF receptor superfamily member 1B, NF-κBp65, and IFN-γ mRNA, while expression of NF-κB inhibitor-alpha (IκB-α) mRNA was significantly decreased (Yang *et al.*, 2020).

Ginsenosides, the major constituents of ginseng with unique biological activities, were shown to promote proliferation of chicken primordial germ cells through protein kinase C (PKC)-involved activation of NF-κB (Ge *et al.*, 2007). Tanshinone IIA (TIIA), a major lipophilic component extracted from the root of *Salvia miltiorrhiza* Bunge used in Chinese medicine, was shown to have a protective effect against pulmonary arterial hypertension-related inflammatory responses (Lee *et al.*, 2018a). Treatment with an extract of *Hypericum perforatum* L., also known as Saint John's wort, at doses of 480-120 mg/kg for 5 days was indicated to reduce infectious bronchitis virus (IBV)-induced injury and reduced the mRNA expression level of IBV in the chicken trachea *in vivo*. In particular, the expression of IL-6, TNF-α, and NF-κB was found to be significantly decreased, but mitochondrial antiviral signalling gene, IFN-α, and

IFN-β mRNA levels were shown to be significantly induced *in vitro* and *in vivo* (Chen *et al.*, 2019).

6.5 Silymarin and NF-κB regulation

The anti-inflammatory activity of phenolic compounds has been demonstrated in a number of *in vitro* and *in vivo* studies and polyphenols may affect inflammation mainly as modulators of inflammatory redox signalling pathways (Gupta *et al.*, 2014). The polyphenolic compounds express anti-inflammatory activity by modulating the expression of pro-inflammatory genes such as cyclooxygenase, lipoxygenase, nitric oxide synthases and several important cytokines, mainly acting through nuclear factor-κB and mitogen-activated protein kinase signalling (Gupta *et al.*, 2014; Stevenson and Hurst, 2007). Due to the large number of studies that have demonstrated regulatory effects of SM/SB on the expression of NF-κB in various *in vitro* and *in vivo* models there is insufficient space in this chapter to analyse all of them, so we will focus only on recent investigations addressing the issue. It is well established that various plant-derived polyphenols can suppress TNF-α activated, NF-κB-associated inflammatory pathways both *in vitro* and *in vivo*. These polyphenols include SM as well as curcumin, resveratrol, genistein, epigallocatechin gallate, flavopiridol, emodin, morin isoliquiritigenin, naringenin, ellagic acid, apigenin, kaempferol, catechins, myricetin, xanthohumol, fisetin, vitexin, escin, mangostin and others (Gupta *et al.*, 2014). SM has long been known to inhibit the activation of inflammatory NF-κB signalling (Ramasamy and Agarwal, 2008). Recent studies have confirmed that the protective anti-inflammatory effects of SM/SB could be mediated by their inhibitory potential on the NF-κB, which is a key transcriptional factor for numerous genes involved in regulation of inflammation, immune system, cell differentiation, survival, apoptosis, etc. Here, we give some examples of participation of SM/SB in NF-κB pathway inhibition.

6.5.1 *In vitro* studies

SB is a potent inhibitor of NF-κB activation. For example, Manna *et al.* (1999) tested SB in a number of *in vitro* human cell experimental systems and found it inhibited TNF-mediated NF-κB activation in a dose-dependent manner with maximum inhibition at 50 μM and it regulated NF-κB 100 times more effectively than aspirin. Furthermore, SB (80 μM) protected glial cells against peroxide-induced ROS formation, ATP depletion, and cell damage (Tsai *et al.*, 2010). Interestingly, the inhibition of peroxide-induced ROS by SB was partially attenuated by inhibitors of NF-κB or PKC, suggesting an involvement of NF-κB and PKC signalling pathways. Similarly, a significant decrease in NF-κB was observed, when peripheral blood mononuclear cells (PBMCs) from pre-eclamptic patients were cultured with SB at 5 μM and 50 μM concentrations and stimulated with LPS (Giorgi *et al.*, 2012). Moreover, SB (50-200 μM) inhibited the nuclear translocation of nuclear factor NF-κB through inhibition of the phosphorylation of IκBα and suppressed NF-κB transcriptional activity in stimulated HMC-1 cells (Kim *et al.*, 2013a). SM is also effective in inhibiting T cell activation and proliferation, by acting on pathways of NF-κB activation/translocation. In particular, in CD4+ splenocytes from C57/Bl6 mice, SM (50 μM) significantly inhibited CD4+ cells proliferation, inhibited IL-2 and IFN-γ production and blocked nuclear translocation of transcription factor NF-κB. Moreover, SM inhibited p65/NF-κB phosphorylation in CD4+ T cell (Gharagozloo *et al.*, 2010).

The significant upregulation of oxidative stress biomarkers including MDA, TNF-α, IFN-γ and IL-1β genes was observed as well as NF-κB, cyclooxygenase-2 (COX-2) and iNOS proteins expression occurred upon heat stress in chicken hepatocytes. Furthermore, AO enzyme (SOD, CAT, GR) activities decreased. SM (259 μM) was able to normalise the expression of all these biomarkers in heat-induced chicken hepatocytes (Oskoueian *et al.*, 2014). SB was clearly shown to inhibit the expression of NF-κB at transcriptional and translational levels (Kang *et al.*, 2019). SB also downregulates the NF-κB pathway and NLRP1/NLRP3 inflammasomes in monocytes from pregnant women with preeclampsia (Matias *et al.*, 2019). However, there is a need for more studies with pure SB at physiologically-relevant concentrations (0.2-2 μM) in order to confirm its modulating effect on the NF-κB pathway.

6.5.2 *In vivo* studies

It has been shown that SB (50 mg/kg/BW) had a protective effect against d-galactose-induced senescence due to promotion of cellular oxidoreductase activities and inhibition of NF-κB activation and ROS production (Wang *et al.*, 2011). Histopathological and immunohistochemical studies in the kidney of rats also shows that SB (75 mg/kg/BW) markedly reduced the toxicity of As and preserved the normal histological architecture of the renal tissue, inhibited the caspase-3 mediated tubular cell apoptosis and decreased the NADPH oxidase, iNOS and NF-κB overexpression by As (Prabu and Muthumani, 2012). In a model of experimental ischemic stroke in male rats, SB (100 mg/kg) significantly downregulated NF-κB in ischemic brain tissue after stroke (Wang *et al.*, 2012). In an experimental nonalcoholic steatohepatitis model, mice fed a methionine-choline deficient diet consistently had increased NF-κB p65 and p50 binding activity, while SB administration (20 mg/kg/BW/i.p.) significantly decreased the activity of both subunits (Salamone *et al.*, 2012).

It was shown that CCl_4 treatment of mice enhanced the NF-κB expression in the liver and induced hepatic fibrosis, while SM (200 mg/kg/BW) reduced the CCl_4-induced hepatic NF-κB and improved CCl_4-induced liver fibrosis (Li *et al.*, 2012). Protective effect of SB (150 mg/kg/BW/intragastric) in the rat model of cerebral ischemia was associated with decreased expression of the Bax, NF-κB protein and Bax, NF-κB mRNA in the brain (Liu *et al.*, 2014). SM is also shown to have NF-κB inhibiting effects. For example, mRNA and protein expressions of NF-κB were significantly up-regulated in D-galactosamine induced hepatotoxic rats and treatment with SM (25 mg/kg/BW) significantly down-regulated the expressions of these genes (Aristatile *et al.*, 2013). Furthermore, it has been shown that the serum levels of transforming growth factor (TGF-β1), NF-κB, and IL-6 were significantly elevated in the samples from cirrhosis rats while SM (50 g/kg) significantly prevented the aforementioned changes (Salama *et al.*, 2013) and SM (250 mg/kg/BW) suppressed NF-κB signalling cascade in alcoholic liver fibrosis in guinea pigs (Abhilash *et al.*, 2013; 2014). In a mouse model of non-alcoholic steatohepatitis SB treatment was reported to alleviate the severity of hepatic inflammation and steatohepatitis due to the inhibition as a result of inhibition of NF-κB-signalling pathway (Lee *et al.*, 2018b). Similarly, SB was reported to alleviate hepatic steatosis and fibrosis in NASH mice by inhibiting oxidative stress and decreasing NF-κB signalling (Ou *et al.*, 2018). Protective role of SB against myocardial ischemia/reperfusion injury-induced cardiac dysfunction was shown to be associated with decreased apoptosis, oxidative stress and inflammatory response through deactivation of NF-κB pathway (Chen *et al.*, 2020). Similarly, SB was reported to attenuate renal fibrosis *in vitro* and *in vivo* via inhibition of NF-κB (Liu *et al.*, 2019a). Overall, SM/SB targets multiple signalling pathways, including NF-κB, towards inhibiting the secretion of pro-inflammatory cytokines. Together these findings suggest that the inhibitory effect of SM/SB on NF-κB signalling in a variety of cells, as well as in *in vivo* studies, could be an important mechanism of its anti-inflammation efficacy, and that targeting this signalling pathway by SB may have potential applications in the clinic and veterinary practice.

6.6 Nrf2 and NF-κB interplay in oxidative stress

Proof of the interaction and cooperative action of Nrf2 and NF-κB was taken from experimental work with various model systems employing plant extracts and individual compounds *in vitro* and *in vivo* using pure chemicals, and some known toxicants to impose oxidative stress (Saha *et al.*, 2020). In our recent review, a central role of Nrf2 in antioxidant defences and vitagene regulation was described in detail (Surai *et al.*, 2019b), and it seems likely that, under oxidative stress, the transcription factors NF-κB and Nrf2 antagonise each other to coordinate a stress response (Tkach *et al.*, 2014; Zhang *et al.*, 2019a,b). For example, deletion of Nrf2 (Nrf2 knockout mice) enhanced inflammation, while Nrf2 upregulation was reported to decrease NF-κB-dependent proinflammatory and immune responses (Sivandzade *et al.*, 2019). Several known Nrf2 activators are able to inhibit the NF-κB pathway. There are many examples showing that activation and repression occur between members of the Nrf2 and NF-κB pathways through various mechanisms (Wakabayashi *et al.*, 2020). Some mechanisms of Nrf2-NF-κB interactions are summarised in Table 6.1.

There is accumulating evidence indicating that various nutrients with AO activities could differently affect transcription factors: increasing expression of Nrf2 and simultaneously decreasing NF-κB expression and activity. This was proven in various model systems employing plant extracts and individual polyphenolics. Firstly, in *in vitro* systems, these include sinomenine (Wu, *et al.*, 2019), aloin (Lee *et al.*, 2019a), urolithin B (Lee *et al.*, 2019b), 4-ethylguaiacol (Zhao *et al.*, 2019), gambogic acid (Ren *et al.*, 2019), and the combination of ascorbic acid and rutin (Gęgotek *et al.*, 2019). There are also a range of *in vivo* studies confirming that various plant-derived compounds,

Table 6.1. Possible mechanisms of Nrf2-NF-κB interactions.[1]

Mechanisms of Nrf2-NF-κB Interactions	**References**
Inhibiting effects of Nrf2 on NF-κB	
Decreasing the intracellular ROS levels. This inhibits oxidative stress-mediated NF-κB activation.	Soares *et al.*, 2004
Preventing the IκB-proteasomal degradation and inhibiting nuclear translocation of NF-κB. In Nrf2-deficient cells an inhibitor of NF-κB activity (IκB) is over-phosphorylated with rapid proteasomal degradation and increased NF-κB activity. Upregulation of Nrf2 induces increase HO-1 levels and induce phase II enzymes expression blocking the degradation of IκB.	Yerra *et al.*, 2013; Thimmulappa, *et al.*, 2006; Bellezza *et al.*, 2012; Chen *et al.*, 2018
Reducing p50 and p65 DNA binding. Nrf2 silencing enhanced p50 and p65 DNA binding and TNF-α-induced proinflammatory gene expression.	Rushworth *et al.*, 2011
Preventing the recruitment of RNA polymerase II to start transcription of NF-κB-regulated genes. Nrf2 binds to regulatory regions of proinflammatory genes in an ARE-independent manner and prevents the recruitment of RNA polymerase II to start transcription of NF-κB-regulated genes.	Kobayashi *et al.*, 2016
Competition between Nrf2 and p65 for binding to the transcriptional co-activator CBP-p300 complex.[1] Overexpression of p65 limits the availability of CBP for Nrf2 interaction. Knockdown of p65 promotes Nrf2 complex formation with CBP.	Kim *et al.*, 2013b; Liu *et al.*, 2008
Degrading IKKβ through ubiquitination by Keap1.	Lee *et al.*, 2009
Inhibiting effects of NF-κB on Nrf2	
Inactivating Nrf2 by inducing cyclooxygenase 2.	Banning and Brigelius-Flohé, 2005; Brigelius-Flohé and Flohé, 2011
Recruiting MAF BZIP Transcription Factor K (MafK)-associated histone deacetylase 3 (HDAC3) activity to the HO-1 enhancer and deacetylating CBP leading to a suppression of its co-activator activity.	Chuang, *et al.*, 2006; Hung *et al.*, 2001
Interacting with CBP, the competent Nrf2 coactivator, and inhibiting the transcription of genes regulated by Nrf2.	Ahmed, *et al.*, 2017; Liu *et al.*, 2008; Yang *et al.*, 2005
Decreasing free CBP, a transcriptional co-activator of Nrf2, and promoting phosphorylation of p65.	Liu *et al.*, 2008
Overexpression of p65 limits the availability of CBR for Nrf2 interaction. Knockdown of p65 promotes Nrf2 complex formation with CBP.	
κB sites in proximal promoter of Nrf2 are believed to be subject to binding and transcription initiation by p65.	Rushworth *et al.*, 2012

[1] CBP = CREB-binding protein, where CREB is a transcription factor.

mainly polyphenols, decrease NF-κB and increase Nrf2 activity/expression in various model systems. These include peiminine (Luo *et al.*, 2019), hesperetin (Muhammad *et al.*, 2019), oxyresveratrol, resveratrol and mulberroside (Jia *et al.*, 2019), salvianolic acid A (Zhang *et al.*, 2019c), naringenin (Abdel-Magied and Shedid, 2019), δ-amyrone (Wang *et al.*, 2019), chrysin, luteolin, apigenin, hesperetin and 3′, 4′-dimethoxy hesperetin (He *et al.*, 2019), luteoloside (Li *et al.*, 2019a), alpinetin (Liu *et al.*, 2019b), amygdalin (Tang *et al.*, 2019), rosmarinic acid (Li *et al.*, 2019b), chiisanoside (Bian *et al.*, 2019), arbutin (Ye *et al.*, 2019), and chicoric acid (Ding *et al.*, 2019). Moreover, the different direction of activation of Nrf2 and NF-κB was also shown to be a result of exposure to various toxic compounds. However, other agents and stimuli, including, but not limited to, ROS, LPS, flow shear stress, oxidised low-density lipoprotein, and cigarette smoke, were reported to activate both Nrf2 and NF-κB pathways (Mauro *et al.*, 2011; Wakabayashi *et al.*, 2020).

The redox outcome of the NF-κB-Nrf2 interaction would depend on the activation/inhibition of various antioxidant and prooxidant enzymes. It is known that some antioxidant enzymes are dependent on both Nrf2 and NF-κB. For example, expression of HO-1 is shown to be regulated by Nrf2, NF-κB, and HIF-1α signalling (Zhang *et al.*, 2019a,b). On the one hand, HO-1 was shown to possess a functional ARE that is activated by Nrf2 (Alam *et al.*, 1999). On the other hand, HO-1 was found to have a functional NF-κB site (Lavrovsky *et al.*, 1994). HO-1 is known to be the stress-inducible enzyme providing AO protection in vertebrate systems, participating in the maintenance of redox balance and being responsible for adaptation to oxidative, inflammatory, and cytotoxic stress (Surai, 2020, Surai and Fisinin, 2016a,b). Similarly, a key catalytic subunit of glutamate-cysteine ligase, the key enzyme of the cellular GSH biosynthetic pathway, also has an ARE and can be activated by Nrf2 (Mulcahy *et al.*, 1997), whereas it also possesses a κB site and can be induced by NF-κB (Kimura *et al.*, 2009).

Since GSH is a key physiological buffer responsible for the redox homeostasis (Muri and Kopf, 2021), regulation of its synthesis via Nrf2 and NF-κB pathways is of great importance for redox homeostasis maintenance. Furthermore, SOD2 is also a target for both NF-κB (Kairisalo *et al.*, 2007) and Nrf2 (Surai *et al.*, 2019b). It is well established that SOD2, a key enzyme of the first line of the AO network, is located in mitochondria and deals with major biological ROS, namely, superoxide radicals, and it is considered to be a major player in the establishment and maintenance of redox homeostasis (Surai *et al.*, 2018). Furthermore, GPx1 and GST expression and activities are also under strict control by NF-κB (Morgan and Liu, 2011) and Nrf2 (Surai, 2018; 2020). The important roles of these AO enzymes in AO defence and redox homeostasis have been previously discussed (Surai, 2018; 2020). It seems likely that another redox balance regulator, namely, Trx, is also regulated by NF-κB (Djavaheri-Mergny *et al.*, 2004; Kairisalo *et al.*, 2007) and Nrf2 (Surai, 2020; Surai and Fisinin, 2016a). It is interesting that HO-1, SOD, and Trx belong to the vitagene family responsible for stress adaptation and redox homeostasis (Surai, 2020; Surai and Fisinin, 2016a,b).

It should also be mentioned that the NF-κB pathway can induce free-radical production via activating ROS-producing enzymes, including NADPH oxidase (Anrather *et al.*, 2006), COX-2 (Wakabayashi *et al.*, 2020), cytochrome p450 enzymes, iNOS, neuronal NOS, and xanthine oxidase/dehydrogenase (Morgan and Liu, 2011). The impact of such ROS production on redox balance and adaptation to stress is still not well established; however, this complicates the interpretation of results related to NF-κB-Nrf2 interactions in biological systems under various stress conditions.

In many cases, activation of various transcription factors, including Nrf2, NF-κB, AP-1, HIF-1α, p53, PPAR-γ, and β-catenin/Wnt, was associated with the oxidative stress (Reuter *et al.*, 2010). Therefore, a complex crosstalk between Nrf2 and NF-κB pathways under various stress conditions (Sivandzade *et al.*, 2019) further complicates interpretation of results related to the relative impact of each pathway on the regulation of stress adaptation. Indeed, as mentioned above, Nrf2 and NF-κB affect each other's expression and activity to coordinate antioxidative and inflammatory responses; however, molecular mechanisms of this interconnection are not yet known (Sivandzade *et al.*, 2019).

It is believed that condition-dependent, stress-associated changes in redox balance and in expressions/activities of transcription factors (e.g. Nrf2/Keap1 and NF-κB/IκB/IKK) are responsible for providing adaptive cell responses to a variety of stress stimuli through orchestrating the optimal expression of protective target genes (Moldogazieva *et al.*, 2018). A hypothetical scheme of the Nrf2-NF-κB crosstalk is shown in Figure 6.3.

In physiological conditions, a delicate balance between Nrf2 and NF-κB expression in various tissues is well coordinated and maintained. It seems likely that increased NF-κB expression as a result of low/moderate stresses can lead to a simultaneous increase in the expression of Nrf2, leading to improved antioxidant defences.

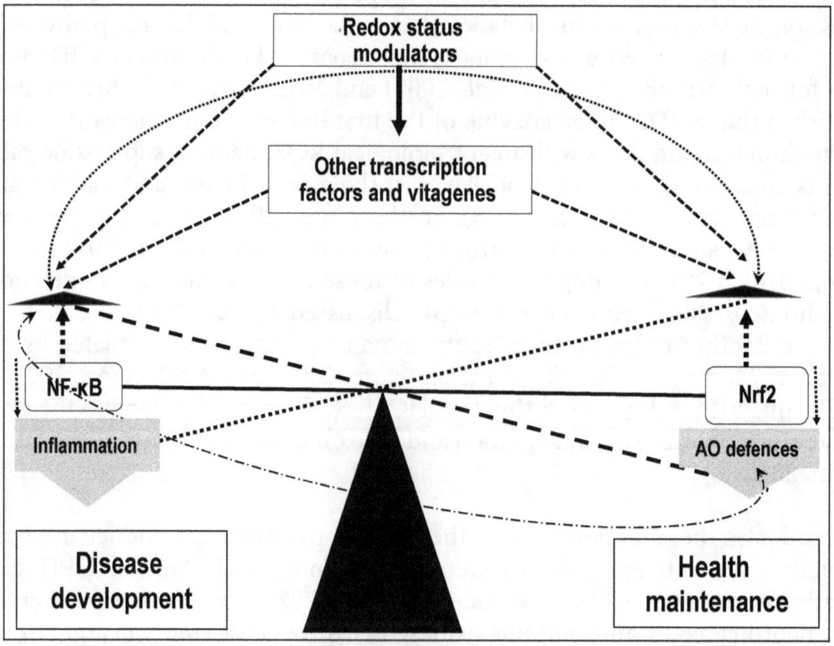

Figure 6.3. Hypothetical Nrf2-NF-κB crosstalk (Surai, 2020; Surai *et al.*, 2019b).

At the same time, decreased NF-κB expression can be observed as a feedback mechanism. This balance is also regulated by other transcription factors and vitagenes. In the case of high oxidative stress, when the ability of the AO defence network to deal with RONS production is overwhelmed, the Nrf2/NF-κB balance would be broken. In such conditions, redox status would be compromised with detrimental consequences to human/animal health. Furthermore, the productive and reproductive performance of poultry and farm animals would be compromised.

6.7 Conclusions

Today, NF-κB is known as a redox-sensitive, inducible nuclear transcription factor that regulates the expression of a number of genes associated with important biological processes, including innate and adaptive immune responses, cell growth, maturation, survival, and adaptive homeostasis establishment via interactions with other transcription factors and vitagenes (Surai, 2020). Intriguingly, NF-κB signalling is an important element in cell adaptation to a diverse array of environmental stimuli, including oxidative stress. These stimuli can be recognised by various receptors, and the subsequent response involves specific adapter proteins. Under normal physiological conditions, the antioxidant defence network and the optimised redox balance in the cell/tissue are responsible for orchestrating important biological processes associated with cell protection, repair, and growth. This includes T-cell maturation, fighting against infections, DNA damage repair, and tissue healing and integrity restoration after injury.

However, under various stress conditions, associated with redox disbalance, aberrant NF-κB activation can lead to detrimental changes, including the development of many age-related diseases. Notably, it was reported that activation of NF-κB is an important mechanism of host defence against infection and stress (Pal *et al.*, 2014). The results from gene knockout experiments clearly showed that mice deficient in NF-κB-mediated transcriptional regulation were susceptible to a variety of infections and were characterised by compromised immunity: specifically, depressed immunoglobulin expression, defective humoral immune responses, and decreased responses to LPS (Sha *et al.*, 1995). It has been recently proposed that NF-κB is a vital regulator of inflammation, indicating that the dynamical attributes and the composition of the nuclear NF-κB complexes cumulatively instruct context-specific inflammatory gene patterns (Chawla *et al.*, 2020). A variety of endogenous and exogenous stimuli have been characterised, including danger, damage, and survival signals from viral and bacterial components, proinflammatory cytokines, DNA damage, growth factors, and other stressors. As mentioned above, the stimuli can be recognised by a range of various receptors with subsequent activation of NF-κB, along with involvement of an array of specific adapter proteins (Zhang *et al.*, 2019a,b).

Nutritional modulation of NF-κB expression and activity was shown to be achieved by using various antioxidants, including selenium, various polyphenols, TAU, retinoic acid, vitamin E, and some probiotics. Under various stress conditions, these nutrients can ameliorate (partly or completely) the increased NF-κB expression and activity imposed by stressors (Surai *et al.*, 2021a). An opportunity to use nutritional/pharmacological means to modulate NF-κB expression and activity should be exploited further and SM is proven to possess NF-κB-modulating properties. Furthermore, other nutrients, including TAU (Surai *et al.*, 2020; 2021b), carnitine (Surai, 2015a,b,c), vitamin E (Surai *et al.*, 2019a), selenium (Surai, 2018; 2021; Surai and Kochish, 2019), carotenoids (Surai and Kochish, 2020), and others (Surai *et al.*, 2017), have been shown to affect antioxidant defences and vitagenes, helping maintain the redox balance in various tissues. There is a need for further research related to interactions of the antioxidant defence network with vitagenes and transcription factors, including NF-κB and Nrf2, which are responsible for the maintenance of redox homeostasis and stress adaptation under various stress conditions in human health and animal/poultry production.

References

Abdel-Magied, N. and Shedid, S.M., 2019. The effect of naringenin on the role of nuclear factor (erythroid-derived 2)-like2 (Nrf2) and haem oxygenase 1 (HO-1) in reducing the risk of oxidative stress-related radiotoxicity in the spleen of rats. Environmental Toxicology 34: 788-795.

Abhilash, P.A., Harikrishnan, R. and Indira, M., 2013. Ascorbic acid is superior to silymarin in the recovery of ethanol-induced inflammatory reactions in hepatocytes of guinea pigs. Journal of Physiology and Biochemistry 69: 785-798.

Abhilash, P.A., Harikrishnan, R. and Indira, M., 2014. Ascorbic acid suppresses endotoxemia and NF-κB signaling cascade in alcoholic liver fibrosis in guinea pigs: A mechanistic approach. Toxicology and Applied Pharmacology 274: 215-224.

Ahmed, S.M., Luo, L., Namani, A., Wang, X.J. and Tang, X., 2017. Nrf2 signaling pathway: Pivotal roles in inflammation. Biochimica et Biophysica Acta. Molecular Basis of Disease 1863: 585-597.

Alam, J., Stewart, D., Touchard, C., Boinapally, S., Choi, A.M. and Cook, J.L., 1999. Nrf2, a Cap'n'Collar transcription factor, regulates induction of the heme oxygenase-1 gene. The Journal of Biological Chemistry 274: 26071-26078.

Anrather, J., Racchumi, G. and Iadecola, C., 2006. NF-kappaB regulates phagocytic NADPH oxidase by inducing the expression of gp91phox. The Journal of Biological Chemistry 281: 5657-5667.

Aristatile, B., Al-Assaf, A.H. and Pugalendi, K.V., 2013. Carvacrol suppresses the expression of inflammatory marker genes in D-galactosamine-hepatotoxic rats. Asian Pacific Journal of Tropical Medicine 6: 205-211.

Awasthee, N., Rai, V., Chava, S., Nallasamy, P., Kunnumakkara, A.B., Bishayee, A., Chauhan, S.C., Challagundla, K.B. and Gupta, S.C., 2019. Targeting IκappaB kinases for cancer therapy. Seminars in Cancer Biology 56: 12-24.

Baker, R.G., Hayden, M.S. and Ghosh, S., 2011. NF-κB, inflammation, and metabolic disease. Cell Metabolism 13: 11-22.

Banning, A. and Brigelius-Flohé, R., 2005. NF-kappaB, Nrf2, and HO-1 interplay in redox-regulated VCAM-1 expression. Antioxidants & Redox Signaling 7: 889-899.

Bellezza, I., Tucci, A., Galli, F., Grottelli, S., Mierla, A.L., Pilolli, F. and Minelli, A., 2012. Inhibition of NF-κB nuclear translocation via HO-1 activation underlies α-tocopheryl succinate toxicity. The Journal of Nutritional Biochemistry 23: 1583-1591.

Bian, X., Liu, X., Liu, J., Zhao, Y., Li, H., Zhang, L., Li, P. and Gao, Y., 2019. Hepatoprotective effect of chiisanoside from Acanthopanax sessiliflorus against LPS/D-GalN-induced acute liver injury by inhibiting NF-κB and activating Nrf2/HO-1 signaling pathways. Journal of the Science of Food and Agriculture 99: 3283-3290.

Brigelius-Flohé, R. and Flohé, L., 2011. Basic principles and emerging concepts in the redox control of transcription factors. Antioxidants & Redox Signaling 15: 2335-2381.

Buelna-Chontal, M. and Zazueta, C., 2013. Redox activation of Nrf2 & NF-κB: a double end sword?. Cellular Signalling 25: 2548-2557.

Cai, D. and Khor, S., 2019. 'Hypothalamic microinflammation' paradigm in aging and metabolic diseases. Cell Metabolism 30: 19-35.

Chawla, M., Roy, P. and Basak, S., 2021. Role of the NF-κB system in context-specific tuning of the inflammatory gene response. Current Opinion in Immunology 68: 21-27.

Chen, H., Muhammad, I., Zhang, Y., Ren, Y., Zhang, R., Huang, X., Diao, L., Liu, H., Li, X., Sun, X., Abbas, G. and Li, G., 2019. Antiviral activity against infectious bronchitis virus and bioactive components of hypericum perforatum L. Frontiers in Pharmacology 10: 1272.

Chen, L.G., Zhang, Y.Q., Wu, Z.Z., Hsieh, C.W., Chu, C.S. and Wung, B.S., 2018. Peanut arachidin-1 enhances Nrf2-mediated protective mechanisms against TNF-α-induced ICAM-1 expression and NF-κB activation in endothelial cells. International Journal of Molecular Medicine 41: 541-547.

Chen, Y.H., Lin, H., Wang, Q., Hou, J.W., Mao, Z.J. and Li, Y.G., 2020. Protective role of silibinin against myocardial ischemia/reperfusion injury-induced cardiac dysfunction. International Journal of Biological Sciences 16: 1972-1988.

Chuang, H.C., Chang, C.W., Chang, G.D., Yao, T.P. and Chen, H., 2006. Histone deacetylase 3 binds to and regulates the GCMa transcription factor. Nucleic Acids Research 34: 1459-1469.

Dayalan Naidu, S., Kostov, R.V. and Dinkova-Kostova, A.T., 2015. Transcription factors Hsf1 and Nrf2 engage in crosstalk for cytoprotection. Trends in Pharmacological Sciences 36: 6-14.

Ding, H., Ci, X., Cheng, H., Yu, Q. and Li, D., 2019. Chicoric acid alleviates lipopolysaccharide-induced acute lung injury in mice through anti-inflammatory and anti-oxidant activities. International Immunopharmacology 66: 169-176.

Djavaheri-Mergny, M., Javelaud, D., Wietzerbin, J. and Besançon, F., 2004. NF-kappaB activation prevents apoptotic oxidative stress via an increase of both thioredoxin and MnSOD levels in TNFalpha-treated Ewing sarcoma cells. FEBS Letters 578: 111-115.

Fan, H., Lv, Z., Gan, L. and Guo, Y., 2018. Transcriptomics-related mechanisms of supplementing laying broiler breeder hens with dietary daidzein to improve the immune function and growth performance of offspring. Journal of Agricultural and Food Chemistry 66: 2049-2060.

Ge, C., Zhang, C., Ye, J., Tang, X. and Wu, Y., 2007. Ginsenosides promote proliferation of chicken primordial germ cells via PKC-involved activation of NF-kappaB. Cell Biology International 31: 1251-1256.

Gęgotek, A., Ambrożewicz, E., Jastrząb, A., Jarocka-Karpowicz, I. and Skrzydlewska, E., 2019. Rutin and ascorbic acid cooperation in antioxidant and antiapoptotic effect on human skin keratinocytes and fibroblasts exposed to UVA and UVB radiation. Archives of Dermatological Research 311: 203-219.

Gharagozloo, M., Velardi, E., Bruscoli, S., Agostini, M., Di Sante, M., Donato, V., Amirghofran, Z. and Riccardi, C., 2010. Silymarin suppress CD4+ T cell activation and proliferation: effects on NF-kappaB activity and IL-2 production. Pharmacological Research 61: 405-409.

Gimeno, I.M. and Schat, K.A., 2018. Virus-induced immunosuppression in chickens. Avian Diseases 62: 272-285.

Giorgi, V.S.I., Peracoli, M.T.S., Peracoli, J.C., Witkin, S.S. and Bannwart-Castro, C.F., 2012. Silibinin modulates the NF-κb pathway and pro-inflammatory cytokine production by mononuclear cells from preeclamptic women. Journal of Reproductive Immunology 95: 67-72.

Giridharan, S. and Srinivasan, M., 2018. Mechanisms of NF-κB p65 and strategies for therapeutic manipulation. Journal of Inflammation Research 11: 407-419.

Gloire, G., Legrand-Poels, S. and Piette, J., 2006. NF-kappaB activation by reactive oxygen species: fifteen years later. Biochemical Pharmacology 72: 1493-1505.

Gloire, G. and Piette, J., 2009. Redox regulation of nuclear post-translational modifications during NF-kappaB activation. Antioxidants & Redox Signaling 11: 2209-2222.

Grilli, M. and Memo, M., 1997. Transcriptional pharmacology of neurodegenerative disorders: novel venue towards neuroprotection against excitotoxicity? Molecular Psychiatry 2: 192-194.

Gupta, S.C., Tyagi, A.K., Deshmukh-Taskar, P., Hinojosa, M., Prasad, S. and Aggarwal, B.B., 2014. Downregulation of tumor necrosis factor and other proinflammatory biomarkers by polyphenols. Archives of Biochemistry and Biophysics 559: 91-99.

Hayden, M.S. and Ghosh, S., 2014. Regulation of NF-κB by TNF family cytokines. Seminars in Immunology 26: 253-266.

He, Y., Xia, Z., Yu, D., Wang, J., Jin, L., Huang, D., Ye, X., Li, X. and Zhang, B., 2019. Hepatoprotective effects and structure-activity relationship of five flavonoids against lipopolysaccharide/d-galactosamine induced acute liver failure in mice. International Immunopharmacology 68: 171-178.

Herscovitch, M., Comb, W., Ennis, T., Coleman, K., Yong, S., Armstead, B., Kalaitzidis, D., Chandani, S. and Gilmore, T.D., 2008. Intermolecular disulfide bond formation in the NEMO dimer requires Cys54 and Cys347. Biochemical and Biophysical Research Communications 367: 103-108.

Hung, H.L., Kim, A.Y., Hong, W., Rakowski, C. and Blobel, G.A., 2001. Stimulation of NF-E2 DNA binding by CREB-binding protein (CBP)-mediated acetylation. The Journal of Biological Chemistry 276: 10715-10721.

Jia, Y.N., Peng, Y.L., Zhao, Y.P., Cheng, X.F., Zhou, Y., Chai, C.L., Zeng, L.S., Pan, M.H. and Xu, L., 2019. Comparison of the hepatoprotective effects of the three main stilbenes from mulberry twigs. Journal of Agricultural and Food Chemistry 67: 5521-5529.

Jones, S.V. and Kounatidis, I., 2017. Nuclear factor-Kappa B and Alzheimer Disease, unifying genetic and environmental risk factors from cell to humans. Frontiers in Immunology 8: 1805.

Kairisalo, M., Korhonen, L., Blomgren, K. and Lindholm, D., 2007. X-linked inhibitor of apoptosis protein increases mitochondrial antioxidants through NF-kappaB activation. Biochemical and Biophysical Research Communications 364: 138-144.

Kang, D.Y., Sp, N., Do Park, K., Lee, H.K., Song, K.D. and Yang, Y.M., 2019. Silibinin inhibits *in vitro* ketosis by regulating HMGCS2 and NF-κB: elucidation of signaling molecule relationship under ketotic conditions. *In vitro* cellular & developmental biology. Animal 55: 368-375.

Kaspers, B. and Göbel, T.W., 2016. The avian immune system. In: Ratcliffe, M.J.H. (ed) Encyclopaedia of immunobiology. Elsevier, Amsterdam, the Netherlands, pp. 498-503.

Kim, B.R., Seo, H.S., Ku, J.M., Kim, G.J., Jeon, C.Y., Park, J.H., Jang, B.H., Park, S.J., Shin, Y.C. and Ko, S.G., 2013a. Silibinin inhibits the production of pro-inflammatory cytokines through inhibition of NF-κB signaling pathway in HMC-1 human mast cells. Inflammation Research 62: 941-950.

Kim, S.W., Lee, H.K., Shin, J.H and Lee, J.K., 2013b. Up-down regulation of HO-1 and iNOS gene expressions by ethyl pyruvate via recruiting p300 to Nrf2 and depriving It from p65. Free Radical Biology & Medicine 65: 468-476.

Kim, W.H., Chaudhari, A.A. and Lillehoj, H.S., 2019. Involvement of T cell immunity in avian Coccidiosis. Frontiers in Immunology 10: 2732.

Kimura, T., Kawasaki, Y., Okumura, F., Sone, T., Natsuki, R. and Isobe, M., 2009. Ethanol-induced expression of glutamate-cysteine ligase catalytic subunit gene is mediated by NF-kappaB. Toxicology Letters 185: 110-115.

Kobayashi, E.H., Suzuki, T., Funayama, R., Nagashima, T., Hayashi, M., Sekine, H., Tanaka, N., Moriguchi, T., Motohashi, H., Nakayama, K. and Yamamoto, M., 2016. Nrf2 suppresses macrophage inflammatory response by blocking proinflammatory cytokine transcription. Nature Communications 7: 11624.

Kopitar-Jerala N., 2015. Innate immune response in brain, NF-Kappa B signaling and cystatins. Frontiers in Molecular Neuroscience 8: 73.

Kurata, S., Matsumoto, M., Tsuji, Y. and Nakajima, H., 1996. Lipopolysaccharide activates transcription of the heme oxygenase gene in mouse M1 cells through oxidative activation of nuclear factor kappa B. European Journal of Biochemistry 239: 566-571.

Lambrou, G.I., Hatziagapiou, K. and Vlahopoulos, S., 2020. Inflammation and tissue homeostasis: the NF-κB system in physiology and malignant progression. Molecular Biology Reports 47: 4047-4063.

Lavrovsky, Y., Schwartzman, M.L., Levere, R.D., Kappas, A. and Abraham, N.G., 1994. Identification of binding sites for transcription factors NF-kappa B and AP-2 in the promoter region of the human heme oxygenase 1 gene. Proceedings of the National Academy of Sciences of the United States of America 91: 5987-5991.

Lee, D.F., Kuo, H.P., Liu, M., Chou, C.K., Xia, W., Du, Y., Shen, J., Chen, C.T., Huo, L., Hsu, M.C., Li, C.W., Ding, Q., Liao, T.L., Lai, C.C., Lin, A.C., Chang, Y.H., Tsai, S.F., Li, L.Y. and Hung, M.C., 2009. KEAP1 E3 ligase-mediated downregulation of NF-kappaB signaling by targeting IKKbeta. Molecular Cell 36: 131-140.

Lee, G., Park, J.S., Lee, E.J., Ahn, J.H. and Kim, H.S., 2019b. Anti-inflammatory and antioxidant mechanisms of urolithin B in activated microglia. Phytomedicine 55: 50-57.

Lee, M.T., Lin, W.C., Wang, S.Y., Lin, L.J., Yu, B. and Lee, T.T., 2018a. Evaluation of potential antioxidant and anti-inflammatory effects of Antrodia cinnamomea powder and the underlying molecular mechanisms via Nrf2- and NF-κB-dominated pathways in broiler chickens. Poultry Science 97: 2419-2434.

Lee, S.J., Nam, M.J., Lee, D.E., Park, J.W., Kang, B.S., Lee, D.S., Lee, H.S. and Kwon, O.S., 2018b. Silibinin ameliorates O-GlcNAcylation and inflammation in a mouse model of nonalcoholic steatohepatitis. International Journal of Molecular Sciences 19: 2165.

Lee, W., Yang, S., Lee, C., Park, E.K., Kim, K.M., Ku, S.K. and Bae, J.S., 2019a. Aloin reduces inflammatory gene iNOS via inhibition activity and p-STAT-1 and NF-κB. Food and Chemical Toxicology 126: 67-71.

Lepetsos, P., Papavassiliou, K.A. and Papavassiliou, A.G., 2019. Redox and NF-κB signaling in osteoarthritis. Free Radical Biology & Medicine 132: 90-100.

Li, C.C., Hsiang, C.Y., Wu, S.L. and Ho, T.Y., 2012. Identification of novel mechanisms of silymarin on the carbon tetrachloride-induced liver fibrosis in mice by nuclear factor-κB bioluminescent imaging-guided transcriptomic analysis. Food and Chemical Toxicology 50: 1568-1575.

Li, Q., Tian, Z., Wang, M., Kou, J., Wang, C., Rong, X., Li, J., Xie, X. and Pang, X., 2019a. Luteoloside attenuates neuroinflammation in focal cerebral ischemia in rats via regulation of the PPARγ/Nrf2/NF-κB signaling pathway. International Immunopharmacology 66: 309-316.

Li, X., Zhao, Y., Tian, B., Jamaluddin, M., Mitra, A., Yang, J., Rowicka, M., Brasier, A.R. and Kudlicki, A., 2014. Modulation of gene expression regulated by the transcription factor NF-κB/RelA. The Journal of Biological Chemistry 289: 11927-11944.

Li, Z., Feng, H., Wang, Y., Shen, B., Tian, Y., Wu, L., Zhang, Q., Jin, M. and Liu, G., 2019b. Rosmarinic acid protects mice from lipopolysaccharide/d-galactosamine-induced acute liver injury by inhibiting MAPKs/NF-κB and activating Nrf2/HO-1 signaling pathways. International Immunopharmacology 67: 465-472.

Lingappan, K., 2018. NF-κB in oxidative stress. Current Opinion in Toxicology 7: 81-86.

Liu, B.N., Han, B.X. and Liu, F., 2014. Neuroprotective effect of pAkt and HIF-1α on ischemia rats. Asian Pacific Journal of Tropical Medicine 7: 221-225.

Liu, G.H., Qu, J. and Shen, X., 2008. NF-kappaB/p65 antagonizes Nrf2-ARE pathway by depriving CBP from Nrf2 and facilitating recruitment of HDAC3 to MafK. Biochimica et Biophysica Acta 1783: 713-727.

Liu, K., Zhou, S., Liu, J., Wang, Y., Zhu, F. and Liu, M., 2019a. Silibinin attenuates high-fat diet-induced renal fibrosis of diabetic nephropathy. Drug design, development and therapy, 13, 3117-3126.

Liu, L., Fu, C., Yan, M., Xie, H., Li, S., Yu, Q., He, S. and He, J., 2016. Resveratrol modulates intestinal morphology and HSP70/90, NF-κB and EGF expression in the jejunal mucosa of black-boned chickens on exposure to circular heat stress. Food & Function 7: 1329-1338.

Liu, T.G., Sha, K.H., Zhang, L.G., Liu, X.X., Yang, F. and Cheng, J.Y., 2019b. Protective effects of alpinetin on lipopolysaccharide/d-Galactosamine-induced liver injury through inhibiting inflammatory and oxidative responses. Microbial Pathogenesis 126: 239-244.

Luo, Z., Zheng, B., Jiang, B., Xue, X., Xue, E. and Zhou, Y., 2019. Peiminine inhibits the IL-1β induced inflammatory response in mouse articular chondrocytes and ameliorates murine osteoarthritis. Food & Function 10: 2198-2208.

Lushchak, V.I., 2011. Adaptive response to oxidative stress: Bacteria, fungi, plants and animals. Comparative Biochemistry and Physiology. Toxicology & Pharmacology 153: 175-190.

Manna, S.K., Mukhopadhyay, A., Van, N.T. and Aggarwal, B.B., 1999. Silymarin suppresses TNF-induced activation of NF-κB, c-Jun N-terminal kinase, and apoptosis. The Journal of Immunology 163: 6800-6809.

Matias, M.L., Gomes, V.J., Romao-Veiga, M., Ribeiro, V.R., Nunes, P.R., Romagnoli, G.G., Peracoli, J.C. and Peracoli, M., 2019. Silibinin downregulates the NF-κB pathway and NLRP1/NLRP3 inflammasomes in monocytes from pregnant women with preeclampsia. Molecules 24: 1548.

Mauro, C., Leow, S.C., Anso, E., Rocha, S., Thotakura, A.K., Tornatore, L., Moretti, M., De Smaele, E., Beg, A.A., Tergaonkar, V., Chandel, N.S. and Franzoso, G., 2011. NF-κB controls energy homeostasis and metabolic adaptation by upregulating mitochondrial respiration. Nature Cell Biology 13: 1272-1279.

Mc Guire, C., Prinz, M., Beyaert, R. and van Loo, G., 2013. Nuclear factor kappa B (NF-κB) in multiple sclerosis pathology. Trends in Molecular Medicine 19: 604-613.

Meng, Q. and Cai, D., 2011. Defective hypothalamic autophagy directs the central pathogenesis of obesity via the IkappaB kinase beta (IKKbeta)/NF-kappaB pathway. The Journal of Biological Chemistry 286: 32324-32332.

Moldogazieva, N.T., Mokhosoev, I.M., Feldman, N.B. and Lutsenko, S.V., 2018. ROS and RNS signalling: adaptive redox switches through oxidative/nitrosative protein modifications. Free Radical Research 52: 507-543.

Morgan, M.J. and Liu, Z.G., 2011. Crosstalk of reactive oxygen species and NF-κB signaling. Cell Research 21: 103-115.

Muhammad, T., Ikram, M., Ullah, R., Rehman, S.U. and Kim, M.O., 2019. Hesperetin, a citrus flavonoid, attenuates LPS-induced neuroinflammation, apoptosis and memory impairments by modulating TLR4/NF-κB signaling. Nutrients 11: 648.

Mulcahy, R.T., Wartman, M.A., Bailey, H.H. and Gipp, J.J., 1997. Constitutive and beta-naphthoflavone-induced expression of the human gamma-glutamylcysteine synthetase heavy subunit gene is regulated by a distal antioxidant response element/TRE sequence. The Journal of Biological Chemistry 272: 7445-7454.

Muri, J. and Kopf, M., 2021. Redox regulation of immunometabolism. Nature Reviews Immunology 21: 363-381.

Nelson, R.H. and Nelson, D.E., 2018. Signal distortion: How intracellular pathogens alter host cell fate by modulating NF-κB dynamics. Frontiers in Immunology 9: 2962.

Niederberger, E. and Geisslinger, G., 2013. Proteomics and NF-κB: an update. Expert Review of Proteomics 10: 189-204.

Oskoueian, E., Abdullah, N., Idrus, Z., Ebrahimi, M., Goh, Y.M., Shakeri, M. and Oskoueian, A., 2014. Palm kernel cake extract exerts hepatoprotective activity in heat-induced oxidative stress in chicken hepatocytes. BMC Complementary and Alternative Medicine 14: 368.

Ou, Q., Weng, Y., Wang, S., Zhao, Y., Zhang, F., Zhou, J. and Wu, X., 2018. Silybin alleviates hepatic steatosis and fibrosis in NASH mice by inhibiting oxidative stress and involvement with the Nf-κB pathway. Digestive Diseases and Sciences 63: 3398-3408.

Pal, S., Bhattacharjee, A., Ali, A., Mandal, N.C., Mandal, S.C. and Pal, M., 2014. Chronic inflammation and cancer: potential chemoprevention through nuclear factor kappa B and p53 mutual antagonism. Journal of Inflammation 11: 23.

Park, Y.H., 2017. The nuclear factor-kappa B pathway and response to treatment in breast cancer. Pharmacogenomics 18: 1697-1709.

Patel, M., Horgan, P.G., McMillan, D.C. and Edwards, J., 2018. NF-κB pathways in the development and progression of colorectal cancer. Translational Research 197: 43-56.

Pedruzzi, L.M., Stockler-Pinto, M.B., Leite Jr. M. and Mafra, D., 2012. Nrf2-keap1 system versus NF-κB: The good and the evil in chronic kidney disease? Biochimie 94: 2461-2466.

Prabu, S.M. and Muthumani, M., 2012. Silibinin ameliorates arsenic induced nephrotoxicity by abrogation of oxidative stress, inflammation and apoptosis in rats. Molecular Biology Reports 39: 11201-11216.

Rabie, N.S. and Amin Girh, Z., 2020. Bacterial vaccines in poultry. Bulletin of the National Research Centre 44: 1-7.

Ramasamy, K. and Agarwal, R., 2008. Multitargeted therapy of cancer by silymarin. Cancer Letters 269: 352-362.

Ren, J., Li, L., Wang, Y., Zhai, J., Chen, G. and Hu, K., 2019. Gambogic acid induces heme oxygenase-1 through Nrf2 signaling pathway and inhibits NF-κB and MAPK activation to reduce inflammation in LPS-activated RAW264.7 cells. Biomedicine & Pharmacotherapy 109: 555-562.

Reuter, S., Gupta, S.C., Chaturvedi, M.M. and Aggarwal, B.B., 2010. Oxidative stress, inflammation, and cancer: how are they linked?. Free Radical Biology & Medicine 49: 1603-1616.

Rushworth, S.A., Shah, S. and MacEwan, D.J., 2011. TNF mediates the sustained activation of Nrf2 in human monocytes. Journal of Immunology 187: 702-707.

Rushworth, S.A., Zaitseva, L., Murray, M.Y.; Shah, N.M., Bowles, K.M. and MacEwan, D.J., 2012. The high Nrf2 expression in human acute myeloid leukaemia is driven by NF-kappaB and underlies its chemo-resistance. Blood 120: 5188-5198.

Saha, S., Buttari, B., Panieri, E., Profumo, E. and Saso, L., 2020. An overview of Nrf2 signaling pathway and its role in inflammation. Molecules 25: 5474.

Sahin, K., Orhan, C., Akdemir, F., Tuzcu, M., Iben, C. and Sahin, N., 2012. Resveratrol protects quail hepatocytes against heat stress: modulation of the Nrf2 transcription factor and heat shock proteins. Journal of Animal Physiology and Animal Nutrition 96: 66-74.

Salama, S.M., Abdulla, M.A., Al Rashdi, A.S. and Hadi, A.H.A., 2013. Mechanism of hepatoprotective effect of Boesenbergia rotunda in thioacetamide-induced liver damage in rats. Evidence-Based Complementary and Alternative Medicine 2013: 157456.

Salamone, F., Galvano, F., Marino, A., Paternostro, C., Tibullo, D., Bucchieri, F., Mangiameli, A., Parola, M., Bugianesi, E. and Volti, G.L., 2012. Silibinin improves hepatic and myocardial injury in mice with nonalcoholic steatohepatitis. Digestive and Liver Disease 44: 334-342.

Salles, A., Romano, A. and Freudenthal, R., 2014. Synaptic NF-kappa B pathway in neuronal plasticity and memory. Journal of Physiology 108: 256-262.

Schijns, V.E.; van de Zande, S.; Lupiani, B.; Reddy, S.M. Practical aspects of poultry vaccination. In: Schat, K.A., Kaspers, B. and Kaiser, P. (eds) Avian immunology. Academic Press, Cambridge, MA, USA, pp. 345-362.

Scott, O. and Roifman, C.M., 2019. NF-κB pathway and the Goldilocks principle: Lessons from human disorders of immunity and inflammation. The Journal of Allergy and Clinical Immunology 143: 1688-1701.

Sehnert, B., Burkhardt, H., Dübel, S. and Voll, R.E., 2020. Cell-type targeted NF-kappaB inhibition for the treatment of inflammatory diseases. Cells 9: 1627.

Sen, R. and Baltimore, D., 1986. Multiple nuclear factors interact with the immunoglobulin enhancer sequences. Cell 46: 705-716.

Sha, W.C., Liou, H.C., Tuomanen, E.I. and Baltimore, D., 1995. Targeted disruption of the p50 subunit of NF-κB leads to multifocal defects in immune responses. Cell 80: 321-330.

Sies, H. and Jones, D.P., 2020. Reactive oxygen species (ROS) as pleiotropic physiological signalling agents. Nature Reviews. Molecular Cell Biology 21: 363-383.

Sivandzade, F., Prasad, S., Bhalerao, A. and Cucullo, L., 2019. NRF2 and NF-κB interplay in cerebrovascular and neurodegenerative disorders: Molecular mechanisms and possible therapeutic approaches. Redox Biology 21: 101059.

Soares, M.P., Seldon, M.P., Gregoire, I.P., Vassilevskaia, T., Berberat, P.O., Yu, J., Tsui, T.Y. and Bach, F.H., 2004. Hemeoxygenase-1 modulates the expression of adhesion molecules associated with endothelial cell activation. Journal of Immunology 172: 3553-3563.

Stevenson, D.E. and Hurst, R.D., 2007. Polyphenolic phytochemicals-just antioxidants or much more?. Cellular and Molecular Life Sciences 64: 2900-2916.

Sun, S.C., 2017. The non-canonical NF-κB pathway in immunity and inflammation. Nature Reviews. Immunology 17: 545-558.

Surai, P.F., 2014. Polyphenol compounds in the chicken/animal diet: from the past to the future. Journal of Animal Physiology and Animal Nutrition 98: 19-31.

Surai, P.F., 2015a. Antioxidant action of carnitine: molecular mechanisms and practical applications. EC Veterinary Science 2: 66-84.

Surai, P.F., 2015b. Carnitine enigma: from antioxidant action to vitagene regulation. Part 1. Absorption, metabolism and antioxidant activities. Journal of Veterinary Science & Medicine 3, 2: 14.

Surai, P.F., 2015c. Carnitine enigma: from antioxidant action to vitagene regulation. Part 2. Transcription factors and practical applications. Journal of Veterinary Science & Medicine 3, 2: 17.

Surai, P.F., 2015d. Silymarin as a natural antioxidant: an overview of the current evidence and perspectives. Antioxidants 4: 204-247.

Surai, P.F., 2018. Selenium in poultry nutrition and health. Wageningen Academic Publishers, Wageningen, The Netherlands.

Surai, P.F., 2020. Vitagene in avian biology and poultry health. Wageningen Academic Publishers, Wageningen, The Netherlands.

Surai, P.F. (Ed), 2021. Selenium in pig nutrition and health. Wageningen Academic Publishers: Wageningen, The Netherlands.

Surai, P.F., Earle-Payne, K. and Kidd, M.T., 2021b. Taurine as a natural antioxidant: From direct antioxidant effects to protective action in various toxicological models. Antioxidants 10: 1876.

Surai, P.F. and Fisinin, V.I., 2016a. Vitagenes in poultry production. Part 3. Vitagene concept development. World's Poultry Science Journal 72, 793-804.

Surai, P.F. and Fisinin, V.I., 2016b. Antioxidant system regulation: from vitamins to vitagenes. In: Watson, R.R. and De Meester, F. (eds) Handbook of cholesterol. Wageningen Academic Publishers, Wageningen, the Netherlands, pp. 451-481.

Surai, P.F. and Kochish, I.I., 2019. Nutritional modulation of the antioxidant capacities in poultry: the case of selenium. Poultry Science 98: 4231-4239.

Surai, P.F. and Kochish, I.I., 2020. Carotenoids in Aviculture. In: Jacob-Lopes, E., Queiroz, M.I. and Zepka, L.Q. (eds) Pigments from microalgae handbook. Springer Nature Switzerland, Cham, Switzerland, pp. 515-540.

Surai, P.F., Kochish, I.I. and Fisinin, V.I., 2017. Antioxidant systems in poultry biology: nutritional modulation of vitagenes. European Journal of Poultry Science 81: 1612-9199.

Surai, P.F., Kochish, I.I., Fisinin, V.I., Grozina, A.A. and Shatskikh E.V., 2018. Molecular mechanisms of chicken gut health maintenance: role of microbiota. Agricultural Technologies, Moscow, Russia.

Surai, P.F., Kochish, I.I., Fisinin, V.I. and Kidd, M.T., 2019b. Antioxidant defence systems and oxidative stress in poultry biology: An update. Antioxidants 8; 235.

Surai, P.F., Kochish, I.I. and Kidd, M.T., 2020. Taurine in poultry nutrition. Animal Feed Science and Technology 260: 114339.

Surai, P.F., Kochish, I.I. and Kidd, M.T., 2021a. Redox homeostasis in poultry: Regulatory roles of NF-κB. Antioxidants 10: 186.

Surai, P.F., Kochish, I.I., Romanov, M.N. and Griffin, D.K., 2019a. Nutritional modulation of the antioxidant capacities in poultry: the case of vitamin E. Poultry Science, 98: 4030-4041.

Tang, F., Fan, K., Wang, K. and Bian, C., 2019. Amygdalin attenuates acute liver injury induced by D-galactosamine and lipopolysaccharide by regulating the NLRP3, NF-κB and Nrf2/NQO1 signalling pathways. Biomedicine & Pharmacotherapy 111: 527-536.

Thimmulappa, R.K., Lee, H., Rangasamy, T., Reddy, S.P., Yamamoto, M., Kensler, T.W. and Biswal, S., 2006. Nrf2 is a critical regulator of the innate immune response and survival during experimental sepsis. The Journal of Clinical Investigation 116: 984-995.

Thoma, A. and Lightfoot, A.P., 2018. NF-κB and inflammatory cytokine signalling: Role in skeletal muscle atrophy. Advances in Experimental Medicine and Biology 1088: 267-279.

Tilborghs, S., Corthouts, J., Verhoeven, Y., Arias, D., Rolfo, C., Trinh, X.B. and van Dam, P.A., 2017. The role of Nuclear Factor-kappa B signaling in human cervical cancer. Critical Reviews in Oncology/Hematology 120: 141-150.

Tkach, K.E., Oyler, J.E. and Altan-Bonnet, G., 2014. Cracking the NF-κB code. Science Signaling 7: pe5.

Tornatore, L., Thotakura, A.K., Bennett, J., Moretti, M. and Franzoso, G., 2012. The nuclear factor kappa B signaling pathway: integrating metabolism with inflammation. Trends in Cell Biology 22: 557-566.

Tsai, M.J., Liao, J.F., Lin, D.Y., Huang, M.C., Liou, D.Y., Yang, H.C., Lee, H.J., Chen, Y.T., Chi, C.W., Huang, W.C. and Cheng, H., 2010. Silymarin protects spinal cord and cortical cells against oxidative stress and lipopolysaccharide stimulation. Neurochemistry International 57: 867-875.

Wakabayashi, N., Slocum, S.L., Skoko, J.J., Shin, S. and Kensler, T.W., 2010. When NRF2 talks, who's listening?. Antioxidants & Redox Signaling 13: 1649-1663.

Wang, G.W., Zhang, X.L., Wu, Q.H., Jin, Y.B., Ning, C.T., Wang, R., Mao, J.X. and Chen, M., 2019. The hepatoprotective effects of Sedum sarmentosum extract and its isolated major constituent through Nrf2 activation and NF-κB inhibition. Phytomedicine 53: 263-273.

Wang, Q., Liu, M., Liu, W.W., Hao, W.B., Tashiro, S.I., Onodera, S. and Ikejima, T., 2012. *In vivo* recovery effect of silibinin treatment on streptozotocin-induced diabetic mice is associated with the modulations of Sirt-1 expression and autophagy in pancreatic β-cell. Journal of Asian Natural Products Research 14: 413-423.

Wang, Q., Zou, L., Liu, W., Hao, W., Tashiro, S.I., Onodera, S. and Ikejima, T., 2011. Inhibiting NF-κB activation and ROS production are involved in the mechanism of silibinin's protection against D-galactose-induced senescence. Pharmacology Biochemistry and Behavior 98: 140-149.

Wang, X. and Hai, C., 2016. Novel insights into redox system and the mechanism of redox regulation. Molecular Biology Reports 43: 607-628.

Wu, J., Ding, J., Yang, J., Guo, X. and Zheng, Y., 2018. MicroRNA roles in the nuclear factor kappa B signaling pathway in cancer. Frontiers in Immunology 9, 546.

Wu, M., Bian, Q., Liu, Y., Fernandes, A.F., Taylor, A., Pereira, P. and Shang, F., 2009. Sustained oxidative stress inhibits NF-kappaB activation partially via inactivating the proteasome. Free Radical Biology & Medicine 46: 62-69.

Wu, Y., Lin, Z., Yan, Z., Wang, Z., Fu, X. and Yu, K., 2019. Sinomenine contributes to the inhibition of the inflammatory response and the improvement of osteoarthritis in mouse-cartilage cells by acting on the Nrf2/HO-1 and NF-κB signaling pathways. International Immunopharmacology 75: 105715.

Yan, J., Zhang, H., Yin, Y., Li, J., Tang, Y., Purkayastha, S., Li, L. and Cai, D., 2014. Obesity- and aging-induced excess of central transforming growth factor-β potentiates diabetic development via an RNA stress response. Nature Medicine 20: 1001-1008.

Yang, H., Magilnick, N., Ou, X. and Lu, S.C., 2005. Tumour necrosis factor alpha induces co-ordinated activation of rat GSH synthetic enzymes via nuclear factor kappaB and activator protein-1. The Biochemical Journal 391: 399-408.

Yang, J.X., Maria, T.C., Zhou, B., Xiao, F.L., Wang, M., Mao, Y.J. and Li, Y., 2020. Quercetin improves immune function in Arbor Acre broilers through activation of NF-κB signaling pathway. Poultry Science 99: 906-913.

Ye, J., Guan, M., Lu, Y., Zhang, D., Li, C. and Zhou, C., 2019. Arbutin attenuates LPS-induced lung injury via Sirt1/Nrf2/NF-κBp65 pathway. Pulmonary Pharmacology & Therapeutics 54: 53-59.

Yerra, V.G., Negi, G., Sharma, S.S. and Kumar, A., 2013. Potential therapeutic effects of the simultaneous targeting of the Nrf2 and NF-κB pathways in diabetic neuropathy. Redox Biology 1: 394-397.

Yu, H., Lin, L., Zhang, Z., Zhang, H. and Hu, H., 2020. Targeting NF-κB pathway for the therapy of diseases: mechanism and clinical study. Signal Transduction and Targeted Therapy 5: 209.

Zhang, C., Tian, Y., Yan, F., Kang, X., Han, R., Sun, G. and Zhang, H., 2014. Modulation of growth and immunity by dietary supplementation with resveratrol in young chickens receiving conventional vaccinations. American Journal of Veterinary Research 75: 752-759.

Zhang, H.F., Wang, J.H., Wang, Y.L., Gao, C., Gu, Y.T., Huang, J., Wang, J.H. and Zhang, Z., 2019c. Salvianolic acid A protects the kidney against oxidative stress by activating the Akt/GSK-3β/Nrf2 signaling pathway and inhibiting the NF-κB signaling pathway in 5/6 nephrectomized rats. Oxidative Medicine and Cellular Longevity 2019: 2853534.

Zhang, L., Xiao, X., Arnold, P.R. and Li, X.C., 2019b. Transcriptional and epigenetic regulation of immune tolerance: roles of the NF-κB family members. Cellular & Molecular Immunology 16: 315-323.

Zhang, L., Yousefzadeh, M.J., Suh, Y., Niedernhofer, L.J. and Robbins, P.D., 2019a. Signal transduction, ageing and disease. Sub-Cellular Biochemistry 91: 227-247.

Zhang, Q., Lenardo, M.J. and Baltimore, D., 2017. 30 years of NF-κB: A blossoming of relevance to human pathobiology. Cell 168: 37-57.

Zhang, X., Zhang, G., Zhang, H., Karin, M., Bai, H. and Cai, D., 2008. Hypothalamic IKKbeta/NF-kappaB and ER stress link overnutrition to energy imbalance and obesity. Cell 135: 61-73.

Zhao, D.R., Jiang, Y.S., Sun, J.Y., Li, H.H., Luo, X.L. and Zhao, M.M., 2019. Anti-inflammatory mechanism involved in 4-ethylguaiacol-mediated inhibition of LPS-induced inflammation in THP-1 cells. Journal of Agricultural and Food Chemistry 67: 1230-1243.

Chapter 7
Silymarin and vitagenes

What is worth doing at all is worth doing well

*Anton Surai[1] and Peter F. Surai[2-7]**
[1]Healthy Food Services, Bristol, UK; [2]Vitagene and Health Research Centre, Bristol, UK; [3]Department of Microbiology and Biochemistry, Faculty of Veterinary Medicine, Trakia University, Stara Zagora, Bulgaria; [4]Department of Animal Nutrition, Faculty of Agricultural and Environmental Sciences, Szent Istvan University, Hungary; [5]Saint-Petersburg State Academy of Veterinary Medicine, St. Petersburg, Russia; [6]Sumy National Agrarian University, Sumy, Ukraine; [7]Odessa National Academy of Food Technologies, Odessa, Ukraine
psurai@feedfood.co.uk

Abstract

Vitagenes are a group of redox-sensitive genes that are strictly involved in stress sensing and creating adaptive stress response to preserve cellular homeostasis by inducing synthesis of an array of protective molecules such as heat shock proteins (HSP), namely HO-1 and HSP70; SOD (SOD1, SOD2 and SOD3); elements of thioredoxin system (Trx, TrxR, Prx and Srx); members of glutathione system (GSH, GR, GPx and Grx) and sirtuins. The vitagene network together with a range of transcription factors represent the major cellular pathway involved in redox balance maintenance, providing an effective protection against oxidative stress and toxic products of RONS metabolism. This chapter presents evidence of protective effects of silymarin (SM) under various stress conditions via prevention of inactivation of the vitagene network. Indeed, SM was shown to preserve stress-compromised SOD, HO-1, HSP70, Trx, TrxR, GSH, GR, GPx, SIRT1, SIRT2 and SIRT3. Protective effects of SM on SOD were proven in various *in vitro* and *in vivo* model systems, including hepatotoxicity induced by CCL4, by metals and by other dietary compounds; neurotoxicity models; cardio-, nephro-, lung, gastric and testicular toxicity models; various stress models; ischemia/reperfusion injury and animal reproduction models. Silymarin was demonstrated to upregulate HO-1 and improve antioxidant defences in Cd-induced toxicity models. SM is also shown to decrease HSP70 expression in stressed cells indicating improved AO defences and decrease stress by other means. It was also proven that the ability of SM to maintain activity of Trx- and GSH- systems in stress conditions is an important element of improving the adaptive ability of animals/humans via the vitagene network. There are also several recent publications showing a regulatory role of SM in the sirtuin functions. Further research is needed to fully understand the molecular mechanisms involved in the vitagene network activation by SM.

Keywords: silymarin, vitagenes, redox homeostasis, stress models

DOI:10.3920/978-90-8686-944-2_007,

7.1 Introduction

The term 'vitagene' was introduced in 1998 by Rattan who wrote 'Our survival and the physical quality of life depends upon an efficient functioning of various maintenance and repair processes. This complex network of the so-called longevity assurance processes is composed of several genes, which may be called *vitagenes*'. Later vitagene concept has been further developed in medical sciences by Calabrese and colleagues (Calabrese *et al.*, 2004; 2007; 2009a,b; 2014) and was adapted to poultry/animal sciences (Surai, 2020a,b; Surai and Fisinin, 2016a,b; Surai *et al.*, 2019; 2021a) and major prosurvival mechanisms controlled by homodynamic vitagene network are shown in Figure 7.1.

7.2 Vitagene family

In accordance with Calabrese *et al.* (2007; 2009a,b; 2014), Surai and Fisinin (2016a,b) and Surai (2016; 2019; 2020a,b,c) the term vitagenes refers to a group of redox-sensitive genes that are strictly involved in stress sensing and preserving cellular adaptive homeostasis and the vitagene family includes:

- Heat shock proteins (HSP): HO-1, HSP70.
- SOD: SOD1, SOD2, SOD3.

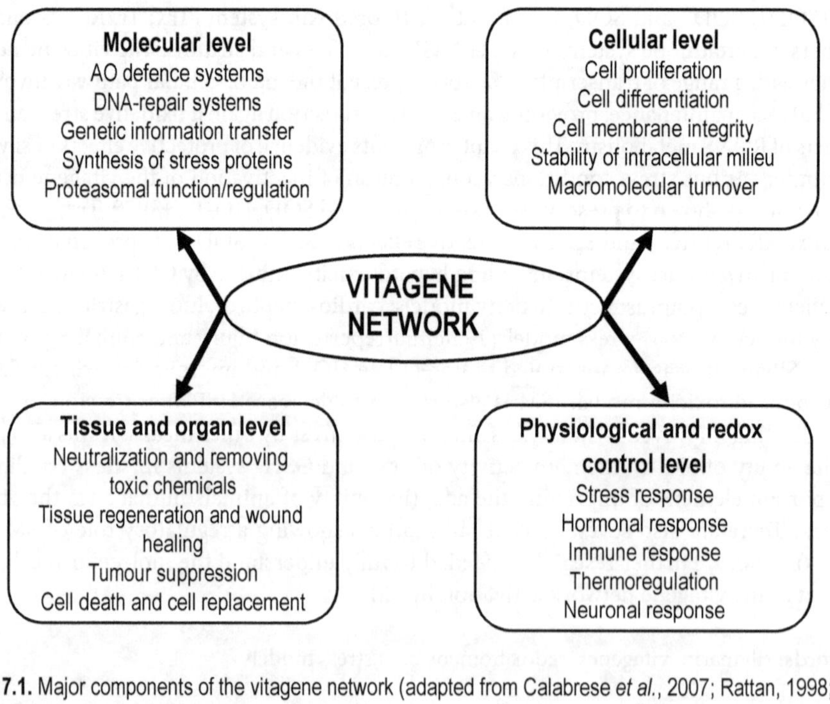

Figure 7.1. Major components of the vitagene network (adapted from Calabrese *et al.*, 2007; Rattan, 1998; Surai, 2018a; 2019; Surai 2020a; Surai and Fisinin, 2016a).

- Thioredoxin system: Trx, TrxR, Prx, Srx.
- Glutathione system: GSH, GR, GPx, Grx.
- Sirtuins: SIRT1, SIRT2, SIRT3, SIRT4, SIRT5, SIRT6, SIRT7.

The products of the above-mentioned genes actively operate in detecting and controlling diverse forms of stress and cell injuries by regulation of synthesis of an array of protective molecules. The cooperative mechanisms of the vitagene network are reviewed in recently published comprehensive reviews (Calabrese *et al.*, 2014; Trovato Salinaro *et al.*, 2014) with a major conclusion indicating an essential regulatory role of the vitagene network in cell and whole organism adaptation to various stresses. Increasing evidences have demonstrated that cellular stress response is mediated via the regulation of pro-survival pathways and vitagene activation with the following synthesis of a range of protective antioxidant molecules is the central event in such an adaptation. The vitagene concept found its acceptance in medical sciences, including neurodegenerative disorders (Calabrese *et al.*, 2004; 2009a; 2017; Ontario *et al.*, 2022; Scuto *et al.*, 2022a; Siracusa *et al.*, 2022), aging and longevity (Calabrese *et al.*, 2007; 2011; 2012; 2014; 2015; Bucciantini *et al.*, 2022), dermatology (Calabrese *et al.*, 2008), free radical-related diseases (Calabrese *et al.*, 2010), osteoporosis and Alzheimer pathology (Cornelius *et al.*, 2013; 2014; Dattilo *et al.*, 2015; Trovato *et al.*, 2016a,b), autism (Calabrese *et al.*, 2016a), vascular dementia (Calabrese *et al.*, 2016b), kidney disorders (Calabrese *et al.*, 2020; Chen *et al.*, 2019) and cancer (Scuto *et al.*, 2021; 2022b).

The vitagene concept in relation to poultry production was further developed in our previous publications (Fisinin and Surai, 2011a,b; Surai, 2015a,b,c; 2016; 2018b; 2020a,b,c; 2022; Surai and Earle-Payne, 2022; Surai and Fisinin, 2012a,b; Surai *et al.*, 2017; 2018; 2019; 2021a,b,c). It seems likely that by upregulating the vitagenes and improving adaptive ability of animals to stress it is possible to decrease negative consequences of various stresses in poultry and farm animal production. By upregulating the vitagenes and improving adaptive ability of animals to stress it is possible to decrease negative consequences of the four major types of stresses in poultry and farm animal production. Furthermore, there is an opportunity to nutritionally modulate the vitagene network by using various natural antioxidants: carnitine (Calabrese *et al.*, 2009b; Surai, 2015a,b), betaine, vitamins A, E, D, C (Surai *et al.*, 2017), TAU (Surai, 2018b; Surai *et al.*, 2018; 2020; 2021b), phytochemicals (Calabrese *et al.*, 2012), including SM (Surai, 2015c) and other nutrients. In this regard, activation of the vitagene network by nutritional means is considered as a fundamental mechanism for improving animal/poultry resistance to various stresses (Surai and Fisinin, 2016a,b; Surai *et al.*, 2017).

As can be seen from Figure 7.2 vitagenes provide optimal conditions for redox signalling, redox homeostasis being major players in cell/organism adaptation to various stresses.

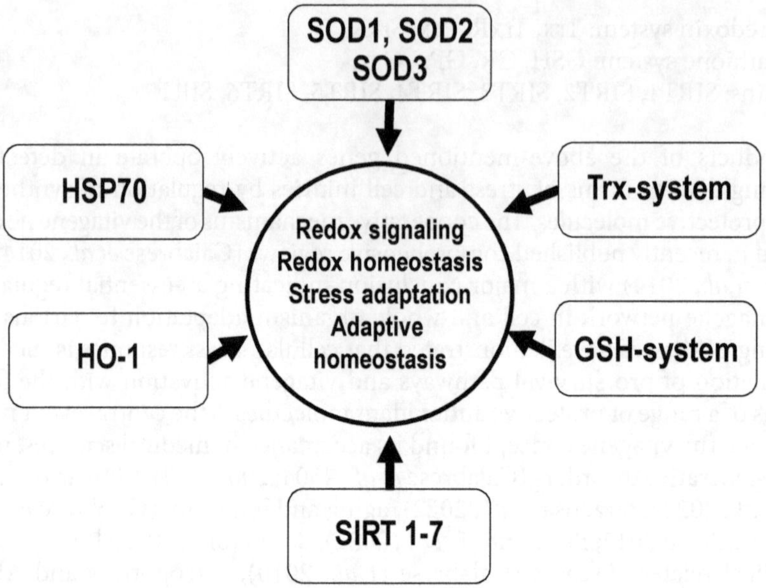

Figure 7.2. Protective roles of vitagenes in adaptive homeostasis.

7.3 Effect of silymarin on vitagene expression

Emerging findings suggest a large number of potential mechanisms of action of SM (polyphenols) in preventing disease, which may be beyond their direct conventional antioxidant activities. It seems likely that SM, similar to other flavonoids, can affect the vitagene network. The recent relevant findings are reviewed below.

7.3.1 SOD

To study protective effects of SM/SB in oxidative stress related conditions various toxic models were used. Growing evidence indicates that toxicants can induce oxidative stress compromising vitagene expression and respective antioxidant enzyme activities, including SOD. By using SM/SB in *in vitro* and *in vivo* toxicological models protective actions of SM/SB were clearly proven.

7.3.1.1 *In vitro* studies

SM (100μM) was shown to attenuate PQ-induced cytotoxicity in macrophages by ameliorating decreased activities of SOD and GPx (Liu *et al.*, 2018). Ochratoxin A-induced oxidative stress in primary chicken hepatocytes was reported to be mitigated by SM as evidenced by a significant attenuation of compromised/decreased SOD activity and GSH content (Yu *et al.*, 2018). In AML12 hepatocytes *in vitro* SB nanoparticles were illustrated to increase SOD2 activity (Durymanov *et al.*, 2020). In trophoblast cells SB was indicated to ameliorate H_2O_2-induced oxidative stress response by activating Nrf2 signalling (increasing the expression levels of HO-1 and quinone oxidoreductase 1) and restoring SOD activity and mitochondrial membrane potential (Guo *et al.*, 2020). SB (1, 5, and 10 μM) was indicated to have protective effects against H_2O_2-induced oxidative damage in SH-SY5Y cells by increasing SOD activity and improving mitochondrial function (Tie *et al.*, 2022). In a model of oxidative stress-stimulated neurotoxicity associated with Alzheimer's disease based on LPS-treated neuron-like cells (SH-SY5Y), inclusion of SB (50 μg/ml) or SB encapsulated into human serum albumin (silibinin-HAS) nanoparticles led to the activation of SOD and CAT, increase of GSH content, and reduction of ROS level, Caspase-3 activity with simultaneous recovery of cell viability (Pan *et al.*, 2021).

7.3.1.2 *In vivo* studies

CCl_4 hepatotoxicity

In a model of CCl_4-induced rat liver damage both SM and TAU were shown to have protective effects by ameliorating decreased activities of AO enzymes (SOD, GPx, GR and GST) in the liver. Interestingly, the combined post-treatment with TAU+SM showed the best protective results in comparison to monotherapy (Abdel-Moneim *et al.*, 2015). In a mouse model of CCl_4-toxicity SM (25 and 50 mg/kg) was found to attenuate decreased activity of SOD and GSH content in the liver (Tung *et al.*, 2019). Similarly, in broiler chickens SM (100 mg/kg) showed protective effects. The protection was associated with restoration of the antioxidant defences in the liver as indicated by amelioration of CCl_4-induced inhibition of the expression of SOD, GPx and CAT (Baradaran *et al.*, 2019).

Metal-induced hepatotoxicity

SM (200 mg/kg) was shown to attenuate lead-induced decrease in SOD and GPx activities in the rat liver (Jalali *et al.*, 2017). Similarly, SM in lower doses (50 and 100 mg/kg) was found to dose-dependently decrease the toxic effects of lead acetate on the liver and kidneys through ameliorating lead-induced decrease in hepatic and renal SOD activity and GSH levels (Abd Eldaim *et al.*, 2021). SB and nano-SB demonstrated protective effects against lead poisoning in Male Wistar rats by increasing the compromised activities of SOD, CAT and concentrations of GSH in serum (Mohammadi *et al.*, 2022). In Cd-treated mice SM was able to ameliorate reduced activities of SOD, GPx and CAT in the testis (Faraji *et al.*, 2019). Similarly, in Cd-treated mice SM (100 mg/kg) mitigated Cd-induced reduction of activities of SOD, GPx and CAT activities (Farjad *et al.*, 2018). In a model of $AlCl_3$-prompted Alzheimer's-like disease in rats SM (200 mg/kg) was observed to partly ameliorate decreased activities of SOD, CAT and concentration GSH and mitigate increased markers of inflammation (TNF-α and IL-1β) reversing most of the histological and ultrastructural changes triggered by $AlCl_3$ in experimental animals (Aboelwafa *et al.*, 2020).

Dietary hepatotoxicity

In HFD mice SM was found to restore HFD-down-regulated activities of antioxidant enzymes (SOD, GPx and CAT) in the plasma and/or liver and showed anti-inflammatory effects as evidenced by decreased expression of NF-κB and inflammatory cytokines, including IL-1β and TNF-α (Feng *et al*, 2016). In a STZ-induced mouse model of diabetes SM was shown to ameliorate STZ-compromised/reduced SOD activity in pancreas (Stolf *et al.*, 2018). In a miniature clinical trial with hepatitis C patients, SM adjunct therapy in combination with sofosbuvir and ribavirin was found to enhance the efficiency of direct-acting antivirals and demonstrated an ameliorative effect on oxidative stress markers including SOD, TAS, GSH, GSSG, and MDA in serum (Ahmed *et al.*, 2022). Milk thistle (*Silybum marianum* L.) showed protective therapeutical effect on nonalcoholic fatty liver disease in type 2 diabetic rats indicative by significantly improved serum SOD activity and decreased lipid peroxidation (MDA) associated with amelioration of detrimental histological changes in the liver (Doostkam *et al.*, 2022).

Other models of hepatotoxicity

In D-galactosamine/LPS-induced hepatotoxicity in rats SB (100 mg/kg) was able to mitigate reduced activities of hepatic SOD, CAT and GSH levels (Hashem *et al.*, 2016). In a similar mouse model of D-galactose/LPS-induced organ damage and inflammation SM (150 mg/kg) was shown to increase the antioxidant defences (SOD, CAT, GSH, GPx, T-AOC), to improve anti-inflammatory status (IL-10, and IL-12), and to decrease lipid peroxidation (MDA) and levels of pro-inflammatory cytokines (IL-6, IL-1β, TNF-α, IFN-γ) in the mouse serum and liver tissues. This was associated with improvement of liver function indexes evidenced by reduction in alanine aminotransferase (ALT) and aspartate aminotransferase (AST) in the mouse serum (Zhao *et al.*, 2021).

In a model of triptolide (TP)-induced acute hepatotoxicity in rats SM was able to ameliorate TP-induced depletions in the activity of the antioxidant enzymes, including SOD, GPx, GST and CAT (Wang *et al.*, 2018). In a model of diclofenac-induced liver toxicity in male rats treatment with SM (100 mg/kg) was reported to significantly increase SOD, GPx and CAT activity and GSH concentration in the liver of diclofenac-treated animals (Heidarian and Nouri, 2021). In a rat model of a thioacetamide (TAA)-induced acute toxicity SM (400 mg/kg) was reported to modulate Keap1-Nrf2/HO-1 signalling and ameliorate decreased SOD activity in the liver (Hussein *et al.*, 2021).

Neurotoxicity models

Treatment with SB was found to increase GSH and SOD activity and reduce lipid peroxidation (MDA) in APP/PS1 mice (double transgenic mice where both mutations are associated with early-onset Alzheimer's disease; Bai *et al.*, 2017). Similarly, in APP/PS1 mice SB treatment was associated with a significant attenuation of the oxidative stress (increased SOD and CAT activities and decreased MDA levels) in the cerebral cortex (Bai *et al.*, 2019). In a 1-methyl-4-phenyl-1,2,3,6-tetrahydropyridine (MPTP)-induced Parkinson's disease mouse model SB (280 mg/kg) was found to ameliorates cognitive deficits by ameliorating decreased SOD activity and restoring mitochondrial membrane potential and improving mitochondrial dynamics in hippocampus (Liu *et al.*, 2021).

Pretreatment of rats with 100, 200 or 300 mg/kg of SM (daily for 5 days) before infusion of 6-hydroxydopamine (6-OHDA) into the central region of the substantia nigra pars copmacta (SNc) showed protective antioxidant effects. In particular, SM was demonstrated to attenuate 6-OHDA-induced reduction in SOD, GPx, GR and CAT activities and GSH levels in rat brain SNc (Haddadi *et al.*, 2018). In cisplatin (CS)-treated mice SB was shown to reduce lipid peroxidation while increasing SOD activity, GSH content and T-AOC in mice brain tissue associated with the improved behavioural abnormalities (Wang *et al.*, 2022). In a CS-induced rat nephrotoxicity and hepatotoxicity model SM supplementation was found to ameliorate/increase CS-compromised SOD activity in the liver and kidney tissue (Doğan *et al.*, 2022).

SM-albumin nanoplex was reported to improve its capability to reduce LPS-induced oxidative stress by restoration of SOD and increase of CAT activity in rat brain tissue (Sohrabi *et al.*, 2019). SM (125 and 159 mg/kg) was indicated to significantly ameliorate brain SOD, GPx, CAT, GSH in docetaxel (DTX)-administered rats. Furthermore, SM markedly up-regulated the expression of Nrf2, and HO-1 while downregulated the expression of NF-κB in the brain and sciatic nerve tissues of DTX-treated rats (Yardım *et al.*, 2021). The administration of SM (160 mg/kg) to arylamide-exposed rats significantly alleviated redox disruptions by restoring SOD, GPx, CAT and decreasing MDA levels in the cerebellum (Elsawy *et al.*, 2021).

Cardio-, nephro-, lung, gastric and testicular toxicity models

In a rat model of cyclophosphamide (CP)-induced cardiotoxicity SM was indicated to ameliorate CP-imposed reduction in cardiac SOD activity (Avci *et al.*, 2017). In a rat model of isoproterenol-prompted myocardial infarction SM and SM liquisolid (with improved solubility) were reported to increase cardiac SOD and reduced lipid peroxidation (MDA; Sheta *et al.*, 2020). SM showed protective effects against gentamicin-induced nephrotoxicity in rats evident by amelioration of compromised renal SOD activity and GSH content (Feng *et al.*, 2016). In PQ-induced lung injury in rats, SM was shown to restore decreased activities of SOD, GPx and CAT in lung tissue and serum simultaneously with upregulation of Nrf2 (Zhao *et al.*, 2015).

In a model of an indomethacin-induced gastric injury in rats SM (50 mg/kg) was reported to suppress oxidative stress by enhancing SOD and GPx activities and upregulating Nrf2. SM also was able to suppress gastric inflammation by decreasing expression of NF-κB, proinflammatory cytokines (TNF-α and IL-6) and reducing myeloperoxidase (MPO) activity (Arafa Keshk *et al.*, 2017). In a varicocele-induced testicular pathogenesis model SM (50 mg/kg) was found to up-regulate testicular SOD, GPx and TAC (Mazhari *et al.*, 2018). SM was also found to ameliorate acrylamide-induced oxidative stress-mediated testicular toxicity in rats via modulation of antioxidant mechanisms including attenuation of diminished testicular activities of antioxidant enzymes (e.g. SOD, GPx and CAT; Alturki *et al.*, 2022).

Various stress models

In a model of the acute restraint stress (ARS) in mice SM (100 and 200 mg/kg) was found to mitigate ARS-induced impairment in SOD and CAT activities in brain hippocampus and cerebral cortex (Thakare *et al.*, 2016). In mice subjected to chronic unpredictable mild stress for 4 weeks, SM (100 mg/kg and 200 mg/kg) was responsible for restoration of antioxidant defence system, including SOD and CAT activities, in cerebral cortex and hippocampus (Thakare *et al.*, 2018). In the serum of male half marathon athletes supplemented with aqueous extract of seeds and leaves of milk thistle a significant increase of serum SOD and CAT activity and GSH levels and reduction in the levels of MDA were reported (Boukazoula and Ayari, 2022).

Ischemia/reperfusion injury
In a model of global cerebral I/R injury in rats SM-loaded chitosan nanoparticles were shown to significantly increased the activities of SOD, GPx, CAT, GR and GSH content in I/R brain. At the same time SM was able to decrease lipid peroxidation (MDA) and inflammatory response (IL-6 and TNF-α) induced by I/R (Moghaddam *et al.*, 2020). SB phytosome treatment was proven to significantly increase SOD activity and GSH levels simultaneously with decreasing MDA, TNF-α and IL-6 levels in both the hippocampus and cortex of the ischemia-reperfusion-injured rats (Pasala *et al.*, 2022).

Animal reproduction models
In Sanjabi ewes treated with SM (2 g/kg feed for 15 d after lambing) increased activities of SOD, GPx and CAT in serum were recorded (Khamisabadi *et al.*, 2020). Micelle silymarin supplementation to sows' diet from day 109 of gestation to entire lactation period was shown to enhance their reproductive performance and affected serum AO parameters including increased serum SOD at parturition and GPx activity and GSH concentration on day 21 of lactation (Zhang *et al.*, 2021a).

7.3.2 HO-1

It was observed that SM/SB can affect HO-1 activity in different model systems. For example, As-intoxicated rats showed a significant up-regulation of myocardial NADPH (NOX) oxidase sub-units such as NOX2 and NOX4 as well as Keap1 and down-regulation of Nrf2 and vitagene HO-1 protein expressions. Pre-administration of SB (75 mg/kg/BW) recovered all these altered parameters to near normalcy in As-induced cardiotoxic rat (Muthumani and Prabu, 2014). Similarly, in a model of liver injury caused by alcohol plus pyrazole, SM administration (50 mg/kg/BW) had a protective effect with a trend in restoring the decreased activity of HO-1 and Nrf2 (Choi *et al.*, 2013). SM (250 mg/kg/BW) possesses substantial protective effect against benzo[a]pyrene (B(a)P)-induced damages by increasing (restoring) HO-1 activity (Kiruthiga *et al.*, 2015). Similarly, *in vitro* SM (500 μM) reduced tert-butyl hydroperoxide-induced hepatocyte toxicity by activating HO-1 gene expression (Cerný *et al.*, 2009). Treatment of primary human dermal fibroblasts with both SM and SB was shown to reduce UVA-stimulated ROS generation, prevent GSH depletion, moderately increased HO-1 level and reduced HSP70 level (Rajnochová Svobodová *et al.*, 2018). It has been also shown that ameliorative effects of SM on HCl-induced acute lung injury in rats was associated with activation of the Nrf-2/HO-1 pathway (Ahmed *et al.*, 2019).

The enzyme HO-1 is an important regulatory molecule present in most mammalian and avian cells. The main function of HO-1 is to break down the pro-oxidant molecule heme into three products; carbon monoxide (CO), biliverdin and free iron and actively participate in the antioxidant defence in the human/animal body (Venditti and Smith, 2014). HO-1 is a stress-inducible protein and can be induced by various oxidative and inflammatory signals. Therefore, HO-1 expression is regarded as an important adaptive cellular mechanism of AO defence in stress conditions (Ambegaokar *et al.*, 2014; Naito *et al.*, 2014). From the data presented above it is clear that SM/SB can upregulate HO-1 and improve antioxidant defences.

7.3.3 HSP

It seems likely that SM/SB can affect HSPs including HSP70. In an *in vitro* system based on CHO-K1 cells treated with As, SM (5 μM) significantly decreased HSP70 expression previously elevated by As (Bongiovanni *et al.*, 2007). In another *in vitro* system based on heat-induced chicken hepatocytes, SM (259 μM) significantly affected HSP70 expression, preventing its alleviation by heat stress (Oskoueian *et al.*, 2014). A similar protective effect of SM (100 mg/kg/BW) on HSP70 was seen in rats given SM for 7 days prior to mesenteric I/R (Demir *et al.*, 2014). It is interesting to note that SB was identified as a novel HSP90 inhibitor (Zhao *et al.*, 2011). Similarly, SM (2 g/kg feed for 15 d after lambing) was shown to decrease expression of HSP70 gene in blood serum of postparturient sanjabi ewes (Khamisabadi, 2020). Therefore, SM/SB can decrease HSP70 expression in stressed cells indicating improved AO defences and decrease stress by other means (e.g. Nrf2-related increased AO synthesis).

7.3.4 Thioredoxin system

SM can show protective effect on other vitagene-dependent antioxidants namely a thioredoxin system. Silybin-phospholipid complex containing vitamin E (Realsil) was administered daily by gavage (15 mg vitamin E and 47 mg SB complexed with phospholipids) to rats fed a choline-deprived or a HFD for 30 days and 60 days, respectively. Realsil was found to be able to maintain Trx concentration in the rat liver fed on a HFD at day 60, while in the control group it dramatically decreased (Grattagliano *et al.*, 2013). In a rat model of D-galactosamine/lipopolysaccharide induced hepatotoxicity SB was able to increase expression of Trx1 and TrxR1 in the liver of experimental animals (Hashem *et al.*, 2016).

SM was shown to attenuate PQ-induced cytotoxicity in macrophage by regulating Trx/ thioredoxin interacting protein (TXNIP) complex (promoted the expression of Trx and antioxidant enzymes and suppress the TXNIP) and inhibiting NLRP3 inflammasome activation and apoptosis (Liu *et al.*, 2018). It is well accepted that the ability of SM to maintain Trx system in stress conditions is an important element of improving the adaptive ability of animals/humans via the vitagene network.

7.3.5 Glutathione system

In the above section devoted to SOD protective effects of SM/SB on main elements of the glutathione system, namely GSH, GPx and GR, have been described. In most model systema SM/SB effects on SOD and the glutathione systems were the same: amelioration of stress-induced deceases in GSH concentration and GPx and GR expressions and activities. A typical example of protective effects of SM on vitagenes and transcription factors is shown in Figure 7.3.

7.3.6 Sirtuins

There are several recent publications showing a regulatory role of SM/SB in the sirtuin functions. A protective effect of SB against chemotherapeutic reagent mitomycin C-induced cell death in A375-S2 cells was studied. It was shown that mitomycin C caused cell apoptosis and over-expression of p53, elevated translocation of p53 into the nucleus, and decreased SIRT1 expression; and these effects were alleviated by SB (100-150 μM) to a large extent (Jiang *et al.*, 2009). SB protected cardiac myocytes against isoproterenol-induced injury through resuming mitochondrial function and regulating the expression of SIRT1 and B-cell lymphoma 2 (Bcl-2) family members (Zhou *et al.*, 2006). Systemic administration of SB (50 mg/kg/BW) reversed STZ-induced downregulation of SIRT1 expression in mice (Wang *et al.*, 2012).

It is important to note that SIRT1 was activated by SM (500 μM) in UV-irradiated human malignant melanoma, A375-S2 cells (Li *et al.*, 2007). However, SB could have

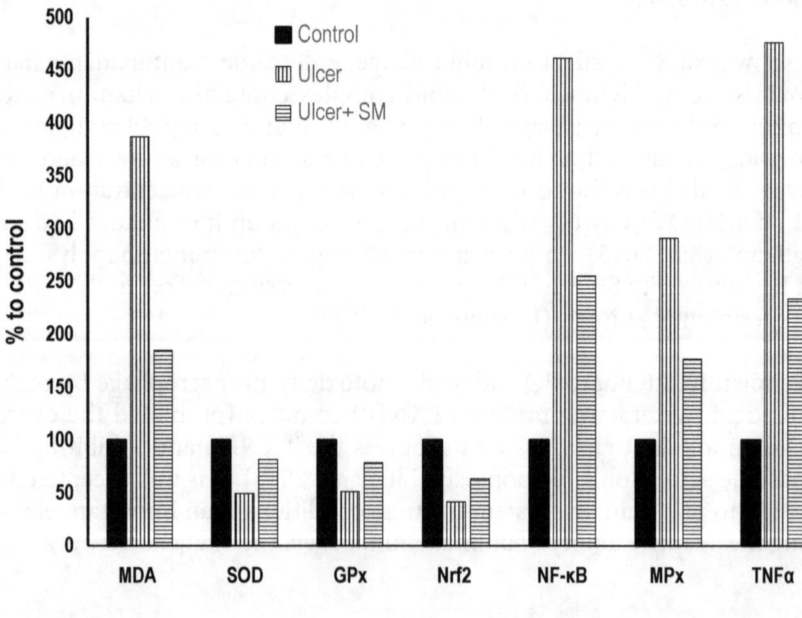

Figure 7.3. Protective effects of SM in experimental gastric ulcer (adapted from Keshk *et al.*, 2017).

completely the opposite action in regulating SIRT1 expression in normal cardiac myocytes and breast cancer MCF-7 cells, where it downregulates SIRT1 and promotes apoptosis (Wang *et al.*, 2008). Similarly, SB treatment downregulated SIRT1 in human lung adenocarcinoma cells (Wu *et al.*, 2014a). In human adipose tissue derived mesenchymal stem cells, SB (10 μM) was observed to increase an SIRT-1, PPARα, PGC-1α, and UCP gene expression (Barbagallo *et al.*, 2016). SB treatment (10, 50 or 10 μM) was reported to increase sirtuin activity in LX-2 cells (Ezhilarasan *et al.*, 2017).

Recent findings indicate that SIRT-mediated signalling pathways are involved in metabolic reprogramming and upregulation of antioxidant defence systems (Wu *et al.*, 2014b). In mice with nonalcoholic fatty liver disease SB was shown to inhibit NLRP3 inflammasome assembly through the NAD^+/SIRT2 pathway (Zhang *et al.*, 2018). Furthermore, SB restored NAD^+ levels and induced the SIRT1/AMPK pathway in non-alcoholic fatty liver (Salomone *et al.*, 2017). Activation of SIRT3 by SB was reported to attenuate mitochondrial dysfunction in CS-induced acute kidney injury (Li *et al.*, 2017). SM (20 mg/kg/day i.p., 4 weeks) was found to increase SIRT1 levels in brain of aged rats (Sarubbo *et al.*, 2018). SM administration (60 or 120 mg/kg) to diabetic rats was indicated to protect against oxidative stress by promoting SIRT1, GPx and CAT expression in the liver tissue (Kheiripour *et al.*, 2018).

In human articular chondrocytes SM was shown to restore the expression of *Sirt1* (Wu *et al.*, 2021). In mice with diet-induced obesity SM was able to activate hepatic SIRT1 pathway to mitigate the disordered glucose metabolism (Feng *et al.*, 2021). In a mouse model of nonalcoholic fatty liver disease SB was reported to increase NAD^+ concentration, to promote SIRT2 expression, and to decrease p65 acetylation both *in vivo* and *in vitro* (Zhang *et al.*, 2021b). Therefore, SM-related activation or prevention of inhibition of sirtuins in stress conditions could be considered as an important adaptive mechanism responsible for maintaining redox homeostasis in the cell and in the whole body.

7.4 Conclusions

The vitagene network represents the major cellular pathway involved in the so called 'programmed cell life' as an opposite to apoptosis, providing an effective protection against oxidative stress and toxic products of RONS metabolism (Calabrese *et al.*, 2009a; 2009b; 2010). In particular, nutritional antioxidants can be neuroprotective through the activation of hormetic pathways under the control of the vitagene protein network (Calabrese *et al.*, 2014). Recently modulatory effect of SM on Nrf2-regulated regulated redox status and NF-κB-mediated inflammation in experimental gastric ulcer have been evaluated (Keshk *et al.*, 2017). As can be seen from Figure 7.3 SM partly prevented decrease in expression of Nrf2 and its target AO (SOD, GPx) and ameliorated increased NF-κB, TNF-α, MDA and activity of MPO. Summarised protective effects of SM/SB via vitagene modulation are shown in Figure 7.4.

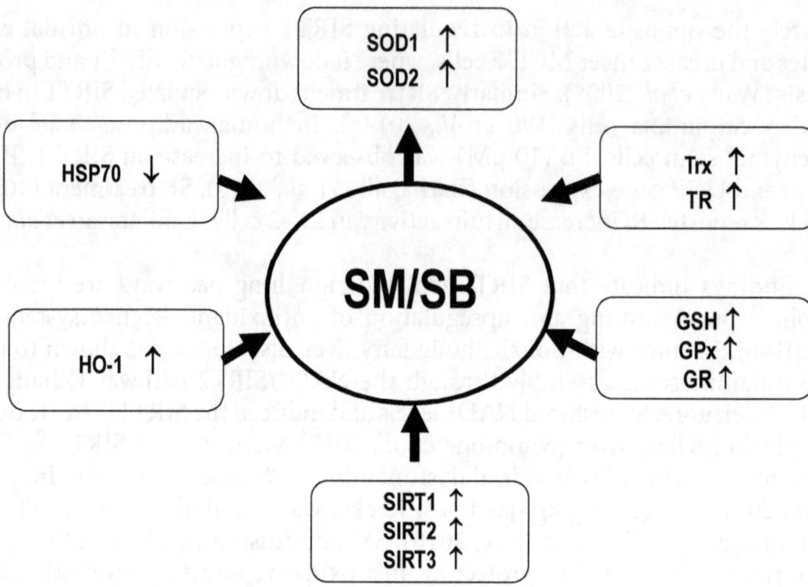

Figure 7.4. Protective effects of SM/SB via vitagene modulation.

The aforementioned results clearly indicate that, similar to other polyphenols, SM, or its active ingredient SB, can affect vitagene network decreasing detrimental consequences of stresses. Further research is needed to fully understand the molecular mechanisms involved in the vitagene network activation by SM/SB.

References

Abd Eldaim, M.A., Barakat, E.R., Alkafafy, M. and Elaziz, S., 2021. Antioxidant and anti-apoptotic prophylactic effect of silymarin against lead-induced hepatorenal toxicity in rats. Environmental Science and Pollution Research International 28: 57997-58006.

Abdel-Moneim, A.M., Al-Kahtani, M.A., El-Kersh, M.A. and Al-Omair, M.A., 2015. Free radical-scavenging, anti-inflammatory/anti-fibrotic and hepatoprotective actions of taurine and silymarin against CCl4 induced rat liver damage. PloS One 10: e0144509.

Aboelwafa, H.R., El-Kott, A.F., Abd-Ella, E.M. and Yousef, H.N., 2020. The possible neuroprotective effect of silymarin against aluminum chloride-prompted Alzheimer's-like disease in rats. Brain Sciences 10: 628.

Ahmed, R.F., Moussa, R.A., Eldemerdash, R.S., Zakaria, M.M. and Abdel-Gaber, S.A., 2019. Ameliorative effects of silymarin on HCl-induced acute lung injury in rats; role of the Nrf-2/HO-1 pathway. Iranian Journal of Basic Medical Sciences 22: 1483-1492.

Ahmed, S., Ullah, N., Parveen, S., Javed, I., Jalil, N., Murtey, M.D., Sheikh, I.S., Khan, S., Ojha, S.C. and Chen, K., 2022. Effect of silymarin as an adjunct therapy in combination with sofosbuvir and ribavirin in hepatitis C patients: A miniature clinical trial. Oxidative Medicine and Cellular Longevity 2022: 9199190.

Alturki, H.A., Elsawy, H.A. and Famurewa, A.C., 2022. Silymarin abrogates acrylamide-induced oxidative stress-mediated testicular toxicity via modulation of antioxidant mechanism, DNA damage, endocrine deficit and sperm quality in rats. Andrologia 54: e14491.

Ambegaokar, S.S. and Kolson, D.L., 2014. Heme oxygenase-1 dysregulation in the brain: implications for HIV associated neurocognitive disorders. Current HIV Research 12: 174-188.

Arafa Keshk, W., Zahran, S.M., Katary, M.A. and Abd-Elaziz Ali, D., 2017. Modulatory effect of silymarin on nuclear factor-erythroid-2-related factor 2 regulated redox status, nuclear factor-κB mediated inflammation and apoptosis in experimental gastric ulcer. Chemico-biological Interactions 273: 266-272.

Avci, H., Epikmen, E.T., Ipek, E., Tunca, R., Birincioglu, S.S., Akşit, H., Sekkin, S., Akkoç, A.N. and Boyacioglu, M., 2017. Protective effects of silymarin and curcumin on cyclophosphamide-induced cardiotoxicity. Experimental and Toxicologic Pathology 69: 317-327.

Bai, D., Jin, G., Yin, S., Zou, D., Zhu, Q., Yang, Z., Liu, X., Ren, L., Sun, Y. and Gan, S., 2017. Antioxidative and anti-apoptotic roles of silibinin in reversing learning and memory deficits in APP/PS1 mice. Neurochemical Research 42: 3439-3445.

Bai, D., Jin, G., Zhang, D., Zhao, L., Wang, M., Zhu, Q., Zhu, L., Sun, Y., Liu, X., Chen, X., Zhang, L., Li, W. and Cui, Y., 2019. Natural silibinin modulates amyloid precursor protein processing and amyloid-β protein clearance in APP/PS1 mice. The Journal of Physiological Sciences 69: 643-652.

Baradaran, A., Samadi, F., Ramezanpour, S.S. and Yousefdoust, S., 2019. Hepatoprotective effects of silymarin on CCl_4-induced hepatic damage in broiler chickens model. Toxicology Reports 6: 788-794.

Barbagallo, I., Vanella, L., Cambria, M.T., Tibullo, D., Godos, J., Guarnaccia, L., Zappalà, A., Galvano, F. and Li Volti, G., 2016. Silibinin regulates lipid metabolism and differentiation in functional human adipocytes. Frontiers in Pharmacology 6: 309.

Bongiovanni, G.A., Soria, E.A. and Eynard, A.R., 2007. Effects of the plant flavonoids silymarin and quercetin on arsenite-induced oxidative stress in CHO-K1 cells. Food and Chemical Toxicology 45: 971-976.

Boukazoula, F. and Ayari, D., 2022. Effect of milk thistle (*Silybum marianum*) supplementation on the serum levels of oxidative stress markers in male half marathon athletes. Biomarkers 27: 461-469.

Bucciantini, M., Leri, M., Scuto, M., Ontario, M., Trovato Salinaro, A., Calabrese, E.J., Calabrese, V. and Stefani, M., 2022. Xenohormesis underlies the anti-aging and healthy properties of olive polyphenols. Mechanisms of Ageing and Development 202: 111620.

Calabrese, V., Boyd-Kimball, D., Scapagnini, G. and Butterfield, D.A., 2004. Nitric oxide and cellular stress response in brain aging and neurodegenerative disorders: the role of vitagenes. *In vivo* 18: 245-267.

Calabrese, V., Calafato, S., Puleo, E., Cornelius, C., Sapienza, M., Morganti, P. and Mancuso, C., 2008. Redox regulation of cellular stress response by ferulic acid ethyl ester in human dermal fibroblasts: role of vitagenes. Clinics in Dermatology 26: 358-363.

Calabrese, V., Cornelius, C., Cuzzocrea, S., Iavicoli, I., Rizzarelli, E. and Calabrese, E.J., 2011. Hormesis, cellular stress response and vitagenes as critical determinants in aging and longevity. Molecular Aspects of Medicine 32: 279-304.

Calabrese, V., Cornelius, C., Dinkova-Kostova, A.T., Iavicoli, I., Di Paola, R., Koverech, A., Cuzzocrea, S., Rizzarelli, E. and Calabrese, E.J., 2012. Cellular stress responses, hormetic phytochemicals and vitagenes in aging and longevity. Biochimica et Biophysica Acta 1822: 753-783.

Calabrese, V., Cornelius, C., Dinkova-Kostova, A.T. and Calabrese, E.J., 2009b. Vitagenes, cellular stress response, and acetylcarnitine: Relevance to hormesis. Biofactors 35: 146-160.

Calabrese, V., Cornelius, C., Mancuso, C., Barone, E., Calafato, S., Bates, T., Rizzarelli, E. and Kostova, A.T., 2009a. Vitagenes, dietary antioxidants and neuroprotection in neurodegenerative diseases. Frontiers in Bioscience 14: 376-397.

Calabrese, V., Cornelius, C., Trovato, A., Cavallaro, M., Mancuso, C., Di Rienzo, L., Condorelli, D., De Lorenzo, A. and Calabrese, E.J., 2010. The hormetic role of dietary antioxidants in free radical-related diseases. Current Pharmaceutical Design 16: 877-883.

Calabrese, V., Dattilo, S., Petralia, A., Parenti, R., Pennisi, M., Koverech, G., Calabrese, V., Graziano, A., Monte, I., Maiolino, L., Ferreri, T. and Calabrese, E.J., 2015. Analytical approaches to the diagnosis and treatment of aging and aging-related disease: redox status and proteomics. Free Radical Research 49: 511-524.

Calabrese, V., Giordano, J., Crupi, R., Di Paola, R., Ruggieri, M., Bianchini, R., Ontario, M.L., Cuzzocrea, S. and Calabrese, E.J., 2017. Hormesis, cellular stress response and neuroinflammation in schizophrenia: Early onset versus late onset state. Journal of Neuroscience Research 95: 1182-1193.

Calabrese, V., Giordano, J., Ruggieri, M., Berritta, D., Trovato, A., Ontario, M.L., Bianchini, R. and Calabrese, E.J., 2016a. Hormesis, cellular stress response, and redox homeostasis in autism spectrum disorders. Journal of Neuroscience Research 94: 1488-1498.

Calabrese, V., Giordano, J., Signorile, A., Laura Ontario, M., Castorina, S., De Pasquale, C., Eckert, G. and Calabrese, E.J., 2016b. Major pathogenic mechanisms in vascular dementia: Roles of cellular stress response and hormesis in neuroprotection. Journal of Neuroscience Research 94: 1588-1603.

Calabrese, V., Guagliano, E., Sapienza, M., Panebianco, M., Calafato, S., Puleo, E., Pennisi, G., Mancuso, C., Butterfield, D.A. and Stella, A.G., 2007. Redox regulation of cellular stress response in aging and neurodegenerative disorders: role of vitagenes. Neurochemical Research 32: 757-773.

Calabrese, V., Scapagnini, G., Davinelli, S., Koverech, G., Koverech, A., De Pasquale, C., Salinaro, A.T., Scuto, M., Calabrese, E.J. and Genazzani, A.R., 2014. Sex hormonal regulation and hormesis in aging and longevity: role of vitagenes. Journal of Cell Communication and Signaling 8: 369-384.

Calabrese, V., Scuto, M., Salinaro, A.T., Dionisio, G., Modafferi, S., Ontario, M.L., Greco, V., Sciuto, S., Schmitt, C.P., Calabrese, E.J. and Peters, V., 2020. Hydrogen sulfide and carnosine: Modulation of oxidative stress and inflammation in kidney and brain axis. Antioxidants 9: 1303.

Černý, D., Canová, N.K., Martínek, J., Hořínek, A., Kmoníčková, E., Zídek, Z. and Farghali, H., 2009. Effects of resveratrol pretreatment on tert-butylhydroperoxide induced hepatocyte toxicity in immobilized perfused hepatocytes: involvement of inducible nitric oxide synthase and hemoxygenase-1. Nitric Oxide 20: 1-8.

Chen, Y.Y., Yu, X.Y., Chen, L., Vaziri, N.D., Ma, S.C. and Zhao, Y.Y., 2019. Redox signaling in aging kidney and opportunity for therapeutic intervention through natural products. Free Radical Biology & Medicine 141: 141-149.

Choi, M.K., Han, J.M., Kim, H.G., Lee, J.S., Lee, J.S., Wang, J.H., Son, S.W., Park, H.J. and Son, C.G., 2013. Aqueous extract of Artemisia capillaris exerts hepatoprotective action in alcohol-pyrazole-fed rat model. Journal of Ethnopharmacology 147: 662-670.

Cornelius, C., Koverech, G., Crupi, R., Di Paola, R., Koverech, A., Lodato, F., Scuto, M., Salinaro, A.T., Cuzzocrea, S., Calabrese, E.J. and Calabrese, V., 2014. Osteoporosis and Alzheimer pathology: Role of cellular stress response and hormetic redox signaling in aging and bone remodeling. Frontiers in Pharmacology 5: 120.

Cornelius, C., Trovato Salinaro, A., Scuto, M., Fronte, V., Cambria, M.T., Pennisi, M., Bella, R., Milone, P., Graziano, A., Crupi, R., Cuzzocrea, S., Pennisi, G. and Calabrese, V., 2013. Cellular stress response, sirtuins and UCP proteins in Alzheimer disease: role of vitagenes. Immunity & Ageing 10: 41.

Dattilo, S., Mancuso, C., Koverech, G., Di Mauro, P., Ontario, M.L., Petralia, C.C., Petralia, A., Maiolino, L., Serra, A., Calabrese, E.J. and Calabrese, V., 2015. Heat shock proteins and hormesis in the diagnosis and treatment of neurodegenerative diseases. Immunity & Ageing 12: 20.

Demir, M., Amanvermez, R., Polat, A.K., Karabıçak, I., Cınar, H., Kesicioğlu, T. and Polat, C., 2014. The effect of silymarin on mesenteric ischemia-reperfusion injury. Medical Principles and Practice 23: 140-144.

Doğan, D., Meydan, İ. and Kömüroğlu, A.U., 2022. Protective effect of silymarin and gallic acid against cisplatin-induced nephrotoxicity and hepatotoxicity. International Journal of Clinical Practice 2022: 6541026.

Doostkam, A., Fathalipour, M., Anbardar, M.H., Purkhosrow, A. and Mirkhani, H., 2022. Therapeutic effects of milk thistle (*Silybum marianum* L.) and artichoke (*Cynara scolymus* L.) on nonalcoholic fatty liver disease in type 2 diabetic rats. Canadian Journal of Gastroenterology & Hepatology 2022: 2868904.

Durymanov, M., Permyakova, A. and Reineke, J., 2020. Pre-treatment with PLGA/silibinin nanoparticles mitigates dacarbazine-induced hepatotoxicity. Frontiers in Bioengineering and Biotechnology 8: 495.

Elsawy, H., Alzahrani, A.M., Alfwuaires, M., Sedky, A., El-Trass, E.E., Mahmoud, O., Abdel-Moneim, A.M. and Khalil, M., 2021. Analysis of silymarin-modulating effects against acrylamide-induced cerebellar damage in male rats: Biochemical and pathological markers. Journal of Chemical Neuroanatomy 115: 101964.

Ezhilarasan, D., Evraerts, J., Sid, B., Calderon, P.B., Karthikeyan, S., Sokal, E. and Najimi, M., 2017. Silibinin induces hepatic stellate cell cycle arrest via enhancing p53/p27 and inhibiting Akt downstream signaling protein expression. Hepatobiliary & Pancreatic Diseases International 16: 80-87.

Faraji, T., Momeni, H.R. and Malmir, M., 2019. Protective effects of silymarin on testis histopathology, oxidative stress indicators, antioxidant defence enzymes and serum testosterone in cadmium-treated mice. Andrologia 51: e13242.

Farjad, E. and Momeni, H.R., 2018. Silymarin ameliorates oxidative stress and enhances antioxidant defense system capacity in cadmium-treated mice. Cell Journal 20: 422-426.

Feng, B., Huang, B., Jing, Y., Shen, S., Feng, W., Wang, W., Meng, R. and Zhu, D., 2021. Silymarin ameliorates the disordered glucose metabolism of mice with diet-induced obesity by activating the hepatic SIRT1 pathway. Cellular Signalling 84: 110023.

Feng, B., Meng, R., Huang, B., Shen, S., Bi, Y. and Zhu, D., 2016. Silymarin alleviates hepatic oxidative stress and protects against metabolic disorders in high-fat diet-fed mice. Free Radical Research 50: 314-327.

Fisinin, V.I. and Surai, P.F., 2011a. Effective protection against stresses in poultry production: from vitamins to vitagenes. Poultry and Poultry Products (Moscow) 5: 23-26.

Fisinin, V.I. and Surai, P.F., 2011b. Effective protection against stresses in poultry production: from vitamins to vitagenes. Poultry and Poultry Products (Moscow) 6: 10-13.

Grattagliano, I., Diogo, C.V., Mastrodonato, M., de Bari, O., Persichella, M., Wang, D.Q., Liquori, A., Ferri, D., Carratù, M.R., Oliveira, P.J. and Portincasa, P., 2013. A silybin-phospholipids complex counteracts rat fatty liver degeneration and mitochondrial oxidative changes. World Journal of Gastroenterology 19: 3007-3017.

Guo, H., Wang, Y. and Liu, D., 2020. Silibinin ameliorates H_2O_2-induced cell apoptosis and oxidative stress response by activating Nrf2 signaling in trophoblast cells. Acta Histochemica 122: 151620.

Haddadi, R., Nayebi, A.M. and Eyvari Brooshghalan, S., 2018. Silymarin prevents apoptosis through inhibiting the Bax/caspase-3 expression and suppresses toll like receptor-4 pathway in the SNc of 6-OHDA intoxicated rats. Biomedicine & Pharmacotherapy 104: 127-136.

Hashem, R.M., Hassanin, K.M., Rashed, L.A., Mahmoud, M.O. and Hassan, M.G., 2016. Effect of silibinin and vitamin E on the ASK1-p38 MAPK pathway in D-galactosamine/lipopolysaccharide induced hepatotoxicity. Experimental Biology and Medicine 241: 1250-1257.

Heidarian, E. and Nouri, A., 2021. Hepatoprotective effects of silymarin against diclofenac-induced liver toxicity in male rats based on biochemical parameters and histological study. Archives of Physiology and Biochemistry 127: 112-118.

Hussein, R.M., Sawy, D.M., Kandeil, M.A. and Farghaly, H.S., 2021. Chlorogenic acid, quercetin, coenzyme Q10 and silymarin modulate Keap1-Nrf2/heme oxygenase-1 signaling in thioacetamide-induced acute liver toxicity. Life Sciences 277: 119460.

Jalali, S.M., Najafzadeh, H. and Bahmei, S., 2017. Protective role of silymarin and D-penicillamine against lead-induced liver toxicity and oxidative stress. Toxicology and Industrial Health 33: 512-518.

Jiang, Y.Y., Wang, H.J., Wang, J., Tashiro, S.I., Onodera, S. and Ikejima, T., 2009. The Protective Effect of silibinin against mitomycin C-induced intrinsic apoptosis in human melanoma A375-S2 cells. Journal of Pharmacological Sciences 111: 137-146.

Keshk, W.A., Zahran, S.M., Katary, M.A. and Ali, D.A.E., 2017. Modulatory effect of silymarin on nuclear factor-erythroid-2-related factor 2 regulated redox status, nuclear factor-κB mediated inflammation and apoptosis in experimental gastric ulcer. Chemico-Biological Interactions 273: 266-272.

Khamisabadi, H., 2020. Effects of silymarin on milk production, liver enzymes, oxidative status and HSP70 gene expression in postparturient Sanjabi ewes. Cellular and Molecular Biology 66: 76-81.

Kheiripour, N., Karimi, J., Khodadadi, I., Tavilani, H., Goodarzi, M.T. and Hashemnia, M., 2018. Silymarin prevents lipid accumulation in the liver of rats with type 2 diabetes via sirtuin1 and SREBP-1c. Journal of Basic and Clinical Physiology and Pharmacology 29: 301-308.

Kiruthiga, P.V., Karthikeyan, K., Archunan, G., Pandian, S.K. and Devi, K.P., 2015. Silymarin prevents benzo (a) pyrene-induced toxicity in Wistar rats by modulating xenobiotic-metabolizing enzymes. Toxicology and Industrial Health 31: 523-541.

Li, L.H., Wu, L.J., Tashiro, S.I., Onodera, S., Uchiumi, F. and Ikejima, T., 2007. Activation of the SIRT1 pathway and modulation of the cell cycle were involved in silymarin's protection against UV-induced A375-S2 cell apoptosis. Journal of Asian Natural Products Research 9: 245-252.

Li, Y., Ye, Z., Lai, W., Rao, J., Huang, W., Zhang, X., Yao, Z. and Lou, T., 2017. Activation of sirtuin 3 by silybin attenuates mitochondrial dysfunction in cisplatin-induced acute kidney injury. Frontiers in Pharmacology 8: 178.

Liu, X., Wang, C., Liu, W., Song, S., Fu, J., Hayashi, T., Mizuno, K., Hattori, S., Fujisaki, H. and Ikejima, T., 2021. Oral administration of silibinin ameliorates cognitive deficits of Parkinson's disease mouse model by restoring mitochondrial disorders in hippocampus. Neurochemical Research 46: 2317-2332.

Liu, Z., Sun, M., Wang, Y., Zhang, L., Zhao, H. and Zhao, M., 2018. Silymarin attenuated paraquat-induced cytotoxicity in macrophage by regulating Trx/TXNIP complex, inhibiting NLRP3 inflammasome activation and apoptosis. Toxicology In Vitro 46: 265-272.

Mazhari, S., Razi, M. and Sadrkhanlou, R., 2018. Silymarin and celecoxib ameliorate experimental varicocele-induced pathogenesis: evidences for oxidative stress and inflammation inhibition. International Urology and Nephrology 50: 1039-1052.

Moghaddam, A.H., Mokhtari Sangdehi, S.R., Ranjbar, M. and Hasantabar, V., 2020. Preventive effect of silymarin-loaded chitosan nanoparticles against global cerebral ischemia/reperfusion injury in rats. European Journal of Pharmacology 877: 173066.

Mohammadi, M., Ariafar, S., Talebi-Ghane, E. and Afzali, S., 2022. Comparative efficacy of silibinin and nano-silibinin on lead poisoning in male Wistar rats. Toxicology 475: 153242.

Muthumani, M. and Prabu, S.M., 2014. Silibinin potentially attenuates arsenic-induced oxidative stress mediated cardiotoxicity and dyslipidemia in rats. Cardiovascular Toxicology 14: 83-97.

Naito, Y., Takagi, T. and Higashimura, Y., 2014. Heme oxygenase-1 and anti-inflammatory M2 macrophages. Archives of Biochemistry and Biophysics 564: 83-88.

Ontario, M.L., Siracusa, R., Modafferi, S., Scuto, M., Sciuto, S., Greco, V., Bertuccio, M.P., Trovato Salinaro, A., Crea, R., Calabrese, E.J., Di Paola, R. and Calabrese, V., 2022. Potential prevention and treatment of neurodegenerative disorders by olive polyphenols and hidrox. Mechanisms of Ageing and Development 203: 111637.

Oskoueian, E., Abdullah, N., Idrus, Z., Ebrahimi, M., Goh, Y.M., Shakeri, M. and Oskoueian, A., 2014. Palm kernel cake extract exerts hepatoprotective activity in heat-induced oxidative stress in chicken hepatocytes. BMC Complementary and Alternative Medicine 14: 368.

Pan, Q., Ban, Y. and Xu, L., 2021. Silibinin-albumin nanoparticles: Characterization and biological evaluation against oxidative stress-stimulated neurotoxicity associated with Alzheimer's disease. Journal of Biomedical Nanotechnology 17: 1123-1130.

Pasala, P.K., Uppara, R.K., Rudrapal, M., Zothantluanga, J.H. and Umar, A.K., 2022. Silybin phytosome attenuates cerebral ischemia-reperfusion injury in rats by suppressing oxidative stress and reducing inflammatory response: *In vivo* and in silico approaches. Journal of Biochemical and Molecular Toxicology 36: e23073.

Rajnochová Svobodová, A., Gabrielová, E., Michaelides, L., Kosina, P., Ryšavá, A., Ulrichová, J., Zálešák, B. and Vostálová, J., 2018. UVA-photoprotective potential of silymarin and silybin. Archives of Dermatological Research 310: 413-424.

Rattan, S.I., 1998. The nature of gerontogenes and vitagenes. Antiaging effects of repeated heat shock on human fibroblasts. Annals of the New York Academy of Sciences 854: 54-60.

Salomone, F., Barbagallo, I., Godos, J., Lembo, V., Currenti, W., Cinà, D., Avola, R., D'Orazio, N., Morisco, F., Galvano, F. and Li Volti, G., 2017. Silibinin restores NAD^+ levels and induces the SIRT1/AMPK pathway in non-alcoholic fatty liver. Nutrients 9: 1086.

Siracusa, R., Voltarelli, V.A., Salinaro, A.T., Modafferi, S., Cuzzocrea, S., Calabrese, E.J., Di Paola, R., Otterbein, L.E. and Calabrese, V., 2022. NO, CO and H_2S: A trinacrium of bioactive gases in the brain. Biochemical Pharmacology 202: 115122.

Sarubbo, F., Ramis, M.R., Kienzer, C., Aparicio, S., Esteban, S., Miralles, A. and Moranta, D., 2018. Chronic silymarin, quercetin and naringenin treatments increase monoamines synthesis and hippocampal Sirt1 levels improving cognition in aged rats. Journal of Neuroimmune Pharmacology 13: 24-38.

Scuto, M., Trovato Salinaro, A., Caligiuri, I., Ontario, M.L., Greco, V., Sciuto, N., Crea, R., Calabrese, E.J., Rizzolio, F., Canzonieri, V. and Calabrese, V., 2021. Redox modulation of vitagenes via plant polyphenols and vitamin D: Novel insights for chemoprevention and therapeutic interventions based on organoid technology. Mechanisms of Ageing and Development 199: 111551.

Scuto, M., Modafferi, S., Rampulla, F., Zimbone, V., Tomasello, M., Spano', S., Ontario, M.L., Palmeri, A., Trovato Salinaro, A., Siracusa, R., Di Paola, R., Cuzzocrea, S., Calabrese, E.J., Wenzel, U. and Calabrese, V., 2022a. Redox modulation of stress resilience by Crocus sativus L. for potential neuroprotective and anti-neuroinflammatory applications in brain disorders: From molecular basis to therapy. Mechanisms of Ageing and Development 205: 111686.

Scuto, M., Ontario, M.L., Salinaro, A.T., Caligiuri, I., Rampulla, F., Zimbone, V., Modafferi, S., Rizzolio, F., Canzonieri, V., Calabrese, E.J. and Calabrese, V., 2022b. Redox modulation by plant polyphenols targeting vitagenes for chemoprevention and therapy: Relevance to novel anti-cancer interventions and mini-brain organoid technology. Free Radical Biology & Medicine 179: 59-75.

Sheta, N.M., Elfeky, Y.A. and Boshra, S.A., 2020. Cardioprotective efficacy of silymarin liquisolid in isoproterenol prompted myocardial infarction in rats. AAPS PharmSciTech 21: 81.

Sohrabi, M.J., Dehpour, A.R., Attar, F., Hasan, A., Mohammad-Sadeghi, N., Meratan, A.A., Aziz, F.M., Salihi, A., Shekha, M.S., Akhtari, K., Shahpasand, K., Hojjati, S., Sharifi, M., Saboury, A.A., Rezayat, S.M., Mousavi, S.E. and Falahati, M., 2019. Silymarin-albumin nanoplex: Preparation and its potential application as an antioxidant in nervous system *in vitro* and *in vivo*. International Journal of Pharmaceutics 572: 118824.

Stolf, A.M., Campos Cardoso, C., Morais, H., Alves de Souza, C.E., Lomba, L.A., Brandt, A.P., Agnes, J.P., Collere, F.C., Galindo, C.M., Corso, C.R., Spercoski, K.M., Locatelli Dittrich, R., Zampronio, A.R., Cadena, S. and Acco, A., 2018. Effects of silymarin on angiogenesis and oxidative stress in streptozotocin-induced diabetes in mice. Biomedicine & Pharmacotherapy 108: 232-243.

Surai, P.F., 2015a. Carnitine Enigma: From antioxidant action to vitagene regulation. Part 2. Transcription factors and practical applications. Journal of Veterinary Science & Medicine 3, 2: 17.

Surai, P.F., 2015b. Antioxidant action of carnitine: molecular mechanisms and practical applications. EC Veterinary Science 2.1: 66-84.

Surai, P.F., 2015c. Silymarin as a natural antioxidant: An overview of the current evidence and perspectives. Antioxidants 4: 204-247.

Surai, P.F., 2016. Antioxidant systems in poultry biology: Superoxide dismutase. Journal of Animal Research and Nutrition 1, 1: 8.

Surai, P.F., 2018a. Selenium in poultry nutrition and health. Wageningen Academic Publishers, Wageningen, The Netherlands.

Surai, P.F., 2018b. Taurine and carnitine in poultry production: from vitagene activation to chicken health maintenance. Ptakhivnitstvo.ua (Ukrainian Poultry Science) 1-2: 12-17.

Surai, P.F., 2019. Vitagenes in poultry production: adaptation to commercially relevant stresses. Suchasne Ptakhivnitstvo (Ukraine) 7-8: 28-32.

Surai, P.F. 2020a. Vitagenes in avian biology and poultry health. Wageningen Academic Publishers: Wageningen, The Netherlands.

Surai, P.F., 2020b. Antioxidants in poultry nutrition and reproduction: An update. Antioxidants 9, 2: 105.

Surai, P.F., 2020c. Superoxide dismutase as a new entrant into the vitagene family in animals/poultry. EC Nutrition 15.3: 01-03.

Surai, P.F., 2022. Silymarin as a vitagene modulator: effects on mitochondria integrity in stress conditions. In: Ostojik, S.M. (ed) Molecular nutrition and mitochondria. Elsevier, Academic Press, London, UK, pp. 535-559.

Surai, P.F. and Earle-Payne, K., 2022. Antioxidant defences and redox homeostasis in animals. Antioxidants 11: 1012.

Surai, P.F., Earle-Payne, K. and Kidd, M.T., 2021b. Taurine as a natural antioxidant: From direct antioxidant effects to protective action in various toxicological models. Antioxidants 10: 1876.

Surai, P.F. and Fisinin, V.I., 2012a. The modern antistress technologies in poultry: From antioxidants to vitagenes. Agricultural Biology (Moscow) 4: 3-13.

Surai, P.F. and Fisinin, V.I., 2012b. Modern methods for fighting stresses in poultry production: from antioxidants to sirtuins and vita-genes. Effectivne Ptakhivnitstvo, Ukraine (Effective Poultry Production) 8: 8-13.

Surai, P.F. and Fisinin, V.I., 2016a. Vitagenes in poultry production. Part 3. Vitagene concept development. Worlds Poultry Science Journal 72: 793-804.

Surai, P.F. and Fisinin, V.I., 2016b. Antioxidant system regulation: From vitamins to vitagenes. In: Watson, R.R. and De Meester, F. (eds) Handbook of cholesterol. Wageningen Academic Publishers, Wageningen, the Netherlands, pp. 451-481.

Surai, P.F., Kochish, I.I. and Fisinin, V.I., 2017. Antioxidant systems in poultry biology: Nutritional modulation of vitagenes. European Journal of Poultry Science 81: 1612-9199.

Surai, P.F., Kochish, I.I., Fisinin, V.I., Grozina, A.A. and Shatskikh, E.V., 2018. Molecular mechanisms of chicken gut health maintenance: role of microbiota. Agricultural Technologies, Moscow, Russia.

Surai, P.F., Kochish, I.I., Fisinin, V.I. and Kidd, M.T., 2019. Antioxidant defence systems and oxidative stress in poultry biology: An update. Antioxidants 8, 7: 235.

Surai, P.F., Kochish, I.I. and Kidd, M.T., 2020. Taurine in poultry nutrition. Animal Feed Science and Technology 260: 114339.

Surai, P.F., Kochish, I.I. and Kidd, M.T., 2021a. Redox homeostasis in poultry: Regulatory roles of NF-κB. Antioxidants 10: 186.

Surai, P.F., Kochish, I.I. and Fisinin, V.I., 2021c. Vitagenes in avian biology: protective functions of sirtuins. In: Maise, K. (ed) Sirtuin biology in medicine. Academic Press, UK, USA, pp. 353-372.

Thakare, V.N., Dhakane, V.D. and Patel, B.M., 2016. Potential antidepressant-like activity of silymarin in the acute restraint stress in mice: Modulation of corticosterone and oxidative stress response in cerebral cortex and hippocampus. Pharmacological Reports 68: 1020-1027.

Thakare, V.N., Patil, R.R., Oswal, R.J., Dhakane, V.D., Aswar, M.K. and Patel, B.M., 2018. Therapeutic potential of silymarin in chronic unpredictable mild stress induced depressive-like behavior in mice. Journal of Psychopharmacology 32: 223-235.

Tie, F., Fu, Y., Hu, N. and Wang, H., 2022. Silibinin protects against H_2O_2-induced oxidative damage in SH-SY5Y cells by improving mitochondrial function. Antioxidants 11: 1101.

Trovato Salinaro, A., Cornelius, C., Koverech, G., Koverech, A., Scuto, M., Lodato, F., Fronte, V., Muccilli, V., Reibaldi, M., Longo, A., Uva, M.G. and Calabrese, V., 2014. Cellular stress response, redox status, and vitagenes in glaucoma: a systemic oxidant disorder linked to Alzheimer's disease. Frontiers in Pharmacology 5: 129.

Trovato, A., Siracusa, R., Di Paola, R., Scuto, M., Fronte, V., Koverech, G., Luca, M., Serra, A., Toscano, M.A., Petralia, A., Cuzzocrea, S. and Calabrese, V., 2016b. Redox modulation of cellular stress response and lipoxin A4 expression by Coriolus versicolor in rat brain: Relevance to Alzheimer's disease pathogenesis. Neurotoxicology 53: 350-358.

Trovato, A., Siracusa, R., Di Paola, R., Scuto, M., Ontario, M.L., Bua, O., Di Mauro, P., Toscano, M.A., Petralia, C., Maiolino, L., Serra, A., Cuzzocrea, S. and Calabrese, V., 2016a. Redox modulation of cellular stress response and lipoxin A4 expression by Hericium Erinaceus in rat brain: relevance to Alzheimer's disease pathogenesis. Immunity & Ageing 13: 23.

Tung, N.T., Tran, C.S., Nguyen, H.A., Nguyen, T.D., Chi, S.C., Pham, D.V., Bui, Q.D. and Ho, X.H., 2019. Formulation and biopharmaceutical evaluation of supersaturatable self-nanoemulsifying drug delivery systems containing silymarin. International Journal of Pharmaceutics 555: 63-76.

Venditti, C.C. and Smith, G.N., 2014. Involvement of the heme oxygenase system in the development of preeclampsia and as a possible therapeutic target. Women's Health 10: 623-643.

Wang, H.J., Tashiro, S.I., Onodera, S. and Ikejima, T., 2008. Inhibition of insulin-like growth factor 1 receptor signaling enhanced silibinin-induced activation of death receptor and mitochondrial apoptotic pathways in human breast cancer MCF-7 cells. Journal of Pharmacological Sciences 107: 260-269.

Wang, L., Huang, Q.H., Li, Y.X., Huang, Y.F., Xie, J.H., Xu, L.Q., Dou, Y.X., Su, Z.R., Zeng, H.F. and Chen, J.N., 2018. Protective effects of silymarin on triptolide-induced acute hepatotoxicity in rats. Molecular Medicine Reports 17: 789-800.

Wang, Q., Liu, M., Liu, W.W., Hao, W.B., Tashiro, S.I., Onodera, S. and Ikejima, T., 2012. *In vivo* recovery effect of silibinin treatment on streptozotocin-induced diabetic mice is associated with the modulations of Sirt-1 expression and autophagy in pancreatic β-cell. Journal of Asian Natural Products Research 14: 413-423.

Wang, X.L., Lin, F.L., Xu, W., Wang, C., Wang, Q.Q. and Jiang, R.W., 2022. Silybin B exerts protective effect on cisplatin-induced neurotoxicity by alleviating DNA damage and apoptosis. Journal of Ethnopharmacology 288: 114938.

Wu, W.T., Chen, Y.R., Lu, D.H., Senatov, F.S., Yang, K.C. and Wang, C.C., 2021. Silymarin modulates catabolic cytokine expression through Sirt1 and SOX9 in human articular chondrocytes. Journal of Orthopaedic Surgery and Research 16: 147.

Wu, Y.T., Wu, S.B. and Wei, Y.H., 2014a. Roles of sirtuins in the regulation of antioxidant defense and bioenergetic function of mitochondria under oxidative stress. Free Radical Research 48: 1070-1084.

Wu, Y.T., Wu, S.B. and Wei, Y.H., 2014b. Metabolic reprogramming of human cells in response to oxidative stress: implications in the pathophysiology and therapy of mitochondrial diseases. Current Pharmaceutical Design 20: 5510-5526.

Yardım, A., Kucukler, S., Özdemir, S., Çomaklı, S., Caglayan, C., Kandemir, F.M. and Çelik, H., 2021. Silymarin alleviates docetaxel-induced central and peripheral neurotoxicity by reducing oxidative stress, inflammation and apoptosis in rats. Gene 769: 145239.

Yu, Z., Wu, F., Tian, J., Guo, X. and An, R., 2018. Protective effects of compound ammonium glycyrrhizin, L-arginine, silymarin and glucurolactone against liver damage induced by ochratoxin A in primary chicken hepatocytes. Molecular Medicine Reports 18: 2551-2560.

Zhang, B., Xu, D., She, L., Wang, Z., Yang, N., Sun, R., Zhang, Y., Yan, C., Wei, Q., Aa, J., Liu, B., Wang, G. and Xie, Y., 2018. Silybin inhibits NLRP3 inflammasome assembly through the NAD+/SIRT2 pathway in mice with nonalcoholic fatty liver disease. FASEB Journal 32: 757-767.

Zhang, Q., Ahn, J.M. and Kim, I.H., 2021a. Micelle silymarin supplementation to sows' diet from day 109 of gestation to entire lactation period enhances reproductive performance and affects serum hormones and metabolites. Journal of Animal Science 99: skab354.

Zhang, R., Xu, D., Zhang, Y., Wang, R., Yang, N., Lou, Y., Zhao, H., Aa, J., Wang, G. and Xie, Y., 2021b. Silybin restored CYP3A expression through the sirtuin 2/nuclear factor κ-B pathway in mouse nonalcoholic fatty liver disease. Drug Metabolism and Disposition 49: 770-779.

Zhao, F., Shi, D., Li, T., Li, L. and Zhao, M., 2015. Silymarin attenuates paraquat-induced lung injury via Nrf2-mediated pathway *in vivo* and *in vitro*. Clinical and Experimental Pharmacology & Physiology 42: 988-998.

Zhao, H., Brandt, G.E., Galam, L., Matts, R.L. and Blagg, B.S., 2011. Identification and initial SAR of silybin: an Hsp90 inhibitor. Bioorganic & Medicinal Chemistry Letters 21: 2659-2664.

Zhao, X., Wang, H., Yang, Y., Gou, Y., Wang, Z., Yang, D. and Li, C., 2021. Protective effects of silymarin against D-Gal/LPS-induced organ damage and inflammation in mice. Drug Design, Development and Therapy 15: 1903-1914.

Zhou, B., Wu, L.J., Li, L.H., Tashiro, S.I., Onodera, S., Uchiumi, F. and Ikejima, T., 2006. Silibinin protects against isoproterenol-induced rat cardiac myocyte injury through mitochondrial pathway after up-regulation of SIRT1. Journal of Pharmacological Sciences 102: 387-395.

Chapter 8
Antitoxic properties of silymarin

Danger foreseen is half avoided

Anton Surai[1] and Peter F. Surai[2-7]*
[1]Healthy Food Services, Bristol, UK; [2]Vitagene and Health Research Centre, Bristol, UK; [3]Department of Microbiology and Biochemistry, Faculty of Veterinary Medicine, Trakia University, Stara Zagora, Bulgaria; [4]Department of Animal Nutrition, Faculty of Agricultural and Environmental Sciences, Szent Istvan University, Hungary; [5]Saint-Petersburg State Academy of Veterinary Medicine, St. Petersburg, Russia; [6]Sumy National Agrarian University, Sumy, Ukraine; [7]Odessa National Academy of Food Technologies, Odessa, Ukraine
psurai@feedfood.co.uk

Abstract

This chapter is devoted to anti-toxic properties of silymarin (SM). In various model systems toxic chemicals were used to impose toxicity, which in many cases was associated with oxidative stress indicative by decreased antioxidant defences (AO enzymes and non-enzymatic antioxidants, total antioxidant activity, etc.) and increased concentrations of oxidative stress markers, including MDA accumulation. In many cases inflammatory responses were also observed. Protective effects of SM were demonstrated in models of chemical toxicity induced by CCl_4, thioacetamide, cisplatin, benzo[a]pyrene, doxorubicin, APAP, pesticides (paraquat and maneb), anti-TB drugs (rifampicin, isoniazid and pyrazinamide), arsenic, cadmium, lead, mercury, aluminium, iron, copper, manganese, fluoride, silver nanoparticles, ethanol and gentamicin. Furthermore, SM was also effective in protection against other 46 chemicals, including 1-methyl-4-phenyl-1,2,3,6-tetrahydropyridine, 6-hydroxydopamine, acrolein, acrylamide, adriamycin, α-amanitin, bisphenol A, bleomicyn, cocaine, cyclophosphamide, cyclosporine A, cyclosporine A, di(2-ethylhexyl)phthalate, diazinon, diethylnitrosamine, diethylnitrosamine, docetaxel, epirubicin, fingolimod, hydrochloric acid, isoniazid, isoniazid, isoproterenol, itraconazole, kainic acid, ketoprofen, L-arginine, lasalocid, methotrexate, methotrexate, microcystin-LR, mycophenolate mofetil, nickel sulphate, N-nitrosodimethylamine, oxaliplatin, phenylhydrazine, polymyxin E, pyrazinamide, pyrogallol, ribavirin, scopolamine, sodium nitrite, sulphur mustard, thiram, triptolide, vancomycin and zidovudine. In addition, protective effects of SM were proven in various clinically-relevant conditions imposing oxidative stress, including gamma radiation, UV-radiation and ischemia/reperfusion. From the data presented above it is clear that SM provides protection against oxidative stress and following toxicity caused by a great number of chemicals and conditions. In general, it seems very likely that protective effects of SM are associated with modulation of vitagenes and transcription factors with following effects on antioxidant enzymes and other antioxidant defence mechanisms.

DOI:10.3920/978-90-8686-944-2_008,

Keywords: silymarin, toxic chemicals, stress models, oxidative stress, vitagenes

8.1 Introduction

The liver is a primary organ involved in biotransformation of food toxicants and drugs. Toxins absorbed from the intestinal tract first enter the liver and very often induce oxidative stress resulting in a variety of liver disorders. Hepatic disorders are mainly caused by toxic chemicals (alcohol), xenobiotics (carbon tetrachloride, chlorinated hydrocarbons), anticancer (doxorubicin, cisplatin), immunosuppressant (cyclosporine), analgesic anti-inflammatory (paracetamol, thioacetamide), anti-tubercular (isoniazid, rifampicin) drugs, radiations (gamma radiations), heavy metals (cadmium, arsenic), mycotoxins (aflatoxin, T-2 toxin, fumonisins, ochratoxins), galactosamine, lipopolysaccharides, etc. (Ingawale *et al.*, 2014). Increasing evidence supports the important role of oxidative stress as a key mechanism of hepatotoxicity. Therefore, the aforementioned toxicants were used in various experimental models to assess antioxidant protective properties of SM/SB. These are especially important, since SM is primarily used in clinical practice to protect, support and repair the liver. The main results are summarised below.

8.2 Various compounds with toxic effects

8.2.1 Carbone tetrachloride

Carbone tetrachloride (CCl_4), an industrial solvent and refrigerant, is strong toxic chemical in the kidney, testicle, brain, heart, lung, other tissues, and particularly in the liver being a powerful hepatoxic, nephrotoxic and prooxidant agent (Unsal *et al.*, 2020). It should be noted that metabolism of CCl_4 via CYP2E1 to highly reactive ROS plays a major role in the mode of action of the toxicant (Manibusan *et al.*, 2007). It is well established that CCl_4 inhibits AO enzymes (SOD, GPx and CAT) and GSH in liver samples (Raj and Gothandam, 2014), increases the secretion of ALT, aspartate transaminase (AST) and ALP due to hepatic injuries caused by ROS (Alkreathy *et al.*, 2014) and enhances TBARS in the liver (Krishnappa *et al.*, 2014) and serum (Shaker *et al.*, 2010). It has been shown that practically all elevated indexes of the oxidative stress caused by CCl_4 were restored almost to the initial physiological levels by SM treatment (25-100 mg/kg/BW) (Abbas *et al.*, 2014; Al-Harbi *et al.*, 2014; Alkreathy *et al.*, 2014; Chang *et al.*, 2014; Krishnappa *et al.*, 2014; Raj and Gothandam, 2014; Shaker *et al.*, 2010; Shine *et al.*, 2014) and hepatic injuries were significantly decreased.

In a rat model of hepatic fibrosis induced by CCl_4, oral administration of SM (200 mg/kg, three times daily), was demonstrated to improve liver integrity (decreased plasma levels of AST and GPT), to ameliorate compromised AO system (SOD and GPx in liver) and to improve hepatic fibrosis, the hepatic levels of hydroxyproline and connective tissue growth factor (Tzeng *et al.*, 2013). Furthermore, SM (0.1-1.0 g/kg diet) had a protective effect against CCl_4-induced liver damage and AO system defences in common carp (Jia *et al.*, 2013). It is important to mention that in a model system based on CCl_4-induced liver fibrosis in mice, microarray analysis showed that SM downregulated the expression levels of cytoskeleton organisation genes and mitochondrion electron-transfer chain genes, such as cytochrome c oxidase, Cox6a2, Cox7a1, and Cox8b genes (Li *et al.*, 2012).

The effects of two different doses of SM (50 and 200 mg/kg) on a CCl_4-induced model of liver fibrosis with a focus on the early stages of liver injury were investigated. Interestingly, SM at 50 mg/kg BW was reported to reduce oxidative stress, hepato-cytolysis, fibrosis, activation of Kupffer cells, and the expression of α-SMA and TGF-β1 with better results than SM at higher (200 mg/kg BW) dose (Clichici *et al.*, 2015). In a mouse model of liver fibrosis caused by injected with $CCl_{4,}$ SM was shown to significantly reduce CCl_4-induced increased expression of pro-inflammatory TNF-α, TGF-β1 and monocyte chemoattractant protein 1 (MCP-1) associated with the decreased numbers of intrahepatic Ly6C^{hi} monocytes (Zhao *et al.*, 2017). Similarly, in rats SM, alone and combined with chlorogenic acid and/or melatonin was reported to protect the liver against CCl_4-induced hepatotoxicity via attenuating inflammation, oxidative DNA damage, apoptosis, and fibrotic changes (Al-Rasheed *et al.*, 2016). SM (200 mg/kg) administered after the CCl_4-induced liver injury in rats was observed to be capable of reducing inflammation and liver fibrosis (Clichici *et al.*, 2016).

In a rat model of CCl_4-induced hepatic fibrosis it was shown that down-regulation of NF-κBp65 mRNA expression and inhibition of phosphorylation of NF-κBp65 (at Ser536) and IκB leading to decreased levels of TNF-α, TGF-β1, matrix metalloproteinase-2 (MMP-2), tissue inhibitor of metalloproteinase-1 (TIMP-1) and vascular endothelial growth factor (VEGF), were implicated in the anti-fibrotic effect of SM. Furthermore, lisinopril was reported to inhibit NF-κB and augments sensitivity to SM in experimental liver fibrosis (Saber *et al.*, 2018).

Protective effects of SM (50 mg/kg) against CCl_4 toxicity in rats was associated with partial restoration of activities of AO enzymes (CAT, SOD, GST), GSH concentration and total AO activity compromised by the toxicant (El Rabey *et al.*, 2021). SM (50 mg/kg BW) and silymarin nanoparticles (SILNPs; 25 or 50 mg/kg) were shown to induce a significant improvement in the AO defences in the liver and kidney, haematological parameters, liver and kidney function/integrity, lipid profile, serum cytokines gene expression, DNA fragmentation and histology of liver and kidney tissue which were compromised by CCl_4 treatment (Aboshanab *et al.*, 2020). In a broiler chicken model remarkable down-regulation in the expression of CAT, GPx, and SOD2 hepatic genes in CCl_4-challenged birds was observed and SM was shown to significantly up-regulate the aforementioned genes (Baradaran *et al.*, 2019).

Interestingly, both SM and TAU at 100 mg/kg (5 times a week for 4 weeks) post-CCl_4-treatments were shown to be able to relieve most of the antioxidant (SOD, GPx, GR, GST and GSH), pro-inflammatory and fibrogenic cytokines (TNF-α, TGF-β1, IL-6, leptin and resistin), and liver injury parameters (serum ALT, AST, ALP and bilirubin; Abdel-Moneim *et al.*, 2015). However, the combination therapy was more effective than single applications in reducing TBARS levels, NO production, hydroxyproline content in fibrotic liver and the activity of serum gamma-glutamyl transferase (GGT). Combined treatment (but not TAU- or SIL-alone) was also shown to be able to effectively prevent CCl_4-induced decrease in adiponectin (the anti-inflammatory cytokine) serum levels.

Furthermore, the combined post-treatment with TAU+SIL (but not monotherapy) normalised serum FFA in CCl_4-treated rats (Abdel-Moneim *et al.*, 2015). The authors suggested that, SM may be used in combination with TAU as an additional adjunct therapy to cure liver diseases such as fibrosis, cirrhosis and viral hepatitis.

8.2.2 Thiacetamide

Thiacetamide (TAA), an organosulphur compound used in the synthesis of organic and inorganic compounds, is a potent hepatotoxicant which requires metabolic activation by the mixed-function oxidases and in the development of TAA-induced toxicity, ROS formation and oxidative stress are thought to play a crucial role (Ingawale *et al.*, 2014; Mustafa *et al.*, 2013). In particular, TAA-induced cirrhosis is associated with oxidative stress in the liver, as indicated by a high level of lipid peroxidation, accompanied by distorted status of antioxidants and redox balance (Fazal *et al.*, 2015). Therefore, TAA-treated animals can be used to evaluate antioxidant protective effects of SM.

SM is shown to have a protective effect against oxidative stress caused by TAA in rats. A significant decrease in TAA-induced liver damage was observed in SM-pre-treated rats indicated by a reduction in serum GPT, AST and alkaline phosphatase (ALP), restoration of the antioxidant system (SOD, CAT, GR, GPx and GST) and decreased lipid peroxidation (Singh *et al.*, 2012a). Increases in hepatic levels of malondialdehyde (MDA) and protein carbonyls in rats associated with TAA administration were partially blocked by SM consumption (Ali *et al.*, 2014).

Since the pregnane X receptor (PXR) is one of the major transcriptional regulators of CYP3A4, inhibitory effects of SM on PXR-mediated CYP3A4 induction (Mooiman *et al.*, 2013) deserves more attention. SB (200 mg/kg for 2 weeks) was shown to ameliorate the loss of CYP3A and PXR in TAA-injured rat liver, and to decrease PXR translocation into the cell nucleus. Interestingly, PXR silencing was demonstrated to weaken the effect of SB on cytoprotection and CYP3A regulation (Xie *et al.*, 2013). Furthermore, GSH depletion and HSP47 gene expressions were also decreased in response to SM administration. Pre-treatment of rats with SM (50 or 100 mg/kg) resulted in the protection against TAA-induced liver dysfunction as indicated by restoration of activity of liver enzymes, including ALT, AST, ALP in serum by reduction of apoptosis and oxidative stress as evidenced by restoration of GPx activity (Teksoy *et al.*, 2020). Furthermore, SM therapy (50 or 100 mg/kg) before TAA treatment is shown to be able to guard kidney tissues against TAA-induced nephrotoxicity (Cengiz, 2018). In a mouse model SM was reported to protect liver and kidney from TAA-induced toxicity by scavenging ROS and activating PI3K-Akt pathway (Ghosh *et al.*, 2016).

8.2.3 Cisplatin

Cisplatin (CS) is the most commonly used chemotherapy drug for the treatment of various cancers and its nephrotoxicity is thought to be associated with ROS overproduction (Dos Santos *et al.*, 2012), decreasing activities of AO enzymes (SOD and GPx), GSH and increasing lipid peroxidation in rat liver (El-Awady *et al.*, 2011; Mansour *et al.*, 2006). CS can also cause structural damages to the liver as indicated by significantly elevated serum activities of lactate dehydrogenase and creatine kinase (El-Awady *et al.*, 2011). Therefore, it is proven that oxidative stress plays an important role in CS-induced renal damage and several dietary antioxidants have been shown to ameliorate this detrimental effect (Gómez-Sierra *et al.*, 2018).

SM (100 mg/kg/BW) significantly prevented the CS-evoked disturbances in the above-mentioned antioxidant indexes (El-Awady *et al.*, 2011; Mansour *et al.*, 2006). Rat pretreatment with SM 2 h before CS is shown to significantly decrease the detrimental pathological changes induced by CS and decrease its toxicity (Abdelmeguid *et al.*, 2010). Furthermore, *in vitro* pre-treatment with 25-200 μM of SM significantly protected against CS-induced cell death in a dose-dependent manner (Ninsontia *et al.*, 2011), inhibited apoptotic cascade and increased cell viability in the HEI-OC1 cells (Cho *et al.*, 2014). Based on the analysis of findings from animal studies presented in a review paper, it was concluded that SM has an ability to significantly protect (or ameliorate) from detrimental effects of drug-induced kidney disease, including CS-induced renal damage (Dashti-Khavidaki *et al.*, 2012).

In a clinical trial study, 60 patients with malignancy, were randomly enrolled in two equal groups. In patients of a control group CS was prescribed, while in an experimental group, SM (140 mg/day) was administrated seven days before CS administration. After two weeks, blood urea nitrogen and serum creatinine were significantly lower in the SM group compared to the control group indicating protective effect of SM against CS-induced nephrotoxicity (Momeni *et al.*, 2015a). SB is considered to be a pharmacological activator of SIRT3 which can provide protective effects against CS-induced tubular cell apoptosis and acute kidney injury by improving mitochondrial function and bioenergetics. The protective effect of SB was SIRT-dependent, since it was shown in wild-type, but not SIRT3-defective, cells and mice (Li *et al.*, 2017b). In a rat model of CS-induced acute renal failure there was a significant improvement in kidney function tests and renal histopathology as a result of using SM as protective mechanism (Ibrahim *et al.*, 2018).

In normal hepatocyte LO2 cells SB (50 μM) was reported to effectively reduce CS and/or toxal-induced hepatotoxicity by protecting DNA from damage leading to restoration of the potential of cell proliferation (Yang *et al.*, 2019). Silymarin-loaded amphiphilic chitosan polymeric micelles with SM concentration of 50 and 100 μg/ml were shown to increase the killing efficacy of CS on the cancer cells. At the same time, they showed the renoprotective effects: increasing cell viability from 29 to 82-96% and reducing cell apoptosis and necrosis induced by CS (Soodvilai *et al.*, 2019).

8.2.4 Benzo[a]pyrene

Benzo[a]pyrene (B[a]P), a polycyclic aromatic hydrocarbon found in coal tar, tobacco smoke and many foods, especially grilled meats is considered to be an environmental contaminant. B[a]P is shown to cause oxidative stress and possess genotoxic activity with the direct intercalation with the DNA leading to mutations (Sampaio *et al.*, 2021). The protective effect of SM/SB (400-500 μM) was shown. It was associated with decreasing DNA damage and apoptosis (Perumal Vijayaraman *et al.*, 2012), preventing protein thiol oxidation and AO enzyme (SOD, GPx, CAT, GR, GST) inhibition in the hemolysate (Kiruthiga *et al.*, 2007), restoring redox status, modulating GSH metabolising enzymes, decreasing formation of protein oxidation products and changing the level of antioxidant enzymes (5mM; Kiruthiga *et al.*, 2010). Furthermore, SM was found to prevent the toxicity induced by B[a]P in human erythrocytes by preserving its membrane integrity (Kiruthiga *et al.*, 2014).

SM (50-250 mg/kg/BW) showed substantial protective effects against B(a)P-induced damages by inhibiting phase I detoxification enzyme CYP1A1 and modulating phase II conjugating enzymes (glutathione-S-transferase, epoxide hydroxylases, uridine diphosphate glucuronosyltransferases, NAD(P)H: quinone oxidoreductase 1, sulfotransferases) in rat liver (Kiruthiga *et al.*, 2015). In general, it seems likely that SM possesses substantial protective effect against B(a)P-induced damages by inhibiting phase I detoxification enzyme CYP1A1 and modulating phase II conjugating enzymes (Kiruthiga *et al.*, 2015). Furthermore, SM (40 μM) is shown to have anti-genotoxic effects: it prevented B[a]P-7,8-dihydrodiol-9,10-epoxide-DNA adduct formation in HepG2 cells by modulating the Nrf2 and PXR signalling pathways (Jee *et al.*, 2020).

8.2.5 Doxorubicin

Doxorubicin (DOX, also called adriamycin) is an effective chemotherapeutic drug widely used for the treatment of patients with cancer. However, its side effect is related to cardiotoxicity, caused by oxidative stress, redox disbalance, mitochondrial dysfunction and apoptosis (Cappetta *et al.*, 2017; Dirks-Naylor, 2013). In general, the precise mechanisms of the cardiotoxicity of DOX are not described yet, but impairment of the antioxidant defence system and oxidative stress associated with mitochondrial dysfunction and cell membrane damage have been suggested as potential etiologic factors (Hosseini and Sahebkar, 2017).

SM, and the constituent flavonolignans SB, silydianin and silychristin were shown to protected rat heart microsomes and mitochondria against iron-dependent DOX-induced lipid peroxidation (Psotová *et al.*, 2002). Similarly, SM and flavonolignans (25, 50 and 100 μM) displayed a dose-dependent cytoprotection against DOX toxicity (100 μM, incubation 8 h). The protective effects of SM, SB, dehydrosilibinin and silychristin were shown to be comparable to that of dexrasoxane, while silydianin showed the best protective effect (Chlopcíková *et al.*, 2004). It has been shown that DOX-induced biochemical and histopathological alterations in rat testis could be prevented and/or protected by SM (50 mg/kg/BW). The SM protective and preventive effects which result in the reduction of DOX-induced carbonyl stress and DNA damage (Malekinejad *et al.*, 2012), decrease in the plasma creatine phosphokinase, LDH, creatinine and urea, myocardial MDA contents and renal tissue contents of MDA have also been shown (El-Shitany *et al.*, 2008). Similarly, SM (16 mg/kg/BW) significantly decreased an oxidative stress in DOX-treated rats by decreasing MDA and DNA fragmentation in the liver (Patel *et al.*, 2010).

A protective influence of SM (60 mg/kg/BW) on the heart and liver tissue against toxicity induced by DOX in rats was associated with a prevention of an increase in AST and CK serum activity (Rašković *et al.*, 2011). SM (injected i.p. at 100 mg/kg dose for 5 days before DOX administration) was reported to significantly protect from DOX-induced toxicities in the rat kidney, heart, and liver as indicated histopathological and electron microscopic examinations (Cecen *et al.*, 2011). Sperm quality was assessed in male rats following DOX administration with or without SM. Administration of SM was shown to significantly reduce DOX-induced sperm abnormalities, DNA fragmentation, nitric oxide concentration associated with a marked increase in total antioxidant power, sperm motility and viability (Shafiei-Roudbari *et al.*, 2017). SM (420 mg/day) showed protective effect in DOX-treated children with acute lymphoblastic leukaemia as evidenced by reduction of early DOX-induced left ventricular systolic function disturbances (Hagag *et al.*, 2019). Synergistic therapeutic effects of SM and Vitis vinifera extract on DOX-induced cardiorenal injury rat model associated with increased Nrf2 expression were shown (Abdelsalam *et al.*, 2019). SM in combination with chlorogenic acid was indicated to protect against hepatotoxicity induced by DOX in rats through inhibiting apoptosis biomarkers, maintaining antioxidant enzyme levels, decreasing pro-inflammatory cytokines as well as regulating liver adenosine monophosphate-activated protein kinase signalling (Abbas *et al.*, 2020). In a randomised, triple blind, placebo-controlled clinical trial, oral administration of SM (140 mg three times a day) was shown to be able to significantly reduce hepatotoxicity severity after 1 month of treatment in non-metastatic breast cancer patients treated with DOX/cyclophosphamide-paclitaxel regimen (Moezian *et al.*, 2022).

8.2.6 Acetaminophen

Acetaminophen, also known as N-acetyl para-aminophenol (APAP) or paracetamol, is one of the most widely used, over the counter analgesic and antipyretic drug and is considered to be safe when used at usual therapeutic doses. However, in overdoses, it is a potent hepatotoxin, causing hepatic and renal tubular necrosis, which can be lethal in human and animal. Its toxicity is associated with AO system dysregulation and oxidative stress (Chowdhury *et al.*, 2020).

In 1992 it was suggested that SM can protect against APAP intoxication through its antioxidant properties (Muriel *et al.*, 1992). During next 30 years research has proven the efficacy of SM in protection against APAP-induced toxicity in various animal models and clinical trials. When APAP-exposed rats were pretreated with SM (200 mg/kg orally for three days), APAP-compromised AO defences in rat brain were effectively re-established indicative by increase in GSH concentrations and increased SOD activity (Nencini *et al.*, 2007). In APAP-induced hepatotoxicity in cats SM (single dose 150 mg/kg, p.o.) was observed to protect liver tissue against oxidative stress (Avizeh *et al.*, 2010). Oral administration of APAP (500 mg/kg for 1 to 3 days) to rats resulted in significant elevation of serum triglycerides, total cholesterol, blood urea nitrogen, serum creatinine, and AST activity. Post-treatment with SM (25 mg/kg from day 4 to 14) offered a significant protection by reversing the metabolic alterations (Gopi *et al.*, 2010). It was suggested that SM could be used as an antidote for patients with APAP-induced acute hepatic injury and delayed treatment (Hau *et al.*, 2010).

A single dose of orally administered SM (150 mg/kg) was shown to significantly attenuated APAP-induced liver damage in rat as indicated by restoration of serum AST, ALT, and ALP and liver histopathology (Kazemifar *et al.*, 2012). SM pretreatment (200 mg/kg, before APAP exposure) was indicated to restore the hepatocyte functional and histopathological alterations induced by APAP in normotensive and hypertensive rats (Freitag *et al.*, 2015). It was suggested that the protective effects of SM against APAP-induced damages could be associated with its antioxidant and anti-inflammatory properties (Bektur *et al.*, 2016).

In rats, APAP overdose was associated with locomotor retardation, excessive self-grooming, working-memory impairment, anxiety, derangement of liver/kidney biochemistry, antioxidant imbalance, and detrimental histological changes in the liver, kidney and cerebral cortex. However, pre-treatment with SM (25 mg/kg for 14 days) was recorded to counteract the behavioural changes, reversed biochemical indices of liver/kidney injury, and improved antioxidant activity (Onaolapo *et al.*, 2017). In a mouse model of APAP-induced toxicity, SM-pretreated mice (100 mg/kg BW, per os, once daily for three days, 2 hours before APAP treatment) was found to significantly reduce APAP-induced liver injury, assessed according to AST and ALT release and histological examination. Furthermore, SM pretreatment significantly reduced superoxide production, as indicated by lower GSSG content, lower HO-1 induction, alleviated nitrosative stress, decreased p-JNK activation (Papackova *et al.*, 2018).

Hepatoprotective actions of ascorbic acid (500 mg/kg), alpha lipoic acid (100 mg/kg) and SM (200 mg/kg) in combination against APAP-induced hepatotoxicity in rats was shown to be increased when compared to individual administration of antioxidants (Abdulrazzaq *et al.*, 2019). In APAP-induced rat model of liver injury oral use of SM loaded onto mesoporous silica nanoparticles (250 mg/kg) was exhibited to have improved protective effects against APAP toxicity in comparison to free SM (Nasr *et al.*, 2019). SM pretreatment (100 mg/kg for 7 days) was demonstrated to have protective effects against APAP-induced hepatotoxicity in adult male albino rats (Ahmad *et al.*, 2019a).

In a domestic pigeon model of APAP-induced toxicity, SM supplementation (35 mg/kg, starting at 12 hours after APAP exposure, for 3 days) was found to decrease the serum levels of ASP, ALT, urea, and uric acid compared with the APAP-treated birds and completely prevented mortality, which was 86% in the control APAP-treated birds (Ihedioha *et al.*, 2020). In a rat model of APAP-induced hepatotoxicity elevated ALT, AST and ALP levels were significantly decreased by SM or SM-solid dispersion (SMD, both 20 mg/kg, three times per day for 5 days), but these decreases were much higher in SMD animals than in those treated with SM (Song *et al.*, 2021a).

8.2.7 Pesticides: Paraquat and maneb

Paraquat (PQ), a cheap and an effective herbicide, is widely used worldwide to remove weeds in cultivated crop fields, while maneb (MB) is a fungicide used in the control of early and late blights on potatoes and tomatoes. However, these pesticides are toxic with a multi-target mechanism causing serious harm to the environment and organisms (Chen *et al.*, 2021). Molecular mechanisms of damaging effects of PQ and maneb have not been fully understood, but oxidative stress and inflammation are among major molecular events of their toxicity.

In MB- and PQ-induced mouse model of Parkinson's disease (PD) SM (40 mg/kg for 9 weeks) was reported to significantly improve MB- and PQ-mediated reductions in locomotor activities, dopamine content, vesicular monoamine transporter 2 (VMAT2) mRNA expression and the expression of p53 protein. Furthermore, SM was found to attenuate the increases in lipid peroxidation, number of degenerating neurons, nitrite content, mRNA expressions and catalytic activities of cytochrome P-450 2E1 and GST and P-p53, Bax and caspase 9 protein expressions (Singhal *et al.*, 2011). In an *in vitro* experiment protective roles of SM against PQ-induced oxidative stress on human A549 adenocarcinoma cell line were investigated. In particular, it was shown that SM (10-100 μg/ml) was able to dramatically prevent cell toxicity and reduce the LDH retention induced by PQ in A549 cells. SM was also reported to induce antioxidant related genes, including Nrf2, NQO1 and HO-1, in the presence of PQ, improving AO defences and alleviating PQ intoxication (Podder *et al.*, 2012).

In MB- and PQ-induced Parkinsonism mouse model, SM (40 mg/kg for 9 weeks) significantly resisted the changes in the expression of genes related to apoptosis, inflammation, cell cycle, cell-signalling, etc. (Singhal *et al.*, 2013). SM (100 mg/kg, intraperitoneally, 2 h before toxicants treatment) was observed to protect MB- and/or PQ-induced hepatotoxicity in rats by reducing oxidative stress (restoration of SOD, GPx activity and GSH concentration, increase of GR activity and decrease of MDA concentration). SM also decreased inflammation (decreased expression of pro-inflammatory TNF-α, IL-1β and iNOS) and modulated xenobiotic metabolising enzymes in the liver of MB- and/or PQ-treated rats (Ahmad *et al.*, 2013). SM also was indicated to attenuate PQ-induced lung injury via Nrf2-mediated pathway *in vivo* and *in vitro* (Zhao *et al.*, 2015) and its protective effects against PQ-induced cytotoxicity in macrophages was associated with regulating Trx/TXNIP complex, inhibiting NLRP3 inflammasome activation and apoptosis (Liu *et al.*, 2018). Therefore, SM is suggested to be employed as a safe and effective therapeutic modality for patients with PQ poisoning (Zakariaei, 2019).

8.2.8 Anti-TB drugs, rifampicin, isoniazid and pyrazinamide

Tuberculosis (TB) is highly endemic in various countries including India. The first-line anti-TB therapy (ATT) involving isoniazid (INH), rifampicin (RIF) and pyrazinamide (PZA) is shown to have side effects and cause hepatotoxicity in approximately 11.5% of Indian patients associated with oxidative stress caused by the drugs and metabolites (Singh *et al.*, 2012a).

Liver toxicity caused by co-administration of anti-TB drugs (ATD), RIF, INH and PZA, in a sub-chronic mode (12 weeks) was associated with a compromised AO system manifested by decreased GSH content, GPx, CAT activities and increased MDA in liver. At the same time increased levels of ALT, AST and ALP, a high bilirubin content in serum were also observed. SM was reported to reverse those abnormal alterations (Tasduq *et al.*, 2005). Similarly, when rats were treated with ATD (INH 25 mg/kg + RIF 50 mg/kg + PYR 140 mg/kg orally) daily for 45 days there was a significant decrease in the AO status as manifested by decreased GPx, GST, GR and GSH in liver tissue in comparison with saline-treated control animals. Treatment with SM (50 mg/kg) was shown to enhance the activities of GST and GPx but did not affect GSH levels compared with control (Victorrajmohan *et al.*, 2005). Treatment of rats with ATD (INH+RIF or INH+RIF+PZA) induced hepatotoxicity as evidenced by increased serum ALT, AST and ALP activities and total bilirubin and histopathological changes in drug-treated animals. Simultaneous administration of SM (200 mg/kg) was found to significantly decrease the biochemical and histological changes induced by the drugs (Eminzade *et al.*, 2008).

In another experiment rats with STZ-induced diabetes, nondiabetic rats and insulin-treated diabetic rats received ATD (INH+RIF+PZA) with or without SM (100 mg/kg/day p.o.) treatment for 45 days. Coadministration of SM was indicated to provide protection against ATD hepatotoxicity in all animals. However, insulin treatment of diabetic animals was reported to increase efficacy of SM-induced hepatoprotection against ATD-induced liver injury. (Srivastava *et al.*, 2008). Furthermore, in an *in vitro* study it was shown that the presence of hepatoprotective drugs, such as SM during treatment of HepG2 cells with ATD drugs could lower the hepatotoxic effect of the latter (Singh *et al.*, 2012b). When INH effects were studied in rabbits its toxicity was manifested by changes in serum bilirubin and ALT, while SM (50 mg/kg/day) normalised those parameters (Jahan *et al.*, 2015). Similarly, INH- and RIF-treated rats showed abnormalities in liver integrity markers which were normalised by SM treatment (Sabina *et al.*, 2019). A total of 1,198 patients from five randomised controlled trials (585 with SM and 613 in placebo groups) that compared SM and placebo to prevent antituberculosis drug-induced liver injury (anti-TB DILI) were included into a meta-analysis. It was indicated that SM significantly reduced the occurrence of anti-TB DILI at week 4 in patients undergoing anti-TB drug-treatments (Tao *et al.*, 2019).

8.2.9 Arsenic

Arsenic, a naturally occurring element widely distributed in the Earth's crust, is widely used in the production of pesticides, herbicides and insecticides and common sources of metal exposure include groundwater contamination, mining and leather tanning (Flora *et al.*, 2011). As-induced toxicity is associated with increased production of ROS, elevation in lipid peroxidation, protein carbonylation and DNA oxidation, and disruption of the cell cycle that results in apoptosis (Rashid *et al.*, 2013). The toxic effect of arsenic was indicated by significantly decrease activities of AO enzymes (SOD, CAT, GPx, GST, GR and glucose 6-phosphate dehydrogenase) along with non-enzymatic antioxidants (GSH, vitamins C and E) and decreased Nrf2 and HO-1 activities in the rat heart (Muthumani and Prabu, 2014).

SB was effective in counteracting all the parameters of oxidative stress. Administration of SB (50-75 mg/kg/BW) exhibited a significant preservation of antioxidant defences by maintaining activity of AO enzymes and non-enzymatic antioxidants in As-treated rats (Jain *et al.*, 2011; Soria *et al.*, 2010). Therefore, administration of SB showed a significant reversal of As-induced toxicity in hepatic tissue including reduction of DNA damage in hepatocytes and histopathological observations of the liver (Muthumani and Prabu, 2012). SM (20 μM) can also compensate the adverse effects of sodium arsenite on the ram sperm plasma membrane, acrosome integrity (Eskandari and Momeni, 2016b) and mitochondrial membrane potential of ram sperm (Eskandari and Momeni, 2016a). In earlier *in vitro* study, it has also been shown that SM had a protective effect on the sodium arsenite-induced stress responses of acute (200 μM $NaAsO_2$ plus 5 μM SM) or sub-chronic (5 μM $NaAsO_2$ plus 0.125 μM SM) arsenic exposure in CHO-K1 cells indicative by decreased GGT activity, reduced diene conjugate formation and reduced HSP70 expression (Bongiovanni *et al.* 2007).

8.2.10 Cadmium

Cadmium (Cd) is considered to be one of the most toxic elements that human beings can be exposed to at work or in the environment. Several epidemiological and experimental data indicate that chronic exposure to Cd in human beings can be associated with variety of different diseases including carcinogenesis. It seems likely that Cd toxicity is multidirectional, and creation of oxidative stress is an important event in the toxicity development. Indeed, Cd exerts its toxic effect by blocking the mitochondrial ETC and compromising AO defences resulting in redox disbalance and oxidative stress associated with macromolecule oxidation, mitochondrial membrane depolarisation, mtDNA mutation, and apoptosis (Genchi *et al.*, 2020).

First publication related to protective effect of SM in Cd toxicity appeared 40 years ago. In Cd and lead poisoning SM was reported to be responsible for the partial but significant prevention of structural damage and histochemical and enzymatic changes in tissues (Barbarino *et al.*, 1981). Pretreatment of J774A.1 cells with SM (50 μM) was reported to inhibit Cd-induced cell damage, including mitochondrial dysfunction, growth arrest, apoptosis and necrosis (Kim and Sharma, 2006). When rats subcutaneously received Cd (3 mg/kg BW/day) followed by oral administration of SB (80 mg/kg BW/day) in 0.1% DMSO for 3 weeks, there was a protective effect of SB related to decreased liver damage (AST, ALT, ALP, LDH, GGT), prevention of oxidative stress (plasma and liver TBARS) and improved antioxidant defences (vitamin E, vitamin C and GSH in plasma and liver). At the histological level SB also showed protective effect on the liver of Cd-treated rats: there was reduction of fatty changes with decrease of inflammation in hepatocytes (Srinivasan and Ramprasath, 2012). Oral administration of SB at 80 mg/kg b. w. was shown to normalise the acetylcholinesterase (AChE) activity and reduced the levels of lipid peroxidation and also restored the antioxidant and ATPases enzymes in the brain of Cd-treated rats (Srinivasan and Ramprasath, 2011).

In a mouse model of Cd toxicity, in the Cd-treated animals there was a significant reduction in serum FRAP, the activity of AO enzymes (SOD, GPx, CAT) and thiol groups compared to the control associated with a significant increase in MDA levels in serum. In SM+Cd group, SM (100 mg/kg BW, i.p., 24 h before the Cd treatment) was found to significantly reverse the reduction of AO enzymes and was able to decrease MDA compared to the Cd group (Farjad and Momeni, 2018). Furthermore, SM was reported to prevent the adverse effects of Cd chloride on testis histopathology, testosterone level, oxidative stress indicators (MDA) and antioxidant defence enzymes (SOD, GPx and CAT) in mice (Faraji *et al.*, 2019).

Supplementing milk thistle (10 g/kg) or SM (250 mg/kg) were shown to ameliorate Cd-induced mortality, organ weights, spermatogenesis, and histopathological lesions in quail (Saleemi *et al.*, 2019). SM was found to protect the structure of kidney in the neonatal rats exposed to maternal Cd toxicity: Cd caused subacute glomerulosclerosis, severe damage to urinary tubules such as tubular necrosis, and severe hyperaemia in the medulla, but SM (100 mg/kg, subcutaneously, 3 days per week for three weeks) was able to preserve those complications (Hamidian *et al.*, 2020).The authors suggested that the administration of SM during pregnancy may be used as a useful and effective way of protecting the maternal Cd toxicity complications in the kidney tissue of neonatal rats. SM (2 μM) was also shown to be able to partly compensate for the caspase-independent apoptosis in the Cd-treated human spermatozoa (Etemadi *et al.*, 2020).

8.2.11 Lead

Lead (Pb) is a nonessential heavy metal pollutant widely distributed in the environment being a major public health concern. Exposure to Pb is known to cause neurotoxicity that ranges from neurodevelopmental disorders to severe neurodegenerative lesions, leading to impairments in learning, memory, cognitive function, etc. This metal can affect a range of cellular pathways regulating cell survival, altering calcium homeostasis, and inducing apoptosis, inflammation, energy metabolism disorders, oxidative stress and autophagy (Fang *et al.*, 2021). Thus, oxidative stress has been identified as the primary contributor in the pathogenesis of Pb exposure (Balali-Mood *et al.*, 2021).

Combined treatment of lead-exposed rats with SM (1 mg/100 g body weight) and Vitamin C (1 mg/100 g body weight) by gastric tube three times per week was shown to impose marked improvement of the biochemical (AST, ALT, ALP, GGT in serum) molecular (DNA fragmentation) and histopathological (fibrosis and apoptosis) findings (Shalan *et al.*, 2005). In lead-treated rats, significant elevation in kidney lead level, decrease in renal GPx and elevation in kidney MDA were observed. Histologically, lead was reported to induce disorganisation and shrinkage of glomeruli with sloughing of epithelium, widening of Bowman's space and inflammatory infiltration in renal medulla. Treatment by SM combined with garlic extract resulted in a significant improvement in the affected parameters. (El-Khishin *et al.*, 2015). In Pb-treated rats, SM (100 mg/kg orally for 8 weeks) was recorded to provide significant protection on the genotoxic effect of Pb and improved the renal histopathological lesions (Alcaraz-Contreras *et al.*, 2016). Pb exposure in rats was shown to induce hepatotoxicity with suppression of liver antioxidant defence system and SM (200-mg/kg, orally for 10 days) was able to alleviate this effect (Jalali *et al.*, 2017). Lead acetate was reported to alter liver structure and function with significant elevation of the activities of serum AST and ALT and serum levels of urea and creatinine, increasing hepatic and renal MDA and reducing GSH content and SOD and CAT activities, increasing caspase-3 mRNA expression and altering liver and kidney tissues' architectures. At the same time, SM (50 or 100 mg/kg BW, 1 h before administration of lead acetate for 10 weeks) was found to ameliorate in a dose-dependent manner the toxic effects of lead acetate on the liver and kidneys: reducing lipid oxidation and pathological changes of hepatic and renal tissue structure, improving antioxidant defence system of liver and kidneys, and decreasing pro-apoptotic gene expression in hepatic tissue (Abd Eldaim *et al.*, 2021).

8.2.12 Mercury

Mercury is one of the most toxic heavy metals detectable in the environment and is involved in nervous tissue damage causing neurotoxicity and neuronal cell death in mammalian species including humans. Mercury toxicity depends on its chemical forms, times, and doses of exposure. Mercury is known to be involved in redox balance dysregulation associated with compromised AO system, calcium homeostasis dysregulation and excess in ROS production leading to oxidative stress and apoptosis. Mercury can bind functional groups (–SH) of cysteine residues and GSH causing inactivation of proteins such as various enzymes, hormones, cofactors, etc. leading to cellular injury. Moreover, methylmercury is believed to exert its toxicity interfering with intracellular signal transmission of multiple receptors. (Cariccio *et al.*, 2019).

In murine macrophages (J774A.1 cell culture) mercury-induced apoptosis was shown to be mediated by ROS-activated p38 MAPK followed by caspase activation. Treatment of cells with mercury at 70 μM increased TNF-α mRNA and induced necrosis and apoptosis. Pretreatment of cultures with SM (5 μM) or SB (2 μM) reduced mercury-induced TNF-α expression and decreased mercury-induced necrosis (Kim and Sharma, 2004).

8.2.13 Aluminium

Aluminium (Al) is the most widely distributed metal in the environment, and it can become a contaminant from anthropogenic sources and through the weathering of rocks and minerals. Al intoxication can occur in animals and human populations and toxic effects of Al are associated with redox disbalance and oxidative stress leading to immunologic alterations, genotoxicity, pro-inflammatory effect, enzymatic dysfunction, metabolic derangement, membrane perturbation, apoptosis, necrosis and dysplasia. The pathological conditions associated with Al toxicosis are desquamative interstitial pneumonia, pulmonary alveolar proteinosis, granulomas, granulomatosis and fibrosis, toxic myocarditis, thrombosis and ischemic stroke, granulomatous enteritis, Crohn's disease, inflammatory bowel diseases, anaemia, Alzheimer's disease, dementia, sclerosis, autism, oligospermia and infertility, hepatorenal disease, pancreatitis, pancreatic necrosis and diabetes mellitus (Igbokwe *et al.*, 2019).

In a study of hepatoprotective effect of Wattakaka volubilis extract on aluminium sulphate induced liver toxicity in rat model SM was used for a comparison as a standard treatment. It was shown that SM administration (25 mg/kg) to $Al_2(SO_4)_3$-treated rats was associated with significant improvement in serum liver integrity marker enzymes (AST, ALT, LDH, GGT). The detrimental effects of $Al_2(SO_4)_3$ on the body weight and liver function such as carbohydrate, protein and nucleic acid metabolism were also improved by SM supplementation (Rani *et al.*, 2014). In a mouse model of ($AlCl_3$-induced) neurotoxicity SB (100 and 200 mg/kg/day, p.o. for 42 days) was found to exert neuroprotective effects against $AlCl_3$-induced cognitive impairment and neurochemical changes including normalisation of AChE and CAT activity, GSH and MDA content, as well as pro-inflammatory cytokines (IL-1β and TNF-α) in the hippocampus (Jangra *et al.*, 2015). In rats challenged with fructose-induced insulin resistance SM (100 mg/kg/day) was found to alleviate the neurotoxic effects of aluminium. The administration of SM was shown to suppress $AlCl_3$-induced memory deficit, oxidative stress, and neuroinflammation in brain tissue of insulin resistant rats by inhibiting $AlCl_3$-induced activation of TLR4 signalling pathway including the downstream activation of NF-κB (Ali *et al.*, 2019). Aluminium chloride was found to induce toxic effect on ram sperm plasma membrane integrity and acrosome integrity and SM (5 μM) added to the diluent was able to protect from the detrimental effects of $AlCl_3$ (Momeni *et al.*, 2015b). Human spermatozoa treated with aluminium chloride were characterised by decreased percentage of intact acrosome and plasma membrane integrity, viability, motility and the total antioxidant capacity in comparison with control group.

Adding SM to the aluminium-treated spermatozoa was reported to significantly compensate the adverse effects of aluminium chloride on those parameters (Aghashahi *et al.*, 2020). In a rat model of aluminium chloride-induced Alzheimer's-like disease SM (200 mg/kg/day for 15 days) was found to mend most previously evoked neuronal damages in the hippocampal tissues of $AlCl_3$-trated rats (Aboelwafa *et al.*, 2020). SM administered to rats (100 and 200 mg/kg) after their exposure to $AlCl3{\cdot}6H_2O$ was shown to improve learning and memory function by inhibiting excessive apoptosis and oxidative stress indicative by restoration of SOD and GPx activity in the brain and serum and decreasing MDA in the tissues (Li *et al.*, 2020).

8.2.14 Iron

Iron is an essential element necessary for almost all forms of life, ranging from bacteria to humans contributing to many important biological processes, including electron transport in mitochondria and energy production, DNA replication, the TCA activity, etc. However, iron is a major catalyser of ROS formation in biological systems. Therefore, excess iron is shown to be detrimental to the body causing oxidative stress associated with an increased risk of neurodegenerative diseases, cancer, and diabetes (Zhang *et al.*, 2022).

Iron overload (2.5% carbonyl-iron diet) caused a dramatic accumulation of MDA-protein adducts into iron-filled periportal hepatocytes that was substantially decreased by SB treatment (100 mg/kg body WT/day for 4 months). Furthermore, SB treatment decreased the iron-induced accumulation of MDA in mitochondria, mitochondrial energy wasting and tissue ATP depletion (Pietrangelo *et al.*, 1995). In a male gerbils model, SB administration (100 mg/kg body WT/day by gavage) was shown to significantly reduce both functional anomalies and the fibrotic process by chelating desferrioxamine chelatable iron (Masini *et al.*, 2000). In acutely iron-dosed gerbils model iron overload in nonparenchymal cells was observed to lead to an activation of hepatic stellate cells and fibrogenesis and was reported to significantly increase the mitochondrial desferrioxamine-chelatable iron pool associated with the impairment of mitochondrial oxidative metabolism and the hepatic ATP decrease. All biochemical and functional derangements were indicated to be prevented by *in vivo* SB administration and block fibrogenesis (Pietrangelo *et al.*, 2002). The iron-chelating potential of SB was demonstrated in patients with hereditary haemochromatosis: consumption of SB with a meal resulted in a reduction in the postprandial increase in serum iron compared with water (Hutchinson *et al.*, 2010).

SB was shown to form a complex with unchelated iron in the ferric form rendering it unavailable for absorption and it is considered as a good candidate in the chelation therapy of chronic iron overload due to (Borsari *et al.*, 2001):

- a very high affinity for ferric ion;
- absence of Fe(III) precipitation or ligand decomposition in a wide pH range;
- ameliorative effects on the severity of fibrosis in iron-induced oxidant stress model.

In general, in thalassemia patients immunity can be compromised as a result of reduction of GSH levels and proliferation of PHA-activated peripheral blood mononuclear cells, detrimental changes which can be corrected by adding SM (5-20 μg/ml) into the incubation medium (Alidoost *et al.*, 2006). Major β-thalassemia (β-TM) is one of the most common inherited haemolytic types of anaemia which is a result of absence or reduced synthesis of β-globin chains of haemoglobin. This defect is associated with red blood cells lysis and chronic anaemia that are usually treated by multiple blood transfusions and iron chelation therapy. Without iron chelation therapy, iron overload would cause oxidative stress leading to various complications in patients. SM is considered to be an important chelating agent in adjuvant therapy of β-TM (Moayedi Esfahani *et al.*, 2015).

In clinical trials SM was shown to be effective at reducing iron overload in β-thalassemia major patients when used in conjunction with desferrioxamine (Gharagozloo *et al.*, 2009; Moayedi *et al.*, 2013). In a rat model of iron overload, SM (200 and 400 mg/kg) was found to be a nephroprotectant possessing protective ability against kidney iron deposition (Nematbakhsh *et al.*, 2013) and SM was reported to have a protective effect similar to deferoxamine on iron overload-induced hepatotoxicity (Najafzadeh *et al.*, 2010). Combined therapy with deferasirox and SM was recorded to be safely used in the treatment of iron-loaded thalassaemic patients (Hagag *et al.*, 2013).

In a 12-week clinical trial in two groups of patients with β-thalassemia major in combined therapy group (n=25), patients received desferrioxamine at the dose of 40 mg/kg/day and SM (420 mg daily), while in SM group (n=5), patients received only SM. Immunological tests were assessed at the beginning and the end of the trial. Interestingly, SM was shown to stimulate cell-mediated immune response as evidenced by decreased serum TNF-α and neopterin as well as increased production of IFN-γ and IL-4 after SM treatment (Gharagozloo *et al.*, 2013). In a crossover, randomised controlled trial effects of SM on inflammatory status of patients with β-thalassemia major and iron overload (one of the main causes of inflammation) were assessed. According to protocol of the study SM (140 mg, 3 times a day) or placebo were prescribed to all patients (n=82) for 12 weeks, and after a 2-week washout period, patients were crossed over to the other group. Compared to the placebo group, SM was shown to significantly decrease C-reactive protein (CRP), IL-6, and raise IL-10 showing clear improvement of inflammatory status in patients treated with SM (Darvishi-Khezri *et al.*, 2021). In the same study the authors also reported a negative change in the serum iron and ferritin levels and a positive change in the total iron-binding capacity level due to SM supplementation (Darvishi-Khezri *et al.*, 2018) and SM was indicated to decrease serum oxidative stress and to enhance serum AO capability (decreased MDA and protein carbonyls, increased GSH) in patients with β-thalassemia major (Darvishi-Khezri *et al.*, 2017). The authors suggested that SM could be given as an adjuvant therapy to standard iron chelators to decrease oxidative stress in patients with β-thalassemia major.

A cross-sectional study was performed on ten β-thalassemia intermedia patients who were treated with a standardised commercial preparation of milk thistle containing 80% of SM at a daily dose of 420 mg orally (140 mg, three times a day) for 6 months (Reisi *et al.*, 2022). It was shown that serum ferritin levels were significantly reduced after 3 and 6 months suggesting that SM is effective iron-chelating agent for the treatment of iron-overloaded conditions. A similar conclusion was drawn earlier as a result of reviewing clinical and experimental studies investigating the use of SM prior to September 1, 2015, using major databases (PubMed, ISI Web of Knowledge, Science Direct, Scopus, Ovid, and Cochrane Library databases): SM may be a useful and important adjuvant for improving multiple organ dysfunctions in patients with β-thalassemia major (Darvishi Khezri *et al.*, 2016).

8.2.15 Copper

Copper (Cu) is a crucial trace element for human and animals involved in regulation of various physiological functions including growth and development, immunocompetence maintenance and signalling in eukaryotic organisms (El Sabry *et al.*, 2021). Copper imbalances (overload or deficiency) have been shown to result in the development of various diseases, including anaemia, neutropenia, thrombocytopenia and carcinogenesis (Ruiz *et al.*, 2021). Of note, copper access leads to increased ROS production and oxidative stress (Chen *et al.*, 2020b).

SM was shown to inhibit *in vitro* the copper-induced oxidation of human LDL in a concentration-dependent manner (Skottová *et al.*, 1999). Similarly, the inhibitory effect of different concentrations of SM (0.01- 1.0 mg/ml) on conjugated diene formation induced by copper ions in human plasma was recorded (Asghar and Masood, 2008). The *in vitro* complexation of SB with Ni^{2+}, Fe^{3+}, Cu^{2+} and Zn^{2+} was found with the strongest interaction observed between SB and Cu^{2+} (Zatloukalová *et al.*, 2011). SM (0.50 mg/ml) was observed to decrease goat heart mitochondria damages caused by copper-ascorbate mixture used to promote lipid peroxidation (Dutta *et al.*, 2014). However, it is not clear from the experimental set up if chelating ability of SM for Cu was involved. Recently, in an *in vitro* study it has been shown that among SM constituents, only 2,3-dehydrosilybin was a potent or moderately active iron and copper chelator, while silybin A, silybin B and silychristin A were less potent or inactive chelators (Tvrdý *et al.*, 2018).

8.2.16 Mn

It is well known that manganese toxicity in animals is associated with increased oxidative stress, apoptosis and inflammation (Karki *et al.*, 2013). Animals exposed to manganese chloride were characterised by a significant increase in TBARS levels associated with a decrease of enzymatic (SOD, CAT and GPx) and non-enzymatic (GSH and ascorbic acid) antioxidants (Chtourou *et al.*, 2010; 2013), increased lipid and protein oxidation (Chtourou *et al.*, 2012), DNA fragmentation and urinary hydrogen peroxide (Chtourou *et al.*, 2014). Co-administration of SM (100 mg/kg/BW) to Mn-treated rats significantly restored antioxidant defences and attenuated oxidative damages observed in the liver, kidney and brain (Chtourou *et al.*, 2010; 2012; 2013; 2014).

8.2.17 Fluoride

Fluoride, an important industrial chemical, could cause damage to cellular processes in different tissues, due to oxidative stress associated with compromised redox balance (Miranda *et al.*, 2018). Furthermore, the proteomic analysis indicated important changes in proteins related to endoplasmic reticulum and mitochondrial oxidative stress, mitochondrial alteration, apoptosis and cellular respiration upon exposure due to fluoride exposure (Pereira Habds *et al.*, 2018). It was indicated that SM can improve damages induced by sodium fluoride in rat cardiac tissue via its antioxidant activity. SM (10 and 20 mg/kg /day), one week prior to sodium fluoride could decrease MDA level, increase SOD and CAT activities in heart tissues of rats treated by sodium fluoride. Vitamin C (10 mg/kg/day) was used as a positive control. The effect of SM (20 mg/Kg) was similar to that of vitamin C (Nabavi *et al.*, 2012).

8.2.18 Silver nanoparticles (AgNPs)

Silver nanoparticles (AgNPs) are known to be an important class of nanomaterials with a wide range of industrial and medical applications. However, the unique properties of AgNPs are associated with a range of hazards to human health due to AgNP-induced stimulation of oxidative stress, genotoxicity and apoptosis (Kim and Ryu, 2013). Based on data on effects of AgNP on mice liver primary cell viability in culture, SM (600 µg/ml) and vitamin E (2,500 µmol/l) were shown to have protective effects against AgNP toxicity and a combination of the two antioxidants were more effective than their individual use (Faedmaleki *et al.*, 2016). Exposure of Nile tilapia to AgNPs was found to cause a reduction in the levels of GPx and SOD activity and an increase in the level of MDA. At the same time free and nanoencapsulated SM treatment (50 or 200 mg kg^{-1} for 50 days prior to exposure to AgNPs) was shown to have protective effects as evidenced by increased GPx activity and reduced MDA levels in tilapia liver compared with controls (Veisi *et al.*, 2021).

8.2.19 Ethanol

Oxidative stress plays an important role in the pathogenesis of alcoholic liver damage. During ethanol metabolism, RONS are formed causing oxidative stress (Galicia-Moreno and Gutiérres-Reyes, 2014). Supplementation with a standardised SM (200 mg/kg/BW) attenuated an oxidative stress caused by acute ethanol administration, including prevention of elevation of serum ALT activity, decrease in hepatic GSH and enhanced lipid peroxidation, and increased hepatic TNF production (Song *et al.*, 2006). Similarly, SM (100-200 mg/kg/BW) effectively protected liver from alcohol-induced oxidative stress as evidenced by reducing ALT and AST activities in serum, increasing SOD and GPx activities and decreasing MDA content in the liver (Zhang *et al.*, 2013b).

SB (100 mg/kg) is shown to ameliorate steatosis and insulin resistance during non-alcoholic fatty liver disease development partly through targeting IRS-1/PI3K/Akt pathway (Zhang *et al.*, 2013a). Furthermore SB (250 mg/kg/BW) normalised alcohol-altered AO parameters in the whole blood hemolysate of mice, including AO enzymes (SOD, CAT, GR, GPx), GSH and TBARS (Das and Mukherjee, 2012). In mouse primary hepatocytes *in vitro* SB (10-40 µM) was not effective in repressing the ethanol-induced hepatocyte injury, whereas SB was shown to reduce acetaldehyde-caused hepatocyte injury through down-regulation of apoptosis and up-regulation of autophagy (Song *et al.*, 2021b).

8.2.20 Gentamicin

Gentamicin (GEN), an antibiotic used to treat bacterial infections, is one of the leading cause of drug-induced nephrotoxicity (Randjelovic *et al.*, 2017). In a model of GEN-induced nephrotoxicity in dogs, protective effect of SM alone (20 mg/kg once daily for 9 days) was indicated: total AOA increased but MDA decreased (Varzi *et al.*, 2007). SM pretreatment (100 mg/kg, oral gavage, 2 h before GEN) was shown to be able to restore nerve growth factor levels and increase tropomyosin-related kinase receptors-A m-RNA expression in cochlear tissue and preserve hair cells of organ. SM also caused significant amelioration in oxidative stress state as indicative by reducing MDA levels and increasing CAT activity (Draz *et al.*, 2015). SM was observed to attenuate GEN-induced renal injury in rats as a result of amelioration of oxidative stress indicative by decreased renal ROS and MDA levels (Ghaznavi *et al.*, 2016).

8.2.21 Other toxicants

The protective effects of similar doses of SM/SB on the antioxidant systems of the body are also shown in pyrogallol toxicity (Gupta *et al.*, 2002; Upadhyay *et al.*, 2007; 2010), bleomicyn-injected mice (Razavi-Azarkhiavi *et al.*, 2014), acrolein toxicity in mice (Taghiabadi *et al.*, 2012), diethylnitrosamine-induced oxidative stress in rats (Parashar *et al.*, 2019; Pradeep *et al.*, 2007), methotrexate-induced nephrotoxicity in rats (Dabak and Kocaman, 2015), ketoprofen-induced hepatotoxicity in rats (Kelany and Abdallah, 2016), isoproterenol prompted cardiotoxicity in rats (Sheta *et al.*, 2020), vancomycin-induced nephrotoxicity in rats (Guzel *et al.*, 2020), docetaxel-induced central and peripheral neurotoxicity in rats (Yardum *et al.*, 2021). The protective effects of SM/SM was demonstrated in cyclosporine A induced hepatorenal toxicity in rat (Vangaveti *et al.*, 2021), pyrazinamide and isoniazid hepatotoxicity (Goh *et al.*, 2020), nickel sulphate-induced reproductive toxicity in male rats (Temamogullari *et al.*, 2021), epirubicin-induced mucosal barrier injury in mice (Sasu *et al.*, 2015), in the liver and pancreas of alloxan-induced diabetic rats (Miranda *et al.*, 2020), microcystin-LR-induced cardiac and pulmonary injuries in mice (Al-Hazmi, 2020), HCl-induced acute lung injury in rats (Ahmed *et al.*, 2019b), kainic acid-induced neurotoxicity in the hippocampus (Kim *et al.*, 2017b), kainic acid-induced excitotoxicity (Lu *et al.*, 2020).

The SM/SB protection was obvious in triptolide-induced acute hepatotoxicity in rats (Wang *et al.*, 2018), thiram cytotoxicity in human, rat and chicken cell cultures (Radko *et al.*, 2017), polymyxin E-induced toxicity in rat kidneys (Hassan *et al.*, 2017), zidovudine and isoniazid-induced hepatotoxicity in rats (Raghu and Karthikeyan, 2016; Ramanathan and Sivanesan, 2017), L-arginine-induced acute pancreatitis in rats (Uçmak *et al.*, 2016), N-nitrosodimethylamine-induced glutathione dysregulation and hepatotoxicity in rats (Ezhilarasan and Karthikeyan, 2016), diazinon-induced hepatotoxicity in rats (Beydilli *et al.*, 2015), itraconazole-induced liver damage in rats (Sozen *et al.*, 2015), mycophenolate mofetil-induced duodenal injuries in rats (Malekinejad *et al.*, 2014).

Furthermore, anti-toxic effects of SM/SM was also demonstrated in acute cocaine toxicity in astroglial, liver and kidney cells (Badisa *et al.*, 2014), di(2-ethylhexyl)phthalate-induced injury in liver FL83B cells (Lo *et al.*, 2014), lasalocid-induced cytotoxicity in chicken and rat cell lines (Radko *et al.*, 2013b) and in HepG2 cells (Radko *et al.*, 2013a), oxaliplatin-induced neuropathy in rats (Di Cesare Mannelli *et al.*, 2012), chemical warfare agent sulphur mustard skin toxicity (Tewari-Singh *et al.*, 2012), anti-viral drug ribavirin (Noshy, *et al.*, 2013), neurotoxin 6-hydroxydopamine (Haddadi *et al.*, 2020), sodium nitrite (Sherif and Al-Gayyar, 2013) and phenylhydrazine (Valenzuela *et al.*, 1985), acrylamide (Elsawy *et al.*, 2021; Li *et al.*, 2017a), α-amanitin (Popp *et al.*, 2020), cyclophosphamide (Avci *et al.*, 2017), scopolamine (El-Marasy *et al.*, 2018), 1-methyl-4-phenyl-1,2,3,6-tetrahydropyridine (Tripathi *et al.*, 2020), fingolimod (Ghiasian *et al.*, 2021), bisphenol A (Lama *et al.*, 2019; Zaulet *et al.*, 2017) toxicity.

8.3 Oxidative stress-related conditions

8.3.1 Gamma radiation

Ionising radiation, a valuable diagnostic and therapeutic tool in medicine, is harmful to human body, due to direct ionisation of cellular structures (e.g. DNA) and/or from the indirect effect through ROS production as a result of water radiolysis (Abdel-Aziz *et al.*, 2021). SM administered 1 h before irradiation, moderated radiation-induced changes in RNA and DNA in liver and bone marrow (days 7 and 14 after administration) and increased total content of DNA in spleen at 30 h after SM treatment (Hakov'a and Misúrová, 1993). Whole-body gamma-irradiation (3 or 6 grays; Gy) revealed that 3 days after radiation exposure antioxidant defences were compromised as evidenced by decrease in GR and GPx activity and GSH concentration in the rat liver tissue associated with liver damages indicative by increased activity of serum AST and ALT. Administration of SM as single (70 mg/kg), fractionated (490 mg/kg) oral doses or as intravenous injection (50 mg/kg) showed significant protection of liver integrity and AO defences (Ramadan *et al.*, 2002). In the *in vitro* liposomal system SM was shown to be able to inhibit lipid peroxidative stress imposed by supra-lethal radiation stress as well as to modulate the level of NF-κB in other model systems (Adhikari *et al.*, 2010). SB was reported to have a strong protective activity to prevent radiation-induced DNA damage under both *in vitro* and *in vivo* conditions.

On the one hand, under *in vitro* conditions of irradiation, SB in a concentration dependent manner (0-200 μM) was found to protect plasmid pBR322 DNA against gamma-radiation-induced strand breaks. SB also provided protection to DNA and reduced ROS formation in lymphocytes exposed to radiation (3 Gy). On the other hand, in mouse studies SB (70 mg/kg for 3 days prior to whole-body gamma-exposure at 7.5 Gy) was reported to show significant protection to radiation-induced mortality and DNA damage in blood leukocytes (Tiwari *et al.*, 2010).

In general, protection against radiation-induced cell-death and DNA damage by SM was attributed to a reduction in ROS production and oxidative stress induced by γ-radiation (Adhikari *et al.*, 2013). Combining SB with ionising radiation (IR) was reported to demonstrate anti-cancer effects by down-regulating endothelial cell proliferation, clonogenicity and tube formation ability and reducing migratory and invasive properties of prostate cancer cells, while IR treatment alone only marginally affected those cell properties (Nambiar *et al.*, 2015b).

It seems likely that SB might be a useful agent for lung cancer patients as a non-toxic complementary approach to alleviate the side effects by thorax irradiation. In C57BL/6 mice given 13 Gy thoracic irradiation, SB treatments (100 mg/kg/day for seven days after irradiation) was shown to increase mouse survival, to reduce the number of inflammatory cells in the bronchoalveolar lavage fluid (BALF), to ameliorate radiation-induced haemorrhage, inflammation and fibrosis in lung tissue and to reduce inflammatory cell infiltration in the respiratory tract (Son *et al.*, 2015). SB (25 μM) was found to strongly enhance IR (2.5-10 Gy)-caused inhibition of colony formation selectively in prostate cancer cells, and prolonged and enhanced IR-caused G2-M arrest, apoptosis, and ROS production (Nambiar *et al.*, 2015a). SB was also demonstrated to inhibit basal cell carcinoma growth via suppression of mitogenic signalling and transcription factors (AP-1 and NF-κB) activation (Tilley *et al.*, 2016).

Survival studies indicated that SM (70 mg/kg body weight administered orally for 3 days) provided maximum protection (67%) against lethal 9 Gy γ-irradiation in mice. The protection was associated with a partial prevention of decrease of AO enzymes activities (SOD, GPx, GR and CAT) in the liver and intestine as well as various degree of protection of haematological and immune system of the irradiated animals (Adhikari and Arora, 2016). Nano-silymarin was shown to provide protection against γ-radiation-induced oxidative stress in cultured human embryonic kidney cells with maximum protection against DNA damage at 10 μg/ml (Adhikari and Arora, 2015). In a randomised, double-blinded, placebo-controlled clinical trial SM (420 mg orally, daily in three divided doses starting at the first day of radiotherapy for 6 weeks), was reported to significantly reduce the severity of radiotherapy induced mucositis and delayed its occurrence in patients with head and neck cancer (Elyasi *et al.*, 2016). SB (100 mg/kg) was demonstrated to attenuate radiation-induced intestinal fibrosis and reverses epithelial-to-mesenchymal transition (Kim *et al.*, 2017a).

Irradiation of 2 Gy γ-rays to the testis of the rats was indicated to dramatically alter spermatogenesis: significantly affected the frequency of spermatogonia, primary spermatocyte, round spermatid, spermatozoa, seminiferous tube and lumen diameters, thickness of the epithelium, Leydig cell nuclear diameter and volume, epithelium height, and apoptotic cells. However, administration of SM (200 mg/kg, 24 h before exposure to the γ-radiation) was shown to significantly improve the mentioned spermatogenesis parameters (Marzban *et al.*, 2017). Similarly, radioprotective effects of SM (50 mg/kg of SM for 7 consecutive days, and one day later, last injections were irradiated by 2 Gy of γ-rays) on the sperm parameters of γ-irradiated mice were also shown (Fatehi *et al.*, 2018).

In a randomised, double-blind, placebo-controlled clinical trial it was proven that topical SM administration can be an effective approach for prevention of acute radiodermatitis in breast cancer patients: prophylactic SM gel application for 5 weeks was able to significantly reduce the severity of radiodermatitis and delay its occurrence (Karbasforooshan *et al.*, 2019). Exposure of rats to 8 Gy of γ-rays imposed severe nephrotoxicity with biochemical and histological detrimental changes. At the same time, treatment of irradiated rats with SM (100 mg/kg daily, for 14 days) was shown to reduce the elevated levels of lipid peroxidation, attenuated the renal dysfunction, decreased the levels of inflammatory and apoptotic markers and normalised the altered renal morphology (Abdel-Magied and Elkady, 2019). Possible roles of SM/SB in radiotherapy-induced toxicities have been reviewed recently and it was concluded that its protective effects were associated with its antioxidant, anti-apoptosis, anti-inflammatory activities, and some other mechanisms (Latacela *et al.*, 2022).

8.3.2 UV radiation

Solar UV radiation is a significant climatic stress for animals leading to various damage to the biological molecules including DNA, proteins and PUFAs, oxidative and genotoxic stress and genome instability (Roy, 2017). Dietary SB (1% dose (w/w) for 2 weeks before a single ultraviolet B (UVB) irradiation at 180 mJ/cm^2) provided protection against UVB-induced damages in skin epidermis and mechanisms of such protection are suggested to include (Gu *et al.*, 2005a,b):

- preventing DNA damage or/and enhancing repair;
- reducing UVB-induced hyperproliferative response;
- inhibiting UVB-caused apoptosis and sunburn cell formation;
- inhibiting UVB-induced MAPK and AKT signalling and increasing p53.

Furthermore, SM (topically applied at 0.5 or 1.0 mg/cm^2) was shown to inhibit UV radiation-induced immunosuppression through augmentation of IL-12 in mice (Meeran *et al.*, 2006). Interestingly, SM (10-20 μg/ml) was observed to protect epidermal keratinocytes from UV radiation-induced apoptosis and DNA damage by nucleotide excision repair mechanism to prevent the harmful effects of UV radiation on the genomic stability of epidermal cells (Katiyar *et al.*, 2011). SM (5-20 μg/ml) was reported to inhibit UV radiation-induced immune suppression through DNA repair-dependent activation of dendritic cells and stimulation of effector T cells (Vaid *et al.*, 2013). Using JB6 cells and SKH-1 hairless mouse skin it was indicated that SB induced a significant increase in IL-12 levels in UVB-irradiated JB6 cells as well as in mouse skin epidermis (Narayanapillai *et al.*, 2014). Taking into account protective roles of IL-12 in reducing UVB-induced DNA damage and apoptosis, the authors suggested that SB can inhibit UVB-induced DNA-damage and apoptosis by enhancing IL-12 expression.

Treatment of irradiated skin epidermal cells (HaCaT, 20 J/cm^2) with SM (0.7-34 mg/l; 4 h) was shown to concentration-dependently diminish ultraviolet A (UVA)-caused oxidative stress: preventing GSH depletion, ROS production, lipid peroxidation, DNA single strand breaks and caspase-3 activity in irradiated cells (Svobodová *et al.*,

2007). The protective action of SM is associated with down-regulation of androgen receptor-, epidermal growth factor receptor-, and NF-κB- mediated signalling (Deep and Agarwal, 2007). SB was reported to protect murine fibroblast L929 cells from UVB-induced apoptosis via inhibition of ATM-p53 pathway and autophagy (Liu *et al.*, 2013). Evidence has been increasingly emerged that p53-mediated GADD45α upregulation is the key mechanism by which SB protects against UVB-induced photodamage (Roy *et al.*, 2012). SB can enhance the repair of UVB-induced DNA damage by activating p53-dependent nucleotide excision repair mechanism in human dermal fibroblasts (Guillermo-Lagae *et al.*, 2015), preventing the harmful effects of UV radiation on the genomic stability of epidermal cells (Katiyar *et al.*, 2011). SM/SB is also shown to affect various signalling pathways including mitogenic, cell cycle, apoptosis, autophagy, p53 and NF-κB and characterised by anti-inflammatory, anti-oxidant, DNA damage repair, immune-modulatory and anti-proliferative properties (Kumar *et al.*, 2015).

Furthermore, by using p53 heterozygous ($p53^{+/-}$) and p53 knockout ($p53^{-/-}$) mice it was clearly demonstrated that absence of the p53 allele predisposed mice to photodamage and photo-carcinogenesis, confirming that SB mediates its protection against UVB-induced photodamage, inflammation and photocarcinogenesis partly through p53 activation (Rigby *et al.*, 2017). In an *in vitro* study treatment of primary human dermal fibroblasts with both SM and SB (3-12 μg/ml) was reported to cause a reduction in UVA-stimulated ROS generation and single-strand breaks production, as well as in the prevention of GSH depletion, a decrease in the activation of caspase-3 and protein level of matrix metalloproteinase-1 associated with moderate increase in HO-1 level and reduced HSP70 level (Rajnochová Svobodová *et al.*, 2018).

In various *in vitro* tests SM was found to possess anti-collagenase (IC_{50}=2.03 mg/l) and anti-elastase activities and was more effective than most of the pure flavonolignans (Vostálová *et al.*, 2019) and the authors considered SM as a suitable candidate for a component of dermatological preparations focusing on the prevention of sunlight-induced damage and (photo)aging. It seems likely that SM has the dual role in UVA-exposed keratinocytes. On the one hand, SM was able to attenuate the UVA-induced ROS generation. On the other hand, SM pre-treatment was shown to increase the cyclobutane pyrimidine dimer photolesions in keratinocytes after UVA exposure (Fidrus *et al.*, 2019).

It was also suggested that SM may be used for sunscreen protection, as well as being effective in protection against skin diseases associated with solar UV radiation-induced inflammation, oxidative stress and immunomodulatory effects (Vaid and Katiyar, 2010). Hydrogel containing SB-loaded pomegranate oil based nanocapsules were shown to exhibit anti-inflammatory effects on skin damage UVB radiation-induced in mice (Marchiori *et al.*, 2017). It seems likely that SB-loaded hydrogel can be introduced as an effective sun-protective product since it effectively reduced the inflammation mediators IL-22 and TNF-α and provided skin protection against UVB (Ali Karami *et al.*, 2021). When immortalised keratinocytes were pre-incubated with different concentrations of milk thistle purified extract and irradiated with increasing doses of solar simulator a protection against the direct DNA damage was observed (Di Caprio *et al.*, 2020). SB was found to up-regulate both oestrogen receptors (ERα and ERβ) pathways in UVB-treated dermal HFF cells and epidermal HaCaT cells, resulting in protection of skin from UVB-damage (Liu *et al.*, 2021).

The photoprotective ability of SB was also suggested to be related to induction of insulin receptor substrate protein 1 (an important regulator of skin homeostasis and physiology) expression in UVA + UVB treated rat skin (Gorgisen *et al.*, 2020). UV-induced oxidative stress is considered to play an important role in pathogenesis of a highly prevalent hyperpigmentation disorder called melasma and the efficacy and safety of topical SM (0.7% and 1.4%) versus hydroquinone 4% in the treatment of melasma were investigated in 42 adult female patients with melasma for 3 months. It was shown that SM was as effective as hydroquinone in decreasing melasma score without any side effects, while hydroquinone treatment was associated with significant adverse effects (Nofal *et al.*, 2019). The authors concluded that SM cream could be an effective and safe treatment modality for melasma.

Importantly, in contrast to the inhibition of apoptosis and p53 expression in UVB-exposed skin cells, SB was indicated to increase these variables in tumours (Gu *et al.*, 2006). Furthermore, SM was reported to sensitise colon cancer cells to radiation: pre-irradiation treatment of HCT-15 and RKO colon cancer cell with SM (20 μg/ml) followed by radiation exposure was shown to inhibit colon cancer cell proliferation and enhances cell death in a time-dependent manner (Lal and Gupta, 2016). Evidence of the beneficial effect of SM/SB in cancer prevention and intervention has been recently reviews and confirmed their strong efficacy against all stages of photocarcinogenesis during nonmelanoma skin cancers growth and progression. Molecular mechanisms of such protection include (Prasad *et al.*, 2020):

- protection from UVB-induced DNA damage;
- initiating DNA damage repair following UVB exposure;
- increase in tumour suppressor p53 levels;
- initiation of p53 mediated-cell cycle arrest or apoptosis based on acute/chronic exposure effects of UVB;
- modulation of survival and mitogenic signalling;
- initiating anti-inflammatory and anti-oxidative responses.

8.3.3 Ischemia

Ischemia-reperfusion (I/R) injury is considered to be an important cause of organ damage and human diseases associated with excessive ROS generation, disturbances of redox status and oxidative stress in various tissues (G Bardallo *et al.*, 2021). Initially, the protective effect of SB (100, 200 and 400 mg/kg, 30-min before occlusion) on ischemic brain was suggested to be a result of the inhibition of 5-lipoxygenase and scavenging of ROS (Rui *et al.*, 1990). Protective actions of SB on myocardial infarction size and I/R-induced arrhythmias were studied in a rat model. It was observed that pretreatment with SB (20, 50, and 80 mg/kg iv) was able to reduce infarct size by 34.7%, 35.0%, and 50.6% respectively at 4 h after ligation.

Furthermore, pretreatment with SB (20 mg/kg) significantly decreased reperfusion-induced arrhythmia (Chen *et al.*, 1992). In a rat model of ischemia, provoked by clamping the afferent vessels to the median and left lateral lobes of the liver for 60 min, followed by removal of the clamp and reperfusion, SM (100 mg/kg BW) administered intravenously at 5 min before both the induction of ischemia and the restoration of blood flow (*in vivo* ischemia) and at 1 h and at 5 min before sacrifice (*in vitro* ischemia) was shown to reduce serum AST and ALT and decreased and the extent of liver necrosis compared with the control group (Wu *et al.*, 1993).

In a rat model of ischemia, pretreatment with SM (25, 50 mg, and 100 mg/kg body weight) significantly decreased post-ischemic mucosal injury as evidenced by decreased ulcer indexes in comparison to control rats. The protective effects of SM were associated with a reduction in the number of neutrophils in the gastric mucosa (Alarcón de la Lastra *et al.*, 1995). In a rat model of liver ischemia, SM (100 mg/kg, intraperitoneally 45 minutes before ischemia) was found to significantly reduced AST and ALT values (by more than 50%) in the treated animals when compared with the ischemic group. Reduced degrees of liver injury (congestion and dissociation and separation of liver cell plates), preservation of tight junctions and reduced superoxide generation in the treated groups were also observed (Oliveira *et al.*, 2001). In comparison to the control group, in rats subjected to I/R, a severe impairment of mitochondrial bioenergetics was reported: state 3 respiration was decreased, while state 4 increased, leading to lower membrane potential and decreased ATP levels. The aforementioned effects of I/R injury on mitochondria were ameliorated in the presence of SM (Rolo *et al.*, 2003).

SM also showed cardioprotective activity in I/R-induced myocardial infarction in Wistar albino rats. For instance, SM administration to rats (100 mg/kg, 250 mg/kg and 500 mg/kg, by gastric gavage for one week) was shown to have protective effects on the endogenous antioxidant enzymes (SOD, CAT, GST), decreased lipid peroxidation, serum marker enzymes (AST, GPT, LDH), suppressed the neutrophil infiltration during I/R and limited the infarct size in rats subjected to 30 min coronary artery occlusion followed by 4 h of reperfusion (Rao and Viswanath, 2007). SM (100 mg/kg for 7 days before I/R) was found to protect rat kidneys against I/R injury as evidenced by significantly ameliorated I/R-induced reduction in serum SOD and GSH and prevented increase in serum and tissue MDA, NO and protein carbonyls (Turgut *et al.*, 2008). Similarly, SM (50 mg/kg or 100 mg/kg) was indicated to prevent I/R-induced tubular dilatation, tubular vacuolisation, pelvic inflammation, interstitial inflammation, perirenal adipose infiltration, tubular necrosis and glomerular necrosis in rat kidney (Senturk *et al.*, 2008).

In an animal model of acute ischemic stroke injury by inducing cerebral I/R in rats, SM dose-dependently (1-10 μg/kg, i.v.) reduced I/R-induced brain infarction by 16-40% and improved neurological deficits in rats with a stroke. This SM action was associated with amelioration of the oxidative and nitrosative stresses and inflammation-mediated tissue injury as a result of mitigation of the activation of proinflammatory transcription factors (e.g. NF-κB and STAT-1) and prevention of proinflammatory cytokine production in stroke-damaged sites (Hou *et al.*, 2010).

In male Wistar rats, pre-treated with SM (200 mg/kg body weight, orally for 15 days) and I/R procedure, SM was reported to slow down the progression of neurodegeneration in focal cerebral ischemia mediated through upregulating the antioxidant status (GSH, GPx, GR and SOD) and lowering the apoptotic responses (Raza *et al*, 2011). In focal ischemic rats SM (200 mg/kg) treatment significantly improved behavioural, biochemical (GSH, SOD, CAT) and histopathological changes, and reduced water content and infarct size (Muley *et al.*, 2012). Anti-inflammatory and anti-apoptotic activities of SB in a model of ischemic brain were investigated. It was demonstrated that SB significantly alleviated neurological deficit, reduced infarct volume, and suppressed brain oedema, which were accompanied with upregulation of Akt, mammalian target of rapamycin (mTOR), HIF-1α, Bcl-2 and downregulation of Bax, NF-κB in ischemic brain tissue after stroke (Wang *et al.*, 2012).

In a rat model of mesenteric I/R injury, SM (100 mg/kg/day for 7 days before I/R) was found to attenuate the oxidative (SOD), inflammatory (TNF-α) and intestinal damage induced by I/R injuries (Demir *et al.*, 2014). In an *in vitro* model of ischemic stroke based on neuronal cells (SH-SY5Y cells and primary mouse cortical neurons) maintained in an oxygen-glucose deprivation condition followed by re-oxygenation, it was shown that SB-mediated neuroprotection is associated with activation of AMPK signalling (Xie *et al.*, 2014). The authors confirmed that pharmacological inhibition or genetic depletion of AMPK were associated with alleviation of the neuroprotective ability of SM in the ischemic stroke model.

The efficacy of SM in a mouse model of renal I/R was investigated. The treatment with SM (100, 30 and 10 mg/kg) was reported to reduce kidney dysfunction, histological damage, neutrophil infiltration and oxidative stress (CAT, SOD1 and SOD2) in a dose dependent manner (Impellizzeri *et al.*, 2015). Furthermore, 2,3-dehydrosilybin (10 μM), a constituent of SM, was shown to ameliorate cardiomyocyte damage following hypoxia/reoxygenation by limiting oxidative stress (Gabrielová *et al.*, 2015). In a lung I/R injury model SM (250 mg/kg/day of SM for 8 days) was demonstrated to markedly improve lung I/R-induced pulmonary vascular dysfunction and lung moisture and decreased inflammation and oxidative stress in rats. In such conditions, SM was reported to inhibit the activation of caspase-3 and caspase-9, HIF-1α and iNOS protein expression in the lung I/R-injury rats (Jin *et al.*, 2016). SM preconditioning (100 mg/kg, 15 min before I/R) was found to protect against hepatic I/R injury in insulin resistant rats via providing antioxidant, anti-inflammatory, and antiapoptotic effects and suppressing H_2S production (Younis *et al.*, 2016). In rats with ischemic surgery SM (200 mg/kg) was indicated to delay neuronal cell death in hippocampus (Hirayama *et al.*, 2016). In a rat model of supra-celiac aorta I/R injury, SM (200 mg/kg) was shown to decrease oxidative stress and damage to the lungs, liver and kidneys in comparison to the control group, while no protection was observed in the myocardium (Koçarslan *et al.*, 2016). Similarly, SB (200 mg/kg daily for 3 consecutive days) was found to promote neuron viability upon H_2O_2 challenge and reduced hypoxia/ischemia injury in the middle cerebral artery occlusion mouse model (Wang *et al.*, 2016).

Hepatic I/R injury in rats was observed to induce remote renal damage while the intravenous administration of SB led to significant nephroprotective action associated with a significant decrease in TNF-α levels in kidneys (Kyriakopoulos *et al.*, 2018). Interestingly, the hepatoprotective effect of SB was associated with the reduction of the expression of Fas/FasL, HMGB-1 and CD45 in liver tissue under I/R conditions (Tsaroucha *et al.*, 2018). Furthermore, SB (30 mg/kg, 30 min before laparotomy and immediately after the beginning of reperfusion) was found to improve liver circulation by preventing sinusoidal congestion, inflammation, and inducing modification of the vasoregulatory gene expression (Akbari-Kordkheyli *et al.*, 2019). In a rat model of I/R in the lower extremities, brain tissue damage was shown to occur and SM (200 mg/kg, i.p.) showed protective effect associated with decreased oxidative stress: reduced serum hydroperoxide levels and increased total free sulfhydryl levels (Karabag and Koçarslan, 2020).

SM-loaded chitosan nanoparticles were shown to effectively prevent oxidative (SOD, GPx, CAT, GR, GSH) and inflammatory (IL-6, TNF-α) damage in the rat brain caused by I/R (Moghaddam *et al.*, 2020). Similarly, collagen nanoparticle-mediated brain SM delivery (10, 100, and 1,000 μg/kg BW) was considered as an effective approach for treating cerebral ischemia and reperfusion-induced brain injury in rats (Rathore *et al.*, 2020). Anti-apoptotic effect of SM-loaded chitosan nanoparticles (15 mg/kg for 14 days before I/R) associated with decreased hippocampal caspase-3 and Bcl-2 expression in rats following cerebral I/R injury were reported (Mokhtari Sangdehi *et al.*, 2022). Furthermore, SB-hydroxypropyl-β-cyclodextrin complex (corresponding to 750 μg of SB) was effective in prevention of apoptosis in rat liver and kidney after hepatic I/R injury (Tsaroucha *et al.*, 2020). SB-mediated cardioprotection in myocardial I/R injury (100 mg/kg, intraperitoneal injection for 7 days before I/R) was reported to be associated with decreased apoptosis, oxidative stress and inflammatory response through deactivation of NF-κB pathway (Chen *et al.*, 2020a).

Adjusting the expression of NLRP3 and NF-κB genes during I/R is considered to be one of the important mechanisms of the protective effects of SB (Zarpou *et al.*, 2021). Recently the hepatoprotective effect of SB after hepatic I/R, including expression of inflammatory factors, in a rat model has been confirmed by immunohistochemistry and qRT-PCR (Betsou *et al.*, 2021). It seems likely that protective effects of SB (60 mg/kg, injection) on liver cells against I/R induced injuries could be also associated with preservation of integrity of mitochondrial membrane (Qajari *et al.*, 2020).

8.4 Conclusions

In various model systems toxic chemicals were used to impose toxicity, which in many cases was associated with oxidative stress indicative by decreased antioxidant defences (AO enzymes and non-enzymatic antioxidants, total antioxidant activity, etc.) and increased concentrations of oxidative stress markers, including MDA accumulation. In many cases inflammatory responses were also observed. Main chemicals used to induce toxicity/oxidative stress included CCl_4, thioacetamide, cisplatin, benzo[a]pyrene, doxorubicin, APAP, pesticides (paraquat and maneb), anti-TB drugs (rifampicin, isoniazid and pyrazinamide), arsenic, cadmium, lead, mercury, aluminium, iron, copper, manganese, fluoride, silver nanoparticles, ethanol and gentamicin. Furthermore, SM/SB was also effective in protection against other 46 chemicals, including 1-methyl-4-phenyl-1,2,3,6-tetrahydropyridine, 6-hydroxydopamine, acrolein, acrylamide, adriamycin, α-amanitin, bisphenol A, bleomicyn, cocaine, cyclophosphamide, cyclosporine A, cyclosporine A, di(2-ethylhexyl)phthalate, diazinon, diethylnitrosamine, diethylnitrosamine, docetaxel, epirubicin, fingolimod, hydrochloric acid, isoniazid, isoniazid, isoproterenol, itraconazole, kainic acid, ketoprofen, L-arginine, lasalocid, methotrexate, methotrexate, microcystin-LR, mycophenolate mofetil, nickel sulphate, N-nitrosodimethylamine, oxaliplatin, phenylhydrazine, polymyxin E, pyrazinamide, pyrogallol, ribavirin, scopolamine, sodium nitrite, sulphur mustard, thiram, triptolide, vancomycin and zidovudine. In addition, protective effects of SM/SB were tested in various clinically-relevant conditions imposing oxidative stress, including gamma radiation, UV-radiation and ischemia/reperfusion (Figure 8.1).

From the data presented above it is clear that SM/SB provides protection against oxidative stress and following toxicity caused by a great number of chemicals and conditions. In general, it seems very likely that protective effects of SM/SB are

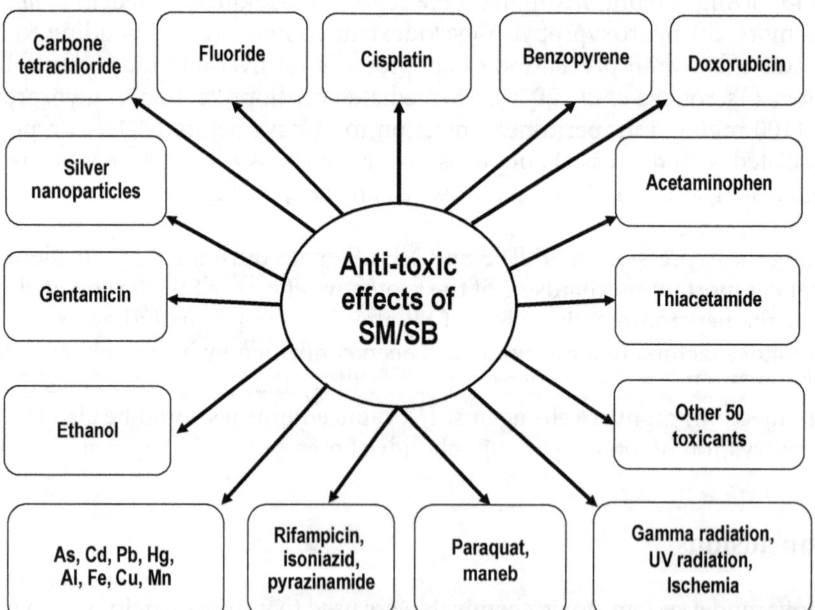

Figure 8.1. Anti-toxic effects of SM/SB.

associated with modulation of vitagenes and transcription factors with following effects on antioxidant enzymes and other antioxidant defence mechanisms. Clearly, the aforementioned data clearly confirmed great potential of SM/SB in clinical practise to decrease side effects of various drugs and to be used as an adjuvant therapy for various clinical conditions. Furthermore, SM/SB can also be effectively used in animal/poultry production to decrease detrimental consequences of various commercially-relevant stress conditions.

References

Abbas, N., Awad, M.M. and Nafea, O.E., 2020. Silymarin in combination with chlorogenic acid protects against hepatotoxicity induced by doxorubicin in rats: possible role of adenosine monophosphate-activated protein kinase pathway. Toxicology Research 9: 771-777.

Abbas, A.T., El-Shitany, N.A., Shaala, L.A., Ali, S.S., Azhar, E.I., Abdel-Dayem, U.A. and Youssef, D.T., 2014. Red Sea Suberea mollis sponge extract protects against CCl4-induced acute liver injury in rats via an antioxidant mechanism. Evidence-Based Complementary and Alternative Medicine 2014: 745606.

Abd Eldaim, M.A., Barakat, E.R., Alkafafy, M. and Elaziz, S., 2021. Antioxidant and anti-apoptotic prophylactic effect of silymarin against lead-induced hepatorenal toxicity in rats. Environmental Science and Pollution Research International 28: 57997-58006.

Abdel-Aziz, N., Elkady, A.A. and Elgazzar, E.M., 2021. Effect of low-dose gamma radiation and lipoic acid on high- radiation-dose induced rat brain injuries. Dose-Response 19: 15593258211044845.

Abdel-Magied, N. and Elkady, A.A., 2019. Possible curative role of curcumin and silymarin against nephrotoxicity induced by gamma-rays in rats. Experimental and Molecular Pathology 111: 104299.

Abdelmeguid, N.E., Chmaisse, H.N. and Abou Zeinab, N.S., 2010. Silymarin ameliorates cisplatin-induced hepatotoxicity in rats: histopathological and ultrastructural studies. Pakistan Journal of Biological Sciences 13: 463-479.

Abdel-Moneim, A.M., Al-Kahtani, M.A., El-Kersh, M.A. and Al-Omair, M.A., 2015. Free radical-scavenging, anti-inflammatory/anti-fibrotic and hepatoprotective actions of taurine and silymarin against CCl4 induced rat liver damage. PloS One 10: e0144509.

Abdelsalam, H.M., Samak, M.A. and Alsemeh, A.E., 2019. Synergistic therapeutic effects of Vitis vinifera extract and silymarin on experimentally induced cardiorenal injury: The pertinent role of Nrf2. Biomedicine and Pharmacotherapy 110: 37-46.

Abdulrazzaq, A.M., Badr, M., Gammoh, O., Abu Khalil, A.A., Ghanim, B.Y., Alhussainy, T.M. and Qinna, N.A., 2019. Hepatoprotective actions of ascorbic acid, alpha lipoic acid and silymarin or their combination against acetaminophen-induced hepatotoxicity in rats. Medicina 55: 181.

Aboelwafa, H.R., El-Kott, A.F., Abd-Ella, E.M. and Yousef, H.N., 2020. The possible neuroprotective effect of silymarin against aluminum chloride-prompted Alzheimer's-like disease in rats. Brain Sciences 10: 628.

Aboshanab, M., El-Nabarawi, M.A., Teaima, M.H., El-Nekeety, A.A., Abdel-Aziem, S.H., Hassan, N.S. and Abdel-Wahhab, M.A., 2020. Fabrication, characterization and biological evaluation of silymarin nanoparticles against carbon tetrachloride-induced oxidative stress and genotoxicity in rats. International Journal of Pharmaceutics 587: 119639.

Adhikari, M., Arora, R., Chawla, R., Sharma, J., Dhaker, A.S., Gupta, D., Dubey, N., Kumar, R., Ivanov, V., Gadjeva, V., Gevrenova, R. and Sharma, R.K., 2010. Evaluation of silymarin as a promising radioprotector. Journal of Biosciences 65: 337-346.

Adhikari, M. and Arora, R., 2015. Nano-silymarin provides protection against γ-radiation-induced oxidative stress in cultured human embryonic kidney cells. Mutation Research. Genetic Toxicology and Environmental Mutagenesis 792: 1-11.

Adhikari, M. and Arora, R., 2016. The flavonolignan-silymarin protects enzymatic, hematological and immune system against γ-radiation-induced toxicity. Environmental Toxicology 31: 641-654.

Adhikari, M., Dhaker, A., Adhikari, J., Ivanov, V., Singh, V., Chawla, R., Kumar, R., Sharma, R., Karamalakova, Y., Gadjeva, V. and Arora, R., 2013. *In vitro* studies on radioprotective efficacy of silymarin against γ-irradiation. International Journal of Radiation Biology 89: 200-211.

Aghashahi, M., Momeni, H.R. and Darbandi, N., 2020. Impact of aluminium toxicity on vital human sperm parameters-Protective effects of silymarin. Andrologia 52: e13742.

Ahmad, I., Shukla, S., Kumar, A., Singh, B.K., Kumar, V., Chauhan, A.K., Singh, D., Pandey, H.P. and Singh, C., 2013. Biochemical and molecular mechanisms of N-acetyl cysteine and silymarin-mediated protection against maneb- and paraquat-induced hepatotoxicity in rats. Chemico-Biological Interactions 201: 9-18.

Ahmad, M.M., Rezk, N.A., Fawzy, A. and Sabry, M., 2019a. Protective effects of curcumin and silymarin against paracetamol induced hepatotoxicity in adult male albino rats. Gene 712: 143966.

Ahmed, R.F., Moussa, R.A., Eldemerdash, R.S., Zakaria, M.M. and Abdel-Gaber, S.A., 2019b. Ameliorative effects of silymarin on HCl-induced acute lung injury in rats; role of the Nrf-2/HO-1 pathway. Iranian Journal of Basic Medical Sciences 22: 1483-1492.

Akbari-Kordkheyli, V., Abbaszadeh-Goudarzi, K., Nejati-Laskokalayeh, M., Zarpou, S. and Khonakdar-Tarsi, A., 2019. The protective effects of silymarin on ischemia-reperfusion injuries: A mechanistic review. Iranian Journal of Basic Medical Sciences 22: 968-976.

Alarcón de la Lastra, A.C., Martín, M.J., Motilva, V., Jiménez, M., La Casa, C. and López, A., 1995. Gastroprotection induced by silymarin, the hepatoprotective principle of *Silybum marianum* in ischemia-reperfusion mucosal injury: role of neutrophils. Planta Medica 61: 116-119.

Alcaraz-Contreras, Y., Mendoza-Lozano, R.P., Martínez-Alcaraz, E.R., Martínez-Alfaro, M., Gallegos-Corona, M.A., Ramírez-Morales, M.A. and Vázquez-Guevara, M.A., 2016. Silymarin and dimercaptosuccinic acid ameliorate lead-induced nephrotoxicity and genotoxicity in rats. Human and Experimental Toxicology 35: 398-403.

Al-Harbi, N.O., Imam, F., Nadeem, A., Al-Harbi, M.M., Iqbal, M. and Ahmad, S.F., 2014. Carbon tetrachloride-induced hepatotoxicity in rat is reversed by treatment with riboflavin. International Immunopharmacology 21: 383-388.

Al-Hazmi, A., 2020. Antioxidant activity of silymarin in microcystin-LR cardiac and pulmonary induced injuries on mice. Pakistan Journal of Biological Sciences 23: 1369-1373.

Ali Karami, M., Sharif Makhmalzadeh, B., Pooranian, M. and Rezai, A., 2021. Preparation and optimization of silibinin-loaded chitosan-fucoidan hydrogel: an *in vivo* evaluation of skin protection against UVB. Pharmaceutical Development and Technology 26: 209-219.

Ali, N.M., Mahmoud, A., Mahmoud, M.F. and El Fayoumi, H.M., 2019. Glycyrrhizic acid and silymarin alleviate the neurotoxic effects of aluminum in rats challenged with fructose-induced insulin resistance: possible role of toll-like receptor 4 pathway. Drug and Chemical Toxicology 42: 210-219.

Ali, S.O., Darwish, H.A. and Ismail, N.A., 2014. Modulatory effects of curcumin, silybin-phytosome and alpha-R-lipoic acid against thioacetamide-induced liver cirrhosis in rats. Chemico-Biological Interactions 216: 26-33.

Alidoost, F., Gharagozloo, M., Bagherpour, B., Jafarian, A., Sajjadi, S.E., Hourfar, H. and Moayedi, B., 2006. Effects of silymarin on the proliferation and glutathione levels of peripheral blood mononuclear cells from beta-thalassemia major patients. International Immunopharmacology 6: 1305-1310.

Alkreathy, H.M., Khan, R.A., Khan, M.R. and Sahreen, S., 2014. CCl4 induced genotoxicity and DNA oxidative damages in rats: hepatoprotective effect of Sonchus arvensis. BMC Complementary and Alternative Medicine 14: 452.

Al-Rasheed, N., Faddah, L., Al-Rasheed, N., Bassiouni, Y.A., Hasan, I.H., Mahmoud, A.M., Mahmoud, R.A. and Yacoub, H.I., 2016. Protective effects of silymarin, alone or in combination with chlorogenic acid and/or melatonin, against carbon tetrachloride-induced hepatotoxicity. Pharmacognosy Magazine 12(Suppl 3): S337.

Asghar, Z. and Masood, Z., 2008. Evaluation of antioxidant properties of silymarin and its potential to inhibit peroxyl radicals *in vitro*. Pakistan Journal of Pharmaceutical Sciences 21: 249-254.

Avci, H., Epikmen, E.T., Ipek, E., Tunca, R., Birincioglu, S.S., Akşit, H., Sekkin, S., Akkoç, A.N. and Boyacioglu, M., 2017. Protective effects of silymarin and curcumin on cyclophosphamide-induced cardiotoxicity. Experimental and Toxicologic Pathology 69: 317-327.

Avizeh, R., Najafzadeh, H., Razijalali, M. and Shirali, S., 2010. Evaluation of prophylactic and therapeutic effects of silymarin and N-acetylcysteine in acetaminophen-induced hepatotoxicity in cats. Journal of Veterinary Pharmacology and Therapeutics 33: 95-99.

Badisa, R.B., Fitch-Pye, C.A., Agharahimi, M., Palm, D.E., Latinwo, L.M. and Goodman, C.B., 2014. Milk thistle seed extract protects rat C6 astroglial cells from acute cocaine toxicity. Molecular Medicine Reports 10: 2287-2292.

Balali-Mood, M., Naseri, K., Tahergorabi, Z., Khazdair, M.R. and Sadeghi, M., 2021. Toxic mechanisms of five heavy metals: mercury, lead, chromium, cadmium and arsenic. Frontiers in Pharmacology 12: 643972.

Baradaran, A., Samadi, F., Ramezanpour, S.S. and Yousefdoust, S., 2019. Hepatoprotective effects of silymarin on CCl_4-induced hepatic damage in broiler chickens model. Toxicology Reports 6: 788-794.

Barbarino, F., Neumann, E., Deaciuc, I., Ghelberg, N.W., Suciu, A., Cotuțiu, C., Racoviță, L., Stroilă, C., Nagy, S., Părău, N., Toader, S. and Brilinschi, C., 1981. Effect of silymarin on experimental liver lesions. Medecine Interne 19: 347-357.

Bektur, N.E., Sahin, E., Baycu, C. and Unver, G., 2016. Protective effects of silymarin against acetaminophen-induced hepatotoxicity and nephrotoxicity in mice. Toxicology and Industrial Health 32: 589-600.

Betsou, A., Lambropoulou, M., Georgakopoulou, A.E., Kostomitsopoulos, N., Konstandi, O., Anagnostopoulos, K., Tsalikidis, C., Simopoulos, C.E., Valsami, G. and Tsaroucha, A.K., 2021. The hepatoprotective effect of silibinin after hepatic ischemia/reperfusion in a rat model is confirmed by immunohistochemistry and qRT-PCR. The Journal of Pharmacy and Pharmacology 73: 1274-1284.

Beydilli, H., Yilmaz, N., Cetin, E.S., Topal, Y., Celik, O.I., Sahin, C., Topal, H., Cigerci, I.H. and Sozen, H., 2015. Evaluation of the protective effect of silibinin against diazinon induced hepatotoxicity and free-radical damage in rat liver. Iranian Red Crescent Medical Journal 17: e25310.

Bongiovanni, G.A., Soria, E.A. and Eynard, A.R., 2007. Effects of the plant flavonoids silymarin and quercetin on arsenite-induced oxidative stress in CHO-K1 cells. Food and Chemical Toxicology 45: 971-976.

Borsari, M., Gabbi, C., Ghelfi, F., Grandi, R., Saladini, M., Severi, S. and Borella, F., 2001. Silybin, a new iron-chelating agent. Journal of Inorganic Biochemistry 85: 123-129.

Cappetta, D., De Angelis, A., Sapio, L., Prezioso, L., Illiano, M., Quaini, F., Rossi, F., Berrino, L., Naviglio, S. and Urbanek, K., 2017. Oxidative stress and cellular response to doxorubicin: A common factor in the complex milieu of anthracycline cardiotoxicity. Oxidative Medicine and Cellular Longevity 2017: 1521020.

Cariccio, V.L., Samà, A., Bramanti, P. and Mazzon, E., 2019. Mercury involvement in neuronal damage and in neurodegenerative diseases. Biological Trace Element Research 187: 341-356.

Cecen, E., Dost, T., Culhaci, N., Karul, A., Ergur, B. and Birincioglu, M., 2011. Protective effects of silymarin against doxorubicin-induced toxicity. Asian Pacific Journal of Cancer Prevention 12: 2697-2704.

Cengiz, M.Z., 2018. Renoprotective effects of *Silybum marianum* (L.) Gaertn (silymarin) on thioacetamide-induced renal injury: Biochemical and histopathological approach. Pakistan Journal of Pharmaceutical Sciences 31: 2137-2141.

Chang, H.C., Chiu, Y.W., Lin, Y.M., Chen, R.J., Lin, J.A., Tsai, F.J., Tsai, C.H., Kuo, Y.C., Liu, J.Y. and Huang, C.Y., 2014. Herbal supplement attenuation of cardiac fibrosis in rats with CCl_4-induced liver cirrhosis. The Chinese Journal of Physiology 57: 41-47.

Chen, H., He, Y., Chen, S., Qi, S. and Shen, J., 2020a. Therapeutic targets of oxidative/nitrosative stress and neuroinflammation in ischemic stroke: Applications for natural product efficacy with omics and systemic biology. Pharmacological Research 158: 104877.

Chen, H., Su, D.F., Zhang, T.H., Ding, H.J., Yang, Y.C. and Chen, S.C., 1992. Effects of silybin on acute myocardial infarction and reperfusion injury in anesthetized rats. Acta Pharmacologica Sinica 13: 69-71.

Chen, J., Jiang, Y., Shi, H., Peng, Y., Fan, X. and Li, C., 2020b. The molecular mechanisms of copper metabolism and its roles in human diseases. European Journal of Physiology 472: 1415-1429.

Chen, J., Su, Y., Lin, F., Iqbal, M., Mehmood, K., Zhang, H. and Shi, D., 2021. Effect of paraquat on cytotoxicity involved in oxidative stress and inflammatory reaction: A review of mechanisms and ecological implications. Ecotoxicology and Environmental Safety 224: 112711.

Chlopcíková, S., Psotová, J., Miketová, P. and Simánek, V., 2004. Chemoprotective effect of plant phenolics against anthracycline-induced toxicity on rat cardiomyocytes. Part I. Silymarin and its flavonolignans. Phytotherapy Research 18: 107-110.

Cho, S.I., Lee, J.E. and Do, N.Y., 2014. Protective effect of silymarin against cisplatin-induced ototoxicity. International Journal of Pediatric Otorhinolaryngology 78: 474-478.

Chowdhury, A., Nabila, J., Adelusi Temitope, I. and Wang, S., 2020. Current etiological comprehension and therapeutic targets of acetaminophen-induced hepatotoxicity. Pharmacological Research 161: 105102.

Chtourou, Y., Fetoui, H., Garoui, E., Boudawara, T. and Zeghal, N., 2012. Improvement of cerebellum redox states and cholinergic functions contribute to the beneficial effects of silymarin against manganese-induced neurotoxicity. Neurochemical Research 37: 469-479.

Chtourou, Y., Fetoui, H., Sefi, M., Trabelsi, K., Barkallah, M., Boudawara, T., Kallel, H. and Zeghal, N., 2010. Silymarin, a natural antioxidant, protects cerebral cortex against manganese-induced neurotoxicity in adult rats. Biometals 23: 985-996.

Chtourou, Y., Garoui, E., Boudawara, T. and Zeghal, N., 2013. Therapeutic efficacy of silymarin from milk thistle in reducing manganese-induced hepatic damage and apoptosis in rats. Human and Experimental Toxicology 32: 70-81.

Chtourou, Y., Garoui, E., Boudawara, T. and Zeghal, N., 2014. Protective role of silymarin against manganese-induced nephrotoxicity and oxidative stress in rat. Environmental Toxicology 29: 1147-1154.

Clichici, S., Olteanu, D., Filip, A., Nagy, A.L., Oros, A. and Mircea, P.A., 2016. Beneficial effects of silymarin after the discontinuation of CCl4-induced liver fibrosis. Journal of Medicinal Food 19: 789-797.

Clichici, S., Olteanu, D., Nagy, A.L., Oros, A., Filip, A. and Mircea, P.A., 2015. Silymarin inhibits the progression of fibrosis in the early stages of liver injury in CCl_4-treated rats. Journal of Medicinal Food 18: 290-298.

Dabak, D.O. and Kocaman, N., 2015. Effects of silymarin on methotrexate-induced nephrotoxicity in rats. Renal Failure 37: 734-739.

Darvishi Khezri, H., Salehifar, E., Kosaryan, M., Aliasgharian, A., Jalali, H. and Hadian Amree, A., 2016. Potential effects of silymarin and its flavonolignan components in patients with β-Thalassemia Major: A comprehensive review in 2015. Advances in Pharmacological Sciences 2016: 3046373.

Darvishi-Khezri, H., Kosaryan, M., Karami, H., Salehifar, E., Mahdavi, M., Alipour, A. and Aliasgharian, A., 2021. Can use of silymarin improve inflammatory status in patients with β-Thalassemia Major? A crossover, randomized controlled trial. Complementary Medicine Research 28: 123-130.

Darvishi-Khezri, H., Salehifar, E., Kosaryan, M., Karami, H., Alipour, A., Shaki, F. and Aliasgharian, A., 2017. The impact of silymarin on antioxidant and oxidative status in patients with β-thalassemia major: A crossover, randomized controlled trial. Complementary Therapies in Medicine 35: 25-32.

Darvishi-Khezri, H., Salehifar, E., Kosaryan, M., Karami, H., Mahdavi, M., Alipour, A. and Aliasgharian, A., 2018. Iron-chelating effect of silymarin in patients with β-thalassemia major: A crossover randomised control trial. Phytotherapy Research 32: 496-503.

Das, S.K. and Mukherjee, S., 2012. Biochemical and immunological basis of silymarin effect, a milk thistle (*Silybum marianum*) against ethanol-induced oxidative damage. Toxicology Mechanisms and Methods 22: 409-413.

Dashti-Khavidaki, S., Shahbazi, F., Khalili, H. and Lessan-Pezeshki, M., 2012. Potential renoprotective effects of silymarin against nephrotoxic drugs: a review of literature. Journal of Pharmacy and Pharmaceutical Sciences 15: 112-123.

Deep, G. and Agarwal, R., 2007. Chemopreventive efficacy of silymarin in skin and prostate cancer. Integrative Cancer Therapies 6: 130-145.

Demir, M., Amanvermez, R., Kamalı Polat, A., Karabıçak, I., Cınar, H., Kesicioğlu, T. and Polat, C., 2014. The effect of silymarin on mesenteric ischemia-reperfusion injury. Medical Principles and Practice 23: 140-144.

Di Caprio, R., Monfrecola, G., Gasparri, F., Micillo, R., Balato, A. and Lembo, S., 2020. Milk thistle and olive extract: old substances with a new mission against sun-induced skin damage. Giornale Italiano di Dermatologia e Venereologia 155: 286-293.

Di Cesare Mannelli, L., Zanardelli, M., Failli, P. and Ghelardini, C., 2012. Oxaliplatin-induced neuropathy: oxidative stress as pathological mechanism. Protective effect of silibinin. The Journal of Pain 13: 276-284.

Dirks-Naylor, A.J., 2013. The role of autophagy in doxorubicin-induced cardiotoxicity. Life Sciences 93: 913-916.

dos Santos, N.A., Carvalho Rodrigues, M.A., Martins, N.M. and dos Santos, A.C., 2012. Cisplatin-induced nephrotoxicity and targets of nephroprotection: an update. Archives of Toxicology 86: 1233-1250.

Draz, E.I., Abdin, A.A., Sarhan, N.I. and Gabr, T.A., 2015. Neurotrophic and antioxidant effects of silymarin comparable to 4-methylcatechol in protection against gentamicin-induced ototoxicity in guinea pigs. Pharmacological Reports 67: 317-325.

Dutta, M.O., Ghosh, A., Rangari., V.I., Jain, G.A., Khobragade, S., Chattopadhyay, A.I., Bhowmick, D.E., Das, T.R. and Bandyopadhyay, D.E., 2014. Silymarin protects against copper-ascorbate induced injury to goat cardiac mitochondria *in vitro*: Involvement of antioxidant mechanism (s). International Journal of Pharmacy and Pharmaceutical Sciences 6: 422-429.

El Rabey, H.A., Rezk, S.M., Sakran, M.I., Mohammed, G.M., Bahattab, O., Balgoon, M.J., Elbakry, M.A. and Bakry, N., 2021. Green coffee methanolic extract and silymarin protect against CCl4-induced hepatotoxicity in albino male rats. BMC Complementary Medicine and Therapies 21: 19.

El Sabry, M.I., Stino, F. and El-Ghany, W., 2021. Copper: benefits and risks for poultry, livestock and fish production. Tropical Animal Health and Production 53: 487.

El-Awady, E., Moustafa, Y.M., Abo-Elmatty, D.M. and Radwan, A., 2011. Cisplatin-induced cardiotoxicity: Mechanisms and cardioprotective strategies. European Journal of Pharmacology 650: 335-341.

El-Khishin, I.A., El-Fakharany, Y. and Abdel Hamid, O.I., 2015. Role of garlic extract and silymarin compared to dimercaptosuccinic acid (DMSA) in treatment of lead induced nephropathy in adult male albino rats. Toxicology Reports 2: 824-832.

El-Marasy, S.A., Abd-Elsalam, R.M. and Ahmed-Farid, O.A., 2018. Ameliorative effect of silymarin on scopolamine-induced dementia in rats. Open access Macedonian Journal of Medical Sciences 6: 1215-1224.

Elsawy, H., Alzahrani, A.M., Alfwuaires, M., Sedky, A., El-Trass, E.E., Mahmoud, O., Abdel-Moneim, A.M. and Khalil, M., 2021. Analysis of silymarin-modulating effects against acrylamide-induced cerebellar damage in male rats: Biochemical and pathological markers. Journal of Chemical Neuroanatomy 115: 101964.

El-Shitany, N.A., El-Haggar, S. and El-Desoky, K., 2008. Silymarin prevents adriamycin-induced cardiotoxicity and nephrotoxicity in rats. Food and Chemical Toxicology 46: 2422-2428.

Elyasi, S., Hosseini, S., Niazi Moghadam, M.R., Aledavood, S.A. and Karimi, G., 2016. Effect of oral silymarin administration on prevention of radiotherapy induced mucositis: A randomized, double-blinded, placebo-controlled clinical trial. Phytotherapy Research 30: 1879-1885.

Eminzade, S., Uraz, F. and Izzettin, F.V., 2008. Silymarin protects liver against toxic effects of anti-tuberculosis drugs in experimental animals. Nutrition and Metabolism 5: 18.

Eskandari, F. and Momeni, H.R., 2016a. Protective effect of silymarin on viability, motility and mitochondrial membrane potential of ram sperm treated with sodium arsenite. International Journal of Reproductive Biomedicine 14: 397-402.

Eskandari, F. and Momeni, H.R., 2016b. Silymarin protects plasma membrane and acrosome integrity in sperm treated with sodium arsenite. International Journal of Reproductive Biomedicine 14: 47-52.

Etemadi, T., Momeni, H.R. and Ghafarizadeh, A.A., 2020. Impact of silymarin on cadmium-induced apoptosis in human spermatozoa. Andrologia 52: e13795.

Ezhilarasan, D. and Karthikeyan, S., 2016. Silibinin alleviates N-nitrosodimethylamine-induced glutathione dysregulation and hepatotoxicity in rats. Chinese Journal of Natural Medicines 14: 40-47.

Faedmaleki, F., Shirazi, F.H., Ejtemaeimehr, S., Anjarani, S., Salarian, A.A., Ahmadi Ashtiani, H. and Rastegar, H., 2016. Study of silymarin and vitamin E protective effects on silver nanoparticle toxicity on mice liver primary cell culture. Acta Medica Iranica 54: 85-95.

Fang, Y., Lu, L., Liang, Y., Peng, D., Aschner, M. and Jiang, Y., 2021. Signal transduction associated with lead-induced neurological disorders: A review. Food and Chemical Toxicology 150: 112063.

Faraji, T., Momeni, H.R. and Malmir, M., 2019. Protective effects of silymarin on testis histopathology, oxidative stress indicators, antioxidant defence enzymes and serum testosterone in cadmium-treated mice. Andrologia 51: e13242.

Farjad, E. and Momeni, H.R., 2018. Silymarin ameliorates oxidative stress and enhances antioxidant defense system capacity in cadmium-treated mice. Cell Journal 20: 422-426.

Fatehi, D., Mohammadi, M., Shekarchi, B., Shabani, A., Seify, M. and Rostamzadeh, A., 2018. Radioprotective effects of silymarin on the sperm parameters of NMRI mice irradiated with γ-rays. Journal of Photochemistry and Photobiology. B, Biology 178: 489-495.

Fazal, Y., Fatima, S.N., Shahid, S.M. and Mahboob, T., 2015. Effects of curcumin on angiotensin-converting enzyme gene expression, oxidative stress and anti-oxidant status in thioacetamide-induced hepatotoxicity. Journal of the Renin-angiotensin-aldosterone System 16: 1046-1051.

Fidrus, E., Ujhelyi, Z., Fehér, P., Hegedűs, C., Janka, E.A., Paragh, G., Vasas, G., Bácskay, I. and Remenyik, É., 2019. Silymarin: friend or foe of UV exposed keratinocytes?. Molecules 24: 1652.

Flora, S.J., 2011. Arsenic-induced oxidative stress and its reversibility. Free Radical Biology & Medicine 51: 257-281.

Freitag, A.F., Cardia, G.F., da Rocha, B.A., Aguiar, R.P., Silva-Comar, F.M., Spironello, R.A., Grespan, R., Caparroz-Assef, S.M., Bersani-Amado, C.A. and Cuman, R.K., 2015. Hepatoprotective effect of silymarin (*Silybum marianum*) on hepatotoxicity induced by acetaminophen in spontaneously hypertensive rats. Evidence-Based Complementary and Alternative Medicine 2015: 538317.

G Bardallo, R., Panisello-Roselló, A., Sanchez-Nuno, S., Alva, N., Roselló-Catafau, J. and Carbonell, T., 2022. Nrf2 and oxidative stress in liver ischemia/reperfusion injury. The FEBS Journal 289: 5463-5479.

Gabrielová, E., Křen, V., Jabůrek, M. and Modrianský, M., 2015. Silymarin component 2,3-dehydrosilybin attenuates cardiomyocyte damage following hypoxia/reoxygenation by limiting oxidative stress. Physiological Research 64: 79-91.

Galicia-Moreno, M. and Gutiérrez-Reyes, G., 2014. The role of oxidative stress in the development of alcoholic liver disease. Revista de Gastroenterologia de Mexico 79: 135-144.

Genchi, G., Sinicropi, M.S., Lauria, G., Carocci, A. and Catalano, A., 2020. The Effects of cadmium toxicity. International Journal of Environmental Research and Public Health 17: 3782.

Gharagozloo, M., Karimi, M. and Amirghofran, Z., 2013. Immunomodulatory effects of silymarin in patients with β-thalassemia major. International Immunopharmacology 16: 243-247.

Gharagozloo, M., Moayedi, B., Zakerinia, M., Hamidi, M., Karimi, M., Maracy, M. and Amirghofran, Z., 2009. Combined therapy of silymarin and desferrioxamine in patients with beta-thalassemia major: a randomized double-blind clinical trial. Fundamental and Clinical Pharmacology 23: 359-365.

Ghaznavi, H., Mehrzadi, S., Dormanesh, B., Tabatabaei, S.M., Vahedi, H., Hosseinzadeh, A., Pazoki-Toroudi, H. and Rashidian, A., 2016. Comparison of the protective effects of melatonin and silymarin against gentamicin-induced nephrotoxicity in rats. Journal of Evidence-based Complementary and Alternative Medicine 21: NP49-NP55.

Ghiasian, M., Nafisi, H., Ranjbar, A., Mohammadi, Y. and Ataei, S., 2021. Antioxidative effects of silymarin on the reduction of liver complications of fingolimod in patients with relapsing-remitting multiple sclerosis: A clinical trial study. Journal of Biochemical and Molecular Toxicology 35: e22800.

Ghosh, S., Sarkar, A., Bhattacharyya, S. and Sil, P.C., 2016. Silymarin protects mouse liver and kidney from thioacetamide induced toxicity by scavenging reactive oxygen species and activating PI3K-Akt pathway. Frontiers in Pharmacology 7: 481.

Goh, Z.H., Tee, J.K. and Ho, H.K., 2020. An evaluation of the *in vitro* roles and mechanisms of silibinin in reducing pyrazinamide- and isoniazid-induced hepatocellular damage. International Journal of Molecular Sciences 21: 3714.

Gómez-Sierra, T., Eugenio-Pérez, D., Sánchez-Chinchillas, A. and Pedraza-Chaverri, J., 2018. Role of food-derived antioxidants against cisplatin induced-nephrotoxicity. Food and Chemical Toxicology 120: 230-242.

Gopi, K.S., Reddy, A.G., Jyothi, K. and Kumar, B.A., 2010. Acetaminophen-induced hepato- and nephrotoxicity and amelioration by silymarin and terminalia chebula in rats. Toxicology International 17: 64-66.

Gorgisen, G., Ozkol, H., Tuluce, Y., Arslan, A., Ecer, Y., Keskin, S., Kaya, Z. and Ragbetli, M.C., 2020. Silibinin and ellagic acid increase the expression of insulin receptor substrate 1 protein in ultraviolet irradiated rat skin. Biotechnic and Histochemistry 95: 641-646.

Gu, M., Dhanalakshmi, S., Mohan, S., Singh, R.P. and Agarwal, R., 2005a. Silibinin inhibits ultraviolet B radiation-induced mitogenic and survival signaling and associated biological responses in SKH-1 mouse skin. Carcinogenesis 26: 1404-1413.

Gu, M., Dhanalakshmi, S., Singh, R.P. and Agarwal, R., 2005b. Dietary feeding of silibinin prevents early biomarkers of UVB radiation-induced carcinogenesis in SKH-1 hairless mouse epidermis. Cancer Epidemiology, Biomarkers and Prevention 14: 1344-1349.

Gu, M., Singh, R.P., Dhanalakshmi, S., Mohan, S. and Agarwal, R., 2006. Differential effect of silibinin on E2F transcription factors and associated biological events in chronically UVB-exposed skin versus tumors in SKH-1 hairless mice. Molecular Cancer Therapeutics 5: 2121-2129.

Guillermo-Lagae, R., Deep, G., Ting, H., Agarwal, C. and Agarwal, R., 2015. Silibinin enhances the repair of ultraviolet B-induced DNA damage by activating p53-dependent nucleotide excision repair mechanism in human dermal fibroblasts. Oncotarget 6: 39594-39606.

Gupta, Y.K., Sharma, M. and Chaudhary, G., 2002. Pyrogallol-induced hepatotoxicity in rats: a model to evaluate antioxidant hepatoprotective agents. Methods and Findings in Experimental and Clinical Pharmacology 24: 497-500.

Guzel, S., Sahinogullari, Z.U., Canacankatan, N., Antmen, S.E., Kibar, D. and Coskun Yilmaz, B., 2020. Potential renoprotective effects of silymarin against vancomycin-induced nephrotoxicity in rats. Drug and Chemical Toxicology 43: 630-636.

Haddadi, R., Eyvari-Brooshghalan, S., Nayebi, A.M., Sabahi, M. and Ahmadi, S.A., 2020. Neuronal degeneration and oxidative stress in the SNc of 6-OHDA intoxicated rats; improving role of silymarin long-term treatment. Naunyn-Schmiedeberg's Archives of Pharmacology 393: 2427-2437.

Hagag, A.A., El Shehaby, W.A., El-Abasy, A.I. and Mabrouk, M.M., 2019. Protective role of silymarin in early doxorubicin-induced cardiac dysfunction in children with scute lymphoblastic leukemia. Infectious Disorders Drug Targets 19: 133-140.

Hagag, A.A., Elfrargy, M.S., Gazar, R.A. and El-Lateef, A.E., 2013. Therapeutic value of combined therapy with deferasirox and silymarin on iron overload in children with Beta thalassemia. Mediterranean Journal of Hematology and Infectious Diseases 5: e2013065.

Hakov'a, H. and Misúrová, E., 1993. The effect of silymarin and gamma radiation on nucleic acids in rat organs. The Journal of Pharmacy and Pharmacology 45: 910-912.

Hamidian, G., Mirdar, S., Raee, P., Asghari, K. and Jarrahi, M., 2020. Silymarin protects the structure of kidney in the neonatal rats exposed to maternal cadmium toxicity: A stereological study. Veterinary Research Forum 11: 143-152.

Hassan, S.S., Thomann, C., Ettarh, R. and Ahmad, Z., 2017. Possible protective role of silybin against polymyxin E-induced toxic effect in rat kidneys: A biochemical approach. Neurourology and Urodynamics 36: 2003-2010.

Hau, D.K., Wong, R.S., Cheng, G.Y., Wong, W.Y., Tong, S.W., Chan, K.W., Leung, A.K., Zhu, G.Y., Lai, P.B., Lau, F.Y., Chui, C.H., Gambari, R. and Fong, D.W., 2010. Novel use of silymarin as delayed therapy for acetaminophen-induced acute hepatic injury. Forschende Komplementarmedizin 17: 209-213.

Hirayama, K., Oshima, H., Yamashita, A., Sakatani, K., Yoshino, A. and Katayama, Y., 2016. Neuroprotective effects of silymarin on ischemia-induced delayed neuronal cell death in rat hippocampus. Brain Research 1646: 297-303.

Hosseini, A. and Sahebkar, A., 2017. Reversal of Doxorubicin-induced cardiotoxicity by using phytotherapy: A review. Journal of Pharmacopuncture 20: 243-256.

Hou, Y.C., Liou, K.T., Chern, C.M., Wang, Y.H., Liao, J.F., Chang, S., Chou, Y.H. and Shen, Y.C., 2010. Preventive effect of silymarin in cerebral ischemia-reperfusion-induced brain injury in rats possibly through impairing NF-κB and STAT-1 activation. Phytomedicine 17: 963-973.

Hutchinson, C., Bomford, A. and Geissler, C.A., 2010. The iron-chelating potential of silybin in patients with hereditary haemochromatosis. European Journal of Clinical Nutrition 64: 1239-1241.

Ibrahim, M.E., Bana, E.E. and El-Kerdasy, H.I., 2018. Role of bone marrow derived mesenchymal stem cells and the protective effect of silymarin in cisplatin-induced acute renal failure in rats. The American Journal of the Medical Sciences 355: 76-83.

Igbokwe, I.O., Igwenagu, E. and Igbokwe, N.A., 2019. Aluminium toxicosis: a review of toxic actions and effects. Interdisciplinary Toxicology 12: 45-70.

Ihedioha, J.I., Anyogu, D.C. and Ogbonna, M.E., 2020. The effects of silymarin on acetaminophen-induced acute hepatic and renal toxicities in domestic pigeons (*Columba livia*). Journal of Avian Medicine and Surgery 34: 348-357.

Impellizzeri, D., Bruschetta, G., Ahmad, A., Crupi, R., Siracusa, R., Di Paola, R., Paterniti, I., Prosdocimi, M., Esposito, E. and Cuzzocrea, S., 2015. Effects of palmitoylethanolamide and silymarin combination treatment in an animal model of kidney ischemia and reperfusion. European Journal of Pharmacology 762: 136-149.

Ingawale, D.K., Mandlik, S.K. and Naik, S.R., 2014. Models of hepatotoxicity and the underlying cellular, biochemical and immunological mechanism(s): a critical discussion. Environmental Toxicology and Pharmacology 37: 118-133.

Jahan, S., Khan, M., Imran, S. and Sair, M., 2015. The hepatoprotective role of silymarin in isoniazid induced liver damage of rabbits. JPMA. The Journal of the Pakistan Medical Association 65: 620-622.

Jain, A., Yadav, A., Bozhkov, A.I., Padalko, V.I. and Flora, S.J., 2011. Therapeutic efficacy of silymarin and naringenin in reducing arsenic-induced hepatic damage in young rats. Ecotoxicology and Environmental Safety 74: 607-614.

Jalali, S.M., Najafzadeh, H. and Bahmei, S., 2017. Protective role of silymarin and D-penicillamine against lead-induced liver toxicity and oxidative stress. Toxicology and Industrial Health 33: 512-518.

Jangra, A., Kasbe, P., Pandey, S.N., Dwivedi, S., Gurjar, S.S., Kwatra, M., Mishra, M., Venu, A.K., Sulakhiya, K., Gogoi, R., Sarma, N., Bezbaruah, B.K. and Lahkar, M., 2015. Hesperidin and silibinin ameliorate aluminum-induced neurotoxicity: Modulation of antioxidants and inflammatory cytokines level in mice Hippocampus. Biological Trace Element Research 168: 462-471.

Jee, S.C., Kim, M. and Sung, J.S., 2020. Modulatory effects of silymarin on benzo [a] pyrene-induced hepatotoxicity. International Journal of Molecular Sciences 21: 2369.

Jia, R., Cao, L., Du, J., Xu, P., Jeney, G. and Yin, G., 2013. The protective effect of silymarin on the carbon tetrachloride (CCl4)-induced liver injury in common carp (Cyprinus carpio). *In vitro* cellular and developmental biology. Animal 49: 155-161.

Jin, Y., Zhao, X., Zhang, H., Li, Q., Lu, G. and Zhao, X., 2016. Modulatory effect of silymarin on pulmonary vascular dysfunction through HIF-1α-iNOS following rat lung ischemia-reperfusion injury. Experimental and Therapeutic Medicine 12: 1135-1140.

Karabag, H. and Koçarslan, S., 2020. Comparison of the effects of thymoquinone and silymarin on the brain of rats having ischemia-reperfusion in the lower extremities. Annali Italiani di Chirurgia 91: 131-136.

Karbasforooshan, H., Hosseini, S., Elyasi, S., Fani Pakdel, A. and Karimi, G., 2019. Topical silymarin administration for prevention of acute radiodermatitis in breast cancer patients: A randomized, double-blind, placebo-controlled clinical trial. Phytotherapy Research 33: 379-386.

Karki, P., Lee, E. and Aschner, M., 2013. Manganese neurotoxicity: a focus on glutamate transporters. Annals of Occupational and Environmental Medicine 25: 4.

Katiyar, S.K., Mantena, S.K. and Meeran, S.M., 2011. Silymarin protects epidermal keratinocytes from ultraviolet radiation-induced apoptosis and DNA damage by nucleotide excision repair mechanism. PloS One 6: e21410.

Kazemifar, A.M., Hajaghamohammadi, A.A., Samimi, R., Alavi, Z., Abbasi, E. and Asl, M.N., 2012. Hepatoprotective property of oral silymarin is comparable to N-acetyl cysteine in acetaminophen poisoning. Gastroenterology Research 5: 190-194.

Kelany, M.E. and Abdallah, M.A., 2016. Protective effects of combined β-caryophyllene and silymarin against ketoprofen-induced hepatotoxicity in rats. Canadian Journal of Physiology and Pharmacology 94: 739-744.

Kim, J. and Sharma, R.P., 2006. Cadmium-induced apoptosis in murine macrophages is antagonized by antioxidants and caspase inhibitors. Journal of Toxicology and Environmental Health. Part A 69: 1181-1201.

Kim, S.H. and Sharma, R.P., 2004. Mercury-induced apoptosis and necrosis in murine macrophages: role of calcium-induced reactive oxygen species and p38 mitogen-activated protein kinase signaling. Toxicology and Applied Pharmacology 196: 47-57.

Kim, J.S., Han, N.K., Kim, S.H. and Lee, H.J., 2017a. Silibinin attenuates radiation-induced intestinal fibrosis and reverses epithelial-to-mesenchymal transition. Oncotarget 8: 69386-69397.

Kim, S., Jung, U.J., Oh, Y.S., Jeon, M.T., Kim, H.J., Shin, W.H., Hong, J. and Kim, S.R., 2017b. Beneficial effects of silibinin against kainic acid-induced neurotoxicity in the hippocampus *in vivo*. Experimental Neurobiology 26: 266-277.

Kim, S. and Ryu, D.Y., 2013. Silver nanoparticle-induced oxidative stress, genotoxicity and apoptosis in cultured cells and animal tissues. Journal of Applied Toxicology 33: 78-89.

Kiruthiga, P.V., Karutha Pandian, S. and Pandima Devi, K., 2014. Silymarin prevents the toxicity induced by benzo(a)pyrene in human erythrocytes by preserving its membrane integrity: an *in vitro* study. Environmental Toxicology 29: 165-175.

Kiruthiga, P.V., Pandian, S.K. and Devi, K.P., 2010. Silymarin protects PBMC against B(a)P induced toxicity by replenishing redox status and modulating glutathione metabolizing enzymes–an *in vitro* study. Toxicology and Applied Pharmacology 247: 116-128.

Kiruthiga, P.V., Shafreen, R.B., Pandian, S.K. and Devi, K.P., 2007. Silymarin protection against major reactive oxygen species released by environmental toxins: exogenous H2O2 exposure in erythrocytes. Basic and Clinical Pharmacology and Toxicology 100: 414-419.

Kiruthiga, P.V., Karthikeyan, K., Archunan, G., Pandian, S.K. and Devi, K.P., 2015. Silymarin prevents benzo(a)pyrene-induced toxicity in Wistar rats by modulating xenobiotic-metabolizing enzymes. Toxicology and Industrial Health 31: 523-541.

Koçarslan, A., Koçarslan, S., Aydin, M.S., Gunay, Ş., Karahan, M.A., Taşkın, A., Üstunel, M. and Aksoy, N., 2016. Intraperitoneal administration of silymarin protects end organs from multivisceral ischemia/reperfusion injury in a rat model. Brazilian Journal of Cardiovascular Surgery 31: 434-439.

Krishnappa, P., Venkatarangaiah, K., Venkatesh, Shivamogga Rajanna, S.K. and Kashi Prakash Gupta, R., 2014. Antioxidant and prophylactic effects of Delonix elata L., stem bark extracts and flavonoid isolated quercetin against carbon tetrachloride-induced hepatotoxicity in rats. BioMed Research International 2014: 507851.

Kumar, R., Deep, G. and Agarwal, R., 2015. An Overview of ultraviolet B radiation-induced skin cancer chemoprevention by silibinin. Current Pharmacology Reports 1: 206-215.

Kyriakopoulos, G., Tsaroucha, A.K., Valsami, G., Lambropoulou, M., Kostomitsopoulos, N., Christodoulou, E., Kakazanis, Z., Anagnostopoulos, C., Tsalikidis, C. and Simopoulos, C.E., 2018. Silibinin improves TNF-α and M30 expression and histological parameters in rat kidneys after hepatic ischemia/reperfusion. Journal of Investigative Surgery 31: 201-209.

Lal, M. and Gupta, D., 2016. Studies on radiation sensitization efficacy by silymarin in colon carcinoma cells. Discoveries 4: e56.

Latacela, G.A., Ramaiah, P., Patra, I., Jalil, A.T., Gupta, R., Madaminov, F.A., Shaker Shafik, S., Al-Gazally, M.E., Ansari, M.J., Kandeel, M., Mustafa, Y.F. and Farhood, B., 2022. The radioprotective potentials of silymarin/silibinin against radiotherapy-induced toxicities: A systematic review of clinical and experimental studies. Current Medicinal Chemistry, https://doi.org/10.2174/0929867330666221124155339.

Lama, S., Vanacore, D., Diano, N., Nicolucci, C., Errico, S., Dallio, M., Federico, A., Loguercio, C. and Stiuso, P., 2019. Ameliorative effect of silybin on bisphenol A induced oxidative stress, cell proliferation and steroid hormones oxidation in HepG2 cell cultures. Scientific Reports 9: 3228.

Li, L., Sun, H.Y., Liu, W., Zhao, H.Y. and Shao, M.L., 2017a. Silymarin protects against acrylamide-induced neurotoxicity via Nrf2 signalling in PC12 cells. Food and Chemical Toxicology 102: 93-101.

Li, Y., Ye, Z., Lai, W., Rao, J., Huang, W., Zhang, X., Yao, Z. and Lou, T., 2017b. Activation of sirtuin 3 by silybin attenuates mitochondrial dysfunction in cisplatin-induced acute kidney injury. Frontiers in Pharmacology 8: 178.

Li, S., Zhang, Q., Ding, Y., Wang, X. and Liu, P., 2020. Flavonoids ameliorate aluminum chloride-induced learning and memory impairments via suppression of apoptosis and oxidative stress in rats. Journal of Inorganic Biochemistry 212: 111252.

Li, C.C., Hsiang, C.Y., Wu, S.L. and Ho, T.Y., 2012. Identification of novel mechanisms of silymarin on the carbon tetrachloride-induced liver fibrosis in mice by nuclear factor-κB bioluminescent imaging-guided transcriptomic analysis. Food and Chemical Toxicology 50: 1568-1575.

Liu, W.W., Wang, F., Li, C., Song, X.Y., Otkur, W., Zhu, Y.Y., Hayashi, T., Mizuno, K., Hattori, S., Fujisaki, H. and Ikejima, T., 2022. Silibinin relieves UVB-induced apoptosis of human skin cells by inhibiting the YAP-p73 pathway. Acta Pharmacologica Sinica 43: 2156-2167.

Liu, Z., Sun, M., Wang, Y., Zhang, L., Zhao, H. and Zhao, M., 2018. Silymarin attenuated paraquat-induced cytotoxicity in macrophage by regulating Trx/TXNIP complex, inhibiting NLRP3 inflammasome activation and apoptosis. Toxicology In Vitro 46: 265-272.

Liu, W., Otkur, W., Zhang, Y., Li, Q., Ye, Y., Zang, L., He, H., Hayashi, T., Tashiro, S., Onodera, S. and Ikejima, T., 2013. Silibinin protects murine fibroblast L929 cells from UVB-induced apoptosis through the simultaneous inhibition of ATM-p53 pathway and autophagy. The FEBS Journal 280: 4572-4584.

Lo, D., Wang, Y.T. and Wu, M.C., 2014. Hepatoprotective effect of silymarin on di(2-ethylhexyl)phthalate (DEHP) induced injury in liver FL83B cells. Environmental Toxicology and Pharmacology 38: 112-118.

Lu, C.W., Lin, T.Y., Chiu, K.M., Lee, M.Y., Huang, J.H. and Wang, S.J., 2020. Silymarin inhibits glutamate release and prevents against kainic acid-induced excitotoxic injury in rats. Biomedicines 8: 486.

Malekinejad, H., Sheikhzadeh, S. and Hobbenaghi, R., 2014. Silymarin attenuates mycophenolate mofetil-induced duodenal disorders in rats. Avicenna Journal of Phytomedicine 4: 170-181.

Malekinejad, H., Janbaz-Acyabar, H., Razi, M. and Varasteh, S., 2012. Preventive and protective effects of silymarin on doxorubicin-induced testicular damages correlate with changes in c-myc gene expression. Phytomedicine 19: 1077-1084.

Manibusan, M.K., Odin, M. and Eastmond, D.A., 2007. Postulated carbon tetrachloride mode of action: a review. Journal of Environmental Science and Health. Part C, Environmental Carcinogenesis and Ecotoxicology Reviews 25: 185-209.

Mansour, H.H., Hafez, H.F. and Fahmy, N.M., 2006. Silymarin modulates Cisplatin-induced oxidative stress and hepatotoxicity in rats. Journal of Biochemistry and Molecular Biology 39: 656-661.

Marchiori, M., Rigon, C., Camponogara, C., Oliveira, S.M. and Cruz, L., 2017. Hydrogel containing silibinin-loaded pomegranate oil based nanocapsules exhibits anti-inflammatory effects on skin damage UVB radiation-induced in mice. Journal of Photochemistry and Photobiology. B, Biology 170: 25-32.

Marzban, M., Anjamshoa, M., Jafari, P., Masoumi, H., Ahadi, R. and Fatehi, D., 2017. Effects of gamma rays on rat testis tissue according to the morphological parameters and immunohistochemistry: radioprotective role of silymarin. Electronic Physician 9: 4524-4532.

Masini, A., Ceccarelli, D., Giovannini, F., Montosi, G., Garuti, C. and Pietrangelo, A., 2000. Iron-induced oxidant stress leads to irreversible mitochondrial dysfunctions and fibrosis in the liver of chronic iron-dosed gerbils. The effect of silybin. Journal of Bioenergetics and Biomembranes 32: 175-182.

Meeran, S.M., Katiyar, S., Elmets, C.A. and Katiyar, S.K., 2006. Silymarin inhibits UV radiation-induced immunosuppression through augmentation of interleukin-12 in mice. Molecular Cancer Therapeutics 5: 1660-1668.

Miranda, L., Agostini, L., Lima, W.G., Camini, F.C. and Costa, D.C., 2020. Silymarin attenuates hepatic and pancreatic redox imbalance independent of glycemic regulation in the alloxan-induced diabetic rat model. Biomedical and Environmental Sciences 33: 690-700.

Miranda, G., Gomes, B., Bittencourt, L.O., Aragão, W., Nogueira, L.S., Dionizio, A.S., Buzalaf, M., Monteiro, M.C. and Lima, R.R., 2018. Chronic exposure to sodium fluoride triggers oxidative biochemistry misbalance in mice: Effects on peripheral blood circulation. Oxidative Medicine and Cellular Longevity 2018: 8379123.

Moayedi Esfahani, B.A., Reisi, N. and Mirmoghtadaei, M., 2015. Evaluating the safety and efficacy of silymarin in β-thalassemia patients: a review. Hemoglobin 39: 75-80.

Moezian, G., Javadinia, S.A., Sales, S.S., Fanipakdel, A., Elyasi, S. and Karimi, G., 2022. Oral silymarin formulation efficacy in management of AC-T protocol induced hepatotoxicity in breast cancer patients: A randomized, triple blind, placebo-controlled clinical trial. Journal of Oncology Pharmacy Practice 28: 827-835.

Moghaddam, A.H., Mokhtari Sangdehi, S.R., Ranjbar, M. and Hasantabar, V., 2020. Preventive effect of silymarin-loaded chitosan nanoparticles against global cerebral ischemia/reperfusion injury in rats. European Journal of Pharmacology 877: 173066.

Mokhtari Sangdehi, S.R., Hajizadeh Moghaddam, A. and Ranjbar, M., 2022. Anti-apoptotic effect of silymarin-loaded chitosan nanoparticles on hippocampal caspase-3 and Bcl-2 expression following cerebral ischemia/reperfusion injury. The International Journal of Neuroscience 132: 1102-1109.

Momeni, A., Hajigholami, A., Geshnizjani, S. and Kheiri, S., 2015a. Effect of silymarin in the prevention of Cisplatin nephrotoxicity, a clinical trial study. Journal of Clinical and Diagnostic Research 9: OC11-OC13.

Momeni, H.R., Sepehri, H. and Yosefi, M., 2015b. Effect of silymarin on plasma membrane and acrosome of sperm treated with aluminum chloride. Journal of Arak University of Medical Sciences 18: 71-80.

Mooiman, K.D., Maas-Bakker, R.F., Moret, E.E., Beijnen, J.H., Schellens, J.H. and Meijerman, I., 2013. Milk thistle's active components silybin and isosilybin: novel inhibitors of PXR-mediated CYP3A4 induction. Drug Metabolism and Disposition: The Biological Fate of Chemicals 41: 1494-1504.

Muley, M.M., Thakare, V.N., Patil, R.R., Kshirsagar, A.D. and Naik, S.R., 2012. Silymarin improves the behavioural, biochemical and histoarchitecture alterations in focal ischemic rats: a comparative evaluation with piracetam and protocatachuic acid. Pharmacology, Biochemistry and Behavior 102: 286-293.

Muriel, P., Garciapiña, T., Perez-Alvarez, V. and Mourelle, M., 1992. Silymarin protects against paracetamol-induced lipid peroxidation and liver damage. Journal of Applied Toxicology 12: 439-442.

Mustafa, H.N., El Awdan, S.A. and Hegazy, G.A., 2013. Protective role of antioxidants on thioacetamide-induced acute hepatic encephalopathy: biochemical and ultrastructural study. Tissue and Cell 45: 350-362.

Muthumani, M. and Prabu, S.M., 2014. Silibinin potentially attenuates arsenic-induced oxidative stress mediated cardiotoxicity and dyslipidemia in rats. Cardiovascular Toxicology 14: 83-97.

Muthumani, M. and Prabu, S.M., 2012. Silibinin potentially protects arsenic-induced oxidative hepatic dysfunction in rats. Toxicology Mechanisms and Methods 22: 277-288.

Nabavi, S.M., Nabavi, S.F., Moghaddam, A.H., Setzer, W.N. and Mirzaei, M., 2012. Effect of silymarin on sodium fluoride-induced toxicity and oxidative stress in rat cardiac tissues. Anais da Academia Brasileira de Ciencias 84: 1121-1126.

Najafzadeh, H., Jalali, M.R., Morovvati, H. and Taravati, F., 2010. Comparison of the prophylactic effect of silymarin and deferoxamine on iron overload-induced hepatotoxicity in rat. Journal of Medical Toxicology 6: 22-26.

Nambiar, D.K., Rajamani, P., Deep, G., Jain, A.K., Agarwal, R. and Singh, R.P., 2015a. Silibinin preferentially radiosensitizes prostate cancer by inhibiting DNA repair signaling. Molecular Cancer Therapeutics 14: 2722-2734.

Nambiar, D.K., Rajamani, P. and Singh, R.P., 2015b. Silibinin attenuates ionizing radiation-induced pro-angiogenic response and EMT in prostate cancer cells. Biochemical and Biophysical Research Communications 456: 262-268.

Narayanapillai, S., Agarwal, C., Deep, G. and Agarwal, R., 2014. Silibinin inhibits ultraviolet B radiation-induced DNA-damage and apoptosis by enhancing interleukin-12 expression in JB6 cells and SKH-1 hairless mouse skin. Molecular Carcinogenesis 53: 471-479.

Nasr, S.S., Nasra, M., Hazzah, H.A. and Abdallah, O.Y., 2019. Mesoporous silica nanoparticles, a safe option for silymarin delivery: preparation, characterization and *in vivo* evaluation. Drug Delivery and Translational Research 9: 968-979.

Nematbakhsh, M., Pezeshki, Z., Moaeidi, B.A., Eshraghi-Jazi, F., Talebi, A., Nasri, H., Baradaran, S., Gharagozloo, M., Safari, T. and Haghighi, M., 2013. Protective role of silymarin and deferoxamine against iron dextran-induced renal iron deposition in male rats. International Journal of Preventive Medicine 4: 286-292.

Nencini, C., Giorgi, G. and Micheli, L., 2007. Protective effect of silymarin on oxidative stress in rat brain. Phytomedicine 14: 129-135.

Ninsontia, C., Pongjit, K., Chaotham, C. and Chanvorachote, P., 2011. Silymarin selectively protects human renal cells from cisplatin-induced cell death. Pharmaceutical Biology 49: 1082-1090.

Nofal, A., Ibrahim, A.M., Nofal, E., Gamal, N. and Osman, S., 2019. Topical silymarin versus hydroquinone in the treatment of melasma: A comparative study. Journal of Cosmetic Dermatology 18: 263-270.

Noshy, M.M., Hussien, N.A. and El-Ghor, A.A., 2013. Evaluation of the role of the antioxidant silymarin in modulating the *in vivo* genotoxicity of the antiviral drug ribavirin in mice. Mutation Research 752: 14-20.

Oliveira, C.P., Lopasso, F.P., Laurindo, F.R., Leitão, R.M. and Laudanna, A.A., 2001. Protection against liver ischemia-reperfusion injury in rats by silymarin or verapamil. Transplantation Proceedings 33: 3010-3014.

Onaolapo, O.J., Adekola, M.A., Azeez, T.O., Salami, K. and Onaolapo, A.Y., 2017. L-Methionine and silymarin: A comparison of prophylactic protective capabilities in acetaminophen-induced injuries of the liver, kidney and cerebral cortex. Biomedicine and Pharmacotherapy 85: 323-333.

Papackova, Z., Heczkova, M., Dankova, H., Sticova, E., Lodererova, A., Bartonova, L., Poruba, M. and Cahova, M., 2018. Silymarin prevents acetaminophen-induced hepatotoxicity in mice. PloS One 13: e0191353.

Parashar, P., Rana, P., Dwivedi, M. and Saraf, S.A., 2019. Dextrose modified bilosomes for peroral delivery: improved therapeutic potential and stability of silymarin in diethylnitrosamine-induced hepatic carcinoma in rats. Journal of Liposome Research 29: 251-263.

Patel, N., Joseph, C., Corcoran, G.B. and Ray, S.D., 2010. Silymarin modulates doxorubicin-induced oxidative stress, Bcl-xL and p53 expression while preventing apoptotic and necrotic cell death in the liver. Toxicology and Applied Pharmacology 245: 143-152.

Pereira, H., Dionizio, A.S., Araujo, T.T., Fernandes, M., Iano, F.G. and Buzalaf, M., 2018. Proposed mechanism for understanding the dose- and time-dependency of the effects of fluoride in the liver. Toxicology and Applied Pharmacology 358: 68-75.

Perumal Vijayaraman, K., Muruganantham, S., Subramanian, M., Shunmugiah, K.P. and Kasi, P.D., 2012. Silymarin attenuates benzo(a)pyrene induced toxicity by mitigating ROS production, DNA damage and calcium mediated apoptosis in peripheral blood mononuclear cells (PBMC). Ecotoxicology and Environmental Safety 86: 79-85.

Pietrangelo, A., Borella, F., Casalgrandi, G., Montosi, G., Ceccarelli, D., Gallesi, D., Giovannini, F., Gasparetto, A. and Masini, A., 1995. Antioxidant activity of silybin *in vivo* during long-term iron overload in rats. Gastroenterology 109: 1941-1949.

Pietrangelo, A., Montosi, G., Garuti, C., Contri, M., Giovannini, F., Ceccarelli, D. and Masini, A., 2002. Iron-induced oxidant stress in nonparenchymal liver cells: mitochondrial derangement and fibrosis in acutely iron-dosed gerbils and its prevention by silybin. Journal of Bioenergetics and Biomembranes 34: 67-79.

Podder, B., Kim, Y.S., Zerin, T. and Song, H.Y., 2012. Antioxidant effect of silymarin on paraquat-induced human lung adenocarcinoma A549 cell line. Food and Chemical Toxicology 50: 3206-3214.

Popp, T., Balszuweit, F., Schmidt, A., Eyer, F., Thiermann, H. and Steinritz, D., 2020. Assessment of α-amanitin toxicity and effects of silibinin and penicillin in different *in vitro* models. Toxicology In Vitro 67: 104921.

Pradeep, K., Mohan, C.V., Gobianand, K. and Karthikeyan, S., 2007. Silymarin modulates the oxidant-antioxidant imbalance during diethylnitrosamine induced oxidative stress in rats. European Journal of Pharmacology 560: 110-116.

Prasad, R.R., Paudel, S., Raina, K. and Agarwal, R., 2020. Silibinin and non-melanoma skin cancers. Journal of Traditional and Complementary Medicine 10: 236-244.

Psotová, J., Chlopcíková, S., Grambal, F., Simánek, V. and Ulrichová, J., 2002. Influence of silymarin and its flavonolignans on doxorubicin-iron induced lipid peroxidation in rat heart microsomes and mitochondria in comparison with quercetin. Phytotherapy Research 16: S63-S67.

Qajari, N.M., Shafaroudi, M.M., Gholami, M. and Khonakdar-Tarsi, A., 2020. Silibinin treatment results in reducing OPA1 and MFN1 genes expression in a rat model hepatic ischemia-reperfusion. Molecular Biology Reports 47: 3271-3280.

Radko, L., Cybulski, W. and Rzeski, W., 2013a. Cytoprotective effect of silybin against lasalocid-induced toxicity in HepG2 cells. Polish Journal of Veterinary Sciences 16: 275-282.

Radko, L., Cybulski, W. and Rzeski, W., 2013b. The protective effect of silybin against lasalocid cytotoxic exposure on chicken and rat cell lines. BioMed Research International 2013: 783519.

Radko, L., Cybulski, W. and Rzeski, W., 2017. The protective effects of silybin on the cytotoxicity of thiram in human, rat and chicken cell cultures. Pesticide Biochemistry and Physiology 143: 154-160.

Raghu, R. and Karthikeyan, S., 2016. Zidovudine and isoniazid induced liver toxicity and oxidative stress: Evaluation of mitigating properties of silibinin. Environmental Toxicology and Pharmacology 46: 217-226.

Raj, S. and Gothandam, K.M., 2014. Hepatoprotective effect of polyphenols rich methanolic extract of Amorphophallus commutatus var. wayanadensis against CCl4 induced hepatic injury in swiss albino mice. Food and Chemical Toxicology 67: 105-112.

Rajnochová Svobodová, A., Gabrielová, E., Michaelides, L., Kosina, P., Ryšavá, A., Ulrichová, J., Zálešák, B. and Vostálová, J., 2018. UVA-photoprotective potential of silymarin and silybin. Archives of Dermatological Research 310: 413-424.

Ramadan, L.A., Roushdy, H.M., Abu Senna, G.M., Amin, N.E. and El-Deshw, O.A., 2002. Radioprotective effect of silymarin against radiation induced hepato-toxicity. Pharmacological Research 45: 447-454.

Ramanathan, R. and Sivanesan, K., 2017. Evaluation of ameliorative ability of silibinin against zidovudine and isoniazid-induced hepatotoxicity and hyperlipidaemia in rats: Role of silibinin in Phase I and II drug metabolism. Chemico-biological Interactions 273: 142-153.

Randjelovic, P., Veljkovic, S., Stojiljkovic, N., Sokolovic, D. and Ilic, I., 2017. Gentamicin nephrotoxicity in animals: Current knowledge and future perspectives. EXCLI Journal 16: 388-399.

Rani, S.U., Chitra, M. and Jainu, M., 2014. Hepatoprotective effect of Wattakaka volubilis extract on Aluminium sulphate induced liver toxicity. International Journal of Pharmaceutical Sciences and Drug Research 6: 169-173.

Rao, P.R. and Viswanath, R.K., 2007. Cardioprotective activity of silymarin in ischemia-reperfusion-induced myocardial infarction in albino rats. Experimental and Clinical Cardiology 12: 179-187.

Rashid, K., Sinha, K. and Sil, P.C., 2013. An update on oxidative stress-mediated organ pathophysiology. Food and Chemical Toxicology 62: 584-600.

Rašković, A., Stilinović, N., Kolarović, J., Vasović, V., Vukmirović, S. and Mikov, M., 2011. The protective effects of silymarin against doxorubicin-induced cardiotoxicity and hepatotoxicity in rats. Molecules 16: 8601-8613.

Rathore, P., Arora, I., Rastogi, S., Akhtar, M., Singh, S. and Samim, M., 2020. Collagen nanoparticle-mediated brain silymarin delivery: An approach for treating cerebral ischemia and reperfusion-induced brain injury. Frontiers in Neuroscience 14: 538404.

Raza, S.S., Khan, M.M., Ashafaq, M., Ahmad, A., Khuwaja, G., Khan, A., Siddiqui, M.S., Safhi, M.M. and Islam, F., 2011. Silymarin protects neurons from oxidative stress associated damages in focal cerebral ischemia: a behavioral, biochemical and immunohistological study in Wistar rats. Journal of the Neurological Sciences 309: 45-54.

Razavi-Azarkhiavi, K., Ali-Omrani, M., Solgi, R., Bagheri, P., Haji-Noormohammadi, M., Amani, N. and Sepand, M.R., 2014. Silymarin alleviates bleomycin-induced pulmonary toxicity and lipid peroxidation in mice. Pharmaceutical Biology 52: 1267-1271.

Reisi, N., Esmaeil, N., Gharagozloo, M. and Moayedi, B., 2022. Therapeutic potential of silymarin as a natural iron-chelating agent in β-thalassemia intermedia. Clinical Case Reports 10: e05293.

Rigby, C.M., Roy, S., Deep, G., Guillermo-Lagae, R., Jain, A.K., Dhar, D., Orlicky, D.J., Agarwal, C. and Agarwal, R., 2017. Role of p53 in silibinin-mediated inhibition of ultraviolet B radiation-induced DNA damage, inflammation and skin carcinogenesis. Carcinogenesis 38: 40-50.

Rolo, A.P., Oliveira, P.J., Moreno, A.J. and Palmeira, C.M., 2003. Protection against post-ischemic mitochondrial injury in rat liver by silymarin or TUDC. Hepatology Research 26: 217-224.

Roy, S., Deep, G., Agarwal, C. and Agarwal, R., 2012. Silibinin prevents ultraviolet B radiation-induced epidermal damages in JB6 cells and mouse skin in a p53-GADD45α-dependent manner. Carcinogenesis 33: 629-636.

Roy, S., 2017. Impact of UV radiation on genome stability and human health. Advances in Experimental Medicine and Biology 996: 207-219.

Rui, Y.C., Zhang, D.Z., Sun, D.X. and Zeng, G.Q., 1990. Effects of silybin on production of oxygen free radical, lipoperoxide and leukotrienes in brain following ischemia and reperfusion. Acta Pharmacologica Sinica 11: 418-421.

Ruiz, L.M., Libedinsky, A. and Elorza, A.A., 2021. Role of copper on mitochondrial function and metabolism. Frontiers in Molecular Biosciences 8: 711227.

Saber, S., Mahmoud, A., Helal, N.S., El-Ahwany, E. and Abdelghany, R.H., 2018. Renin-angiotensin system inhibition ameliorates CCl_4-induced liver fibrosis in mice through the inactivation of nuclear transcription factor kappa B. Canadian Journal of Physiology and Pharmacology 96: 569-576.

Sabina, E.P., Peter, S.J. and Geetha, A., 2019. A comparison of hepatoprotective activity of bacoside to silymarin treatment against a combined Isoniazid and Rifampin-induced hepatotoxicity in female Wistar rats. Journal of Histotechnology 42: 128-136.

Saleemi, M.K., Tahir, M.W., Abbas, R.Z., Akhtar, M., Ali, A., Javed, M.T., Fatima, Z., Zubair, M., Bhatti, S.A. and Zahoor Ul Hassan, 2019. Amelioration of toxicopathological effects of cadmium with silymarin and milk thistle in male Japanese quail (Coturnix japonica). Environmental Science and Pollution Research International 26: 21371-21380.

Sampaio, G.R., Guizellini, G.M., da Silva, S.A., de Almeida, A.P., Pinaffi-Langley, A., Rogero, M.M., de Camargo, A.C. and Torres, E., 2021. Polycyclic aromatic hydrocarbons in foods: Biological effects, legislation, occurrence, analytical methods and strategies to reduce their formation. International Journal of Molecular Sciences 22: 6010.

Sasu, A., Herman, H., Mariasiu, T., Rosu, M., Balta, C., Anghel, N., Miutescu, E., Cotoraci, C. and Hermenean, A., 2015. Protective effects of silymarin on epirubicin-induced mucosal barrier injury of the gastrointestinal tract. Drug and Chemical Toxicology 38: 442-451.

Senturk, H., Kabay, S., Bayramoglu, G., Ozden, H., Yaylak, F., Yucel, M., Olgun, E.G. and Kutlu, A., 2008. Silymarin attenuates the renal ischemia/reperfusion injury-induced morphological changes in the rat kidney. World Journal of Urology 26: 401-407.

Shafiei-Roudbari, S.K., Malekinejad, H., Janbaz-Aciabar, H. and Razi, M., 2017. Crosstalk between E2F1 and P53 transcription factors in doxorubicin-induced DNA damage: evidence for preventive/protective effects of silymarin. The Journal of Pharmacy and Pharmacology 69: 1116-1124.

Shaker, E., Mahmoud, H. and Mnaa, S., 2010. Silymarin, the antioxidant component and *Silybum marianum* extracts prevent liver damage. Food and Chemical Toxicology 48: 803-806.

Shalan, M.G., Mostafa, M.S., Hassouna, M.M., El-Nabi, S.E. and El-Refaie, A., 2005. Amelioration of lead toxicity on rat liver with Vitamin C and silymarin supplements. Toxicology 206: 1-15.

Sherif, I.O. and Al-Gayyar, M.M., 2013. Antioxidant, anti-inflammatory and hepatoprotective effects of silymarin on hepatic dysfunction induced by sodium nitrite. European Cytokine Network 24: 114-121.

Sheta, N.M., Elfeky, Y.A. and Boshra, S.A., 2020. Cardioprotective efficacy of silymarin liquisolid in isoproterenol prompted myocardial infarction in rats. AAPS PharmSciTech 21: 81.

Shine, V.J., Latha, P.G., Suja, S.N., Anuja, G.I., Raj, G. and Rajasekharan, S.N., 2014. Ameliorative effect of alkaloid extract of Cyclea peltata (Poir.) Hook. f. and Thoms. roots (ACP) on APAP/CCl4 induced liver toxicity in Wistar rats and *in vitro* free radical scavenging property. Asian Pacific Journal of Tropical Biomedicine 4: 143-151.

Singh, M., Sasi, P., Gupta, V.H., Rai, G., Amarapurkar, D.N. and Wangikar, P.P., 2012a. Protective effect of curcumin, silymarin and N-acetylcysteine on antitubercular drug-induced hepatotoxicity assessed in an *in vitro* model. Human and Experimental Toxicology 31: 788-797.

Singh, K., Singh, N., Chandy, A. and Manigauha, A., 2012. *In vivo* antioxidant and hepatoprotective activity of methanolic extracts of Daucus carota seeds in experimental animals. Asian Pacific Journal of Tropical Biomedicine 2: 385-388.

Singhal, N.K., Chauhan, A.K., Jain, S.K., Shanker, R., Singh, C. and Singh, M.P., 2013. Silymarin- and melatonin-mediated changes in the expression of selected genes in pesticides-induced Parkinsonism. Molecular and Cellular Biochemistry 384: 47-58.

Singhal, N.K., Srivastava, G., Patel, D.K., Jain, S.K. and Singh, M.P., 2011. Melatonin or silymarin reduces maneb- and paraquat-induced Parkinson's disease phenotype in the mouse. Journal of Pineal Research 50: 97-109.

Skottová, N., Krecman, V. and Simánek, V., 1999. Activities of silymarin and its flavonolignans upon low density lipoprotein oxidizability *in vitro*. Phytotherapy Research 13: 535-537.

Son, Y., Lee, H.J., Rho, J.K., Chung, S.Y., Lee, C.G., Yang, K., Kim, S.H., Lee, M., Shin, I.S. and Kim, J.S., 2015. The ameliorative effect of silibinin against radiation-induced lung injury: protection of normal tissue without decreasing therapeutic efficacy in lung cancer. BMC Pulmonary Medicine 15: 68.

Song, I.S., Nam, S.J., Jeon, J.H., Park, S.J. and Choi, M.K., 2021a. Enhanced bioavailability and efficacy of silymarin solid dispersion in rats with acetaminophen-induced hepatotoxicity. Pharmaceutics 13: 628.

Song, X.Y., Li, R.H., Liu, W.W., Hayashi, T., Mizuno, K., Hattori, S., Fujisaki, H. and Ikejima, T., 2021b. Effect of silibinin on ethanol- or acetaldehyde-induced damage of mouse primary hepatocytes *in vitro*. Toxicology In Vitro 70: 105047.

Song, Z., Deaciuc, I., Song, M., Lee, D.Y., Liu, Y., Ji, X. and McClain, C., 2006. Silymarin protects against acute ethanol-induced hepatotoxicity in mice. Alcoholism, Clinical and Experimental Research 30: 407-413.

Soodvilai, S., Tipparos, W., Rangsimawong, W., Patrojanasophon, P., Soodvilai, S., Sajomsang, W. and Opanasopit, P., 2019. Effects of silymarin-loaded amphiphilic chitosan polymeric micelles on the renal toxicity and anticancer activity of cisplatin. Pharmaceutical Development and Technology 24: 927-934.

Soria, E.A., Eynard, A.R. and Bongiovanni, G.A., 2010. Modulation of early stress-related biomarkers in cytoplasm by the antioxidants silymarin and quercetin using a cellular model of acute arsenic poisoning. Basic and Clinical Pharmacology and Toxicology 107: 982-987.

Sozen, H., Celik, O.I., Cetin, E.S., Yilmaz, N., Aksozek, A., Topal, Y., Cigerci, I.H. and Beydilli, H., 2015. Evaluation of the protective effect of silibinin in rats with liver damage caused by itraconazole. Cell Biochemistry and Biophysics 71: 1215-1223.

Srinivasan, R. and Ramprasath, C., 2012. Beneficial role of silibinin in monitoring the cadmium induced hepatotoxicity in Albino Wistar rats. Recent Research in Science and Technology 4: 46-52.

Srinivasan, R. and Ramprasath, C., 2011. Protective role of silibinin in cadmium induced changes of acetylcholinesterase, ATPases and oxidative stress in brain of albino Wistar rats. Journal of Ecobiotechnology 3: 34-39.

Srivastava, R.K., Sharma, S., Verma, S., Arora, B. and Lal, H., 2008. Influence of diabetes on liver injury induced by antitubercular drugs and on silymarin hepatoprotection in rats. Methods and Findings in Experimental and Clinical Pharmacology 30: 731-737.

Svobodová, A., Zdarilová, A., Malisková, J., Mikulková, H., Walterová, D. and Vostalová, J., 2007. Attenuation of UVA-induced damage to human keratinocytes by silymarin. Journal of Dermatological Science 46: 21-30.

Taghiabadi, E., Imenshahidi, M., Abnous, K., Mosafa, F., Sankian, M., Memar, B. and Karimi, G., 2012. Protective effect of silymarin against acrolein-induced cardiotoxicity in mice. Evidence-based Complementary and Alternative Medicine 2012: 352091.

Tao, L., Qu, X., Zhang, Y., Song, Y. and Zhang, S.X., 2019. Prophylactic therapy of silymarin (milk thistle) on antituberculosis drug-induced liver injury: A meta-analysis of randomized controlled trials. Canadian Journal of Gastroenterology and Hepatology 2019: 3192351.

Tasduq, S.A., Peerzada, K., Koul, S., Bhat, R. and Johri, R.K., 2005. Biochemical manifestations of anti-tuberculosis drugs induced hepatotoxicity and the effect of silymarin. Hepatology Research 31: 132-135.

Teksoy, O., Sahinturk, V., Cengiz, M., İnal, B. and Ayhancı, A., 2020. The protective effects of silymarin on thioacetamide-induced liver damage: Measurement of miR-122, miR-192 and miR-194 levels. Applied Biochemistry and Biotechnology 191: 528-539.

Temamogullari, F., Atessahin, A., Cebi Sen, C., Yumusak, N. and Dogru, M.S., 2021. Protective role of silibinin over nickel sulfate-induced reproductive toxicity in male rats. Polish Journal of Veterinary Sciences 24: 29-34.

Tewari-Singh, N., Jain, A.K., Inturi, S., Agarwal, C., White, C.W. and Agarwal, R., 2012. Silibinin attenuates sulfur mustard analog-induced skin injury by targeting multiple pathways connecting oxidative stress and inflammation. PloS One 7: e46149.

Tilley, C., Deep, G., Agarwal, C., Wempe, M.F., Biedermann, D., Valentová, K., Kren, V. and Agarwal, R., 2016. Silibinin and its 2,3-dehydro-derivative inhibit basal cell carcinoma growth via suppression of mitogenic signaling and transcription factors activation. Molecular Carcinogenesis 55: 3-14.

Tiwari, P., Kumar, A., Ali, M. and Mishra, K.P., 2010. Radioprotection of plasmid and cellular DNA and Swiss mice by silibinin. Mutation Research 695: 55-60.

Tripathi, M.K., Rasheed, M., Mishra, A.K., Patel, D.K. and Singh, M.P., 2020. Silymarin protects against impaired autophagy associated with 1-Methyl-4-phenyl-1,2,3,6-tetrahydropyridine-induced Parkinsonism. Journal of Molecular Neuroscience 70: 276-283.

Tsaroucha, A.K., Korovesis, G.N., Valsami, G., Lambropoulou, M., Kollaras, V., Anagnostopoulos, C., Kostomitsopoulos, N., Zerbini, E. and Simopoulos, C., 2020. Silibinin-hydroxypropyl-β-cyclodextrin (SLB-HP-β-CD) complex prevents apoptosis in liver and kidney after hepatic ischemia-reperfusion injury. Food and Chemical Toxicology 145: 111731.

Tsaroucha, A.K., Valsami, G., Kostomitsopoulos, N., Lambropoulou, M., Anagnostopoulos, C., Christodoulou, E., Falidas, E., Betsou, A., Pitiakoudis, M. and Simopoulos, C.E., 2018. Silibinin effect on Fas/FasL, HMGB1 and CD45 expressions in a rat model subjected to liver ischemia-reperfusion injury. Journal of Investigative Surgery 31: 491-502.

Turgut, F., Bayrak, O., Catal, F., Bayrak, R., Atmaca, A.F., Koc, A., Akbas, A., Akcay, A. and Unal, D., 2008. Antioxidant and protective effects of silymarin on ischemia and reperfusion injury in the kidney tissues of rats. International Urology and Nephrology 40: 453-460.

Tvrdý, V., Catapano, M.C., Rawlik, T., Karlíčková, J., Biedermann, D., Křen, V., Mladěnka, P. and Valentová, K., 2018. Interaction of isolated silymarin flavonolignans with iron and copper. Journal of Inorganic Biochemistry 189: 115-123.

Tzeng, J.I., Chen, M.F., Chung, H.H. and Cheng, J.T., 2013. Silymarin decreases connective tissue growth factor to improve liver fibrosis in rats treated with carbon tetrachloride. Phytotherapy Research 27: 1023-1028.

Uçmak, F., Ekin, N., İbiloğlu, İ., Arslan, S., Kaplan, İ. and Şenateş, E., 2016. Prophylactic administration of silybin ameliorates L-Arginine-induced acute pancreatitis. Medical Science Monitor 22: 3641-3646.

Unsal, V., Cicek, M. and Sabancilar, İ., 2020. Toxicity of carbon tetrachloride, free radicals and role of antioxidants. Reviews on Environmental Health 36: 279-295.

Upadhyay, G., Kumar, A. and Singh, M.P., 2007. Effect of silymarin on pyrogallol- and rifampicin-induced hepatotoxicity in mouse. European Journal of Pharmacology 565: 190-201.

Upadhyay, G., Tiwari, M.N., Prakash, O., Jyoti, A., Shanker, R. and Singh, M.P., 2010. Involvement of multiple molecular events in pyrogallol-induced hepatotoxicity and silymarin-mediated protection: evidence from gene expression profiles. Food and Chemical Toxicology 48: 1660-1670.

Vaid, M. and Katiyar, S.K., 2010. Molecular mechanisms of inhibition of photocarcinogenesis by silymarin, a phytochemical from milk thistle (*Silybum marianum* L. Gaertn.) (Review). International Journal of Oncology 36: 1053-1060.

Vaid, M., Prasad, R., Singh, T., Elmets, C.A., Xu, H. and Katiyar, S.K., 2013. Silymarin inhibits ultraviolet radiation-induced immune suppression through DNA repair-dependent activation of dendritic cells and stimulation of effector T cells. Biochemical Pharmacology 85: 1066-1076.

Valenzuela, A., Barría, T., Guerra, R. and Garrido, A., 1985. Inhibitory effect of the flavonoid silymarin on the erythrocyte hemolysis induced by phenylhydrazine. Biochemical and Biophysical Research Communications 126: 712-718.

Vangaveti, S., Das, P. and Kumar, V.L., 2021. Metformin and silymarin afford protection in cyclosporine A induced hepatorenal toxicity in rat by modulating redox status and inflammation. Journal of Biochemical and Molecular Toxicology 35: e22614.

Varzi, H.N., Esmailzadeh, S., Morovvati, H., Avizeh, R., Shahriari, A. and Givi, M.E., 2007. Effect of silymarin and vitamin E on gentamicin-induced nephrotoxicity in dogs. Journal of Veterinary Pharmacology and Therapeutics 30: 477-481.

Veisi, S., Johari, S.A., Tyler, C.R., Mansouri, B. and Esmaeilbeigi, M., 2021. Antioxidant properties of dietary supplements of free and nanoencapsulated silymarin and their ameliorative effects on silver nanoparticles induced oxidative stress in Nile tilapia (Oreochromis niloticus). Environmental Science and Pollution Research International 28: 26055-26063.

Victorrajmohan, C., Pradeep, K. and Karthikeyan, S., 2005. Influence of silymarin administration on hepatic glutathione-conjugating enzyme system in rats treated with antitubercular drugs. Drugs in R&D 6: 395-400.

Vostálová, J., Tinková, E., Biedermann, D., Kosina, P., Ulrichová, J. and Rajnochová Svobodová, A., 2019. Skin protective activity of silymarin and its flavonolignans. Molecules 24: 1022.

Wang, C., Wang, Z., Zhang, X., Zhang, X., Dong, L., Xing, Y., Li, Y., Liu, Z., Chen, L., Qiao, H., Wang, L. and Zhu, C., 2012. Protection by silibinin against experimental ischemic stroke: up-regulated pAkt, pmTOR, HIF-1α and Bcl-2, down-regulated Bax, NF-κB expression. Neuroscience Letters 529: 45-50.

Wang, L., Huang, Q.H., Li, Y.X., Huang, Y.F., Xie, J.H., Xu, L.Q., Dou, Y.X., Su, Z.R., Zeng, H.F. and Chen, J.N., 2018. Protective effects of silymarin on triptolide-induced acute hepatotoxicity in rats. Molecular Medicine Reports 17: 789-800.

Wang, M., Li, Y.J., Ding, Y., Zhang, H.N., Sun, T., Zhang, K., Yang, L., Guo, Y.Y., Liu, S.B., Zhao, M.G. and Wu, Y.M., 2016. Silibinin prevents autophagic cell death upon oxidative stress in cortical neurons and cerebral ischemia-reperfusion injury. Molecular Neurobiology 53: 932-943.

Wu, C.G., Chamuleau, R.A., Bosch, K.S. and Frederiks, W.M., 1993. Protective effect of silymarin on rat liver injury induced by ischemia. Virchows Archiv B, Cell Pathology Including Molecular Pathology 64: 259-263.

Xie, Y., Hao, H.P., Wang, H., Wang, Z.X. and Wang, G.J., 2013. Reversing effects of silybin on TAA-induced hepatic CYP3A dysfunction through PXR regulation. Chinese Journal of Natural Medicines 11: 645-652.

Xie, Z., Ding, S.Q. and Shen, Y.F., 2014. Silibinin activates AMP-activated protein kinase to protect neuronal cells from oxygen and glucose deprivation-reoxygenation. Biochemical and Biophysical Research Communications 454: 313-319.

Yang, Z., Pan, Q., Zhang, D., Chen, J., Qiu, Y., Chen, X., Zheng, F. and Lin, F., 2019. Silibinin restores the sensitivity of cisplatin and taxol in A2780-resistant cell and reduces drug-induced hepatotoxicity. Cancer Management and Research 11: 7111-7122.

Yardım, A., Kucukler, S., Özdemir, S., Çomaklı, S., Caglayan, C., Kandemir, F.M. and Çelik, H., 2021. Silymarin alleviates docetaxel-induced central and peripheral neurotoxicity by reducing oxidative stress, inflammation and apoptosis in rats. Gene 769: 145239.

Younis, N.N., Shaheen, M.A. and Mahmoud, M.F., 2016. Silymarin preconditioning protected insulin resistant rats from liver ischemia-reperfusion injury: role of endogenous H2S. The Journal of Surgical Research 204: 398-409.

Zakariaei, Z., 2019. Silymarin as a promising potential therapeutic agent for treatment of patients with paraquat poisoning: An issue that merits further research. Advanced Journal of Emergency Medicine 4: e16.

Zarpou, S., Mosavi, H., Bagheri, A., Malekzadeh Shafaroudi, M. and Khonakdar-Tarsi, A., 2021. NF-κB and NLRP3 gene expression changes during warm hepatic ischemia-reperfusion in rats with and without silibinin. Gastroenterology and Hepatology From Bed to Bench 14: 267-275.

Zatloukalová, M., Křen, V., Gažák, R., Kubala, M., Trouillas, P., Ulrichová, J. and Vacek, J., 2011. Electrochemical investigation of flavonolignans and study of their interactions with DNA in the presence of Cu(II). Bioelectrochemistry (Amsterdam, Netherlands) 82: 117-124.

Zaulet, M., Kevorkian, S., Dinescu, S., Cotoraci, C., Suciu, M., Herman, H., Buburuzan, L., Badulescu, L., Ardelean, A. and Hermenean, A., 2017. Protective effects of silymarin against bisphenol A-induced hepatotoxicity in mouse liver. Experimental and Therapeutic Medicine 13: 821-828.

Zhang, S., Xin, W., Anderson, G.J., Li, R., Gao, L., Chen, S., Zhao, J. and Liu, S., 2022. Double-edge sword roles of iron in driving energy production versus instigating ferroptosis. Cell Death and Disease 13: 40.

Zhang, Y., Hai, J., Cao, M., Zhang, Y., Pei, S., Wang, J. and Zhang, Q., 2013a. Silibinin ameliorates steatosis and insulin resistance during non-alcoholic fatty liver disease development partly through targeting IRS-1/PI3K/Akt pathway. International Immunopharmacology 17: 714-720.

Zhang, W., Hong, R. and Tian, T., 2013b. Silymarin's protective effects and possible mechanisms on alcoholic fatty liver for rats. Biomolecules and Therapeutics 21: 264-269.

Zhao, F., Shi, D., Li, T., Li, L. and Zhao, M., 2015. Silymarin attenuates paraquat-induced lung injury via Nrf2-mediated pathway *in vivo* and *in vitro*. Clinical and Experimental Pharmacology and Physiology 42: 988-998.

Zhao, X.A., Chen, G.M., Liu, Y., Chen, Y.X., Wu, H.Y., Chen, J., Xiong, Y.L., Tian, C., Wang, G.Y., Jia, B., Xia, J., Wang, J., Yan, X.M., Zhang, Z.P., Huang, R. and Wu, C., 2017. Inhibitory effect of silymarin on CCl_4-induced liver fibrosis by reducing Ly6C^{hi} monocytes infiltration. International Journal of Clinical and Experimental Pathology 10: 11941-11951.

Part III.
Silymarin in immunity, inflammation and gut health

No pain, no gain

Chapter 9
Silymarin and immunity

Adapt the remedy to the disease

Peter F. Surai[1-6] and Anton Surai[7]*
[1]Vitagene and Health Research Centre, Bristol, UK; [2]Department of Microbiology and Biochemistry, Faculty of Veterinary Medicine, Trakia University, Stara Zagora, Bulgaria; [3]Department of Animal Nutrition, Faculty of Agricultural and Environmental Sciences, Szent Istvan University, Hungary; [4]Saint-Petersburg State Academy of Veterinary Medicine, St. Petersburg, Russia; [5]Sumy National Agrarian University, Sumy, Ukraine; [6]Odessa National Academy of Food Technologies, Odessa, Ukraine
[7]Healthy Food Services, Bristol, UK
psurai@feedfood.co.uk

Abstract

This chapter is devoted to regulatory actions of silymarin (SM) in maintaining optimal immune response under various stress conditions. Main principles of interactions between innate and adaptive arms of immunity are described with a special attention to redox homeostasis maintenance as the main mechanism of maintaining high immunocompetence in human and farm animals. Immunomodulating properties of SM are considered in relation to phagocyte functions and activity. Regulatory effects of SM on dendrites and mast cells are described. It was demonstrated that SM effects on immunity are dose- and condition-dependent. On the one hand, SM can stimulate both cellular and humoral immune functions, improving B-lymphocyte blastogenesis and T-lymphocyte proliferation. On the other hand, SM can inhibit proliferation of T lymphocytes and splenocytes. The most interesting findings are related to restoration of stress-compromised lymphocyte functions, especially Treg cell proliferation as well as suppression of damages to healthy tissues. Molecular mechanisms of immunomodulating properties are considered with a special emphasis to immunoreceptor integrity. Immunomodulation by SM, together with data on SM regulatory actions in inflammation and gut health built a basis for further expansion of research in this exciting field of science to make a further step forward in SM application in clinical practise and veterinary medicine as well as in nutrition of human and farm animals and poultry. Indeed, antioxidant properties of SM, vitagene-modulating properties and its involvement in redox homeostasis are key elements in maintaining optimal immune-communications between various cell types responsible for high immunocompetence under various stress conditions.

Keywords: silymarin, immunity, immunoreceptors, immunocommunication, oxidative stress

DOI:10.3920/978-90-8686-944-2_009, © Wageningen Academic Publishers, 2023

9.1 Introduction

Human and animal defence against various diseases depends on the efficacy of the immune system responsible for elimination of foreign substances (e.g. parasites, bacteria, moulds, yeast, fungi, viruses and various macromolecules) or the creation of specific inhospitable conditions within the host for a wide range of pathogens. This protective capacity is based on the effective immune system which is considered to be an important determinant of human/animal health and wellbeing. In that sense, a remarkable ability of components of the immune system to distinguish between self and non-self is a great achievement of human/animal evolution.

It is believed that almost all nutrients in the diet play a crucial role in maintaining an 'optimal' immune response, and both insufficient and excessive their intake can have negative consequences on the immune status and susceptibility to a variety of pathogens. Immunocompetence can be presented as a 'violin music'. One can have a best violoncellist in the world with a Stradivari violin in the hands, however, before the violin is properly tuned there is no music, just noise. On the one hand, overreacted immune system is associated with allergy and other immune conditions. Furthermore, to maintain such an increased immune reactivity important nutrients are used. On the other hand, an underreacting immune system is also a problem, since it is not able to adequately protect the body from invaders, including microbes, viruses, etc. Only well-tuned immune system can do a great job of the optimal health protection. Information has been actively accumulated for the last 20 years indicating that SM has immunomodulating properties (Palit *et al.*, 2021). Therefore, in this chapter a short introduction to innate and acquired immunity with a following review of immunomodulating properties of SM/SB will be presented.

9.2 Natural immunity

There are two major types of immune function: natural (innate) and acquired (adaptive) immunity (Figure 9.1). Natural immunity, called the innate immune system, includes protective physical barriers (e.g. skin, mucus coat of the GI tract), specific molecules (e.g. agglutinins, precipitins, defensins, acute-phase proteins, lysozyme, etc.), innate immune cells, including dendritic cells (DC), macrophages, neutrophils/heterophils, mast cells, natural killer (NK) cells, and natural killer T (NKT) cells representing the first line of defence against pathogens and foreign agents (Table 9.1).

Protective mechanisms of innate immune system are summarised in Figure 9.2.

9.3 Adaptive immunity

Acquired or specific immunity includes cell-mediated and humoral immunity (Figure 9.3). There are two major types of lymphocytes, T cells and B cells. The adaptive immune system is characterised by its diverse repertoire of antigen-specific

Table 9.1. Key elements of the immune system (adapted from Surai, 2006; 2018; 2021).

Cells	Significance
Monocytes, macrophages	Phagocytosis, synthesis of cytokines, including IL-1, IL-6, IL-8, and other substances
Neutrophils	Phagocytosis of bacteria, viruses and toxins
Eosinophils	Destruction of parasites
Basophils	Initiation of inflammatory processes
Dendritic cells	Antigen processing and presentation, lymphocyte activation, cytokine secretion
Mast cells	Release of inflammatory mediators
B cells (B lymphocytes)	Immunoglobulin (antibody) production (by plasma cells), antigen presentation and antigen-specific memory B cells formation; 10% of total lymphocytes
T helper cells (Helper T lymphocytes)	Antigen-specific, produce cytokines: IL-2, IL-3, IL-4, IL-5, IL-9 and IL-10; 55% of total lymphocytes
Cytotoxic T cells (T lymphocytes)	Destruction of tumour cells and virus-infected cells; antigen-specific, 25% of total lymphocytes
Regulatory T cells (T lymphocytes), formerly known as suppressor T cells	Modulation of the immune system, maintaining tolerance to self-antigens, resistance to autoimmune diseases and to chronic inflammation; immunosuppressive; about 5% of peripheral CD4+ T lymphocytes
Natural killer cells	Destruction of tumour cells and virus-infected cells, 10% of total lymphocytes
Macromolecules	
Immunoglobulins	Binding foreign cells and proteins; promotion of their ingestion by phagocytes (opsonisation); activating complement system
Interferons (IFN-α; IFN-β;IFN-γ)	Activation of macrophages (γ-interferon); inhibition of viral replication
Complement system: a set of over 20 soluble glycoproteins	Destruction of foreign cells
Interleukins	Regulation of specific types of leukocytes
Leukotrienes	Promotion of inflammatory process
Lysozymes	Dissolution of bacterial membranes
Collectines- a group of carbohydrate-binding proteins	Act as opsonins in nonadaptive immune response to pathogen
Acute phase proteins- a group of plasma proteins produced in the liver in response to microbial stimulus	Maximise activation of the complement system

receptors (TCR and BCR) expressed by T and B lymphocytes respectively and ability to form and retain immunological memory lasting over decades (Poon and Farber, 2020). Therefore, humoral immunity is based on B-cell activities and mediated by antibodies (immunoglobulins) released into the blood stream. They are responsible for specific recognition and elimination of various antigens: they bind and remove from the host invading organisms/substances and opsonise antigens to be recognised by phagocytes. It is also generally accepted that cell-mediated immunity is based on T cells action (Figure 9.3).

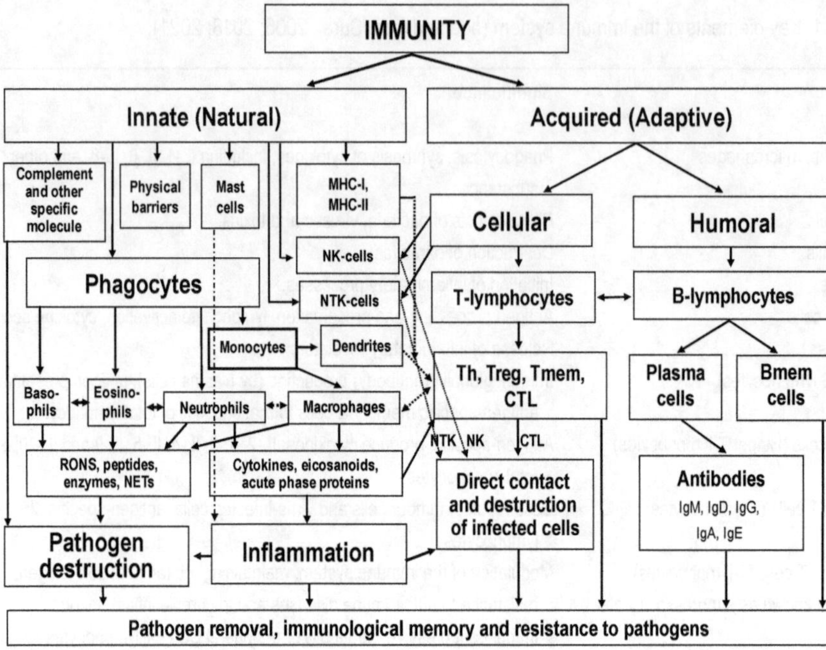

Figure 9.1. General scheme of the immune system (adapted from Surai 2002; 2006; 2018; 2020; 2021) (only three immunoglobulin classes: IgA, IgM and IgY have been identified in the chicken).

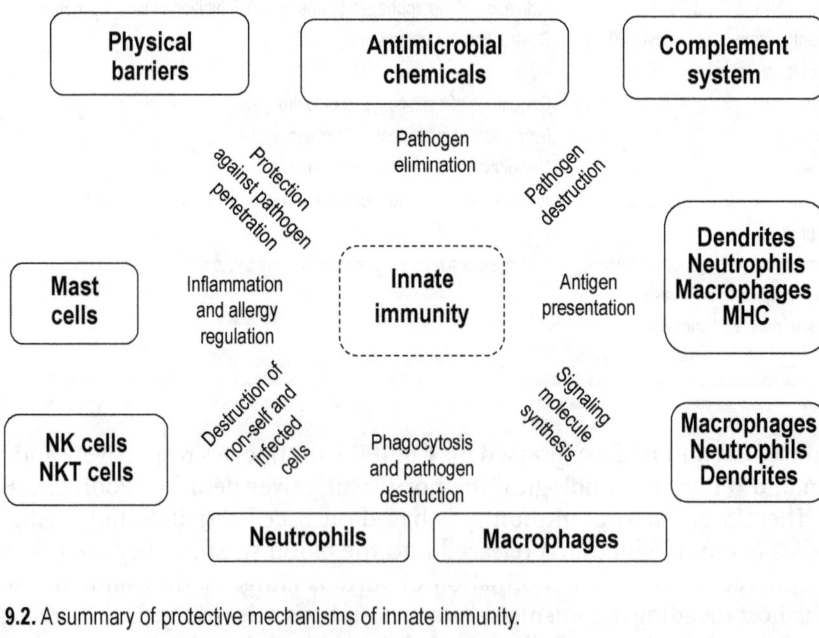

Figure 9.2. A summary of protective mechanisms of innate immunity.

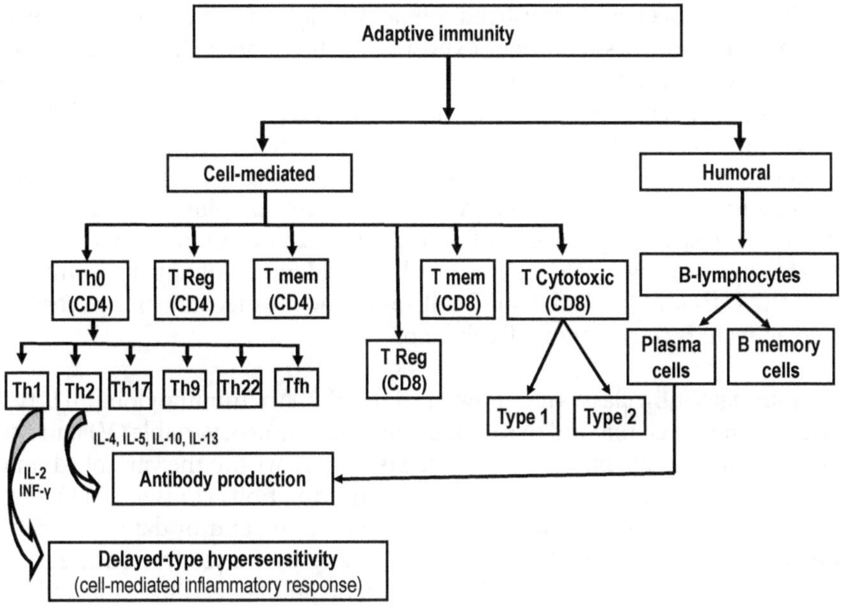

Figure 9.3. General scheme of adaptive immune system (adapted from Surai, 2006; 2018).

9.3.1 Humoral immunity

As mentioned above humoral immunity is based on B-lymphocyte activities. B cells are demonstrated to mature in the bone marrow in mammals and in the bursa of Fabricius in birds (interestingly, the name 'B' cells came from 'bursa' showing a great contribution of avian species to general immunology). After respective activation by an antigen B cells can act as antigen presenting cells (APC) or develop into plasma cells, producing immunoglobulins/antibodies, or into memory B-cells. It is known that B-cell activation takes place as a result of recognising protein epitopes in the form of soluble proteins or proteins associated with surfaces of cells or pathogens by B-cell receptor (BCR) together with an additional signal from a Th2 CD4+ T cell (Kaiser, 2011). It should be mentioned that such an antibody response is effective only against extracellular pathogens and intracellular pathogens are dealt with by T-lymphocytes. Each B cell is shown to expresses a unique BCR that can recognise a particular epitope on a particular antigen, and a typical human B cell could have up to 100,000 of these clonal BCRs on its surface (Kaiser, 2011).

When a pathogen antigen enters the body for the first time, a process called clonal selection takes place with lymphocytes bearing receptors specific for that antigen are activated and responded. As a result, depending on antigen nature the selected B- or T-cells multiply to generate daughter cells expressing the same antigen-specific BCR or TCR. During this so called primary immune response the daughter cells are converted into the short-lived effector cells (e.g. cytotoxic T lymphocytes or plasma cells) able to kill/eliminate pathogen and long-lived memory cells that can be found in the tissues in a resting state until a subsequent exposure to the same pathogen activates them. When the particular pathogen enters the body second time, it is quickly met by an army of antigen-specific memory cells that undergo rapid differentiation into effector cells resulting in a stronger and faster secondary immune response eliminating the pathogen before it can cause damages. Furthermore, during the secondary response, new populations of memory cells are also produced helping maintain long-term immunity to the specific pathogen (Tak Mak *et al.*, 2014). Of note, naive B cells can be activated by a pathogen via either a T cell-dependent, involving direct interactions between Th2 cells and the B cell, or T cell-independent mechanism by cross-linking BCRs, to activate B cells without T cell help.

Main immunoglobulin classes are shown in Table 9.2. An immunoglobulin is typically built with two heavy chains and two light chains consisting of variable (V) and constant (C) domains and the site binding an antigen is located within the variable domains of both chains. Immunoglobulins have several main functions (Kaiser, 2011):

- to bind to pathogens, preventing them from entering and/or damaging cells.
- to opsonise a pathogen, stimulating its uptake by polymorphonuclear (PMN) cells/leucocytes such as macrophages or neutrophils, leading to its subsequent destruction: Fcγ receptors are widely expressed on PMN cells and stimulate phagocytosis of Ig-opsonised pathogens.
- to stimulate pathogen destruction directly by activating complement.

Certain immunoglobulin subclasses are demonstrated to predominate during Th1 responses and involved in opsonising process, whereas other subclasses predominate during Th2 responses and are considered to be neutralising immunoglobulins (Kaiser, 2011). It should be mentioned that immunoglobulins are characterised by great diversity which is controlled by several mechanisms:

- domain variability;
- V(D)J recombination;

Table 9.2. Main immunoglobulin classes (adapted from Surai, 2006; 2018).

Immunoglobulin	Characteristics
IgG1; IgG2; IgG3; IgG4	Largest quantity; provide the bulk of immunity to the most blood borne infectious agents; the only antibody class to cross the placenta to provide humoral immunity to the infant; vaccination asks the immune system to produce IgG specific for a particular antigen
IgA	A first line of defence against microbes entering through mucosal surfaces directly communicating with the environment; synthesised by plasma cells; prevents colonisation of mucosal surfaces by pathogens
IgM	The first antibody produced in an immune response in large quantity
IgD	Present in humans, not documented in animals; functions as an antigen receptor on B cells
IgE	Involved in allergy development and in immediate hypersensitivity syndromes such as hay fever and asthma

- somatic hypermutation;
- affinity maturation; and
- class switching.

9.3.2 Cell-mediated immunity

Since antibodies do not work inside cells, an immune strategy to intracellular invaders is based on the function of T cells able to destroy whole infected or abnormal cells in a process called cell-mediated immune response. In general, four major types of T cells can be distinguished, including

- Cytotoxic T-cells (CTL) responsible for killing abnormal cells;
- T helper (Th) cells providing the signals to activate the adaptive immune responses;
- T regulatory (Treg) cells responsible for a regulation of immune responses including stopping further immune response, once the pathogen is eradiated;
- T memory (Tmem) cells giving an opportunity to immune system to 'remember' the pathogen for a long time to react quickly and effectively to its next appearance.

Cell-mediated immunity is based on specific antigen recognition by thymus-derived T-lymphocytes which can recognise specific antigens through interactions between surface TCR and peptide-bound major histocompatibility complex (MHC) molecules on APCs. The key T cell functions are activated and regulated by a complex, multi-component molecular systems at the T cell surface including the eight-subunit T cell antigen receptor (TCR), a co-receptor (CD4 or CD8) and a costimulatory receptor (CD28) with various additional cell-surface molecules (e.g. cytokine receptors and inhibitory receptors) affecting (positively or negatively) the strength, quality and duration of activating signals (Chandler *et al.*, 2020). Conventional T cells are divided into two main groups CD4+ helper (Th) and CD8+ cytotoxic T (CTL) cells. It is commonly acknowledged that T lymphocytes arise in the bone marrow and migrate to the thymus for maturation. At the same time somatically rearranged gene segments appear leading to the expression of a unique antigen-binding structure called TCR responsible for monitoring all cells of the body and destroying any cell posing a threat to the organism (Andersen *et al.*, 2006). The initial categorisation of T cells based on their biological properties has created two major categories with CD8+ cytotoxic killer and CD4+ Th cells. Later various subsets of Th cells were identified, including Th1, Th2, Th9, Th17, Th22, T follicular helper cells (Tfh), etc (Tuzlak *et al.*, 2021). Therefore, as a result of TCR stimulation and the synergistic effect of cytokines, naive CD4+ T cells differentiate into several distinguished cell subtypes, including Th1, Th2, Th9, Th17, Th22, Tfh and Treg, which are defined by their distinct cytokine production profiles and functions:

- Th1 (in response to intracellular pathogens and some viruses, produce IFN-γ, IL-2, and TNF-α to activate macrophages, NK cells and CD8+ cytotoxic T cells and to induce cell-mediated immunity with pro-inflammatory responses and phagocyte-dependent protective responses).
- Th2 (produce IL-4, IL-5, IL-10, and IL-13 to induce humoral immunity with antibody production. Eosinophil activation, and inhibition of several macrophage functions take place providing phagocyte-independent protective responses).

- Th9 cells are potent producers of IL-9, a pleiotropic cytokine which depending on conditions can have both protective and disease-promoting effects. Th9 cells are shown to participate in host-pathogen interaction, antitumor immunity, and immune-mediated diseases, such as autoimmune inflammatory diseases and allergic conditions, including asthma, allergic rhinitis, atopic dermatitis and food allergies. Th9 cells are considered to be a subpopulation of Th2 cells, phenotypically and functionally differing from them participating in the induction of inflammation. Polarisation of naive CD4 T cells with IL-4 and TGF-β can lead to the development of Th9 cells. Interestingly, TGF-β can induce Th2 cells and Th17 cells to produce IL-9 (Wang *et al.*, 2020).
- Th17 cells are identified as a lineage (distinct from Th1 and Th2 subsets) responsible for production of inflammatory factors such as IL-17A, IL-17F, and IL-22, to protect the host from extracellular pathogen infection and autoimmune diseases. In peripheral blood of healthy population, Th17 cells are quite rare comprising only 0.64-1.4% among CD4+ T cells (Wang *et al.*, 2020). Th17 cells are implicated in a number of chronic inflammatory diseases such as psoriasis, rheumatoid arthritis and Crohn's disease.
- Th22 cells are a subset of $CD4^+$ T cells formed in the presence of cytokine mixture including TNF-α, IL-6, IL-12, IL-21, IL-23. Th22 cells are characterised by the production of IL-22 and expression of aryl hydrocarbon receptor (AHR). Th22 cells provide mucosal defence, tissue repair, and wound healing. IL-22 induces expression of pro-inflammatory mediators, including TNF-α, IL-1β, IL-6, IL-8, IL-1, GM-CSF, and G-CSF, increases the expression of tissue regeneration genes, stimulates the production of antimicrobial peptides, cell proliferation and stimulates epithelial cell survival. (Doulabi *et al.*, 2022).
- T follicular helper cells (Tfh) are a specialised subset of CD4+ T cells that are located close to the B cell zone in secondary lymphoid structures and differentiating independently of other Th subsets from naive CD4+ T cells. Tfh cells play a significant role in the adaptive immune response, providing critical help to B cells within the germinal centres (GC) of secondary lymphoid organs. As a result, B cells that receive sufficient help from Tfh cells form antibody-producing long-lived plasma and memory B cells that provide effective and efficient protection against particular pathogen (Law *et al.*, 2020).
- Treg are designated as a subset of CD4+ T lymphocytes expressing CD25 (IL-2 receptor α-chain) on their surface and the transcription factor Foxp3 intracellularly. They represent approximately 5% of peripheral CD4+ T lymphocytes. Treg (regulatory CD4+Treg) cells participating in maintaining immune tolerance and resistance to excessive inflammatory responses. The main cytokines secreted by Treg cells are shown to include IL-10, TGF-β, and IL-35 and they are involved in peripheral immunosuppression, resistance to autoimmune diseases and to chronic inflammation. It seems likely that Treg cells induce immune tolerance by producing inhibitory cytokines, inhibiting the function of activated T cells and inhibiting the activity of APC (Zhang *et al.*, 2021).

Th cells have different functions and cytokine repertoire. Recently, based on target cells of the Th response a new nomenclature was proposed (Tuzlak *et al.*, 2021):

- Type 1 Th cell response associated with primarily activation and attraction of mononuclear phagocytes including monocytes, macrophages and DCs.
- Type 2 Th cell response targeting B cells and polymorphonucleated granulocytes including mast cells, basophils and eosinophils.
- Type 3 Th cell response associated with non-hematopoietic cells at barrier tissue sites, including epithelial cells and stromal cells.

It is generally accepted that activated CD8+ CTLs kill infected cells and tumour cells by secreting proinflammatory cytokines and cytotoxic mediators (Poon and Farber, 2020). Interestingly, CD8 + T cells have been shown to regulate established T cell and B cell responses (Lees, 2020) via

- direct cytotoxicity;
- modulation of lymphocyte survival factors;
- modulation of lymphocyte differentiation;
- modulation of ongoing antigen presentation; and
- the induction of additional regulatory populations.

Therefore, it seems likely that CD8+ Treg are of great importance for immune homeostasis maintenance. Once a job of antigen clearance is done by expanded clones of antigen-specific T cells, most of them undergo apoptosis, while a small proportion of T cells differentiate into memory T cells providing effective long-term immunosurveillance and enhanced immune responses to the same antigens. Diverse memory T cell subsets can be found in blood and in every tissue site (Poon and Farber, 2020). Due to this cell-mediated immunity, cells infected with a foreign agent, for example virus, are destroyed via a direct contact between an activated T-cell and target (infected) cell and cell-mediated immunity is responsible for delayed-type hypersensitivity reactions, foreign graft rejections, resistance to many pathogenic microorganisms and tumour immunosurveillance (Kaser *et al.*, 2011).

Therefore, adaptive immunity is based on a tightly regulated interplay between antigen-presenting cells and T and B lymphocytes. They facilitate pathogen-specific immunologic effector pathways, formation of immunologic memory, and regulation of host immune homeostasis. Interactions between T and B-cells, as well as antigen presenting cells, are responsible for the development of specific immunity. These defence mechanisms of specific immunity are induced or stimulated by exposure to foreign substances, are specific for distinct macromolecules and increase in magnitude with each successive exposure to a particular macromolecule (Miles and Calder, 1998).

In comparison to natural immunity, specific immunity takes longer to develop, but is highly specific for antigens and has memory (Table 9.3). These two parts of the immune system work together through direct cell contact and through interactions involving such chemical mediators as cytokines and chemokines (Figure 9.4).

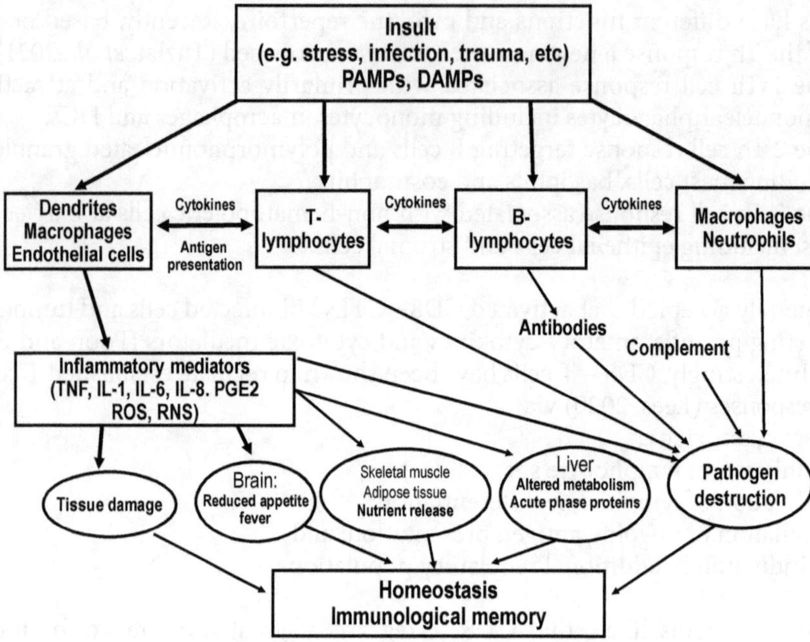

Figure 9.4. The natural and adaptive immunity interactions (adapted from Surai, 2006; 2018; 2021).

Therefore, the human/animal immune system requires the co-operation of macrophages, bursa-derived B-lymphocytes and thymus-derived T-lymphocytes with various other types of cells. The immune response involves cellular proliferation (T-lymphocytes), enhanced protein synthesis (including immunoglobulin synthesis by B-lymphocytes and acute phase protein synthesis by liver) and inflammatory mediator production. Physiological changes resulting from stimulation of the immune system include fever, anorexia and loss of tissue components (Grimble, 1997). The two arms of the immune system (innate and acquired) are complementary, and they operate in an integrated fashion to provide an effective protection of the host. As mentioned above, on the one hand, antigen is recognised and presented to the cells of the acquired immune system by innate immune cells. On the other hand, innate immune system cells (T helpers) regulate the bactericidal activity of phagocytes (e.g. macrophages and neutrophils/heterophils). The innate immune system provides a rapid response to novel pathogens, but such a protective action can be metabolically and physiologically quite costly to the host. The acquired immune system can respond in a much more pathogen-specific fashion with minimal impact on the host but depends on the interactions with the innate immune system (Korver, 2012; Rahe *et al.*, 2017; Table 9.3).

Effect and role of human/animal immune system in modern life and animal production systems is difficult to overestimate. Banning feed grade antibiotics in Europe has made immune system competence the major factor determining efficiency of poultry/animal

Table 9.3. Key features of innate and adaptive immunity (adapted from Surai, 2006; 2018).

	Innate	**Adaptive**
Appearance in evolution	Primitive organisms	Vertebrates
Induction time	Fast (hours to days)	Slow (days to decades)
Recognises	Common pathogen-associated molecular patterns (PAMPs) and damage-associated molecular patterns (DAMPs)	Unique epitopes on each pathogen/antigen
Cellular components	Phagocytes (macrophages and neutrophils); NK cells; NKT cells; mast cells; dendritic cells	T and B cells
Generation of specificity	Encoded in germline; has some specificity, no memory	Somatic rearrangement; highly specific and has memory
Effector mechanisms	Complement (Alternative pathway); cytokines; RONS; NETosis; granule proteases; defensins; chemokines; cell-mediated cytotoxicity	Antibodies; cytotoxic T cells (CTL); classical complement activation; antibody-dependent cell-mediated cytotoxicity; cytokines; chemokines
Soluble mediators	Macrophage-derived cytokines	Lymphocyte-derived cytokines
Characteristic transcription factors	NF-κB (+JNK/AP-1)	Jak/STAT, NF-κB, etc.
Physiological barriers	Skin Mucosal membranes	
Chemical protectants	Lysosyme Stomach acid	Antibodies in mucosal secretions
Additional protectants	Commensal bacteria	

production. Molecular immunology is developing very quickly and mechanisms of immunocompetence have received substantial attention (Domínguez-Andrés *et al.*, 2023; Özcan and Boyman, 2022; Zheng *et al.*, 2022) and nutritional modulation of resistance to diseases (Colitti *et al.*, 2019; Kidd and Surai, 2022; Venter *et al.*, 2020) is a frontline for future research.

Among different nutrients playing an important role in modulating immune response natural antioxidants, including polyphenolics (Sharma *et al.*, 2020; Martínez *et al.*, 2019) are shown to be very promising. However, antioxidant roles in animal and human immune system modulation received only limited attention. Mechanisms of nutritional modulation of resistance to infectious diseases were divided by Klasing (1998) into seven categories and the antioxidant status of the host is a critical consideration in the optimal functioning of the immune system. In the next sections effect of SM/SB on natural and adaptive immunity will be considered with a specific emphasis to possible molecular mechanisms of their immunomodulatory actions.

9.4 Silymarin and phagocyte functions

Phagocytosis is the process by which leukocytes and other cells ingest particulate ligands whose size exceeds about 1 μm. By ingesting microbial pathogens, phagocytes perform two important immune functions: initiate a microbial death pathway and build a bridge (send specific signals) between the natural and adaptive immune responses (Greenberg and Grinstein, 2002). Phagocytes are responsible not only for removal of pathogens, but also are involved in inflammation creating hostile conditions for the pathogens. It seems likely, that SM/SB can be considered as a fine tuner of phagocyte functions preventing excessive pro-inflammatory cytokines production and decreasing neutrophile infiltration. Recent findings have shown that SM can modulate the immune system by inhibition of neutrophil immigration, mast cell immobilisation, prostaglandin production, leukotriene synthesis; and NF-κB expression and pro-inflammatory cytokine (e.g. TNF-α and others) induction (Nazemian *et al.*, 2010). In particular, it was suggested that inhibitory effects of SM on neutrophil function may contribute significantly to its gastroprotective actions in an I/R mucosal injury model (De la Lastra *et al.*, 1995). SM was shown to reduce oedema as a result of significant reduction of the number of neutrophils and inhibition of neutrophil migration into the inflamed site and accumulation in inflammatory exudates following intraperitoneal injection in mice of carrageenan, a specific inducer of cytopathic effect on macrophages (De La Puerta *et al.*, 1996).

SB (10-50 μM) is reported to inhibit the calcium, phosphatidylserine- and diacylglycerol-dependent protein kinase C translocation and the NADPH oxidase activity in PMA-stimulated human neutrophils leading to decreased apoptosis (Varga *et al.* 2004). In a mouse model of chemically-induced irritant contact dermatitis SM was demonstrated to block neutrophil accumulation into the ear induced by various irritants (Han *et al.*, 2007). In an I/R-induced myocardial infarction model SM improved AO defences, decreased lipid peroxidation, suppressed the neutrophil infiltration and limited the infarct size in albino rats (Rao and Viswanath, 2007). SM was found to prevent sepsis-induced acute lung and brain injury as a result of its promotion of AO defences, decreasing the release of inflammatory regulators and inhibiting neutrophil infiltration (Toklu *et al.*, 2008). In cats, oral administration of a SB-phosphatidylcholine complex was shown to significantly improve the redox balance by increasing lymphocyte and granulocyte GSH content and phagocytic function (a percentage of phagocytic cells that were optimally responded; Webb *et al.*, 2009).

In bronchoalveolar lavage fluid (BALF) of cigarette smoke-exposed mice, the numbers of total cells, macrophages, and neutrophils, along with the MPO activity (a marker of neutrophil accumulation) were remarkably decreased due to SM treatment (25, 50 mg/kg/day, 1 h before CS exposure; Li *et al.*, 2015). Furthermore, SM also dose-dependently downregulated levels of pro-inflammatory cytokines including TNF-α, IL-1β, and IL-8 and improved AO defences (ameliorated decrease of SOD and abolished the increase of MDA) in BALF of mice with CS-induced airway inflammation (Li *et al.*, 2015). In a mouse model of kidney ischemia and reperfusion, the treatment with SM reduced kidney dysfunction, histological damage, neutrophil infiltration and oxidative stress in a dose dependent manner (Impellizzeri *et al.*, 2015).

In PQ-induced lung rat injury model, PQ significantly increased inflammatory cell infiltration, shown by increased numbers of neutrophils and macrophages in BALF. This effect was successfully ameliorated by SM exposure (Zhao *et al.*, 2015). In cerulein-induced acute pancreatitis in mice SM treatment inhibited pancreas and lung injury and neutrophil infiltration (Kim *et al.*, 2020). In mice with myocardial I/R injury SB was observed to reduce cardiomyocytes apoptosis, to attenuate mitochondrial impairment and endoplasmic reticulum (ER) stress, to alleviates ROS generation, neutrophil infiltration and cytokines release (Chen *et al.*, 2020). In warm hepatic I/R in rats SB was shown to ameliorate inflammatory liver tissue injuries, including neutrophil and macrophage infiltration and hepatocyte degeneration (Zarpou *et al.*, 2021).

As mentioned above phagocytes play an important role in natural immunity. Among 6 major specific rationales for modulating macrophage function analysed by Klasing (1998a), mitigation of immunosuppression arising from infectious diseases, dietary toxins or stress could be affected by dietary antioxidants. SM was found to protect mice against LPS-induced sepsis as evidenced by improvement of rate of survival of LPS-treated mice from 6 to 38%. SM was demonstrated to dose-dependently inhibit the LPS-induced expression and production of IL-1β and PGE2 in isolated mouse peritoneal macrophages and RAW 264.7 cells and to suppress LPS-induced DNA binding activity of NF-κB/Rel in RAW 264.7 cells (Kang *et al.*, 2004). SB (50 μg/ml) was demonstrated to suppress LPS-induced macrophage activation including inhibition of iNOS, TNF-α, and IL-1β expression by blocking p38 MAPK in RAW 264.7 cells (Youn *et al.*, 2013).

The pretreatment of mouse macrophages with SM (100 μM) was shown to reduce PQ-induced cytotoxicity, enhance the expression of Trx and antioxidant enzymes (SOD and GPx), suppress oxidative stress and inhibit the TXNIP and NLRP3 inflammasome activation, pro-inflammatory cytokines secretion and apoptosis (Liu *et al.*, 2018). SM was indicated to acts as a protector against high glucose (HG)-related stress by lowering hyperglycaemia and suppressing HG- and inflammasome-mediated IL-1β expressions to improve insulin resistance.

On the one hand, oral administration of SM (100 mg/kg) was associated with reduced hyperglycaemia in the mouse model of diabetes. On the other hand, in cultured macrophages, SM (5-20 μg/ml) was reported to decrease HG-enhanced expressions of iNOS and LPS-stimulated NO production. Furthermore, in LPS-treated macrophages SM dose-dependently ameliorated the enhanced IL-1β secretions in the presence of HG or palmitate (Lu *et al.*, 2018). SB (50 and 100 μM) was found to induce macrophage M2 polarisation in RAW264.7 cells and inhibited Th17 cell differentiation *in vitro* (Tong *et al.*, 2018). Treatment of differentiating mouse embryonic stem cells with SB was shown to dose-dependently increased the number of $CD18^+$, $CD45^+$, and $CD68^+$ cells, reflecting leukocyte/macrophage differentiation. This was associated with

SB-induced activation of phosphoinositide 3-kinase (PI3K), AKT (protein kinase B), signal transducer and activator of transcription 3 (STAT3), increase expression of hypoxia-induced factor-1α (HIF-1α) and vascular endothelial growth factor receptor 2 (VEGFR2) and enhancement of intracellular nitric oxide (Sharifpanah *et al.*, 2019). In a rat model of acute respiratory distress syndrome SM (100-200 mg/kg) was found to ameliorate LPS-induced histological changes of the lungs, and to reduce infiltration of lymphocytes, macrophages, and neutrophils (Zhu and Sun, 2018). Interestingly, immunomodulatory effects of two SM isomers (isosilybin A and silydianin) in a Balb/c mouse model of allergic asthma was shown as evidenced by reduced eosinophilic infiltration of lungs, IL-4 and IL-5 levels in BALF, IL-4 and IL-5 gene expressions (Nasab *et al.*, 2020).

It should be mentioned that depending on conditions inhibitory effects of SM/SB on neutrophils and macrophages could be beneficial or detrimental. Upon arrival into the sites of infectious or sterile inflammation, neutrophils are known to be activated by various inflammatory mediators with the following release of important factors with antimicrobial and pro-inflammatory actions, including cytokines, chemokines, ROS, granule proteases and NETs. The neutrophils are known to be short-lived cells and after performing their job they usually undergo apoptosis in tissues with following their clearance by macrophages leading to resolution of inflammation (Subramanian *et al.*, 2016). However, decreasing efficacy of neutrophils/macrophages in cytokine and other communicating molecules production could also have a detrimental effects. Therefore, regulatory roles of SM/SB on neutrophil/macrophage functions with their preventive roles in over-inflammation could be considered as an important part of health promoting properties of these phytochemicals/botanicals (Figure 9.5).

9.5 Silymarin and dendrites

Dendritic cells (DCs), discovered in 1973 Ralph Steinman and Zanvil Cohn, are professional antigen-presenting cells connecting innate and adaptive immunity (Bošnjak *et al.*, 2022). First, DCs capture antigens, mature, digest the antigen and migrate to lymphoid tissues to present foreign material to naïve T cells and to activate them. The nature of the antigen/pathogen would determine further fate of the T-cells. They would differentiate either into pathogen-specific cytotoxic $CD8^+$ T cells able to effectively destroy infected cells or into $CD4^+$ T helper cells regulating inflammation and orchestrating antibody production by B cells. Importantly, DCs also mediate induction of tolerance by presenting self-antigens or harmless environmental antigens and induce differentiation and maturation of regulatory T cells responsible for suppressing immune response when pathogen id destroyed and maintaining immune homeostasis by inactivation of self-reactive immune cells (Bošnjak *et al.*, 2022).

Inhibitory/immunosuppressive effects of SB on the phenotypic and functional maturation of murine bone marrow-derived DCs *in vitro* and *in vivo* have been reported (Lee *et al.*, 2007). The authors showed that *in vivo* SB was able to strongly inhibit CD80, CD86, MHC class I, and MHC class II expression on the surface of DCs

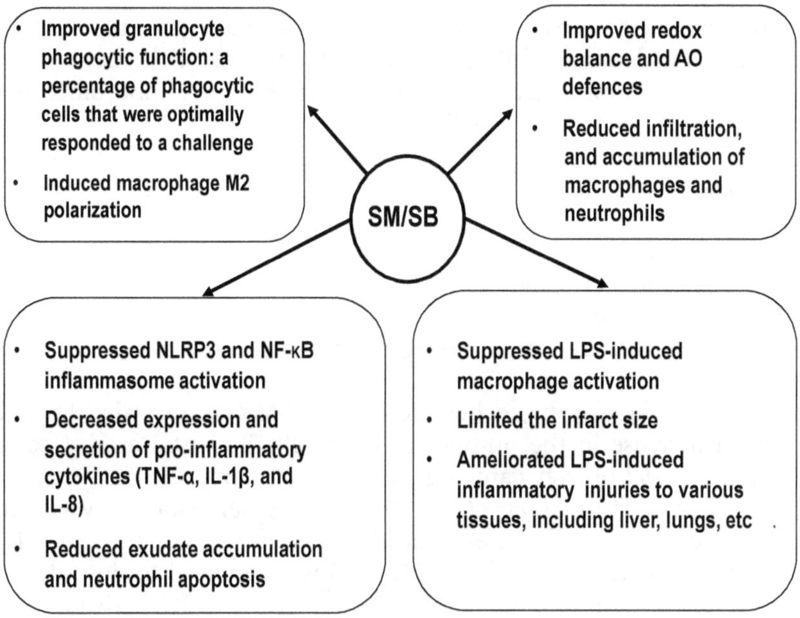

Figure 9.5. Regulatory roles of SM/SB on phagocyte functions.

leading to the impairments of LPS-induced IL-12 expression of DCs. Furthermore, SB was discovered to affect the capability of DC for Th1/Th2 polarisation through the regulation of costimulatory molecules expression and IL-12 production in DC (Lee *et al.*, 2007).

In experimental mouse autoimmune encephalomyelitis, SB treatment (5, 10, and 20 mg/kg) was shown to blocks the migration of inflammatory cells into the CNS, to suppress DCs activation, to repress Th17 cell polarisation/differentiation and to ameliorate the disease severity and significantly reduce inflammation and demyelination of the central nervous system (Yang and Shi, 2021). SB was reported to have immunosuppressive activity by inhibiting the maturation and activation of human DC and therefore it can be used as adjuvant therapy in the treatment of autoimmune diseases (Pagano *et al.*, 2022). Therefore, data on regulatory roles of SM/SB in DCs are quite limited. However, taking into account the importance of intestinal DCs in the initiation of tolerance, the induction of protective immune responses against pathogens and the maintenance of physiological homeostasis to the gut microbiota (Luciani *et al.*, 2022) there is a need for a new research in this exciting area.

9.6 Silymarin and mast cells

As mentioned above mast cells play important and diverse roles in responding to external threats. However, these cells have light and dark sides, and their over-activation can lead to chronic inflammation, tissue damages and pathogenic tissue remodelling contributing to a wide range of diseases (Kolkhir *et al.*, 2022). Therefore, appropriate control of mast cell activation and functioning is of paramount importance in modern human medicine and veterinary medicine.

The anti-inflammatory effects of SM are also based on multiple activities (Jeong *et al.*, 2005) including:

- mast cell stabilisation;
- inhibition of neutrophil migration;
- Kupffer cell inhibition;
- inhibition of leukotrienes, and prostaglandin formation.

In a rat model of CCl_4-induced hepatic fibrosis SM was recorded to ameliorate CCl_4-induced increase in the number of mast cells in portal areas (Jeong *et al.*, 2005). In a rat model of liver carcinogenesis SM was found to attenuate mast cell recruitment (Ramakrishnan *et al.*, 2009). SB supplementation was shown to ameliorate 1,2 dimethyl hydrazine-induced increased number of mast cells in the colon of rats (Sangeetha and Nalini, 2015). SB was reported to dose-dependently reduce histamine release from rat peritoneal mast cells (RPMC) activated by various antigens (compound 48/80 or anti-DNP IgE) and suppressed the NF-κB expression and secretion of pro-inflammatory cytokines, such as TNF-α and IL-6 in RPMC (Choi and Yan, 2009). In *Schistosoma mansoni*-infected mice SM was indicated to reduce number of mast cells and improved AO defences (GSH level; El-Lakkany *et al.*, 2012). SB (0.05-0.4mM) was demonstrated to inhibit the production of pro-inflammatory cytokines (TNF-α, IL-6, and IL-8) through suppression of NF-κB signalling pathway (the phosphorylation of IκBα and suppressed NF-κB transcriptional activity) in HMC-1 human mast cells (Kim *et al.*, 2013).

Topical treatment of mouse skin with SM was reported to prevent UVB-induced immunosuppression and the protective effect of SM was associated with inhibition of IL-10 expression and activation of synthesis of IL-12 in skin and lymph nodes (Meeran *et al.*, 2006). Furthermore, the production of IFN-γ and IL-2 (Th1-type cytokines) was significantly increased in CD8+ T cells from SM-treated UVB-irradiated mice whereas the levels of IL-4 and IL-10 (Th2 immune suppressive cytokines) produced by CD4+ T cells were significantly suppressed (Vaid *et al.*, 2013). At early stages in mouse model of basal cell carcinoma SB was found to suppress UV radiation-induced mast cells recruitment and expression of bone morphogenetic protein 2 in the skin (Rigby *et al.*, 2019). In mice with *Mesocestoides vogae* (Cestoda) infection co-administration of SM was found to suppress the infiltration of mast cells into liver and to elevate the therapeutic effect of praziquantel through modulation of specific antibody profiles, Th1/Th2/Tregs cytokines and down-regulation of fibrogenesis (Hrckova *et al.*, 2020). Therefore, the aforementioned data indicate that SM/SB can regulate mast cell functions in various model systems. In particular, in many cases anti-inflammatory properties of SM/SB are key activities in relation to immunoregulation including mast cell homeostasis.

9.7 Silymarin and lymphocyte functions

SB was shown to have a dose-dependent inhibition of *in vitro* lymphocyte blastogenesis induced by lectins (phytohemagglutinin, PHA; Concanavalin A, ConA; and pokeweed) and by anti-CD3 monoclonal antibody (Meroni *et al.*, 1988). The authors suggested that SB effect on lymphocytes is membrane-associated. SB (50 mg/kg BW) was found to restore cellular immune response including lymphocyte proliferation and cytokine activity compromised by partial hepatectomy in male rats (Horvath *et al.*, 2001). SM showed immunostimulatory properties *in vitro* by dose-dependent increase in lymphocyte proliferation in both mitogen (ConA) and mixed lymphocyte culture assays associated with an increase in IFN-γ, IL-4 and IL-10 cytokines in the mixed lymphocyte culture (Wilasrusmee *et al.*, 2002).

It seems likely that *in vivo* parenteral exposure to SM leads to suppression of T-lymphocyte function at low doses and stimulation of inflammatory processes at higher doses. When male BABL/c mice were treated with SM (10, 50 or 250 mg/kg, i.p.) daily for five days the absolute number of CD3+ T-lymphocytes and the expression of IL-2 and IL-4 were reduced with concomitant reduction in CD4+ and CD8+ T-cell populations only in the 10 mg/kg group. In the same group there was an increase in PHA-induced T-lymphocyte proliferation. At the same time LPS-induced B-lymphocyte blastogenesis was increased due to exposure to 10 and 50 mg/kg of SM. Furthermore, SM dose-dependently increased expression of TNF-α, iNOS, IL-1β and IL-6 mRNA (Johnson *et al.*, 2003). SB is considered as an immune-response modifier suppressing T cell-dependent liver injury. In the mouse model of concanavalin A (ConA)-induced, T cell-dependent hepatitis SB (injected in four doses of 25 mg/kg, i.p., 72, 48, 24, and 1 h before challenge with ConA) was found to significantly suppress ConA-induced liver disease by ameliorating intrahepatic activation of NF-κB and inhibiting intrahepatic expression of TNF, IFN-γ, IL-4, IL-2, and iNOS, and augmenting synthesis of IL-10 (Schümann *et al.*, 2003).

To test the hypothesis that exposure to SM can modulate differentiation and cell selection in the thymus via alterations in gene expression, mice were treated with 0, 10, 50 or 250 mg/kg of SM intraperitoneally once daily for five days. It was shown that SM treatment was associated with increased the absolute numbers of CD4 + and CD8 + positive T-lymphocytes, with the decreased expressions of IL-2 and IL-4, while MHC II expression did not change (Johnson *et al.*, 2002).

SM (10 and 20 μg/ml) was observed to dose-dependently inhibit the proliferation and secretion of TNF-α, IFN-γ, and IL-2 by PBMC stimulated with anti-CD3 and to suppressed T-cell TNF-α and IFN-γ cytokine secretion in response to tetanus and Candida protein antigens. This was consistent with inhibitory SM (20, 50 and 100 μg/ml) action on NF-κB transcriptional activation after T-cell receptor-mediated stimulation of Jurkat T cells. Furthermore, SM was able to inhibit proliferation of CD4(+) T cells and CD8(+) T cells in response to various antigens (Morishima *et al.*, 2010). SB (100 and 200 μM) provided protection to lymphocyte DNA as evidenced by reduction in DNA damage and micronuclei formation, which showed correlation to the extent of intracellular ROS reduction (Tiwari *et al.*, 2010). High-dose oral SM (420 mg three times a day or 700 mg three times a day) was shown to exerts modest nonspecific immunomodulatory effects in patients with chronic hepatitis C infection. In fact, *C. albicans*-induced T-cell IFN-γ expression and PHA-induced T-cell proliferation were inhibited by SM therapy and a trend towards augmentation of interferon-induced ISG15 expression was also observed due to high-dose SM consumption (Adeyemo *et al.*, 2013).

SM was reported to inhibit cell proliferation through G1 cell cycle arrest and also through the suppression of the mTOR signalling pathway in human activated T lymphocytes *in vitro* (Gharagozloo *et al.*, 2013). The ability of SM to inhibit T cell proliferation and pro-inflammatory cytokine secretion *in vitro* was also confirmed experimentally with naive CD4+ T cell isolated from PBMC, activated with PHA/anti-CD28 and treated with 100 μM SM for 72 hr (Gharagozloo *et al.*, 2013). The authors also showed that SM inhibited ERK1/2 and P38 pathway activation in T cells stimulated through TCR engagement. In *in vitro* experiments effects of SM on gene expressions of T cell transcription factors and cytokines were investigated. Treatment of splenocytes with SM (30 μg/ml) was shown to decrease IFN-γ and IL-17 gene expressions and to increase IL-10 and TGF-β gene expression. At the same time treatment of cells with 20 μg/ml of SM significantly decreased gene expression of the nuclear hormone receptor retinoic acid-related orphan receptor gamma t (RORγt) and increased Foxp3 mRNA levels. SM (20 and 30 μg/ml) was also shown to stimulate the differentiation of naive CD4+ CD25− T cells to CD4+ CD25+ Foxp3+ Tregs and Tregs generated in the presence of SM were reported to express higher amounts of Foxp3 protein on a per cell basis compared to those from untreated cultures (Namdari *et al.*, 2018).

Treatment of ovalbumin (Ova)-immunised mice with SM (100 mg/kg for 2 weeks) was found to increase percentage of Tregs, but decreased proportions of Th1 and Th17 cells. Furthermore, *ex vivo* Ova challenge of splenocytes from Ova-immunised mice treated with SM was indicated to decrease proliferation of splenocytes, IFN-γ and IL-17 expressions simultaneously with increased TGF-β expressions in $CD4^{+}T\text{-}bet^{+}$, $CD4^{+}ROR\gamma t^{+}$ and $CD4^{+}Foxp3^{+}$ T cells, respectively (Namdari *et al.*, 2018). SM (50, 100, 150 μM) was able to restore regulatory T cells (Tregs) function in multiple sclerosis patients *in vitro*. Indeed, SM (100 μM) was found to promote Treg proliferation Furthermore, IL-10, TGF-β levels, and FOXP3, JAK3, and STAT5 gene expressions were enhanced by SM dose and time dependently (Shariati *et al.*, 2019). SM (50, 100 and 150 μM) was reported to increase the proliferation of Tregs the TGF-β1 production by Tregs (Keyhanmehr *et al.*, 2019). SM was reported to protect enzymatic (CAT, GPx and SOD), haematological, and immune system against γ-radiation-induced toxicity as evidenced by an increased CD4:CD8 ratio and amelioration of radiation-induced decrease in regulatory T-cells (Adhikari and Arora, 2016).

The immunomodulatory effects of SM were studied in BALB/c mice. SM was injected (i.p.) daily (50, 100 and 150 mg/kg) for 14 consecutive days. The low dose of SM

(50 mg/kg) was shown to stimulate both cellular and humoral immune functions in the treated animals. SM at higher dose (100 mg/kg) could affect delayed type hypersensitivity responses and lymphoproliferation. However, SM at the highest dose (150 mg/kg) did not affect non-functional/functional parameters of mice immune system (Karimi *et al.*, 2018).

In a rat model SM was reported to mitigate LPS-induced lung impairments by down-regulating inflammation. In particular, the SM treatment mitigated LPS-induced increase in proinflammatory cytokines (IFN-γ, IL-6 and TNF-α) and decrease in anti-inflammatory cytokine IL-10 in broncho-alveolar lavage fluid. In addition, SM pretreatment was responsible for partial inactivation of multiple MAPK signalling pathways in the lungs (Zhu and Sun, 2018).

A summary of the regulatory effects of SM/SB on lymphocyte functions are shown in Figure 9.6. It seems likely that SM/SB effects on immunity are dose- and condition-dependent. On the one hand, SM/SB can stimulate both cellular and humoral immune functions, improving B-lymphocyte blastogenesis and T-lymphocyte proliferation. On the other hand, SM can inhibit proliferation of T lymphocytes and splenocytes. The most interesting findings are related to restoration of stress-compromised lymphocyte functions, especially Treg cell proliferation as well as suppression of damages to healthy tissues. Therefore, anti-inflammatory actions of SM are of great importance and they will be considered in detail in the next chapter.

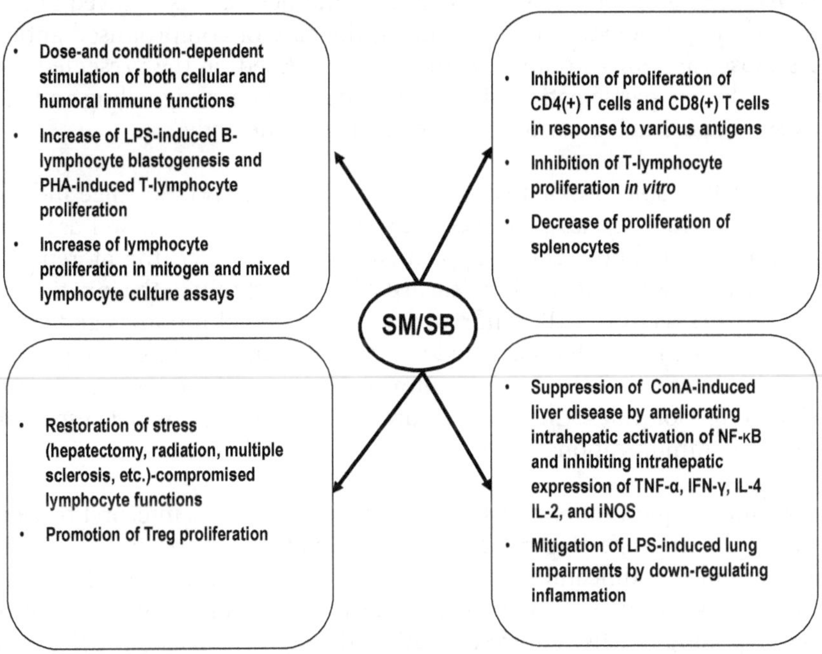

Figure 9.6. Regulatory roles of SM/SB on lymphocyte functions.

9.8 Molecular mechanisms of silymarin immunomodulation

Information has been actively accumulated for the last 20 years indicating that antioxidants are among major immunomodulating agents (Surai, 2002; 2006; 2018; 2020; 2021). If we imagine that immune system is an army fighting against invaders (microorganisms, viruses, etc.) than we would expect them to use signalling devices (similar to mobile phones) to receive and send signals to each other. Remarkably enough, major immune cells (macrophages, neutrophils, dendrites, NK cells, T- and B-lymphocytes) have on their surface something like 'mobile phones' called receptors. Those receptors are extremely sensitive to communicating molecules, but they are also sensitive to redox balance and to damages by free radicals and their expression and integrity can be easily compromised/damaged. In such a situation without proper communication all those huge armies of immune cells would become useless.

Without proper communications, those cells can start fighting each other as well as eventually destroying immunocompetence. Furthermore, if we present immune cells (phagocytes) as 'soldiers' using chemical weapon to kill enemy, then special ammunition protecting them from their own weapon would be a crucial element for effective battle. In the case of immune cells such ammunition is represented by natural antioxidants with HSP, HO-1, SOD, thioredoxin- and glutathione systems and sirtuins being major defences. It seems likely that if not properly protected, phagocyte/macrophage functions could be compromised including initial overproduction of free radicals with consecutive damages to specific enzymatic systems resulting in decreasing efficiency of oxidative burst and apoptosis. Redox balance/homeostasis is believed to be major regulator of the phagocyte functions and in the case of compromised antioxidant defences those functions would be compromised. Based on the presented model it is clear that the SM participating in the antioxidant defence, signalling and adaptive homeostasis is a crucial factor of immune defence in the body.

It was shown that spleen oxidative stress induced by a HFD in mice induced the decreased expression of genes associated with antioxidant defence, as well as Fc receptor and an antioxidant (lipoic acid) supplementation attenuated the aforementioned changes (Cui *et al.*, 2012). It has been learned a lot recently about the innate receptors, such as TLR, that activate APCs in response to microbial products and initiate an immune response. It is well established that the immune response is regulated by a very complex interactions between immune cells via cytokine system as well as via other signalling molecules. Clearly, there are many various cytokines responsible for immune cell communications.

The most difficult question remains to answer is 'how do cells interpret these signals to modulate the immune response?'. A key aspect of the answer lies at the receptor and the multiple modifications and regulatory proteins that collectively shape a cytokine response (Delgoffe *et al.*, 2011). For example, for an optimal and appropriate immune response, T cells require activation through the TCR, which recognises specific antigen presented in the context of MHC (Williams and Kwon, 2004). This recognition also confers the ability of T cell responses to distinguish between 'self' and 'nonself.' Engagement of the TCR, throughout the lifetime of the T cell, controls the survival, proliferation, and/or differentiation of T cells.

Thus, signalling through the TCR has important consequences for proper immune response and the effectiveness of that response. Receptor expression can be dynamically modulated by the cell, based on cell type, stimulation, and cytokine activity. Some receptors are constitutively expressed, while others require additional signals in order to be upregulated and properly expressed. In addition, a lot of cytokine receptors are formed from multiple chains that have distinct modes of regulation. Furthermore, cells can temporally modulate the expression of certain receptors thereby altering the cytokines to which a particular cell is responsive (Delgoffe *et al.*, 2011). As a result of cytokine stimulation, cells can become activated and differentiate and most of the physiologic outcomes observed in the immune system are mediated by cytokines. It seems likely that T-cell activation requires two distinct signals: the first signal (recognition) relies on the interaction between the TCR and an MHC-peptide complex, while the second signal is provided by the cross-linking between co-stimulatory molecules on activated T cells and compromise or loss of one or more of such regulatory and/or co-stimulatory molecules can be detrimental for immunocompetence (Pizzi *et al.*, 2016).

The immune response to pathogens is characterised by a biphasic response: the initial non-specific innate immune response and the subsequent pathogen-specific adaptive immune response. It is well established that the innate immune response is mediated mainly by macrophages, dendritic cells and neutrophils/heterophils, and occurs rapidly after these cells encounter a pathogen, while the adaptive immune response is controlled by T and B cells, which takes place several days after pathogen invasion (Kingeter and Lin, 2012). It is necessary to underline that the innate immune response is crucial for the development of the adaptive immune response. First, phagocytic cells such as dendritic cells and/or macrophages perform antigen presentation functions. They engulf extracellular pathogens, or infected host cells, and present PAMPs to T cells. In this way, the innate immune system indicates to the cells of the adaptive immune system presence of pathogen and the appropriate pathogen-specific adaptive lymphocytes are activated (Kingeter and Lin, 2012).

Therefore, signal transduction pathways are triggered resulting in the activation of various transcription factors, such as NF-κB, responsible for the production of pro-inflammatory cytokines and chemokines, which are involved in further regulation of the immune response. In this scenario immune cell receptor expression and integrity are major determinants of human/animal immunocompetence. We can consider immunocompetence as an effective communication between all types of cells of the immune system.

It should be mentioned that both the innate and adaptive immunity are closely related and there is a complex interplay between innate and adaptive responses. The innate immune system can be considered as an effector arm of the adaptive response. For example, interactions between T cells and macrophages are of great importance. T cell responses are associated with the production of IFN-γ, a cytokine possessing the ability to activate macrophages, increasing their capacity to phagocytose and kill invading microorganisms.

Similarly, macrophages express Fc receptors that bind immunoglobulin (produced by B cells) and enhance recognition and engulfment of foreign pathogen-derived material. There is also a close interactions between T cells and goblet cells resulting in increased secretion of defensins and altered mucus composition (Juul-Madsen *et al.*, 2008). Initial encounter of pathogens with the innate system leads not only to the destruction of the pathogens but also initiates a cascade of important immunological events, including recruitment of various immune components, as well as induction and modulation of the adaptive immune system. In such interactions immune receptors are of great importance and their integrity and protection in stress conditions is a key for effective immunocompetence. For example, in the cellular innate immune system up to 100 different receptors are expressed at a relatively high frequency (Juul-Madsen *et al.*, 2008) and each receptor is usually expressed on millions of innate and adaptive immune cells.

Optimal redox status and antioxidant defences are needed for increase lymphocyte proliferation, expression of the high-affinity IL-2R, cytolytic T lymphocyte efficacy/activity, and NK-cell function, enhancing resistance to infections through modulation of interleukin production and subsequently the Thl/Th2 response. It seems likely that vitagene-regulating nutrients including SM can upregulate the expression or protect from disruptions/damages by RONS receptors for IL-2 and other cytokines on the surface of activated lymphocytes and NK cells. This event favours the interaction of this cytokine with its respective receptors (Surai, 2002; 2006; 2018; Puertollano *et al.*, 2011).

9.9 RONS, redox homeostasis and immunocommunication

Over the last decade crucial roles of RONS and redox balance in regulating T- and B-cell functions was well recognised. In particular, the redox balance is believed to be regulated by dithiol/disulphide equilibrium and additional components of the antioxidant defence system encoded by vitagenes including thioredoxin, thioredoxin reductase, NADPH, SOD, CAT, peroxiredoxins, glutaredoxins, etc. (Patwardhan *et al.*, 2020). The redox balance in general was shown to be able to affect/determine the phenotype and effector functions of T cells (Ginn-Pease and Whisler, 1998; Gostner *et al.*, 2013; Moshfegh and Case, 2021; Saksida *et al.*, 2021; Weyand *et al.*, 2018). T cell activation is believed to depend on the redox balance at the site of their action and it is associated with ROS production in mitochondria. Furthermore, defects in mitochondria ETC are associated with impaired TCR-dependent RONS production and defects in antigen specific proliferation (Patwardhan *et al.*, 2020). In particular, RONS are considered to be essential for T lymphocyte activation, expansion and effector function (Gambhir *et al.*, 2019; Moro-García *et al.*, 2018).

In general, T cell activation is associated with a range of important changes. For example, during T cell activation mitochondria are characterised by elevated membrane potential (Wherry, 2011), metabolic re-programming (Wang *et al.*, 2011) and located to the immunological synapse (Quintana *et al.*, 2007). On the one hand, macrophage derived RONS are shown to induce Tregs in an NADPH oxidase dependent fashion (Kraaij *et al.*, 2010). On the other hand, there is also an activation of NADPH oxidase in T cells (Jackson *et al.*, 2004) with Duox1 (NOX family member) being responsible for TCR-mediated H_2O_2 production and involved in TCR signalling (Kwon *et al.*, 2010) with simultaneous changes in antioxidant defence mechanisms (Gambhir *et al.*, 2019; Sukumar *et al.*, 2016). Therefore, the activity of a range of cytokine receptors is shown to be affected by redox sensitive disulphide bonds and this could be an important mechanism controlling the levels of responses of cells to exogenous cytokines (Metcalfe *et al.*, 2012), associated with redox balance in the cell reflecting efficacy of antioxidant defence and adaptive vitagene-related signalling (Surai, 2020; Surai *et al.*, 2019; 2021).

Disulphide bonds are known to be important determinants of protein structure and function. In particular, they can sense and control changes in the redox environment. They also regulate protein folding, structural stabilisation, activity, localisation and interactions and therefore disturbances of protein disulphide bonds lead to various detrimental consequences to cellular/body homeostasis, including immune system dysregulation. In particular, oxidative stress-induced disulphide formation and thiol-disulphide exchange-mediated reduction of allosteric disulphides could affect immune cell structure and functions (Bechtel and Weerapana, 2017). Protein disulphide bonds serve not only structural role, but they also control the function of the mature protein in which they reside. On the one hand, structural disulphides are shown to be formed during protein folding and they are involved in the folding process and responsible for stability of the resultant protein architecture. On the other hand, functional disulphides can be divided into two groups, namely catalytic disulphides present in specific enzymes (e.g. protein-disulphide isomerase; PDI) or antioxidant compounds (e.g. thioredoxin), and responsible for manipulation of disulphides in other proteins and allosteric disulphides inducing changes in the tertiary structure and controlling the function of the protein in which they are located (Chiu and Hogg, 2019).

Allosteric disulphide bond formation or cleavage can switch the structure and function of a protein (Kuroi *et al.*, 2020). These so called 'allosteric disulphides' allowing post-translation modification of proteins, have been shown to control various physiological processes, including the immune response (Chiu and Hogg, 2019). Modification of these disulphide bonds is believed to cause conformational changes of the protein and altering its activity and function a process observed as a result of the entry of several enveloped viruses into their host cells, e.g. HIV, hepatitis C virus and Newcastle disease virus (Stegmann *et al.*, 2013). These labile disulphide bonds are common, with several classes of proteins being identified including integrins, receptors, transporters and cell-cell recognition proteins (Metcalfe *et al.*,

2011). The importance of disulphide bonds and central role for redox chemistry at the cell surface in creating and adequate immune response have been reviewed and analysed by Metcalfe *et al.* (2012) summarising that:

- disulphide bonds in integrins maintain their low affinity state and functional activity and their activities can be modulated by reducing agents;
- anti-microbial activity of defensins can be increased by reduction of disulphide bonds;
- IL-4 contains a disulphide bond susceptible to mild reduction;
- there are some redox-sensitive ligands for cell surface receptors;
- vaccination is associated with increase in the number of free thiols in lymph nodes;
- activation of T cells by dendritic cells is associated with secretion of Trx into the extracellular space, where it can catalyse reduction of disulphide bonds on the surface of immune cells, including T cells;
- Trx1 is shown to reduce disulphide bonds in the TNF receptor family member CD30 leading to altered cytokine binding and signalling;
- the Cys183-Cys232 disulphide bond in mouse CD132 (an important part of the receptor for several cytokines, including IL-4, IL-21, IL-7, IL-9, IL-15) is shown to be susceptible to reduction by enzymes such as gamma interferon-inducible lysosomal thiol reductase, protein disulphide isomerase and antioxidant thioredoxin, which are commonly secreted during immune activation;
- the Cys183-Cys232 disulphide bond is indicated to be reduced in an *in vivo* LPS-induced acute model of inflammation;
- reduction of the Cys183-Cys232 disulphide in CD132 was reported to inhibit IL-2 binding to the receptor complex (Metcalfe *et al.*, 2012).

Increased levels of oxidative stress associated with several diseases are counteracted by the integrated antioxidant defence system which includes activities of various oxidoreductase enzymes, such as Trx, playing a role of effective reductases of allosteric disulphide bonds in proteins (Gurjar *et al.*, 2019). The immune cells possess an important capacity to produce ROS and various inflammatory compounds as a part of their functional activities. However, as a result of oxidative stress leading to redox disbalance cell signalling/communications can be compromised leading to compromised immune response and over-inflammation, a situation observed in adult mice with premature aging (Garrido *et al.*, 2019). For example, in carp head kidney lymphocyte models, TCRγ knockdown was shown to significantly increase the mRNA expression of IFN-γ, IL-1β, IL-8, IL-10, Nrf2 and NF-κB. It simultaneously decreased the mRNA expression of SOD and CAT and reduced the activities of GPx, T-AOC, CAT and SOD and increased the content of MDA and H_2O_2 (Yang *et al.*, 2020). Interestingly, RONS are also involved in BCR signalling and BCR stimulation was reported to result in extracellular ROS generation by NADPH oxidase enzymatic complex with following participation in a range of cellular events leading to the B cell activation and signalling (Bertolotti *et al.*, 2012).

It was suggested that BCR, TCR and other Ig family members evolved the H_2O_2-generating activity to facilitate and amplify their signalling output (Reth, 2002). The authors suggested that the second messenger H_2O_2 is the molecule that communicates between BCR and TLR receptor systems, while BCR coreceptors could also be involved by increasing H_2O_2 production around the activated BCR. There is also a possibility that activated macrophages can function as APCs for T cell priming as a result of H_2O_2 diffusing from the macrophage to the T cell during their close interaction phase (Reth, 2002). Therefore, ROS, especially H_2O_2, play an important role as secondary messengers in cell communication, including immune-communication. However, an excessive ROS production and oxidative stress are responsible for damages to immunoreceptors leading to disruption of receptor functions and immunosuppression. A summary of the effect of compromised antioxidant system on immune system is shown in Figure 9.7.

9.10 Vitagene-immunity interactions and silymarin

Importance of the vitagene network for immunity is related to several biological features (Surai, 2018; 2020):

- Phagocyte cells produce RONS in physiological conditions and use them as a weapon to kill pathogens.
- Immunocommunication between various immune cells is considered to be key element of effective immunocompetence. Since many immune receptors are redox-sensitive, antioxidant defence and adaptive redox homeostasis represent major mechanisms of immune system regulation.
- Redox equilibrium in the immune cells is related to their activity (activation, inactivation and apoptosis).
- Disease challenge represent major stress associated with oxidative stress.

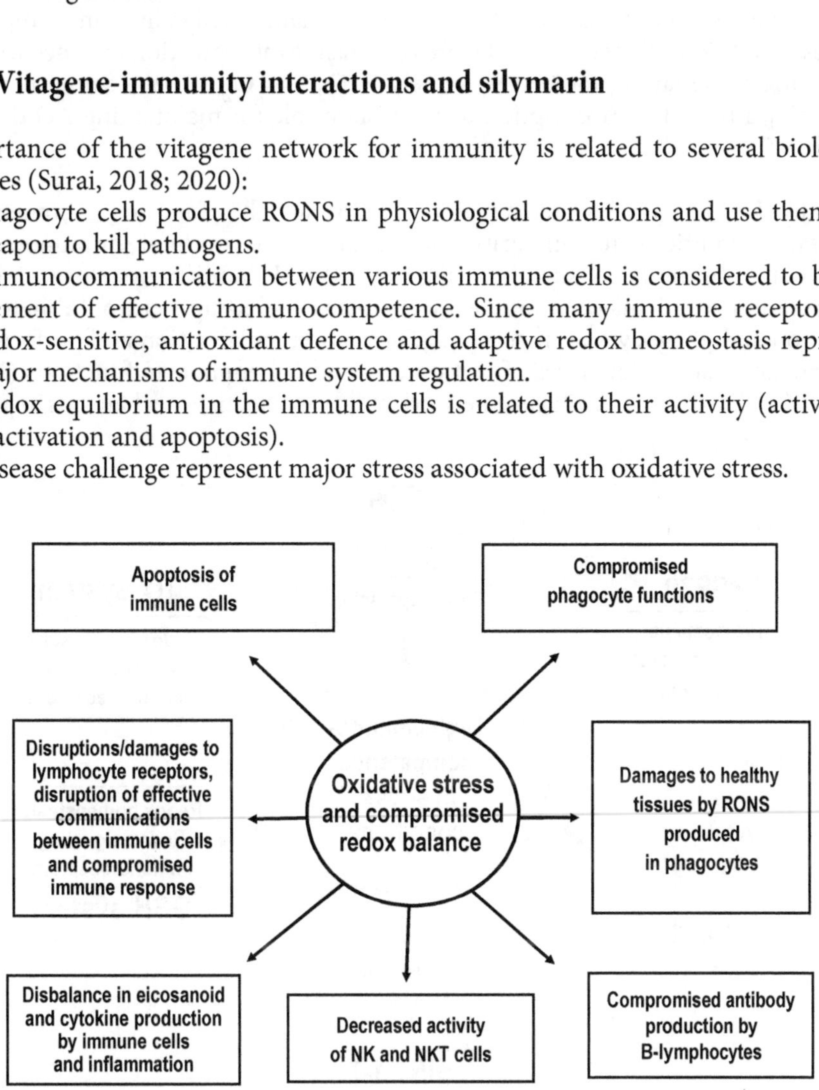

Figure 9.7. Oxidative stress and the immune system (adapted from Surai, 2020).

Vitagene are responsible for synthesis of a range protective molecules, including HSP70, HO-1, SOD, elements of Trx-system and GSH-systems and sirtuins. These protective molecules provide optimal redox balance for cell signalling, including immunocommunication. Furthermore, vitagene-encoded molecules prevent receptor damages/altered expression and provide environment for their optimal expression. Therefore, increased expression of vitagenes in stress conditions is considered to be an important mechanism of maintaining high immunocompetence in stress conditions. Details of controlling functions of vitagenes on immunity are shown in Figure 9.8.

It is important to mention that vitagenes act in concert providing optimal conditions for cell signalling and stress adaptation. This helps maintain high immunocompetence in stress conditions. First of all, SODs are responsible for regulation of concentrations of two major signalling molecules namely H_2O_2 and O_2^-. At the same time SOD could play a role of a transcription factor responsible for maintaining AO defences (Figure 9.9).

Secondly, Trx- and GSH-systems maintain redox signalling and redox homeostasis, necessary conditions for integrity maintenance and optimal immunoreceptor expression and immune cell signalling (Figure 9.10). GSH- and Trx-systems are involved in regulation of all major immune mechanisms including neutrophil/heterophil activation and phagocytosis, macrophage activation, polarisation and performance, dendrite and natural killer cells functions, T- and B-lymphocyte functions (Morris *et al.*, 2022). Furthermore, vitagene network builds an effective mechanisms to provide

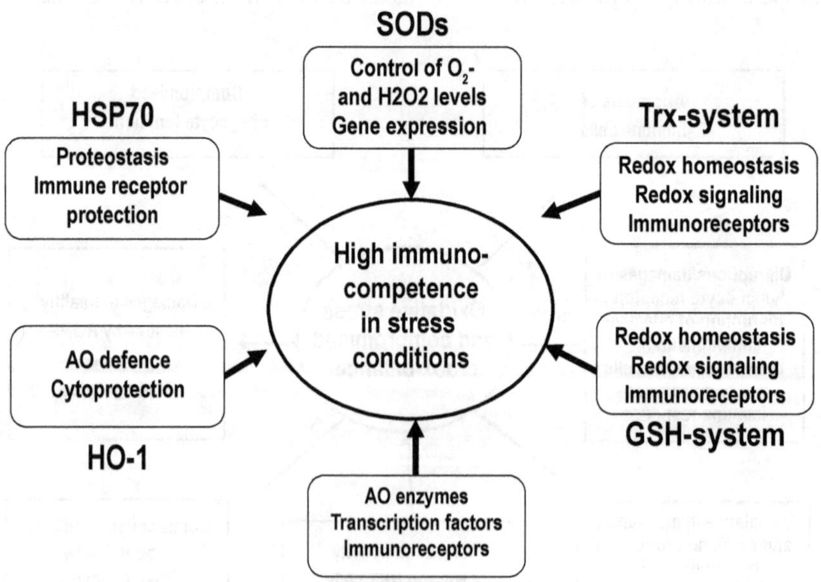

Figure 9.8. Regulating roles of vitagenes in immunocompetence.

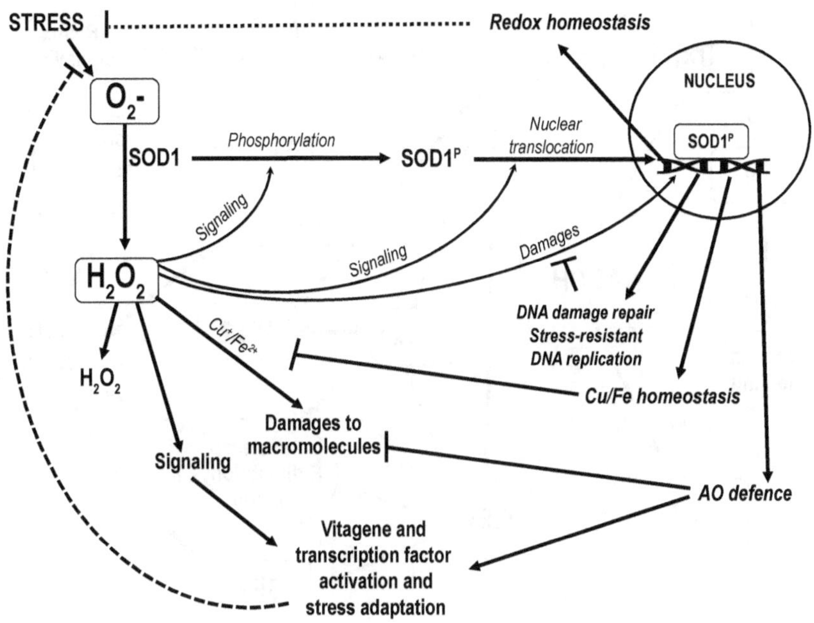

Figure 9.9. SOD as a transcription factor (adapted from Surai, 2020; Tsang *et al.*, 2014).

immune cell communications in stressful conditions and therefore maintaining effective immune defence (Surai, 2020).

Thirdly, HSP70 is responsible for proteostasis and integrity of immunoreceptors in stress conditions. Fourthly, HO-1 is involved in AO defence and cell signalling providing additional defence for immune cells under conditions of high RONS production. Finally, SIRTs regulate expression and activity of many transcription factors, AO enzymes orchestrating optimal AO defence, cell signalling and immunocompetence. Vitagenes are responsible for integrity of immune receptors and their optimal expression, effective immune cell signalling and high immunocompetence under stressful conditions of human life and commercial animal/poultry production.

Redox mechanisms, including control of RONS production and elimination by various cellular mechanisms, including Nrf2 and vitagene (SOD, glutathione and thioredoxin systems) activation are responsible for immune cell integrity, performance and survival (Morris *et al.*, 2022). Furthermore, redox homeostasis is involved in regulation of various immune functions (Morris *et al.*, 2022), including:

- Phagocytosis;
- macrophage and Th cell polarisation;
- metabolic reprogramming of immune cells;
- production of pro- and anti-inflammatory cytokines;
- chemotaxis;
- immune training and tolerance;

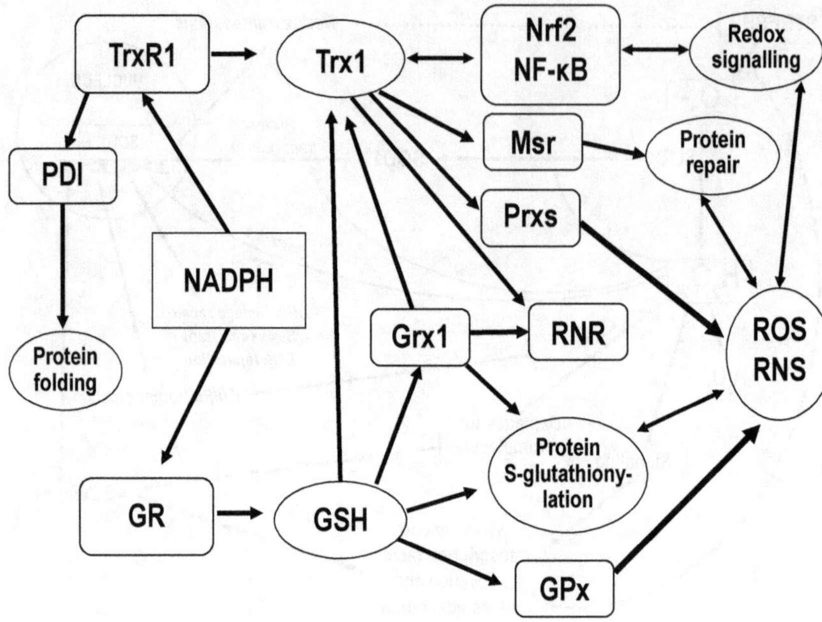

Figure 9.10. Glutathione and thioredoxin systems in animal cells (adapted from Surai, 2020).

- pathogen sensing;
- TLR activity;
- antiviral and antibacterial effects; and
- endotoxin tolerance.

Therefore, taking into account vitagene-, Nrf2- and NF-κB-modulating properties of SM it is possible to suggest that they form the basis for explaining how SM can affect immune system and immunocompetence.

9.11 Conclusions

The aforementioned data clearly showed regulatory roles of SM in animal/poultry and human immunocompetence maintenance. This, together with data on SM/SB regulatory actions in inflammation (Chapter 10) and gut health (Chapter 11), builds a basis for further expansion of research in this exciting field of science and makes a further step forward in SM/SB application in clinical practise and veterinary medicine as well as in nutrition of human and farm animals and poultry. Improved antioxidant defences and adaptive homeostasis are important targets for vitagene activation. Furthermore, involvement of SM in AO defences and redox balance maintenance help maintaining optimal immune-communications between various cell types responsible for high immunocompetence under various stress conditions.

References

Adeyemo, O., Doi, H., Rajender Reddy, K. and Kaplan, D.E., 2013. Impact of oral silymarin on virus- and non-virus-specific T-cell responses in chronic hepatitis C infection. Journal of Viral Hepatitis 20: 453-462.

Adhikari, M. and Arora, R., 2016. The flavonolignan-silymarin protects enzymatic, hematological, and immune system against γ-radiation-induced toxicity. Environmental Toxicology 31: 641-654.

Andersen, M.H., Schrama, D., Thor Straten, P. and Becker, J.C., 2006. Cytotoxic T cells. The Journal of investigative dermatology, 126(1), 32-41.

Bechtel, T.J. and Weerapana, E., 2017. From structure to redox: The diverse functional roles of disulfides and implications in disease. Proteomics 17: 6.

Bertolotti, M., Sitia, R. and Rubartelli, A., 2012. On the redox control of B lymphocyte differentiation and function. Antioxidants and Redox Signaling 16: 1139-1149.

Bošnjak, B., Do, K., Förster, R. and Hammerschmidt, S.I., 2022. Imaging dendritic cell functions. Immunological Reviews 306: 137-163.

Chandler, N.J., Call, M.J. and Call, M.E., 2020. T cell activation machinery: Form and function in natural and engineered immune receptors. International Journal of Molecular Sciences 21: 7424.

Chen, Y.H., Lin, H., Wang, Q., Hou, J.W., Mao, Z.J. and Li, Y.G., 2020. Protective role of silibinin against myocardial ischemia/reperfusion injury-induced cardiac dysfunction. International Journal of Biological Sciences 16: 1972-1988.

Chiu, J. and Hogg, P.J., 2019. Allosteric disulfides: Sophisticated molecular structures enabling flexible protein regulation. Journal of Biological Chemistry 294: 2949-2960.

Choi, Y.H. and Yan, G.H., 2009. Silibinin attenuates mast cell-mediated anaphylaxis-like reactions. Biological and Pharmaceutical Bulletin 32: 868-875.

Colitti, M., Stefanon, B., Gabai, G., Gelain, M.E. and Bonsembiante, F., 2019. Oxidative stress and nutraceuticals in the modulation of the immune function: Current knowledge in animals of veterinary interest. Antioxidants 8: pii: E28.

Cui, S., Pan, X.J., Ge, C.L., Guo, Y.T., Zhang, P.F., Yan, T.T., Zhou, J.Y., He, Q.X., Cheng, L.H., Wang, G.J., Hao, H.P. and Wang, H., 2021. Silybin alleviates hepatic lipid accumulation in methionine-choline deficient diet-induced nonalcoholic fatty liver disease in mice via peroxisome proliferator-activated receptor α. Chinese Journal of Natural Medicines 19: 401-411.

de la Lastra, C.A., Martin, M.J., Motilva, V., Jimenez, M., La Casa, C. and Lopez, A., 1995. Gastroprotection induced by silymarin, the hepatoprotective principle of *Silybum marianum* in ischemia-reperfusion mucosal injury: role of neutrophils. Planta Medica 61: 116-119.

De La Puerta, R., Martinez, E., Bravo, L. and Ahumada, M.C., 1996. Effect of silymarin on different acute inflammation models and on leukocyte migration. Journal of Pharmacy and Pharmacology 48: 968-970.

Delgoffe, G.M., Murray, P.J. and Vignali, D.A., 2011. Interpreting mixed signals: the cell's cytokine conundrum. Current Opinion in Immunology 23: 632-638.

Domínguez-Andrés, J., Dos Santos, J.C., Bekkering, S., Mulder, W., van der Meer, J., Riksen, N.P., Joosten, L. and Netea, M.G., 2023. Trained immunity: adaptation within innate immune mechanisms. Physiological Reviews 103: 313-346.

Doulabi, H., Masoumi, E., Rastin, M., Foolady Azarnaminy, A., Esmaeili, S.A. and Mahmoudi M., 2022. The role of Th22 cells, from tissue repair to cancer progression. Cytokine 149:155749.

El-Lakkany, N.M., Hammam, O.A., El-Maadawy, W.H., Badawy, A.A., Ain-Shoka, A.A. and Ebeid, F.A., 2012. Anti-inflammatory/anti-fibrotic effects of the hepatoprotective silymarin and the schistosomicide praziquantel against Schistosoma mansoni-induced liver fibrosis. Parasites and Vectors 5: 9.

Gambhir, L., Sharma, V., Kandwal, P. and Saxena, S., 2019. Perturbation in cellular redox homeostasis: Decisive regulator of T cell mediated immune responses. International Immunopharmacology 67: 449-457.

Garrido, A., Cruces, J., Ceprián, N., Vara, E. and de la Fuente, M., 2019. Oxidative-inflammatory stress in immune cells from adult mice with premature aging. International Journal of Molecular Sciences 20: 769.

Gharagozloo, M., Jafari, S., Esmaeil, N., Javid, E.N., Bagherpour, B. and Rezaei, A., 2013a. Immunosuppressive effect of silymarin on mitogen-activated protein kinase signalling pathway: the impact on T cell proliferation and cytokine production. Basic and Clinical Pharmacology and Toxicology 113: 209-214.

Ginn-Pease, M.E., and Whisler, R.L., 1998. Redox signals and NF-kappaB activation in T cells. Free Radical Biology & Medicine 25: 346-361.

Gostner, J.M., Becker, K., Fuchs, D. and Sucher, R., 2013. Redox regulation of the immune response. Redox Report 18: 88-94.

Greenberg, S. and Grinstein, S., 2002. Phagocytosis and innate immunity. Current Opinion in Immunology 14: 136-145.

Grimble, R.F., 1997. Effect of antioxidative vitamins on immune function with clinical applications. International Journal for Vitamin and Nutrition Research 67: 312-320.

Gurjar, S.A., Wheeler, J.X., Wadhwa, M., Thorpe, R., Kimber, I., Derrick, J.P., Dearman, R.J. and Metcalfe, C., 2019. The impact of thioredoxin reduction of allosteric disulfide bonds on the therapeutic potential of monoclonal antibodies. Journal of Biological Chemistry 294: 19616-19634.

Han, M.H., Yoon, W.K., Lee, H., Han, S.B., Lee, K., Park, S.K., Yang, K.H., Kim, H.M. and Kang, J.S., 2007. Topical application of silymarin reduces chemical-induced irritant contact dermatitis in BALB/c mice. International Immunopharmacology 7: 1651-1658.

Horváth, M.E., González-Cabello, R., Blázovics, A., van der Looij, M., Barta, I., Müzes, G., Gergely, P. and Fehér, J., 2001. Effect of silibinin and vitamin E on restoration of cellular immune response after partial hepatectomy. Journal of Ethnopharmacology 77: 227-232.

Hrčková, G., Kubašková, T.M., Reiterová, K. and Biedermann, D., 2020. Co-administration of silymarin elevates the therapeutic effect of praziquantel through modulation of specific antibody profiles, Th1/Th2/Tregs cytokines and down-regulation of fibrogenesis in mice with Mesocestoides vogae (Cestoda) infection. Experimental Parasitology 213: 107888.

Impellizzeri, D., Bruschetta, G., Ahmad, A., Crupi, R., Siracusa, R., Di Paola, R., Paterniti, I., Prosdocimi, M., Esposito, E. and Cuzzocrea, S., 2015. Effects of palmitoylethanolamide and silymarin combination treatment in an animal model of kidney ischemia and reperfusion. European Journal of Pharmacology 762: 136-149.

Jackson, S.H., Devadas, S., Kwon, J., Pinto, L.A. and Williams, M.S., 2004. T cells express a phagocyte-type NADPH oxidase that is activated after T cell receptor stimulation. Nature Immunology 5: 818-827.

Jeong, D.H., Lee, G.P., Jeong, W.I., Do, S.H., Yang, H.J., Yuan, D.W., Park, H.Y., Kim, K.J. and Jeong, K.S., 2005. Alterations of mast cells and TGF-beta1 on the silymarin treatment for CCl4-induced hepatic fibrosis. World Journal of Gastroenterology 11: 1141-1148.

Johnson, V.J., He, Q., Osuchowski, M.F. and Sharma, R.P., 2003. Physiological responses of a natural antioxidant flavonoid mixture, silymarin, in BALB/c mice: III. Silymarin inhibits T-lymphocyte function at low doses but stimulates inflammatory processes at high doses. Planta Medica 69: 44-49.

Johnson, V.J., Osuchowski, M.F., He, Q. and Sharma, R.P., 2002. Physiological responses to a natural antioxidant flavonoid mixture, silymarin, in BALB/c mice: II. Alterations in thymic differentiation correlate with changes in c-myc gene expression. Planta Medica 68: 961-965.

Juul-Madsen, H.R., Viertlboeck, B., Smith, A.L. and Gobel, T.W.F., 2008. Avian innate immune responses. In: Davison, F., Kaspers, B. and Schat, K.A. (eds) Avian immunology. Elsevier, Amsterdam, the Netherlands, pp. 107-128.

Kaiser, P. 2011. Immune system. In: Bishop, S.C., Axford, R.F.E., Nicholas, F.W. and Owen, J.B. (eds) Breeding for disease resistance in farm animals. CAB International, Wallingford, UK, pp. 15-37.

Kang, J.S., Jeon, Y.J., Park, S.K., Yang, K.H. and Kim, H.M., 2004. Protection against lipopolysaccharide-induced sepsis and inhibition of interleukin-1beta and prostaglandin E2 synthesis by silymarin. Biochemical Pharmacology 67: 175-181.

Karimi, G., Hassanzadeh-Josan, S., Memar, B., Esmaeili, S.A. and Riahi-Zanjani, B., 2018. Immunomodulatory effects of silymarin after subacute exposure to mice: A tiered approach immunotoxicity screening. Journal of Pharmacopuncture 21: 90-97.

Keyhanmehr, N., Motedayyen, H. and Eskandari, N., 2019. The effects of silymarin and Cyclosporine A on the proliferation and cytokine production of regulatory T cells. Immunological Investigations 48: 533-548.

Kidd, M.T. and Surai, P.F., 2022. Nutritional strategies to boost immune response in poultry. In: de Wit, S. (ed) Optimizing poultry flock health. Burleigh Dodds Science Publishing, Cambridge, UK, pp. 1-43.

Kim, B.R., Seo, H.S., Ku, J.M., Kim, G.J., Jeon, C.Y., Park, J.H., Jang, B.H., Park, S.J., Shin, Y.C. and Ko, S.G., 2013. Silibinin inhibits the production of pro-inflammatory cytokines through inhibition of NF-κB signaling pathway in HMC-1 human mast cells. Inflammation Research 62: 941-950.

Kim, M.J., Kim, D.U., Choi, J.W., Kim, D.G., Song, H.J., Bae, G.S. and Park, S.J., 2020. Silymarin attenuates the severity of Cerulein-induced acute pancreatitis. Pancreas 49: 89-95.

Kingeter, L.M. and Lin, X., 2012. C-type lectin receptor-induced NF-κB activation in innate immune and inflammatory responses. Cell Molecular Immunology 9: 105-112.

Klasing, K.C., 1998. Nutritional modulation of resistance to infectious diseases. Poultry Science 77: 1119-1125.

Kolkhir, P., Elieh-Ali-Komi, D., Metz, M., Siebenhaar, F. and Maurer, M., 2022. Understanding human mast cells: lesson from therapies for allergic and non-allergic diseases. Nature reviews. Immunology 22: 294-308.

Korver, D.R., 2012. Implications of changing immune function through nutrition in poultry. Animal Feed Science and Technology 173: 54-64.

Kraaij, M.D., Savage, N.D., van der Kooij, S.W., Koekkoek, K., Wang, J., van den Berg, J.M., Ottenhoff, T.H., Kuijpers, T.W., Holmdahl, R., van Kooten, C. and Gelderman, K.A., 2010. Induction of regulatory T cells by macrophages is dependent on production of reactive oxygen species. Proceedings of the National Academy of Sciences 107: 17686-17691.

Kuroi, K., Kamijo, M., Ueki, M., Niwa, Y., Hiramatsu, H. and Nakabayashi, T., 2020. Time-resolved FTIR study on the structural switching of human galectin-1 by light-induced disulfide bond formation. Physical Chemistry Chemical Physics 22: 1137-1144.

Kwon, J., Shatynski, K.E., Chen, H., Morand, S., De Deken, X., Miot, F., Leto, T.L. and Williams, M.S., 2010. The nonphagocytic NADPH oxidase Duox1 mediates a positive feedback loop during T cell receptor signaling. Science Signaling 3: ra59.

Law, H., Venturi, V., Kelleher, A. and Munier, C., 2020. Tfh cells in health and immunity: Potential targets for systems biology approaches to vaccination. International Journal of Molecular Sciences 21: 8524.

Lee, J.S., Kim, S.G., Kim, H.K., Lee, T.H., Jeong, Y.I., Lee, C.M., Yoon, M.S., Na, Y.J., Suh, D.S., Park, N.C., Choi, I.H., Kim, G.Y., Choi, Y.H., Chung, H.Y. and Park, Y.M., 2007. Silibinin polarizes Th1/Th2 immune responses through the inhibition of immunostimulatory function of dendritic cells. Journal of Cellular Physiology 210: 385-397.

Lees, J.R., 2020. CD8+ T cells: The past and future of immune regulation. Cellular Immunology 357: 104212.

Li, D., Xu, D., Wang, T., Shen, Y., Guo, S., Zhang, X., Guo, L., Li, X., Liu, L. and Wen, F., 2015. Silymarin attenuates airway inflammation induced by cigarette smoke in mice. Inflammation 38: 871-878.

Liu, Z., Sun, M., Wang, Y., Zhang, L., Zhao, H. and Zhao, M., 2018. Silymarin attenuated paraquat-induced cytotoxicity in macrophage by regulating Trx/TXNIP complex, inhibiting NLRP3 inflammasome activation and apoptosis. Toxicology In Vitro 46: 265-272.

Lu, C.P., Huang, C.Y., Wang, S.H., Chiu, C.H., Li, L.H., Hua, K.F. and Wu, T.H., 2018. Improvement of hyperglycemia in a murine model of insulin resistance and high glucose- and inflammasome-mediated IL-1β expressions in macrophages by silymarin. Chemico-Biological Interactions 290: 12-18.

Luciani, C., Hager, F.T., Cerovic, V. and Lelouard, H., 2022. Dendritic cell functions in the inductive and effector sites of intestinal immunity. Mucosal Immunology 15: 40-50.

Martínez, G., Mijares, M.R. and De Sanctis, J.B., 2019. Effects of flavonoids and its derivatives on immune cell responses. Recent Patents on Inflammation and Allergy Drug Discovery 13: 84-104.

Meeran, S.M., Katiyar, S., Elmets, C.A. and Katiyar, S.K., 2006. Silymarin inhibits UV radiation-induced immunosuppression through augmentation of interleukin-12 in mice. Molecular Cancer Therapeutics 5: 1660-1668.

Meroni, P.L., Barcellini, W., Borghi, M.O., Vismara, A., Ferraro, G., Ciani, D. and Zanussi, C., 1988. Silybin inhibition of human T-lymphocyte activation. International Journal of Tissue Reactions 10: 177-181.

Metcalfe, C., Cresswell, P. and Barclay, A.N., 2012. Interleukin-2 signalling is modulated by a labile disulfide bond in the CD132 chain of its receptor. Open Biology 2: 110036.

Metcalfe, C., Cresswell, P., Ciaccia, L., Thomas, B. and Barclay, A.N., 2011. Labile disulfide bonds are common at the leucocyte cell surface. Open Biology 1: 110010.

Miles, E.A. and Calder, P.C., 1998. Modulation of immune function by dietary fatty acids. Proceedings of the Nutrition Society 57: 277-292.

Morishima, C., Shuhart, M.C., Wang, C.C., Paschal, D.M., Apodaca, M.C., Liu, Y., Sloan, D.D., Graf, T.N., Oberlies, N.H., Lee, D.Y., Jerome, K.R. and Polyak, S.J., 2010. Silymarin inhibits *in vitro* T-cell proliferation and cytokine production in hepatitis C virus infection. Gastroenterology 138: 671-681.

Moro-García, M.A., Mayo, J.C., Sainz, R.M. and Alonso-Arias, R., 2018. Influence of inflammation in the process of T lymphocyte differentiation: Proliferative, metabolic, and oxidative changes. Frontiers in Immunology 9: 339.

Morris, G., Gevezova, M., Sarafian, V. and Maes, M., 2022. Redox regulation of the immune response. Cellular and Molecular Immunology 19: 1079-1101. https://doi.org/10.1038/s41423-022-00902-0.

Moshfegh, C.M. and Case, A.J., 2021. The redox-metabolic couple of T lymphocytes: Potential consequences for hypertension. Antioxidants and Redox Signaling 34: 915-935.

Namdari, H., Izad, M., Rezaei, F. and Amirghofran, Z., 2018. Differential regulation of CD4+ T cell subsets by silymarin *in vitro* and in ovalbumin immunized mice. Daru 26: 215-227.

Nasab, E.M., Athari, S.M., Ghafarzade, S., Nasab, A.M. and Athari, S.S., 2020. Immunomodulatory effects of two silymarin isomers in a Balb/c mouse model of allergic asthma. Allergologia et Immunopathologia 48: 646-653.

Nazemian, F., Karimi, G., Moatamedi, M., Charkazi, S., Shamsara, J. and Mohammadpour, A.H., 2010. Effect of silymarin administration on TNF-α serum concentration in peritoneal dialysis patients. Phytotherapy Research 24: 1654-1657.

Özcan, A. and Boyman, O., 2022. Mechanisms regulating neutrophil responses in immunity, allergy, and autoimmunity. Allergy 77: 3567-3583. https://doi.org/10.1111/all.15505.

Pagano, M.T., Fecchi, K., Pierdominici, M., Ortona, E. and Peruzzu, D., 2022. Human monocyte-derived dendritic cells are the pharmacological target of the immunosuppressant flavonoid silibinin. International Journal of Molecular Sciences 23: 10417.

Palit, P., Mukhopadhyay, A. and Chattopadhyay, D., 2021. Phyto-pharmacological perspective of silymarin: A potential prophylactic or therapeutic agent for COVID-19, based on its promising immunomodulatory, anti-coagulant and anti-viral property. Phytotherapy Research 35: 4246-4257.

Patwardhan, R.S., Singh, B., Pal, D., Checker, R., Bandekar, M., Sharma, D. and Sandur, S.K., 2020. Redox regulation of regulatory T-cell differentiation and functions. Free Radical Research 54: 947-960.

Pizzi, M., Boi, M., Bertoni, F. and Inghirami, G., 2016. Emerging therapies provide new opportunities to reshape the multifaceted interactions between the immune system and lymphoma cells. Leukemia 30: 1805-1815.

Poon, M. and Farber, D.L., 2020. The whole body as the system in systems immunology. IScience 23: 101509.

Puertollano, M.A., Puertollano, E., De Cienfuegos, G.Á. and De Pablo, M.A., 2011. Dietary antioxidants: immunity and host defense. Current Topics in Medicinal Chemistry 11: 1752-1766.

Quintana, A., Schwindling, C., Wenning, A.S., Becherer, U., Rettig, J., Schwarz, E.C. and Hoth, M., 2007. T cell activation requires mitochondrial translocation to the immunological synapse. Proceedings of the National Academy of Sciences 104: 14418-14423.

Rahe, M.C. and Murtaugh, M.P., 2017. Mechanisms of adaptive immunity to porcine reproductive and respiratory syndrome virus. Viruses 9: pii: E148.

Ramakrishnan, G., Jagan, S., Kamaraj, S., Anandakumar, P. and Devaki, T., 2009. Silymarin attenuated mast cell recruitment thereby decreased the expressions of matrix metalloproteinases-2 and 9 in rat liver carcinogenesis. Investigational New Drugs 27: 233-240.

Rao, P.R. and Viswanath, R.K., 2007. Cardioprotective activity of silymarin in ischemia-reperfusion-induced myocardial infarction in albino rats. Experimental and Clinical Cardiology 12: 179-187.

Reth, M., 2002. Hydrogen peroxide as second messenger in lymphocyte activation. Nature Immunology 3: 1129-1134.

Rigby, C., Deep, G., Jain, A., Orlicky, D.J., Agarwal, C. and Agarwal, R., 2019. Silibinin inhibits ultraviolet B radiation-induced mast cells recruitment and bone morphogenetic protein 2 expression in the skin at early stages in Ptch(+/-) mouse model of basal cell carcinoma. Molecular Carcinogenesis 58: 1260-1271.

Sangeetha, N. and Nalini, N., 2015. Silibinin modulates caudal-type homeobox transcription factor (CDX2), an intestine specific tumor suppressor to abrogate colon cancer in experimental rats. Human and Experimental Toxicology 34: 56-64.

Saksida, T., Jevtić, B., Djedović, N., Miljković, Đ. and Stojanović, I., 2021. Redox regulation of tolerogenic dendritic cells and regulatory T cells in the pathogenesis and therapy of autoimmunity. Antioxidants and Redox Signaling 34: 364-382.

Schümann, J., Prockl, J., Kiemer, A.K., Vollmar, A.M., Bang, R. and Tiegs, G., 2003. Silibinin protects mice from T cell-dependent liver injury☆. Journal of Hepatology 39: 333-340.

Shariati, M., Shaygannejad, V., Abbasirad, F., Hosseininasab, F., Kazemi, M., Mirmosayyeb, O. and Esmaeil, N., 2019. Silymarin restores regulatory t cells (TREGS) function in multiple sclerosis (MS) patients *in vitro*. Inflammation 42: 1203-1214.

Sharifpanah, F., Ali, E.H., Wartenberg, M. and Sauer, H., 2019. The milk thistle (*Silybum marianum*) compound silibinin stimulates leukopoiesis from mouse embryonic stem cells. Phytotherapy Research 33: 452-460.

Sharma, S. and Naura, A.S., 2020. Potential of phytochemicals as immune-regulatory compounds in atopic diseases: A review. Biochemical Pharmacology 173: 113790.

Stegmann, M., Metcalfe, C. and Barclay, A.N., 2013. Immunoregulation through membrane proteins modified by reducing conditions induced by immune reactions. European Journal of Immunology 43: 15-21.

Subramanian, P., Mitroulis, I., Hajishengallis, G. and Chavakis, T., 2016. Regulation of tissue infiltration by neutrophils: role of integrin α3β1 and other factors. Current Opinion in Hematology 23: 36.

Sukumar, M., Liu, J., Mehta, G.U., Patel, S.J., Roychoudhuri, R., Crompton, J.G., Klebanoff, C.A., Ji, Y., Li, P., Yu, Z. and Whitehill, G.D., 2016. Mitochondrial membrane potential identifies cells with enhanced stemness for cellular therapy. Cell Metabolism 23: 63-76.

Surai, P.F., 2002. Natural antioxidants in avian nutrition and reproduction. Nottingham University Press, Nottingham, UK.

Surai, P.F., 2006. Selenium in nutrition and health. Nottingham University Press, Nottingham, UK.

Surai, P.F., 2018. Selenium in poultry nutrition and health. Wageningen Academic Publishers, Wageningen, The Netherlands.

Surai, P.F., 2020. Vitagene in avian biology and poultry health. Wageningen Academic Publishers, Wageningen, The Netherlands.

Surai, P.F. (Ed.), 2021. Selenium in Pig Nutrition and Health. Wageningen Academic Publishers, Wageningen, The Netherlands.

Surai, P.F., Kochish, I.I., Fisinin, V.I. and Kidd, M.T., 2019. Antioxidant defence systems and oxidative stress in poultry biology: An update. Antioxidants 8; 235.

Surai, P.F., Kochish, I.I. and Kidd, M.T., 2021. Redox homeostasis in poultry: Regulatory roles of NF-κB. Antioxidants 10: 186.

Tak Mak, Mary Saunders and Bradley Jett, 2014. MAK: Primer to the immune response. Elsevier Inc. Amsterdam, The Netherlands.

Tiwari, P., Kumar, A., Ali, M. and Mishra, K.P., 2010. Radioprotection of plasmid and cellular DNA and Swiss mice by silibinin. Mutation Research 695: 55-60.

Toklu, H.Z., Akbay, T.T., Velioglu-Ogunc, A., Ercan, F., Gedik, N., Keyer-Uysal, M. and Sener, G., 2008. Silymarin, the antioxidant component of *Silybum marianum*, prevents sepsis-induced acute lung and brain injury. Journal of Surgical Research 145: 214-222.

Tong, W.W., Zhang, C., Hong, T., Liu, D.H., Wang, C., Li, J., He, X.K. and Xu, W.D., 2018. Silibinin alleviates inflammation and induces apoptosis in human rheumatoid arthritis fibroblast-like synoviocytes and has a therapeutic effect on arthritis in rats. Scientific Reports 8: 3241.

Tsang, C.K., Liu, Y., Thomas, J., Zhang, Y. and Zheng, X.S., 2014. Superoxide dismutase 1 acts as a nuclear transcription factor to regulate oxidative stress resistance. Nature Communications 5: 1-11.

Tuzlak, S., Dejean, A.S., Iannacone, M., Quintana, F.J., Waisman, A., Ginhoux, F., Korn, T. and Becher, B., 2021. Repositioning T_H cell polarization from single cytokines to complex help. Nature Immunology 22: 1210-1217.

Vaid, M., Prasad, R., Singh, T., Elmets, C.A., Xu, H. and Katiyar, S.K., 2013. Silymarin inhibits ultraviolet radiation-induced immune suppression through DNA repair-dependent activation of dendritic cells and stimulation of effector T cells. Biochemical Pharmacology 85: 1066-1076.

Varga, Z., Ujhelyi, L., Kiss, A., Balla, J., Czompa, A. and Antus, S., 2004. Effect of silybin on phorbol myristate acetate-induced protein kinase C translocation, NADPH oxidase activity and apoptosis in human neutrophils. Phytomedicine 11: 206-212.

Venter, C., Eyerich, S., Sarin, T. and Klatt, K.C., 2020. Nutrition and the immune system: A complicated tango. Nutrients 12: 818.

Wang, R., Dillon, C.P., Shi, L.Z., Milasta, S., Carter, R., Finkelstein, D., McCormick, L.L., Fitzgerald, P., Chi, H., Munger, J. and Green, D.R., 2011. The transcription factor Myc controls metabolic reprogramming upon T lymphocyte activation. Immunity 35: 871-882.

Wang, W., Sung, N., Gilman-Sachs, A. and Kwak-Kim, J., 2020. T Helper (Th) cell profiles in pregnancy and recurrent pregnancy losses: Th1/Th2/Th9/Th17/Th22/Tfh Cells. Frontiers in Immunology 11: 2025.

Webb, C.B., McCord, K.W. and Twedt, D.C., 2009. Assessment of oxidative stress in leukocytes and granulocyte function following oral administration of a silibinin-phosphatidylcholine complex in cats. American Journal of Veterinary Research 70: 57-62.

Weyand, C.M., Shen, Y. and Goronzy, J.J., 2018. Redox-sensitive signaling in inflammatory T cells and in autoimmune disease. Free Radical Biology & Medicine 125: 36-43.

Wherry, E.J., 2011. T cell exhaustion. Nature Immunology 12: 492-499.

Wilasrusmee, C., Kittur, S., Shah, G., Siddiqui, J., Bruch, D., Wilasrusmee, S. and Kittur, D.S., 2002. Immunostimulatory effect of *Silybum marianum* (milk thistle) extract. Medical Science Monitor 8: BR439-43.

Williams, M.S. and Kwon, J., 2004. T cell receptor stimulation, reactive oxygen species, and cell signaling. Free Radical Biology & Medicine 37: 1144-1151.

Yang, H.L. and Shi, X.W., 2021. Silybin alleviates experimental autoimmune encephalomyelitis by suppressing dendritic cell activation and Th17 cell differentiation. Frontiers in Neurology 12: 659678.

Yang, J., Gong, Y., Cai, J., Zheng, Y., Liu, H. and Zhang, Z., 2020. Chlorpyrifos induces redox imbalance-dependent inflammation in common carp lymphocyte through dysfunction of T-cell receptor γ. Journal of Fish Diseases 43: 423-430.

Youn, C.K., Park, S.J., Lee, M.Y., Cha, M.J., Kim, O.H., You, H.J., Chang, I.Y., Yoon, S.P. and Jeon, Y.J., 2013. Silibinin inhibits LPS-induced macrophage activation by blocking p38 MAPK in RAW 264.7 cells. Biomolecules and Therapeutics 21: 258-263.

Zarpou, S., Mosavi, H., Bagheri, A., Malekzadeh Shafaroudi, M. and Khonakdar-Tarsi, A., 2021. NF-κB and NLRP3 gene expression changes during warm hepatic ischemia-reperfusion in rats with and without silibinin. Gastroenterology and Hepatology From Bed to Bench 14: 267-275.

Zhang, W., Liu, X., Zhu, Y., Liu, X., Gu, Y., Dai, X. and Li, B., 2021. Transcriptional and posttranslational regulation of Th17/Treg balance in health and disease. European Journal of Immunology 51: 2137-2150.

Zhao, F., Shi, D., Li, T., Li, L. and Zhao, M., 2015. Silymarin attenuates paraquat-induced lung injury via Nrf2-mediated pathway *in vivo* and *in vitro*. Clinical and Experimental Pharmacology and Physiology 42: 988-998.

Zheng, B., Yang, Y., Chen, L., Wu, M. and Zhou, S., 2022. B-cell receptor repertoire sequencing: Deeper digging into the mechanisms and clinical aspects of immune-mediated diseases. iScience 25: 105002.

Zhu, Z. and Sun, G., 2018. Silymarin mitigates lung impairments in a rat model of acute respiratory distress syndrome. Inflammopharmacology 26: 747-754.

Chapter 10

Silymarin and inflammation: from understanding molecular mechanisms to practical applications

A disease known is half cured

Anton Surai[1] and Peter F. Surai[2-7]*
[1]Healthy Food Services, Bristol, UK; [2]Vitagene and Health Research Centre, Bristol, UK; [3]Department of Microbiology and Biochemistry, Faculty of Veterinary Medicine, Trakia University, Stara Zagora, Bulgaria; [4]Department of Animal Nutrition, Faculty of Agricultural and Environmental Sciences, Szent Istvan University, Hungary; [5]Saint-Petersburg State Academy of Veterinary Medicine, St. Petersburg, Russia; [6]Sumy National Agrarian University, Sumy, Ukraine; [7]Odessa National Academy of Food Technologies, Odessa, Ukraine
psurai@feedfood.co.uk

Abstract

Inflammation is a defence mechanism employed by humans and animals to create hostile conditions for pathogens and to prevent the spread of tissue infection. The task of acute inflammation is the elimination of infectious agents, repair of affected or injured tissues with the following inflammation resolution terminating the inflammatory response and re-establishing the tissue homeostasis. However, in some cases due to delay or misregulation of the inflammation resolution, as a result of various stresses and redox balance alterations, inflammation proceeds from the acute phase to chronic inflammation leading to a variety of chronic illnesses. Pro-inflammatory stress includes a number of universal components including oxidative stress response, DNA damage response, unfolded protein response, heat shock response, autophagy modulation, formation of inflammasome, non-coding RNA response, inducible networks of signalling pathways formation, epigenetic changes. The data presented in this chapter based on *in vitro* and *in vivo* studies clearly proved that silymarin (SM) has a great potential as an anti-inflammation agent. In particular, in *in vitro* studies SM was able to downregulate NF-κB and respective proinflammatory cytokines and chemokines (TNF-α, IL-1β, IL-6, IL-12, IL-23, CCL4, CXCL10) as well as RONS. At the same time SM upregulated anti-inflammatory cytokines (IL-4, IL-10, IL-13, TGF-β, etc.) and lipid mediators responsible for resolution of inflammation. Anti-inflammatory properties of SM were demonstrated in *in vitro* model systems with immune (macrophages and monocytes) and non-immune (epithelial, skin, bone, connective tissue and cancer) cells. Similar anti-inflammatory effects of SM were shown in various *in vivo* models, including nonalcoholic fatty liver disease, toxicity models, ischemia/reperfusion models, ageing and exercising models, stress-induced injuries, wound healing and many other model systems. Therefore, it seems likely that regulatory roles of SM in inflammation could be considered as a key element of health-promoting properties of

Peter F. Surai and Anton Surai **Silymarin puzzle**
DOI:10.3920/978-90-8686-944-2_010, © Wageningen Academic Publishers, 2023

this phytochemical mixture and further research should pay more attention to the protective anti-inflammatory actions of SM.

Keywords: silymarin, inflammation, NF-κB, cytokines, redox homeostasis

10.1 Introduction

Inflammation is a defence mechanism employed to create hostile conditions for pathogens and to prevent the spread of tissue infection. The task of acute inflammation is the elimination of infectious agents, repair of affected or injured tissues to their normal structural and functional state with the following termination of the inflammatory response and re-establishment of the homeostatic state (resolution; Lei *et al.*, 2015). However, in some cases inflammation resolution is delayed or compromised and inflammation proceeds from the acute phase to chronic inflammation leading to a variety of chronic illnesses, including (Lei *et al.*, 2015):

- atherosclerosis;
- obesity;
- cancer;
- chronic obstructive pulmonary disease;
- asthma;
- inflammatory bowel disease;
- multiple sclerosis;
- neurodegenerative disease (Alzheimer's disease, Parkinson's disease, amyotrophic lateral sclerosis); and
- autoimmune disorders such as rheumatoid arthritis, systemic lupus erythematosus, psoriasis, and celiac disease.

There is a range of inflammatory factors in human life and animal/production (Table 10.1) leading very often to excessive inflammation and various diseases.

10.2 Molecular mechanisms of inflammation

It is known that inflammatory responses are initiated as a result of host recognition of inflammatory signals in the form of either PAMPs or damage-associated molecular patterns (DAMPs), by a range of pattern recognition receptors (PRR; Liu *et al.*, 2022) of the innate immune system, including surface Toll-like receptors (TLRs) and cytoplasmic NOD (nucleotide-binding oligomerisation-domain) like receptors (NLRs). It is believed that each TLR recognises a specific PAMP:

- TLR2 recognises peptidoglycan and lipoteichoic acid;
- TLR3 recognises double-stranded RNA;
- TLR4 recognises lipopolysaccharide;
- TLR5 recognises flagellin; and
- TLR9 recognises CpG rich microbial DNA sequences (Broom and Kogut, 2018).

Table 10.1. Inflammatory factors in human and poultry (adapted from Surai, 2020; Yu *et al.*, 2022a).

Category	Proinflammatory factors	
	Human	**Poultry**
Physical factors	Radiation, UV, hyperthermia, hypothermia, trauma	Hyperthermia, hypothermia, trauma, increased stoking density
Chemical factors	Asbestos, heavy metals, organic toxicants, lipopolysaccharides, dust	Heavy metals, mycotoxins, dust
Biological factors	Bacterial infection, virus infection, fungal infection	Bacterial infection, virus infection, fungal infection
Unhealthy lifestyle	Smoking, alcohol, high-calorie diet, stress, sedentary lifestyle	Stress, sedentary lifestyle (cage housing)
Chronic diseases	Obesity, diabetes, hyperglycaemia	Chronic Respiratory Disease
Pathologic tissues	Apoptotic cells, ischemia, hypoxia	Apoptotic cells, hypoxia
Anaphylaxis	Allergens, autoimmune diseases	Allergens

As a result of activation of TLRs or NLRs, inflammation-associated signalling pathways are induced leading to the production of inflammatory cytokines, chemokines and prostaglandins.

Of note, inflammatory immune cells, including neutrophils, macrophages, lymphocytes, and mast cells are core components of the inflammatory response (Figure 10.1). Once activated, these cells can release a large range of cytokines and chemokines (Yu *et al.*, 2022a), including

- TNF-α;
- IL-6;
- IFN-γ;
- NO;
- monocyte chemotactic protein-1 (MCP-1); and
- chemokine ligand 10 (CXCL10).

Neutrophils are the first immune cells to arrive to the place of infection or injury. They are leaked from blood vessels as a result of vasodilatation due to secretion of vasoactive amines (histamine and serotonin) by mast cells, basophils and platelets. The neutrophils are responsible for induction of re-localisation and activation of macrophages at the site of infection or injury. The production of various communicating molecules, including cytokines by activated neutrophils and macrophages drives the process of inflammation. In particular, LPS, IFN-γ, and TNF-α promote the activation of a range transcription factors and enzymes (Yu *et al.*, 2022a), including

- NF-κB;
- STAT;
- iNOS;
- AP-1;

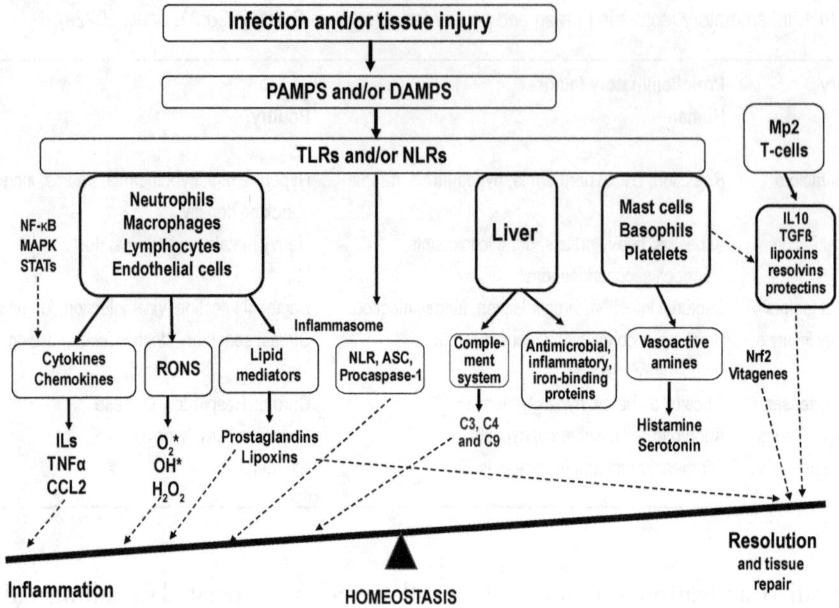

Figure 10.1. Inflammation and resolution (adapted from Broom and Kogut, 2018; Jain *et al.*, 2015; Robinson *et al.*, 2016; Yu *et al.*, 2022a).

- HIF1-α;
- COX-2; and
- NLRP3 inflammasome.

Once the pathogen is neutralised or injury repaired/healed and cellular debris are removed, the acute inflammatory response is normally terminated, which is known as the resolution of inflammation (Yu *et al.*, 2022a; Figure 10.1).

In general, the inflammatory process is associated with an oxidative stress. On the one hand, RONS production in macrophages (so called oxidative burst) is an essential process and they are used as a powerful weapon to kill pathogens and therefore, activated macrophages are very efficient at recognising, phagocytosing and killing pathogens in phagolysosomes (Austermann *et al.*, 2022). On the other hand, excess or uncontrolled RONS production could damage phagocyte cells and decrease their protective efficiency.

However, RONS also play a signalling roles in macrophage polarisation and inflammation resolution. Therefore, if the inflammation is not properly controlled and not timely terminated it can become a chronic state detrimentally affecting tissue integrity and wound healing. This is associated with the transcription factor NF-κB which regulates expression and synthesis of inflammatory mediators (Liu *et al.*, 2022). However, once the infection is eliminated, NF-κB activity should drop to its basal level, however, in pathological inflammatory processes an incorrect termination of NF-κB signalling is observed (Juráňová *et al.*, 2019). Anti-inflammatory properties of SM/SB have been extensively studied in various *in vitro* and *in vivo* model systems with appropriate inflammation markers/indexes, including cytokines, chemokines, lipid mediators as well as transcription factors (e.g. NF-κB) used.

10.3 Silymarin and inflammation: *In vitro* studies

Anti-inflammatory properties of SM/SB have been demonstrated using various *in vitro* systems based on cultivated cells including immune cells and other types of cells. Macrophages and monocytes are vital players of the innate immune response and major regulators of inflammation. They participate in innate immunity by phagocytosis and initiation of inflammation, triggering the adaptive immune response, resolution of inflammation and the reestablishment of homeostasis (Austermann *et al.*, 2022).

10.3.1 Macrophages

Macrophages (MPs) are important immune cells playing a critical role in tissue development/homeostasis and are responsible for the tissue surveillance detecting infection or injury as well as monitoring tissue changes (Austermann *et al.*, 2022). The recognition of multiple stimuli by MPs is due to the expression of a variety of receptors including cytokine receptors, PRRs, and phagocytosis receptors (Degboé *et al.*, 2022).

Depending on conditions/environmental signals, macrophages can exhibit various activated phenotypes, including the M1 and M2 phenotypes. It is well accepted that M1 macrophages are pro-inflammatory secreting important cytokines, chemokines and RONS, including TNF-α, IL-1β, IL-6, IL-12, IL-23, CCL4, CXCL10, ROS and NO leading to inflammation, inducing phagocytosis and oxidative burst to kill pathogens. In great contrast, M2 macrophages produce anti-inflammatory cytokines (e.g. IL-4, IL-10, IL-13, TGF-β, etc.), lipid mediators (lipoxins, resolvins, protectins, etc.) and are responsible for resolution of inflammation (Austermann *et al.*, 2022; Kapellos and Iqbal, 2016). Therefore, initially there is a macrophage phenotype switch from homeostatic function to proinflammatory phenotype to deal with infection. However, once the pathogen is eliminated a switch to an anti-inflammatory/pro-resolving phenotype to terminate the inflammatory response/resolve inflammation and re-establish homeostasis should take place (Austermann *et al.*, 2022).

In general, M1/M2 classification of MPs is already out of date, since it does not take into account the diversity of the stimuli activating MPs *in vivo*, and complexity of the physiological or the pathophysiological contexts *in vivo* (Degboé *et al.*, 2022). However, for a simplicity of this issue in relation to regulatory roles of SM/SB in inflammation, we will keep main principles of polarisation as they were previously described with understanding that a misregulation of this macrophage polarisation leads to over-inflammation and development of various inflammation-related states/diseases.

There is a range of studies employing macrophages and LPS as a stimulating antigen to demonstrate anti-inflammatory properties of SM/SB. For example, SM (50 g/ml) was found to inhibit morphological changes in LPS-stimulated RAW264.7 mouse macrophages by inhibiting NF-κB pathway including suppression of the nuclear translocation and transactivation activities of NF-κB (Kim *et al.*, 2015). In cultured macrophages, SM (~10-40 μM) was reported to reduce LPS-induced NO generation and IL-1β expression (Lu *et al.*, 2018). In the same model system, SB (40 μM) was shown to suppress inflammatory indexes (NF-κB, IL-6 and TNF-α) and the protective effect was more pronounced when the combination of SB and thymol (40 μM and 120 μM, respectively) was used (Chen *et al.*, 2020a). Similarly, enhanced anti-inflammatory effects of SB and capsaicin combination in LPS-induced RAW264.7 cells was associated with inhibiting NF-κB and MAPK activation (Zheng *et al.*, 2022).

In a model of toxicant-induced macrophage injury the pretreatment on mouse macrophages with SM (100 μM) was indicated to reduce PQ-induced cytotoxicity, enhance the expression of Trx and antioxidant enzymes (SOD and GPx), suppress oxidative stress and inhibit the TXNIP and NLRP3 inflammasome activation and decrease proinflammatory cytokine (IL-1β and IL-18) secretion (Liu *et al.*, 2018). SB was able to prevent assembly of the NLRP3 inflammasome complex in mice through the NAD+/SIRT2 pathway (Zhang *et al.*, 2018). Other stimulating antigens/agents were also used. For instance, in *H. pylori* stimulated macrophages, SB (103.6 μM) was shown to inhibit production of pro-inflammatory cytokines, including TNF-α, IL-10 and IL-6 by 100%, 70.3% and 33.9%, respectively (Bittencourt *et al.*, 2020).

In general, primary mouse macrophages treated by SM promoted M2 polarisation associated with decreased levels of pro-inflammatory cytokines (TNF-α and IL-1β) and increased concentrations of anti-inflammatory (IL-10) cytokines (Azadpour *et al.*, 2021). SB was reported to inhibit inflammation by inducing M2-type macrophage polarisation associated with promotion of the secretion of anti-inflammatory factors (CD206, IL-10) and inhibition of the secretion of inflammatory factors (IL-1β, iNOS; Xu *et al.*, 2022).

10.3.2 Mononuclear cells

Monocytes comprise about 5-10% of all blood immune cells, being bone-marrow-derived mononuclear cells with a life span of about 1-3 days and they differentiate into inflammatory macrophages or dendritic cells during an inflammatory process (Austermann *et al.*, 2022). SB demonstrated anti-inflammatory and anti-fibrotic effects on CD14+/- human monocytes challenged by *Paracoccidioides brasiliensis* (Pb18) as a result of inhibition of p65 NF-κB activation (Bannwart *et al.*, 2010). In mononuclear cells (lymphocytes and monocytes) obtained from preeclamptic women SB (50 μM) was able to inhibit LPS-stimulated NF-κB activation as well as the production of inflammatory cytokines including TNF-α and IL-1β (Giorgi *et al.*,

2012b). SB (50-200 μM) was shown to inhibit the production of pro-inflammatory cytokines (TNF-α, IL-6, and IL-8) through inhibition of NF-κB signalling pathway in HMC-1 human mast cells (Kim *et al.*, 2013). Similarly, SB dose-dependently reduced histamine release from rat peritoneal mast cells (RPMC) activated by compound 48/80 or anti-DNP IgE. SB also inhibited the secretion of pro-inflammatory cytokines, such as TNF-α and IL-6 in RPMC (Choi and Yan, 2009).

In LPS-stimulated peripheral blood mononuclear cells from healthy donors SM (0.1 mM) demonstrated the ability to reduce the production of the key proinflammatory cytokines including TNF-α, IL-1α, IL-1β, IL-6, and IFN-γ (Fordham *et al.*, 2014). In the same study, SM showed an inhibitory effects on chemokine production, including CCL2 (responsible for monocyte recruitment and promotion of CD4+ and CD8+ T cell migration), CCL5 (involved in monocyte chemotaxis) and MIP-1 (important chemokine for monocytes, T cells, MPs, DCs, and neutrophils). Reduction in the aforementioned chemokines could affect recruitment of monocytes and neutrophils to sites of local inflammation and reduce inflammation (Fordham *et al.*, 2014). The authors confirmed that anti-inflammatory action of SM was associated with reduced NF-κB activation.

Anti-inflammatory effects of SM were also shown to appear with prolonged (i.e. 24 h) SM exposure, with suppression of multiple pro-inflammatory mRNAs and signalling pathways including NF-κB and FOXO (Lovelace *et al.*, 2015). The authors also demonstrated that SM inhibition of both mTOR and NF-κB was partially AMPK dependent, while SM inhibition of mTOR needed the DNA damage inducible transcript 4. Furthermore, SM showed broad anti-inflammatory and immunoregulatory activity in primary human immune cells. SM treatment (80 μM) was demonstrated to have suppressing effects on pro-inflammatory cytokine expression and production in non-activated and PAMP-activated primary human monocytes and modulated non-activated and cytokine- and TCR-activated mucosal-associated invariant T cells (Lovelace *et al.*, 2017). The authors also showed that SM inhibited the expression of T cell activation and exhaustion markers on CD4+ and CD8+ T cells obtained from chronically-infected, HIV-positive patients. Therefore, SM can modulate multiple metabolic pathways leading to suppression of inflammation in diverse immune cell types, independently on the inflammatory insult or stimulus.

In an *in vitro* study with equine peripheral blood mononuclear cells SB (10 and 50 μM) was shown to have anti-inflammatory effects indicative by amelioration of LPS-induced increased levels of proinflammatory cytokines such as TNF-α, IL-1β, IL-6 and IL-8 (Gugliandolo *et al.*, 2020). Transcriptional profiling, metabolomics, and signalling studies performed in T cell lines and human liver indicated that anti-inflammatory effects of SM was associated with suppression of expression of various pro-inflammatory cytokines and signalling pathways including NF-κB and FOXO (Lovelace *et al.*, 2015).

In T lymphocytes from female and male healthy donors SB was reported to reduce expression of the pro-inflammatory cytokines IL-17 and TNF-α, through ERβ binding and upregulation of ERβ expression (Dupuis *et al.*, 2018). *In vitro* treatment of monocytes from preeclamptic women with SB (50 μM) was shown to downregulate the endogenous activation of NF-κB and to reduce the synthesis of the pro-inflammatory cytokines, including IL-1β, IL-6, IL-8, IL-12p70, IL-23, and TNF-α, in comparison to cultures not treated with SB. Furthermore, SB was reported to induce *in vitro* M2-like phenotype polarisation in monocytes from preeclamptic women. (Gomes *et al.*, 2020).

10.3.3 Epithelial cells

In human bronchial epithelial cells SM (10-20 μM) was shown to attenuate cigarette smoke-induced upregulation of inflammatory cytokines TNF-α, IL-6 and IL-8. Similarly, SM treatment was able to decrease levels of TNF-α in cigarette smoke-exposed mice (Li *et al.*, 2016). When HepG2 cells (nontumorigenic cells with high proliferation rates and an epithelial-like morphology) were exposed to sera from obese individuals SM was observed to inhibit obesity-induced growth and ROS production associated with decreased production of proinflammatory IL-6 and IL-1β (Miethe *et al.*, 2017). In silica dioxide nanoparticles-stimulated NCI-H292 airway epithelial cells, SB was demonstrated to ameliorate elevated inflammatory indexes including expression of TNF-α, IL-6, and IL-1β in association with the reduction of TXNIP, MAPKs, and AP-1 expression (Lim *et al.*, 2020). Human umbilical vein endothelial cells (HUVECs) pretreatment with SB was indicated to reduce TNF-α-induced gene expression of the proinflammatory genes IL-6 and MCP-1 (Speciale *et al.*, 2021).

10.3.4 Skin cells

SB (10 μM *in vitro* and 1 mg with topical application) was reported to ameliorate sulphur mustard analogue-induced skin injury (skin cells and SKH-1 hairless mouse skin) by targeting multiple pathways connecting oxidative stress and inflammation, including NF-κB and AP-1 (Tewari-Singh *et al.*, 2012). Exposure of LPS-challenged human dermal fibroblasts to an active component of SM namely 2,3-dehydrosilybin (DHS, 10 and 15 μM) was reported to dose-dependently diminish IL-6 and IL-8 secretion into the surroundings, but upregulated IL-8 mRNA associated with NF-κB and AP-1 activation (Juráňová *et al.*, 2019). It is well accepted that LPS treatment of keratinocytes can induce inflammatory response and release of pro-inflammatory cytokines (IL-1α and IL-6) and the chemokine IL-8. Therefore, in human epidermal keratinocytes SB (15 μM) was shown to downregulate the LPS-induced production of proinflammatory IL-1α, IL-6 and IL-8 (Frankova *et al.*, 2021).

10.3.5 Bone cells

In vitro SB was able to suppress the IL-1β-induced inflammatory markers including production of NO, PGE2, TNF-α and IL-6 as well as decreased expression of COX-2, iNOS and NF-κB (Zheng *et al.*, 2017). In an *in vitro* study with osteoblasts SB (0.42 mM) was recorded to affect intracellular signalling leading to reprogramming genes related to inflammatory response (Fernandes *et al.*, 2019). In IL-1β- stimulated human primary chondrocytes, SM (25 μM) was reported to downregulate expression of proinflammatory NOS, IL-1β, TNF-α, matrix metalloproteinase-3 (MMP-3), MMP-9 and to restore the expression of SIRT1 (Wu *et al.*, 2021). SB was found to protect against osteoarthritis (OA) through suppressing the inflammatory response and cartilage matrix degradation *in vitro* (in human OA chondrocytes) and *in vivo* (in mice OA models).

10.3.6 Connective tissue cells

The production of inflammatory cytokines (TNF-α, IL-1β and IL-6) in rheumatoid arthritis fibroblast-like synoviocytes and a collagen-induced arthritis rat model were shown to be effectively inhibited by SB (50-150 mg/kg) due to inhibiting the NF-κB pathway (Tong *et al.*, 2018). Furthermore, pretreatment of fibroblast cells with SM was shown to improve AO defences, prevented oxidative stress and decreased H_2O_2-induced injury (Sharifi *et al.*, 2013). It should be mentioned that effect of SM could be condition-dependent. For example, the prolonged exposure of LPS-challenged human dermal fibroblasts to a SM component namely 2,3-dehydrosilybin (DHS) showed both beneficial and detrimental effects. On the one hand, DHS was able to diminish IL-6 and IL-8 secretion. On the other hand, DHS significantly upregulated IL-8 mRNA associated with NF-κB and AP-1 activation (Juráňová *et al.*, 2019). Furthermore, in various *in vitro* assays DHS was able to significantly reduce NO production and TNF-α and IL-6 release in a dose-dependent manner (Dobiasová *et al.*, 2020).

10.3.7 Cancer cells

SB treatment (50-200 μM) of human colorectal cancer cells (SW480, LoVo, and HT29) was shown to inhibit TNF-α-induced NF-κB activation together with decreased nuclear levels of both p65 and p50 sub-units. At the same time SB significantly increased IκBα level and decreased phospho-IκBα. Furthermore, oral SB supplementation also inhibited NF-κB pathway in SW480 (COX-2 negative) and LoVo (COX-2 positive) tumour xenografts in nude mice (Raina *et al.*, 2013). *In vitro* treatment of THP-1 cells with SB led to inhibition of caspase-1 cleavage and IL-1β and TNF-α production (Zhang *et al.*, 2017). Adding SB to the medium clearly showed a protective anti-inflammatory effect in monosodium urate-activated THP-1 cells. The effect was associated with diminished inflammation-related gene expression of NLRP1/NLRP3 inflammasomes and TLR4/NF-κB pathway as well as with inhibition of inflammatory cytokine (IL-1β, IL-18 and TNF-α) production (Matias *et al.*, 2019). In human gastric cancer MKN-1 cells and in the stomach of C57BL/6 mice infected by *H. pylori* SB demonstrated anti-inflammatory effects through suppression of NF-κB and STAT3 and subsequently, decreased expression of COX-2 and iNOS (Cho *et al.*, 2021).

10.3.8 Other cell types

In a model of blue light-emitting diode-induced retinal ganglion cells damage, SB (50 and 100 μM) was found to have a significant protective anti-inflammatory effect as evidenced by decreasing expression of IL-1β, IL-6 and TNF-α and increasing expression of IL-10 in the cells associated with the activation of MEK/ERK/CREB pathway (Shen *et al.*, 2019). SB-mediated cardioprotective effect in myocardial I/R injury was shown to be related to decreased oxidative stress, apoptosis, and inflammatory response through downregulation of NF-κB pathway. During hypoxia/reperfusion in H9C2 cells (embryonic rat cardiomyocytes), SB was able to suppress NF-κB signalling by inhibiting IκBα degradation, IKKα phosphorylation and p65 NF-κB nuclear translocation (Chen *et al.*, 2020b).

10.4 Silymarin and inflammation: *In vivo* studies

Attenuation of inflammation by SM/SB treatment has been shown in various disease models, and the protective effects were associated mainly with suppression of NF-κB pathway, and downregulation of pro-inflammatory cytokines, including TNF-α and IL-1β (Saliou *et al.*, 2001; Kim *et al.*, 2013). Furthermore, SM/SB can activate transcriptional factors (e.g. Nrf2) regulating cellular defence against inflammatory and oxidative challenges (Podder *et al.*, 2012; Zhao *et al.*, 2021). SB was tested in the mouse model of concanavalin A (ConA)-induced, T cell-dependent hepatitis and proved to have immunomodulating properties *in vivo* inhibiting intrahepatic expression of proinflammatory molecules, including TNF-α, INF-γ, IL-4, IL-2, iNOS, NF-κB, and augmenting synthesis of anti-inflammatory IL-10 (Schümann *et al.*, 2003).

10.4.1 Nonalcoholic fatty liver disease/steatohepatitis/diet-induced obesity

NAFLD is tightly associated with metabolic syndrome and type 2 diabetes having important links to inflammation. The disease includes a range of pathological conditions ranging from relatively benign steatosis in the form ectopic lipid storage in the liver, to nonalcoholic steatohepatitis (NASH) with inflammation as a major important factor in tissue remodelling and functional impairment with possible progression to hepatocellular carcinoma (Thibaut *et al.*, 2022). Furthermore, parenchymal cell injury and death are believed to trigger inflammation and tissue fibrosis (Itoh *et al.*, 2020). In a mouse model of experimental nonalcoholic steatohepatitis SB (20 mg/kg intraperitoneally for 4 weeks) was found to modulate lipid homeostasis and to inhibit NF-κB activation in the liver (Salamone *et al.*, 2012). In non-alcoholic steatohepatitis induced by HFD and in fat-laden human hepatocytes *in vitro* SM was shown to decrease hepatic inflammation, oxidative stress, and apoptosis (Marin *et al.*, 2017). In a similar model system, SB was reported to mitigate O-linked β-N-acetylglucosamine (O-GlcNA)-cylation associated with NF-κB-signalling pathway and resulted in decreased inflammation (Lee *et al.*, 2018) and to improve AO defences including upregulation of Nrf2, to suppress NF-κB signalling and expression of proinflammatory cytokines leading to amelioration of hepatic steatosis and fibrosis (Ou *et al.*, 2018). In mice with nonalcoholic fatty liver disease caused by HFD, SB was reported to inhibit NLRP3 inflammasome assembly through the NAD^+/SIRT2 pathway, since the anti-inflammatory effect of SB was blocked by SIRT2 silencing or by the SIRT2 inhibitor AGK2 (Zhang *et al.*, 2018), suppressing liver inflammation and inhibiting NF-κB translocation into the nucleus through elevation of SIRT2 expression and promotion of p65 deacetylation (Zhang *et al.*, 2021).

In a model of HFD-induced obesity mice, SM (60 mg/kg) was demonstrated to decrease inflammation (TNF-α, IL-1β and IL-6) and ameliorated liver damage and insulin resistance (Gu *et al.*, 2016). SM treatment was also reported to ameliorate insulin resistance, dyslipidaemia and inflammation in liver of diet-induced obesity in mice associated with inhibited NF-κB signalling (Guo *et al.*, 2016). In HFD-induced obesity model in mice, SB was reported to ameliorate adipose tissue inflammation (decreased expression of IL-1β and TNF-α and increased expression of IL-10 and adiponectin) and mitigate obesity and its complications (Alsaggar *et al.*, 2020). In a mouse model of dietary-induced obesity, milk thistle seed cold press oil was shown to improve antioxidant defences (SOD1, HO-1 and SIRT1), attenuate markers of inflammation (IL-6 and NF-κB) and metabolic syndrome (Shen *et al.*, 2020).

10.4.2 Toxicity models

10.4.2.1 CCl4

Carbone tetrachloride (CCl_4), an important industrial solvent and refrigerant production intermediate, is characterised by high toxicity and usually causes oxidative stress in the liver. The metabolism of CCl_4 via CYP2E1 with the production of ROS is considered to be an important mechanism of its toxicity. In general, CCl_4 is known to compromise the antioxidant defence network of vital body tissues as a result of inhibition of AO enzymes (SOD, GPx and CAT), decreasing GSH in liver samples, leading to oxidative stress and hepatic injuries with the enhancement of lipid peroxidation in various tissues including the liver and serum (Surai *et al.*, 2021). Accumulating evidence indicates that inflammatory responses exacerbate chemical-induced hepatotoxicity (Luster *et al.*, 2000).

SM (50 mg/kg BW for 10 weeks) was shown to reduce inflammation (IL-6, MAPK, NF-κB), and liver fibrosis in CCl_4-treated rats (Clichici *et al.*, 2016). Similarly, SM (100 mg/kg) showed anti-inflammatory (IL-6) and antioxidant (GSH and MDA) protective effects in a rat model of CCl_4-induced liver fibrosis (Sokar *et al.*, 2017). SM (200 mg/kg) was found to protect the liver against CCl_4-induced hepatotoxicity as a result of attenuation of inflammation, oxidative DNA damage, apoptosis, and fibrosis (Al-Rasheed *et al.*, 2016), ameliorating CCl_4-induced increased expression of TNF-α, TGF-β1 and MCP-1 simultaneously with decreasing intrahepatic monocytes (Zhao *et al.*, 2017). In rat model of chemically-induced (the diethylnitrosamine/2-acetylaminofluorene/CCl_4) renal carcinogenesis SM and SB were shown to regulate various transcription factors, including inhibition of NF-κB and proinflammatory cytokines (IL-6), inhibition of PI3K/Akt signalling, activation of Nrf2 and PPARγ expressions, and suppression of apoptosis (Yassin *et al.*, 2021). Furthermore, SM and SB supplementation reduced IL-6 levels and increased the level of IL-4 and protected against chemically-induced renal carcinogenesis by inhibiting p65 and

IκBα phosphorylation, indicating further inhibition of NF-κB by them (Yassin *et al.*, 2021). Furthermore, in a mouse model of CCl_4-induced liver toxicity a synergistic hepatoprotective effect of combined administration of Lachnum polysaccharide (LEP-2b) with SM associated with decreased hepatic inflammation (TNF-α, IL-6 and IL-1β) and enhances the AO defences (SOD, CAT, GPx, GSH, MDA and T-AOC) was observed (Ye *et al.*, 2021). In this study, compared to single therapy, a combining high dose LEP-2b with SM showed the highest protective effect against acute liver injury.

10.4.2.2 Other toxicants

SM (100 mg/kg, intraperitoneally, 2 h before toxicant treatment) was shown to ameliorate maneb (MB)- and PQ-induced changes in the catalytic activities/ expressions of proinflammatory molecules including iNOS, TNF-α, and IL-1β in rats (Ahmad *et al.*, 2013). By maintaining oxidant-antioxidant/redox balance (GSH, GST and CAT) and regulating inflammatory mediators (TNF-α and IL-6) SM was found to alleviate bleomycin-induced pulmonary toxicity and lipid peroxidation in mice (Razavi-Azarkhiavi *et al.*, 2014). It was indicated that 12-O-tetradecanoylphorbol-13-acetate-stimulated skin inflammation in experimental mice was downregulated (IL-1β, IL-6, TNF-α, COX-2 and NF-κB) by SB dose-dependently (Liu *et al.*, 2015). In a model of bisphenol A (BPA)-induced hepatotoxicity in mouse liver, SM (200 mg/kg for 10 days) ameliorated BPA-induced level of pro-inflammatory cytokines (IL-6 and TNF-α) and reduced ultrastructural injuries (Zaulet *et al.*, 2017). In a rat model of triptolide-induced acute hepatotoxicity in rats, SM (50, 100 and 200 mg/kg for 7 days) was shown to dose-dependently suppress the production of pro-inflammatory cytokines including TNF-α, IL-6 and IL-1β in the liver (Wang *et al.*, 2018). SM (100 mg/kg, once daily for three days) was observed to prevent APAP-induced hepatotoxicity in mice. This was associated with decreased inflammation as evidenced by reduction in APAP-induced neutrophil infiltration and suppressed expression of inflammatory markers, including TNF-α, IL-1β, IL-12 and iNOS (Papackova *et al.*, 2018). In a model of cyclosporine A-induced hepatorenal toxicity in rat SM (50 and 200 mg/kg for 21 days) was found to dose-dependently ameliorate functional damage to liver and kidneys with improvement of AO defences and reduced inflammation markers (Vangaveti *et al.*, 2021). SM was shown to protect against docetaxel-induced brain and sciatic nerve injuries by enhancing the antioxidant defence system (GSH, SOD, CAT, GPx, HO-1 and Nrf2) and suppressing inflammation (NF-κB and TNF-α) and apoptosis (upregulated Bcl-2; Yardim *et al.*, 2021). SM in combination with chlorogenic acid was indicated to protect against hepatotoxicity induced by doxorubicin in rats as a result of maintaining antioxidant enzyme activities, decreasing pro-inflammatory cytokines (TNF-α and IL-1β), reducing NF-κB levels and apoptosis biomarkers (Abbas *et al.*, 2020). In an acute liver toxicity model induced by TAA in rats, SM treatment (400 mg/kg, p.o.) was associated with decreased oxidative stress (decreased ROS, MDA and NO levels and increased GSH content, SOD and HO activities, enhanced Nrf2 expression). Furthermore, SM also decreased the expression level of proinflammatory TNF-α in the liver tissues of TAA-treated rats (Hussein *et al.*, 2021). In addition, SB is shown to inhibits abrin (a potent bio-warfare agent)-induced hepatotoxicity by ameliorating oxidative stress, and inhibiting inflammation in mice (Saxena *et al.*, 2022).

10.4.3 Ischemia/Reperfusion models

In a mouse model of renal I/R, SM reduced kidney dysfunction, histological damage, neutrophil infiltration and oxidative stress in a dose dependent manner. Furthermore, palmitoylethanolamide (PEA)+SM demonstrated a significant potentiated effect leading to inhibition of NF-κB and apoptosis pathways indicating that PEA+SM were able to ameliorate renal inflammation (Impellizzeri *et al.*, 2015). In rats SM treatment (250 mg/kg/day for 8 days) was shown to suppress I/R-induced inflammation (Il-1β, IL-6, TNF-α and NF-κB) and oxidative stress (SOD and MDA) in the lung (Jin *et al.*, 2016a). In a model of cerebral I/R injury in rats SM-loaded chitosan nanoparticles were found to significantly reduce inflammation (IL-6 and TNF-α) and improve AO defences (SOD, CAT, GPx, GR, GSH) in I/R brain (Moghaddam *et al.*, 2020). In a model of hepatic warm I/R injury in rats, SB protected the liver by decreasing inflammation (decreased expression of eNOS and neutrophil infiltration) and inhibiting hepatocyte vacuolisation and degeneration (Akbari-Kordkheyli *et al.*, 2019). In the same model system SB was shown to ameliorate inflammatory liver tissue injuries, including neutrophil and macrophage infiltration, cytoplasmic vacuolation, hepatocyte degeneration, vascular endothelial damages, and sinusoid dilation. SB also ameliorated I/R-induced induction of NF-κB and NLRP3 (Zarpou *et al.*, 2021).

10.4.4 Ageing and exercising models

Anti-aging effects of SM were tested using the *Caenorhabditis elegans* model system. The obtained results indicated that *C. elegans* treated with 25 μM and 50 μM S concentration were characterised by an increase in mean lifespan by 10.1% and 24.8% respectively compared to untreated control. Furthermore, SM treated aged animals demonstrated better locomotion rate, higher response to stimuli and improved tolerance to stress compared to untreated control. In addition, SM treatment increased resistance of animals to Alzheimer's disease development (Kumar *et al.*, 2015). In a model of the senescence-accelerated mice, SB treatment (100 and 200 mg/kg for 6 weeks) was found to significantly ameliorate microglial activation associated with down-regulation of the proinflammatory cytokine IL-6 and inflammation-associated proteins, iNOS and COX-2 (Jin *et al.*, 2016b). In hippocampus of old male rats, SM (20 mg/kg/day i.p., 4 weeks) was shown to increase expression of SIRT1 and decreased expression of NF-κB providing anti-inflammatory effects (Sarubbo *et al.*, 2018).

In rats subjected to regular exercise training SM consumption improved muscle recovery, inflammation, and damaged tissue, and promoted hypertrophy, vascularisation, and muscle fibre shape/appearance (Vargas-Mendoza *et al.*, 2020). Similarly, in rats subjected to 8-week exercise training, administration of SM (100 mg) was associated with increased alveolar and bronchial muscle size, improvement in vascularisation and reduction in lung tissue inflammation (Vargas-Mendoza *et al.*, 2021).

10.4.5 Stress-induced injuries

SM was shown to attenuate inflammation and oxidative stress induced by cigarette smoke in mice indicative by a decreased secretion of TNF-α, IL-1β, and IL-8 in bronchoalveolar lavage fluid (Li *et al.*, 2015). In cigarette smoke-induced and LPS-induced chronic obstructive pulmonary disease model mice SB was found to inhibit the neutrophilic airway inflammation and reduced MPO expression (Park *et al.*, 2016). SB (10 or 20 mg/kg) markedly ameliorated the cigarette smoke-induced increase in inflammatory cell count in the bronchoalveolar lavage fluid and significantly reduced levels of proinflammatory mediators (IL-1β, IL-6 and TNF-α) in mice (Ko *et al.*, 2017).

In peritoneal dialysis patients SM was observed to be a useful treatment of inflammation as evidenced by decreased serum TNF-α (Nazemian *et al.*, 2010). Modulatory effect of SM on inflammatory mediators in experimentally induced benign prostatic hyperplasia were shown. In particular, testosterone-treated rats demonstrated inflammation and hyperplasia. However, co-treatment with SM significantly alleviated these pathological changes by attenuating testosterone-induced nuclear NF-κB, cyclooxygenase-II (COX-II), and iNOS upregulation (Atawia *et al.*, 2014). In mice SB treatment (100 mg/day) was reported to ameliorate the radiation-induced lung injury associated with reduction of inflammation (reducing the number of inflammatory cells in the bronchoalveolar lavage fluid) and fibrosis (Son *et al.*, 2015).

In a mouse model of restraint stress, SM (100 mg/kg) was shown to ameliorate oxidative stress and decreased mRNA levels of pro-inflammatory mediators including TNF-α, IL-1β, IL-6, and CCL2 in liver and serum (Kim *et al.*, 2016). In a rat model of acute respiratory distress syndrome SM (50, 100, and 200 mg/kg) was demonstrated to ameliorate lung impairments by down-regulating inflammation as evidenced by prevention of stress-induced activation of proinflammatory cytokines (TNF-α, IFN-γ and IL-6) simultaneously with activation of anti-inflammatory IL-10 in broncho-alveolar lavage fluid (Zhu and Sun, 2018). In a chronic unpredictable stress model SB was reported to ameliorate stress-induced changes in inflammatory (serum IL-1β, TNF-α), antioxidant (GSH and SOD) and behaviour (memory function) indexes in mice (Garikapati *et al.*, 2018).

In mice topical application of SB prior to UVB or immediately after UVB exposure (5 days per week for 8 weeks) was shown to be associated with inhibition of the UVB-induced inflammatory markers (NF-κB, TNF-α, COX2 and iNOS) in skin tissue (Rigby *et al.*, 2017). In a model of skin protection against UVB damage SB-loaded hydrogel was found to have anti-inflammatory effects as indicated by significantly reduced levels of the inflammation mediators such as IL-22 and TNF-α (Ali Karami *et al.*, 2021). In a mouse model of LPS-induced lung injury and inflammation, SB was reported to suppress airway inflammatory cell (macrophages, T cells and neutrophils) recruitment, inhibited NF-κB signalling and reduced production of proinflammatory cytokines, including IL-1β and TNF-α in bronchoalveolar fluid and serum (Zhang *et al.*, 2017).

In a model of mild traumatic brain injury, SM was shown to decrease neuroinflammation as evidenced by the decreased levels of TNF-α protein (a marker of inflammation) in the mouse prefrontal cortex and hippocampus (Kosari-Nasab *et al.*, 2018). In male mice with mild traumatic brain injury SM (50 mg/kg/day for 20 days) significantly reduced TNF-α in the hippocampus but was not effective in female mice (Shokouhi *et al.*, 2020). In a mouse model of multiple-organ damage induced by D-galactose/lipopolysaccharide, SM-treated mice (75 mg/kg BW and 150 mg/kg BW) demonstrated improvement of liver function (reduced ALT and AST in the serum). At the same time SM treatment was associated with improved AO defences (increased the SOD, CAT, GSH, GPx, T-AOC activities and expression of SOD1, SOD2, CAT, GPx, IL-10, Nrf2, HO-1, NQO1, Trx, and IκB-α). In addition, SM reduced inflammation (increased IL-10 and IL-12 and reduced IL-6, IL-1β and TNF-α concentrations and expressions in addition to decreased expression of NF-κB, NLRP3, COX2, and p38) in the mouse liver (Zhao *et al.*, 2021). In a model of varicocele (VCL)-induced detrimental impact in rat testicular tissue, SM (50 mg/kg, orally) was indicated to partly ameliorate VCL-induced down-regulation of testicular TAC, SOD, GPx and to mitigate increased COX2 and iNOS expression as well as NO content (Mazhari *et al.*, 2018).

The silymarin pluronic-lecithin organogel formulation was shown to significantly relieve inflammatory symptoms of atopic dermatitis such as redness, swelling, and inflammation (Mady *et al.*, 2016). Furthermore, SM pretreatment was responsible for partial inactivation of multiple mitogen-activated protein kinase signalling pathways in the lungs of LPS-treated rats (Zhu and Sun, 2018). Therefore, in a rat model SM was able to mitigate LPS-induced lung impairments by down-regulating inflammation. In a model of irritant contact dermatitis in mice hydrogel containing SB nanocapsules was found to possess effective anti-inflammatory action as indicated by decreased the ear oedema and reduced leukocyte infiltration in damaged tissue (Rigon *et al.*, 2019). In a model of HCl-induced acute lung injury in rats SM showed anti-inflammatory action as evidenced by normalisation of leukocyte count, decreased COX-2 expression and reversed the inflammatory lung changes simultaneously with improved antioxidant defences as indicated by up-regulation of Nrf2 and HO-1 (Ahmed *et al.*, 2019). SM + curcumin loaded albumin nanoparticles coated by chitosan showed anti-inflammatory effects (decreased IL-6 in the lung and reduced CRP in serum) in mouse model of oleic acid-induced lung injury (Hanafy and El-Kemary, 2022). In a rat model of extrahepatic cholestasis, SM loaded gold nanoparticles were shown to improve liver function by enhancing antioxidant defences and decreasing oxidative stress, inflammation and fibrosis (Clichici *et al.*, 2020).

10.4.6 Wound healing

It seems likely that effective control of inflammatory reactions could help in wound healing. For instance, topical application of SM was found to improve the morphological, biochemical and biomechanical properties of experimentally-induced wound defects in rats (Oryan *et al.*, 2012). The authors reported that SM significantly enhanced alignment of the healing tissue, increased maturity of the collagen fibres and fibroblasts and improved the ultimate tensile strength and stress of the healing tissue. In an experiment studying topical administration of SM on excision wound healing in rats, it was confirmed that SM significantly reduced inflammation and improved epithelialisation and in full-thickness wounds in rats (Sharifi *et al.*, 2012). This was associated with acceleration of episiotomy wound healing rate and decreasing pain severity (Toomari *et al.*, 2021). Interestingly, in patients with second degree-burn the 4-week adjuvant treatment with oral SM led to the full and faster wound recovery (Mahmoodi-Nesheli *et al.*, 2018). It is known that preadipocyte migration is a vital process in the adipocyte tissue wound healing. Interestingly, SB-induced autophagy mediated by PPARα-SIRT1-AMPK pathway is involved in the regulation of type I collagen-enhanced migration in murine 3T3-L1 preadipocytes by down-regulating phosphorylated NF-κB p65 (Liu *et al.*, 2019). In a model of experimental Achilles tendon injury in the rat SM consumption led to optimal healing process as evidenced by significantly improved tissue healing indices, functional index and biomechanical properties (Soleimani *et al.*, 2021).

10.4.7 Other *in vivo* model systems

In a mouse ovalbumin (OVA)-induced asthma model, SB was indicated to protect against OVA-induced airway inflammation as a result of downregulation of NF-κB activity (Choi *et al.*, 2012). SB treatment was shown to polarise the Th1/Th2 immune balance toward the Th1-dominant direction and this could be beneficial in prevention/treatment of IgE-mediated allergy (Kuo and Jan, 2009). SB was observed to Ag-nonspecifically down-regulate the secretion of pro-inflammatory Th1 cytokines, to up-regulate the anti-inflammatory Th2 cytokines *in vitro* and to dose-dependently inhibit the production of Th1 cytokines *ex vivo* (Min *et al.*, 2007). SM administration was associated with reduction of sepsis-induced oxidative damage in lung tissues and inhibition of the release of inflammatory mediators (Toklu *et al.*, 2008). In a Balb/c mouse model of allergic asthma two SM isomers (isosilybin A and silydianin) showed anti-inflammatory effects associated with reduction of eosinophilic infiltration of lungs, IL-4 and IL-5 levels and gene expression in bronchoalveolar lavage fluid (Nasab *et al.*, 2020). In newly diagnosed and IFN-β_{1b}-treated multiple sclerosis patients SM inhibited Th1 proliferating activity and inhibited T-bet gene expression and IFN-γ production by these cells (Navabi *et al.*, 2019). In experimental autoimmune encephalomyelitis, an animal model of multiple sclerosis, SB was shown to suppress DC activation and to inhibit pathogenic Th17 inflammatory cell responses, significantly decreasing inflammation and demyelination of the central nervous system of experimental mice (Yang and She, 2021). In mouse model of Mayaro virus infection SM treatment ameliorated virus-induced increased pro-inflammatory cytokines and liver inflammation (Ferraz *et al.*, 2021). In silico capability of SB interact with the SARS-CoV-2 main target proteins was investigated. Computational analysis showed that SB can form a stable complex with SARS-CoV-2 spike protein RBD, possesses good negative binding affinity with main proteases (Mpro) interacting with many residues on the active site of Mpro. It was concluded that SB can inhibit viral entry and replication (Speciale *et al.*, 2021).

In a model of STZ-induced diabetes in mice SM was found to improve antioxidant defences and to decrease inflammation indexes including pancreatic TNF-α and inflammatory cells infiltration in islets (Stolf *et al.*, 2018). In STZ-induced diabetic nephropathy model rats, SM (100, 300 and 900 μg/kg) in nanoliposome form ameliorated oxidative stress as indicative by improved SOD, CAT and GPx activity in kidney. SM also mitigated STZ-induced elevated expression of inflammatory indicators (IL-8, IL-10, TNF-α, IL-6, TGF-β and ICAM-1) in renal tissue. Furthermore, SM decreased the expression of p-STAT3 and p-JAK2 while increased the expression of SOCS1 (Chen *et al.*, 2021). The authors concluded that in diabetic rats with STZ-induced kidney injury SM nanoliposomes were able to mitigate oxidative stress, inflammation and renal fibrosis. In type 2 diabetic zebrafish model, a combined treatment with metformin and SB was reported to reduce the expression of inflammatory genes (IL-1β and TNF-α) and ameliorating the intestinal inflammation (Mohammadi *et al.*, 2020). In an atherosclerotic model with diabetes based on ApoE-/- mice fed with high-fat diet, co-administration of SB with Clopidogrel significantly reduced the inflammation, aortic lesion and endothelial dysfunction in aorta roots (Zhang *et al.*, 2022).

In ischemic brain tissue after experimental stroke in rats, SB was shown to significantly downregulate Bax and NF-κB, upregulate Akt, mTOR, HIF-1α, Bcl-2 associated with alleviation of neurological deficit, reduced infarct volume, and suppressed brain oedema (Wang *et al.*, 2012). In the 1-methyl-4-phenylpyridinium ion (MPP(+))-treated rat model of Parkinson's disease (PD) *in vivo* animals received intraperitoneal (i.p.) injections 10, 50, or 100 mg/kg of SB, starting 1 day before MPP(+) injection. It was found that 100 mg/kg of SB attenuated the MPP(+)-induced neurotoxicity in the substantia nigra in a dose-dependent manner and prevented the MPP(+)-induced increased levels of inflammatory molecules including TNF-α, IL-1β and iNOS (Jung *et al.*, 2014). In a mouse model of Alzheimer's disease, SB encapsulated in macrophage-derived exosomes had improved brain targeting ability and, after entering the brain, alleviated astrocyte inflammation-mediated neuronal damage by reducing the secretion of proinflammatory cytokines (IL-6, IL-1β and TNF-α) and downregulating the protein expression involved in NF-κB signalling (Huo *et al.*, 2021).

A single i.p. injection of SB to rats, before the induction of acute pancreatitis with L-arginine, was shown to mitigate oxidative stress parameters in serum and to demonstrate anti-inflammatory action as evidenced by prevention of histopathological changes in the pancreas (Uçmak *et al.*, 2016). In a model of experimental gastric ulcer in rats, SM (50 mg/kg orally) pretreatment was found to inhibit gastric inflammation as evidenced by decreased MPO, TNF- α and IL-6 levels and NF-κB expression. This was associated with improvement of the AO defences indicative by increased SOD, GPx activities and up-regulation of Nrf2 (Arafa Keshk *et al.*, 2017).

In a model of *Aspergillus fumigatus*-induced early inflammatory response in pulmonary microvascular endothelial cells SB pre-treatment and post-treatment were shown to down-regulate expression of proinflammatory factors and adhesion molecules (IL-6, IL-1β and ICAM-1) simultaneously with inhibition of *A. fumigatus*-induced p38 MAPK activation (Song *et al.*, 2017). Inhibitory effects of SB on inflammatory signalling, collagen deposition, and epithelial-mesenchymal trans-differentiation suggested that it could be used for treatment of pulmonary inflammation and fibrosis. This was proven in mouse model of pulmonary fibrosis where SB effectively alleviated inflammatory indexes, including IL-1β, IL-6, and TNF-α in the fibrotic tissue (Ali *et al.*, 2021).

In human foetal membranes, SB (200 μM) was found to significantly decrease LPS-stimulated expression of IL-6 and IL-8, COX-2, and prostaglandins PGE2 and PGF2α. Similarly, preterm foetal membranes with active infection treated with SB showed a decrease in IL-6, IL-8 and MMP-9 expression (Lim *et al.*, 2014). There was increased endogenous activation of NF-κB as well as TNF-α and IL-1β release by PBMC in the preeclampsia group compared with the normotensive pregnant women. SB was shown to reduce the levels of NF-κB and expression of pro-inflammatory TNF-α and IL-1β in preeclamptic women (Giorgi *et al.*, 2012a). Therefore, SB demonstrated an anti-inflammatory activity as evidenced by inhibition of the spontaneous and LPS-stimulated NF-κB activation as well as the production of inflammatory cytokines in patients with preeclampsia (Giorgi *et al.*, 2012a).

Furthermore, SB was found to show AO and anti-inflammatory activities in monocytes from preeclamptic pregnant women as evidenced by inhibition of the *in vitro* endogenous release of ROS and pro-inflammatory cytokine (TNF-α) production (Cristofalo *et al.*, 2013). In pregnant preeclamptic women SB was indicated to downregulate the NF-κB pathway including decreasing expression of IL-1β, IL-18 and TNF-α and NLRP1/NLRP3 inflammasomes in monocytes (Matias *et al.*, 2019). SB (100 μM) was shown to downregulate the expression of the Th1 and Th17 profiles by modulation of transcription factors including decreasing inflammatory STAT1/STAT4/T-bet and STAT3/RORγt and increasing anti-inflammatory STAT6/GATA-3 and STAT5/FoxP3 transcription factors in pregnant women with preeclampsia. This led to decreased release of inflammatory cytokines and higher levels of anti-inflammatory IL-10 and TGF-β (Ribeiro *et al.*, 2022).

Similarly, thalassemia patients were shown to be characterised by increased inflammation (decreased expression of anti-inflammatory IL-10 and increased concentrations of pro-inflammatory TGF-β and IL-23) and SM treatment demonstrated anti-inflammatory actions in such conditions (Balouchi *et al.*, 2014). Earlier studies showed a redox disbalance (a reduction of GSH concentration) associated with decreased proliferation of PHA-activated PBMC obtained from beta-thalassemia major patients. Interestingly, treatment with SM was able to restore both GSH levels and PBMC proliferation (Alidoost *et al.*, 2006). In patients with β-Thalassemia Major SM (140 mg, 3 times a day for 12 weeks) was found to improve inflammatory status as evidenced by decreased CRP and IL-6 and raised IL-10 (Darvishi-Khezri *et al.*, 2021). In the nigrostriatal dopaminergic system *in vivo* SB was shown to suppress the prothrombin kringle-2-induced production of proinflammatory molecules including iNOS, IL-1β and TNF-α in the mouse substantia nigra (Leem *et al.*, 2019).

A double-blind clinical trial with patients with painful knee osteoarthritis SM (300 mg/day for 8 weeks) was recorded to significantly reduce serum levels of IL-1α, IL-8 and complement proteins C3 and C4 in comparison to the pre-treatment levels (Hussain *et al.*, 2009). In a rat model of experimental colitis SB was shown to be effective in preventing intestinal inflammation and ameliorating the degree of colonic tissue injury as a result of suppressing NF-κB activity and neutrophil infiltration/activation in inflamed colon in addition to a decreased expression of proinflammatory cytokines including TNF-α and IL-1β (Esmaily *et al.*, 2011). An understanding of the functional roles of macrophages, their interactions with microbiota in relation to the intestinal inflammation is of great importance (Han *et al.*, 2021). Since intestinal inflammation is a driving force of many different diseases and is responsible for decreased productive and reproductive performance of poultry and farm animals (Akhtar *et al.*, 2021) the possible protective role of SM in the gut deserves more attention.

In a model of colitis-associated tumorigenesis in mice SB (750 mg/kg body weight by gavage) was shown to inhibit the production of inflammatory cytokines (IL-1β, IL-6 and TNF-α) and to ameliorate the impairment of colonic mucosal barrier (Zheng *et al.*, 2018). Combinations of indole-3-carbinol and SB were indicated to suppress inflammation-driven mouse lung tumorigenesis by modulating critical cell cycle regulators (Song *et al.*, 2015).

10.5 Conclusions

Inflammation is known to be a defence mechanism responsible for creation of hostile conditions for pathogens and for prevention of the spread of tissue infection, as well as for cell/tissue homeostasis maintenance. However, in the case of misregulation of inflammation, as a result of various stresses and redox balance alterations, inflammatory response could cause damages to various tissues and organs (Surai, 2020). Human health complications associated with inflammation and oxidative stress include a range of various diseases including obesity, metabolic syndrome, type-2 diabetes, atherosclerosis and other cardiovascular diseases, chronic kidney disease as well as auto-immune diseases (Menzel *et al.*, 2021). Similarly, low grade chronic inflammation in poultry/animal production systems (Cardoso Dal Pont, 2020) are also of great importance for health maintenance and for achieving high productive and reproductive performance (Broom and Kogut, 2018; Kogut *et al.*, 2018).

Pro-inflammatory stress includes a number of universal components, such as (Gusev and Zhuravleva, 2022; Surai, 2020):

- oxidative stress response;
- DNA damage response;
- unfolded protein response;

- heat shock response;
- autophagy modulation;
- formation of inflammasome;
- non-coding RNA response;
- inducible networks of signalling pathways formation; and
- epigenetic changes.

Accumulating evidence indicates that phytochemicals/polyphenols possess anti-inflammatory properties proven in both *in vitro* and *in vivo* inflammatory disease models being promising candidates for the treatment of several inflammatory diseases. The main anti-inflammatory mechanism of polyphenolic action is attributed to an inhibition of TLR4/NF-κB-mediated signalling pathways and the downregulation of expression of pro-inflammatory mediators (Yu *et al.*, 2022b). Therefore, SM/SB as one of the most widely studied phytochemical with antioxidant and anti-inflammatory properties (Surai, 2015) has received tremendous attention for the last 30 years. The data presented above based on *in vitro* and *in vivo* studies clearly proved that SM/SB has a great potential as an anti-inflammation agent. In particular, in *in vitro* studies SM/SB was able to downregulate NF-κB and respective proinflammatory cytokines and chemokines (TNF-α, IL-1β, IL-6, IL-12, IL-23, CCL4, CXCL10) as well as RONS (Figure 10.2).

At the same time SM/SB upregulated anti-inflammatory cytokines (IL-4, IL-10, IL-13, TGF-β, etc.) and lipid mediators responsible for resolution of inflammation. This was clearly demonstrated with immune (macrophages and monocytes) and non-immune

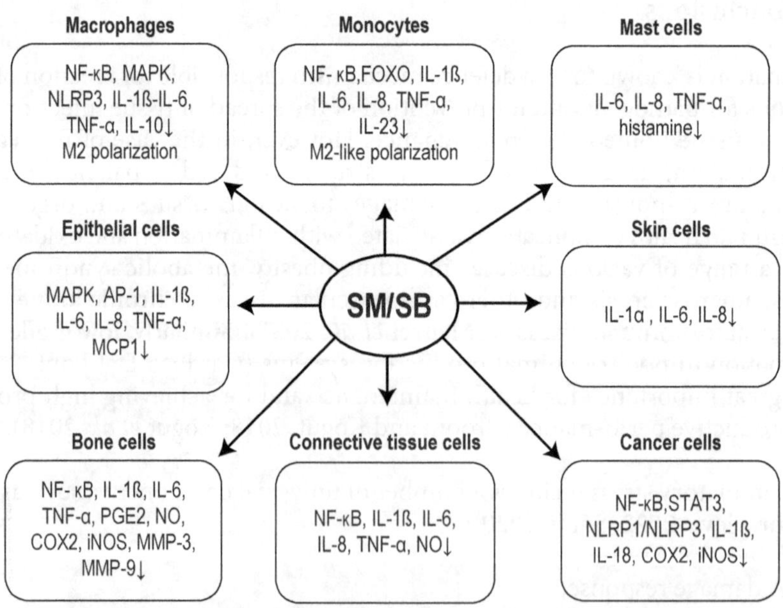

Figure 10.2. Anti-inflammatory action of SM/SB in various *in vitro* systems.

(epithelial, skin, bone, connective tissue and cancer) cells. Similar anti-inflammatory effects of SM/SB were demonstrated in various *in vivo* models, including nonalcoholic fatty liver disease, toxicity models, ischemia/reperfusion models, ageing and exercising models, stress-induced injuries, wound healing and many other model systems. Therefore, it seems likely that regulatory roles of SM/SB in inflammation could be considered as a key element of health-promoting properties of these phytochemicals and further research should pay more attention to the protective anti-inflammatory actions of SM/SB.

References

Abbas, N., Awad, M.M. and Nafea, O.E., 2020. Silymarin in combination with chlorogenic acid protects against hepatotoxicity induced by doxorubicin in rats: possible role of adenosine monophosphate-activated protein kinase pathway. Toxicology Research 9: 771-777.

Ahmad, I., Shukla, S., Kumar, A., Singh, B.K., Kumar, V., Chauhan, A.K., Singh, D., Pandey, H.P. and Singh, C., 2013. Biochemical and molecular mechanisms of N-acetyl cysteine and silymarin-mediated protection against maneb- and paraquat-induced hepatotoxicity in rats. Chemico-Biological Interactions 201: 9-18.

Ahmed, R.F., Moussa, R.A., Eldemerdash, R.S., Zakaria, M.M. and Abdel-Gaber, S.A., 2019. Ameliorative effects of silymarin on HCl-induced acute lung injury in rats; role of the Nrf-2/HO-1 pathway. Iranian Journal of Basic Medical Sciences 22: 1483-1492.

Akbari-Kordkheyli, V., Abbaszadeh-Goudarzi, K., Nejati-Laskokalayeh, M., Zarpou, S. and Khonakdar-Tarsi, A., 2019. The protective effects of silymarin on ischemia-reperfusion injuries: A mechanistic review. Iranian Journal of Basic Medical Sciences 22: 968-976.

Akhtar, M., Chen, Y., Ma, Z., Zhang, X., Shi, D., Khan, J.A. and Liu, H., 2021. Gut microbiota-derived short chain fatty acids are potential mediators in gut inflammation. Animal Nutrition 8: 350-360.

Ali Karami, M., Sharif Makhmalzadeh, B., Pooranian, M. and Rezai, A., 2021. Preparation and optimization of silibinin-loaded chitosan-fucoidan hydrogel: an *in vivo* evaluation of skin protection against UVB. Pharmaceutical Development and Technology 26: 209-219.

Ali, S.A., Saifi, M.A., Godugu, C. and Talla, V., 2021. Silibinin alleviates silica-induced pulmonary fibrosis: Potential role in modulating inflammation and epithelial-mesenchymal transition. Phytotherapy Research 35: 5290-5304.

Alidoost, F., Gharagozloo, M., Bagherpour, B., Jafarian, A., Sajjadi, S.E., Hourfar, H. and Moayedi, B., 2006. Effects of silymarin on the proliferation and glutathione levels of peripheral blood mononuclear cells from beta-thalassemia major patients. International Immunopharmacology 6: 1305-1310.

Al-Rasheed, N., Faddah, L., Al-Rasheed, N., Bassiouni, Y.A., Hasan, I.H., Mahmoud, A.M., Mohamad, R.A. and Yacoub, H.I., 2016. Protective effects of silymarin, alone or in combination with chlorogenic acid and/or melatonin, against carbon tetrachloride-induced hepatotoxicity. Pharmacognosy Magazine 12(Suppl 3): S337-S345.

Alsaggar, M., Bdour, S., Ababneh, Q., El-Elimat, T., Qinna, N. and Alzoubi, K.H., 2020. Silibinin attenuates adipose tissue inflammation and reverses obesity and its complications in diet-induced obesity model in mice. BMC Pharmacology and Toxicology 21: 8.

Arafa Keshk, W., Zahran, S.M., Katary, M.A. and Abd-Elaziz Ali, D., 2017. Modulatory effect of silymarin on nuclear factor-erythroid-2-related factor 2 regulated redox status, nuclear factor-κB mediated inflammation and apoptosis in experimental gastric ulcer. Chemico-Biological Interactions 273: 266-272.

Atawia, R.T., Mosli, H.H., Tadros, M.G., Khalifa, A.E., Mosli, H.A. and Abdel-Naim, A.B., 2014. Modulatory effect of silymarin on inflammatory mediators in experimentally induced benign prostatic hyperplasia: emphasis on PTEN, HIF-1α, and NF-κB. Naunyn-Schmiedeberg's Archives of Pharmacology 387: 1131-1140.

Austermann, J., Roth, J. and Barczyk-Kahlert, K., 2022. The good and the bad: Monocytes' and macrophages' diverse functions in inflammation. Cells 11: 1979.

Azadpour, M., Farajollahi, M.M., Dariushnejad, H., Varzi, A.M., Varezardi, A. and Barati, M., 2021. Effects of synthetic silymarin-PLGA nanoparticles on M2 polarization and inflammatory cytokines in LPS-treated murine peritoneal macrophages. Iranian Journal of Basic Medical Sciences 24: 1446-1454.

Balouchi, S., Gharagozloo, M., Esmaeil, N., Mirmoghtadaei, M. and Moayedi, B., 2014. Serum levels of TGFβ, IL-10, IL-17, and IL-23 cytokines in β-thalassemia major patients: the impact of silymarin therapy. Immunopharmacology and Immunotoxicology 36: 271-274.

Bannwart, C.F., Nakaira-Takahagi, E., Golim, M.A., de Medeiros, L.T., Romão, M., Weel, I.C. and Peraçoli, M.T., 2010. Downregulation of nuclear factor-kappa B (NF-kappaB) pathway by silibinin in human monocytes challenged with Paracoccidioides brasiliensis. Life Sciences 86: 880-886.

Bittencourt, M., Rodrigues, R.P., Kitagawa, R.R. and Gonçalves, R., 2020. The gastroprotective potential of silibinin against Helicobacter pylori infection and gastric tumor cells. Life Sciences 256: 117977.

Broom, L.J. and Kogut, M.H., 2018. Inflammation: friend or foe for animal production?. Poultry Science 97: 510-514.

Cardoso Dal Pont, G., Farnell, M., Farnell, Y. and Kogut, M.H., 2020. Dietary factors as triggers of low-grade chronic intestinal inflammation in poultry. Microorganisms 8: 139.

Chen, J., Li, D.L., Xie, L.N., Ma, Y.R., Wu, P.P., Li, C., Liu, W.F., Zhang, K., Zhou, R.P., Xu, X.T., Zheng, X. and Liu, X., 2020a. Synergistic anti-inflammatory effects of silibinin and thymol combination on LPS-induced RAW264.7 cells by inhibition of NF-κB and MAPK activation. Phytomedicine 78: 153309.

Chen, Y.H., Lin, H., Wang, Q., Hou, J.W., Mao, Z.J. and Li, Y.G., 2020b. Protective role of silibinin against myocardial ischemia/reperfusion injury-induced cardiac dysfunction. International Journal of Biological Sciences 16: 1972-1988.

Chen, Y., Chen, L. and Yang, T., 2021. Silymarin nanoliposomes attenuate renal injury on diabetic nephropathy rats via co-suppressing TGF-β/Smad and JAK2/STAT3/SOCS1 pathway. Life Sciences 271: 119197.

Cho, K., Lee, H.G., Piao, J.Y., Kim, S.J., Na, H.K. and Surh, Y.J., 2021. Protective effects of silibinin on Helicobacter pylori-induced gastritis: NF-κB and STAT3 as potential targets. Journal of Cancer Prevention 26: 118-127.

Choi, Y.H. and Yan, G.H., 2009. Silibinin attenuates mast cell-mediated anaphylaxis-like reactions. Biological and Pharmaceutical Bulletin 32: 868-875.

Choi, Y.H., Jin, G.Y., Guo, H.S., Piao, H.M., Li, L.C., Li, G.Z., Lin, Z.H. and Yan, G.H., 2012. Silibinin attenuates allergic airway inflammation in mice. Biochemical and Biophysical Research Communications 427: 450-455.

Clichici, S., David, L., Moldovan, B., Baldea, I., Olteanu, D., Filip, M., Nagy, A., Luca, V., Crivii, C., Mircea, P., Katona, G. and Filip, G.A., 2020. Hepatoprotective effects of silymarin coated gold nanoparticles in experimental cholestasis. Materials Science and Engineering. C, Materials for Biological Applications 115: 111117.

Clichici, S., Olteanu, D., Filip, A., Nagy, A.L., Oros, A. and Mircea, P.A., 2016. Beneficial effects of silymarin after the discontinuation of CCl4-induced liver fibrosis. Journal of Medicinal Food 19: 789-797.

Cristofalo, R., Bannwart-Castro, C.F., Magalhães, C.G., Borges, V.T., Peraçoli, J.C., Witkin, S.S. and Peraçoli, M.T., 2013. Silibinin attenuates oxidative metabolism and cytokine production by monocytes from preeclamptic women. Free Radical Research 47: 268-275.

Darvishi-Khezri, H., Kosaryan, M., Karami, H., Salehifar, E., Mahdavi, M., Alipour, A. and Aliasgharian, A., 2021. Can use of silymarin improve inflammatory status in patients with β-Thalassemia Major? A crossover, randomized controlled trial. Complementary Medicine Research 28: 123-130.

Degboé, Y., Poupot, R. and Poupot, M., 2022. Repolarization of unbalanced macrophages: Unmet medical need in chronic inflammation and cancer. International Journal of Molecular Sciences 23: 1496.

Dobiasová, S., Řehořová, K., Kučerová, D., Biedermann, D., Káňová, K., Petrásková, L., Koucká, K., Václavíková, R., Valentová, K., Ruml, T., Macek, T., Křen, V. and Viktorová, J., 2020. Multidrug resistance modulation activity of silybin derivatives and their anti-inflammatory Potential. Antioxidants 9: 455.

Dupuis, M.L., Conti, F., Maselli, A., Pagano, M.T., Ruggieri, A., Anticoli, S., Fragale, A., Gabriele, L., Gagliardi, M.C., Sanchez, M., Ceccarelli, F., Alessandri, C., Valesini, G., Ortona, E. and Pierdominici, M., 2018. The natural agonist of estrogen receptor β Silibinin plays an immunosuppressive role representing a potential therapeutic tool in rheumatoid arthritis. Frontiers in Immunology 9: 1903.

Esmaily, H., Vaziri-Bami, A., Miroliaee, A.E., Baeeri, M. and Abdollahi, M., 2011. The correlation between NF-κB inhibition and disease activity by coadministration of silibinin and ursodeoxycholic acid in experimental colitis. Fundamental and Clinical Pharmacology 25: 723-733.

Fernandes, C., Veiga, M.R., Peracoli, M. and Zambuzzi, W.F., 2019. Modulatory effects of silibinin in cell behavior during osteogenic phenotype. Journal of Cellular Biochemistry 120: 13413-13425.

Ferraz, A.C., Almeida, L.T., da Silva Caetano, C.C., da Silva Menegatto, M.B., Souza Lima, R.L., de Senna, J., de Oliveira Cardoso, J.M., Perucci, L.O., Talvani, A., Geraldo de Lima, W., de Mello Silva, B., Barbosa Reis, A., de Magalhães, J.C. and Lopes de Brito Magalhães, C., 2021. Hepatoprotective, antioxidant, anti-inflammatory, and antiviral activities of silymarin against mayaro virus infection. Antiviral Research 194: 105168.

Fordham, J.B., Naqvi, A.R. and Nares, S., 2014. Leukocyte production of inflammatory mediators is inhibited by the antioxidants phloretin, silymarin, hesperetin, and resveratrol. Mediators of Inflammation 2014: 938712.

Frankova, J., Juranova, J., Biedermann, D. and Ulrichova, J., 2021. Influence of silymarin components on keratinocytes and 3D reconstructed epidermis. Toxicology in Vitro 74: 105162.

Garikapati, D.R., Shaik, P.B. and Penchalaiah, H., 2018. Evaluate neuroprotective effect of silibinin using chronic unpredictable stress (cus) model. International Journal of Physiology, Pathophysiology and Pharmacology 10: 184-191.

Giorgi, V.S., Bannwart-Castro, C.F., Peracoli, J.C. and Peracoli, M.T., 2012b. Silibinin modulates NF-κB pathway and proinflammatory cytokines production by mononuclear cells of preeclamptic women. Pregnancy Hypertension 2: 275-276.

Giorgi, V.S., Peracoli, M.T., Peracoli, J.C., Witkin, S.S. and Bannwart-Castro, C.F., 2012a. Silibinin modulates the NF-κB pathway and pro-inflammatory cytokine production by mononuclear cells from preeclamptic women. Journal of Reproductive Immunology 95: 67-72.

Gomes, V.J., Nunes, P.R., Matias, M.L., Ribeiro, V.R., Devides, A.C., Bannwart-Castro, C.F., Romagnoli, G.G., Peraçoli, J.C., Peraçoli, M. and Romao-Veiga, M., 2020. Silibinin induces *in vitro* M2-like phenotype polarization in monocytes from preeclamptic women. International Immunopharmacology 89(Pt A): 107062.

Gu, M., Zhao, P., Huang, J., Zhao, Y., Wang, Y., Li, Y., Li, Y., Fan, S., Ma, Y.M., Tong, Q., Yang, L., Ji, G. and Huang, C., 2016. Silymarin ameliorates metabolic dysfunction associated with diet-Induced obesity via activation of Farnesyl X receptor. Frontiers in Pharmacology 7: 345.

Guo, Y., Wang, S., Wang, Y. and Zhu, T., 2016. Silymarin improved diet-induced liver damage and insulin resistance by decreasing inflammation in mice. Pharmaceutical Biology 54: 2995-3000.

Gusev, E. and Zhuravleva, Y., 2022. Inflammation: A new look at an old problem. International Journal of Molecular Sciences 23: 4596.

Gugliandolo, E., Crupi, R., Biondi, V., Licata, P., Cuzzocrea, S. and Passantino, A., 2020. Protective effect of silibinin on lipopolysaccharide-induced inflammatory responses in equine peripheral blood mononuclear cells, an *in vitro* study. Animals 10: 2022.

Han, X., Ding, S., Jiang, H. and Liu, G., 2021. Roles of macrophages in the development and treatment of gut inflammation. Frontiers in Cell and Developmental Biology 9: 625423.

Hanafy, N. and El-Kemary, M.A., 2022. Silymarin/curcumin loaded albumin nanoparticles coated by chitosan as muco-inhalable delivery system observing anti-inflammatory and anti COVID-19 characterizations in oleic acid triggered lung injury and *in vitro* COVID-19 experiment. International Journal of Biological Macromolecules 198: 101-110.

Huo, Q., Shi, Y., Qi, Y., Huang, L., Sui, H. and Zhao, L., 2021. Biomimetic silibinin-loaded macrophage-derived exosomes induce dual inhibition of Aβ aggregation and astrocyte activation to alleviate cognitive impairment in a model of Alzheimer's disease. Materials Science and Engineering. C, Materials for Biological Applications 129: 112365.

Hussain, S.A., Jassim, N.A., Numan, I.T., Al-Khalifa, I.I. and Abdullah, T.A., 2009. Anti-inflammatory activity of silymarin in patients with knee osteoarthritis. A comparative study with piroxicam and meloxicam. Saudi Medical Journal 30: 98-103.

Hussein, R.M., Sawy, D.M., Kandeil, M.A. and Farghaly, H.S., 2021. Chlorogenic acid, quercetin, coenzyme Q10 and silymarin modulate Keap1-Nrf2/heme oxygenase-1 signaling in thioacetamide-induced acute liver toxicity. Life Sciences 277: 119460.

Impellizzeri, D., Bruschetta, G., Ahmad, A., Crupi, R., Siracusa, R., Di Paola, R., Paterniti, I., Prosdocimi, M., Esposito, E. and Cuzzocrea, S., 2015. Effects of palmitoylethanolamide and silymarin combination treatment in an animal model of kidney ischemia and reperfusion. European Journal of Pharmacology 762: 136-149.

Itoh, M., Ogawa, Y. and Suganami, T., 2020. Chronic inflammation as a molecular basis of nonalcoholic steatohepatitis: role of macrophages and fibroblasts in the liver. Nagoya Journal of Medical Science 82: 391-397.

Jain, P., Pandey, R. and Shukla, S.S., 2015. Inflammation: Natural resources and its applications. Springer, New Delhi, India.

Jin, G., Bai, D., Yin, S., Yang, Z., Zou, D., Zhang, Z., Li, X., Sun, Y. and Zhu, Q., 2016b. Silibinin rescues learning and memory deficits by attenuating microglia activation and preventing neuroinflammatory reactions in SAMP8 mice. Neuroscience Letters 629: 256-261.

Jin, Y., Zhao, X., Zhang, H., Li, Q., Lu, G. and Zhao, X., 2016a. Modulatory effect of silymarin on pulmonary vascular dysfunction through HIF-1α-iNOS following rat lung ischemia-reperfusion injury. Experimental and Therapeutic Medicine 12: 1135-1140.

Jung, U.J., Jeon, M.T., Choi, M.S. and Kim, S.R., 2014. Silibinin attenuates MPP^+-induced neurotoxicity in the substantia nigra *in vivo*. Journal of Medicinal Food 17: 599-605.

Juráňová, J., Aury-Landas, J., Boumediene, K., Baugé, C., Biedermann, D., Ulrichová, J. and Franková, J., 2019. Modulation of skin inflammatory response by active components of silymarin. Molecules 24: 123.

Kapellos, T.S. and Iqbal, A.J., 2016. Epigenetic control of macrophage polarisation and soluble mediator gene expression during inflammation. Mediators of Inflammation 2016: 6591703.

Kim, B.R., Seo, H.S., Ku, J.M., Kim, G.J., Jeon, C.Y., Park, J.H., Jang, B.H., Park, S.J., Shin, Y.C. and Ko, S.G., 2013. Silibinin inhibits the production of pro-inflammatory cytokines through inhibition of NF-κB signaling pathway in HMC-1 human mast cells. Inflammation Research 62: 941-950.

Kim, E.J., Lee, M.Y. and Jeon, Y.J., 2015. Silymarin inhibits morphological changes in LPS-stimulated macrophages by blocking NF-κB pathway. The Korean Journal of Physiology and Pharmacology 19: 211-218.

Kim, S.H., Oh, D.S., Oh, J.Y., Son, T.G., Yuk, D.Y. and Jung, Y.S., 2016. Silymarin prevents restraint stress-induced acute liver injury by ameliorating oxidative stress and reducing inflammatory response. Molecules 21: 443.

Ko, J.W., Shin, N.R., Park, S.H., Lee, I.C., Ryu, J.M., Kim, H.J., Cho, Y.K., Kim, J.C. and Shin, I.S., 2017. Silibinin inhibits the fibrotic responses induced by cigarette smoke via suppression of TGF-β1/Smad 2/3 signaling. Food and Chemical Toxicology 106(Pt A): 424-429.

Kogut, M.H., Genovese, K., Swaggerty, C.L., He, H. and Broom, L., 2018. Inflammatory phenotypes in the intestine of poultry: not all inflammation is created equal. Poultry Science 97: 2339-2346.

Kosari-Nasab, M., Shokouhi, G., Ghorbanihaghjo, A., Abbasi, M.M. and Salari, A.A., 2018. Anxiolytic- and antidepressant-like effects of silymarin compared to diazepam and fluoxetine in a mouse model of mild traumatic brain injury. Toxicology and Applied Pharmacology 338: 159-173.

Kumar, J., Park, K.C., Awasthi, A. and Prasad, B., 2015. Silymarin extends lifespan and reduces proteotoxicity in C. elegans Alzheimer's model. CNS and Neurological Disorders Drug Targets 14: 295-302.

Kuo, F.H. and Jan, T.R., 2009. Silibinin attenuates antigen-specific IgE production through the modulation of Th1/Th2 balance in ovalbumin-sensitized BALB/c mice. Phytomedicine 16: 271-276.

Lee, S.J., Nam, M.J., Lee, D.E., Park, J.W., Kang, B.S., Lee, D.S., Lee, H.S. and Kwon, O.S., 2018. Silibinin ameliorates O-GlcNAcylation and inflammation in a mouse model of nonalcoholic steatohepatitis. International Journal of Molecular Sciences 19: 2165.

Leem, E., Oh, Y.S., Shin, W.H., Jin, B.K., Jeong, J.Y., Shin, M., Kim, D.W., Jang, J.H., Kim, H.J., Ha, C.M., Jung, U.J., Moon, G.J. and Kim, S.R., 2019. Effects of silibinin against prothrombin Kringle-2-induced neurotoxicity in the nigrostriatal dopaminergic system *in vivo*. Journal of Medicinal Food 22: 277-285.

Lei, Y., Wang, K., Deng, L., Chen, Y., Nice, E.C. and Huang, C., 2015. Redox regulation of inflammation: old elements, a new story. Medicinal Research Reviews 35: 306-340.

Li, D., Hu, J., Wang, T., Zhang, X., Liu, L., Wang, H., Wu, Y., Xu, D. and Wen, F., 2016. Silymarin attenuates cigarette smoke extract-induced inflammation via simultaneous inhibition of autophagy and ERK/p38 MAPK pathway in human bronchial epithelial cells. Scientific Reports 6: 37751.

Li, D., Xu, D., Wang, T., Shen, Y., Guo, S., Zhang, X., Guo, L., Li, X., Liu, L. and Wen, F., 2015. Silymarin attenuates airway inflammation induced by cigarette smoke in mice. Inflammation 38: 871-878.

Lim, R., Morwood, C.J. Lim, J.O., Shin, N.R., Seo, Y.S., Nam, H.H., Ko, J.W., Jung, T.Y., Lee, S.J., Kim, H.J., Cho, Y.K., Kim, J.C., Lee, I.C., Kim, J.S. and Shin, I.S., 2020. Silibinin attenuates silica dioxide nanoparticles-induced inflammation by suppressing TXNIP/MAPKs/AP-1 signaling. Cells 9: 678.

Lim, R., Morwood, C.J., Barker, G. and Lappas, M., 2014. Effect of silibinin in reducing inflammatory pathways in *in vitro* and *in vivo* models of infection-induced preterm birth. PloS One 9: e92505.

Liu, W., Li, Y., Zheng, X., Zhang, K. and Du, Z., 2015. Potent inhibitory effect of silibinin from milk thistle on skin inflammation stimuli by 12-O-tetradecanoylphorbol-13-acetate. Food and Function 6: 3712-3719.

Liu, X., Xu, Q., Long, X., Liu, W., Zhao, Y., Hayashi, T., Hattori, S., Fujisaki, H., Ogura, T., Tashiro, S.I., Onodera, S., Yamato, M. and Ikejima, T., 2019. Silibinin-induced autophagy mediated by PPARα-sirt1-AMPK pathway participated in the regulation of type I collagen-enhanced migration in murine 3T3-L1 preadipocytes. Molecular and Cellular Biochemistry 450: 1-23.

Liu, D., Zhong, Z. and Karin, M., 2022. NF-κB: A double-edged sword controlling inflammation. Biomedicines 10: 1250.

Liu, Z., Sun, M., Wang, Y., Zhang, L., Zhao, H. and Zhao, M., 2018. Silymarin attenuated paraquat-induced cytotoxicity in macrophage by regulating Trx/TXNIP complex, inhibiting NLRP3 inflammasome activation and apoptosis. Toxicology in Vitro 46: 265-272.

Lovelace, E.S., Maurice, N.J., Miller, H.W., Slichter, C.K., Harrington, R., Magaret, A., Prlic, M., De Rosa, S. and Polyak, S.J., 2017. Silymarin suppresses basal and stimulus-induced activation, exhaustion, differentiation, and inflammatory markers in primary human immune cells. PloS One 12: e0171139.

Lovelace, E.S., Wagoner, J., MacDonald, J., Bammler, T., Bruckner, J., Brownell, J., Beyer, R.P., Zink, E.M., Kim, Y.M., Kyle, J.E., Webb-Robertson, B.J., Waters, K.M., Metz, T.O., Farin, F., Oberlies, N.H. and Polyak, S.J., 2015. Silymarin suppresses cellular inflammation by inducing reparative stress signaling. Journal of Natural Products 78: 1990-2000.

Lu, C.P., Huang, C.Y., Wang, S.H., Chiu, C.H., Li, L.H., Hua, K.F. and Wu, T.H., 2018. Improvement of hyperglycemia in a murine model of insulin resistance and high glucose- and inflammasome-mediated IL-1β expressions in macrophages by silymarin. Chemico-Biological Interactions 290: 12-18.

Luster, M.I., Simeonova, P.P., Gallucci, R.M., Matheson, J.M. and Yucesoy, B., 2000. Immunotoxicology: role of inflammation in chemical-induced hepatotoxicity. International Journal of Immunopharmacology, 22(12), 1143-1147.

Mady, F.M., Essa, H., El-Ammawi, T., Abdelkader, H. and Hussein, A.K., 2016. Formulation and clinical evaluation of silymarin pluronic-lecithin organogels for treatment of atopic dermatitis. Drug Design, Development and Therapy 10: 1101-1110.

Mahmoodi-Nesheli, M., Alizadeh, S., Solhi, H., Mohseni, J. and Mahmoodi-Nesheli, M., 2018. Adjuvant effect of oral silymarin on patients' wound healing process caused by thermal injuries. Caspian Journal of Internal Medicine 9: 341-346.

Marin, V., Gazzin, S., Gambaro, S.E., Dal Ben, M., Calligaris, S., Anese, M., Raseni, A., Avellini, C., Giraudi, P.J., Tiribelli, C. and Rosso, N., 2017. Effects of oral administration of silymarin in a juvenile murine model of non-alcoholic steatohepatitis. Nutrients 9: 1006.

Matias, M.L., Gomes, V.J., Romao-Veiga, M., Ribeiro, V.R., Nunes, P.R., Romagnoli, G.G., Peracoli, J.C. and Peracoli, M., 2019. Silibinin downregulates the NF-κB pathway and NLRP1/NLRP3 inflammasomes in monocytes from pregnant women with preeclampsia. Molecules 24: 1548.

Mazhari, S., Razi, M. and Sadrkhanlou, R., 2018. Silymarin and celecoxib ameliorate experimental varicocele-induced pathogenesis: evidences for oxidative stress and inflammation inhibition. International Urology and Nephrology 50: 1039-1052.

Menzel, A., Samouda, H., Dohet, F., Loap, S., Ellulu, M.S. and Bohn, T., 2021. Common and novel markers for measuring inflammation and oxidative stress Ex Vivo in research and clinical practice – Which to use regarding disease outcomes?. Antioxidants 10: 414.

Miethe, C., Nix, H., Martin, R., Hernandez, A.R. and Price, R.S., 2017. Silibinin reduces the impact of obesity on invasive liver cancer. Nutrition and Cancer 69: 1272-1280.

Min, K., Yoon, W.K., Kim, S.K. and Kim, B.H., 2007. Immunosuppressive effect of silibinin in experimental autoimmune encephalomyelitis. Archives of Pharmacal Research 30: 1265-1272.

Moghaddam, A.H., Mokhtari Sangdehi, S.R., Ranjbar, M. and Hasantabar, V., 2020. Preventive effect of silymarin-loaded chitosan nanoparticles against global cerebral ischemia/reperfusion injury in rats. European Journal of Pharmacology 877: 173066.

Mohammadi, H., Manouchehri, H., Changizi, R., Bootorabi, F. and Khorramizadeh, M.R., 2020. Concurrent metformin and silibinin therapy in diabetes: assessments in zebrafish (Danio rerio) animal model. Journal of Diabetes and Metabolic Disorders 19: 1233-1244.

Nasab, E.M., Athari, S.M., Ghafarzade, S., Nasab, A.M. and Athari, S.S., 2020. Immunomodulatory effects of two silymarin isomers in a Balb/c mouse model of allergic asthma. Allergologia et Immunopathologia 48: 646-653.

Navabi, F., Shayganneja, V., Abbasirad, F., Vaez, E., Hosseininasab, F., Kazemi, M., Mirmosayyeb, O., Alsahebfosoul, F. and Esmaeil, N., 2019. Immunoregulatory effects of silymarin on proliferation and activation of Th1 cells isolated from newly diagnosed and IFN-β_{1b}-treated MS patients. Inflammation 42: 54-63.

Nazemian, F., Karimi, G., Moatamedi, M., Charkazi, S., Shamsara, J. and Mohammadpour, A.H., 2010. Effect of silymarin administration on TNF-α serum concentration in peritoneal dialysis patients. Phytotherapy Research 24: 1654-1657.

Oryan, A., Tabatabaei Naeini, A., Moshiri, A., Mohammadalipour, A. and Tabandeh, M.R., 2012. Modulation of cutaneous wound healing by silymarin in rats. Journal of Wound Care 21: 457-464.

Ou, Q., Weng, Y., Wang, S., Zhao, Y., Zhang, F., Zhou, J. and Wu, X., 2018. Silybin alleviates hepatic steatosis and fibrosis in NASH mice by inhibiting oxidative stress and involvement with the Nf-κB pathway. Digestive Diseases and Sciences 63: 3398-3408.

Papackova, Z., Heczkova, M., Dankova, H., Sticova, E., Lodererova, A., Bartonova, L., Poruba, M. and Cahova, M., 2018. Silymarin prevents acetaminophen-induced hepatotoxicity in mice. PloS One 13: e0191353.

Park, J.W., Shin, N.R., Shin, I.S., Kwon, O.K., Kim, J.S., Oh, S.R., Kim, J.H. and Ahn, K.S., 2016. Silibinin inhibits neutrophilic inflammation and mucus secretion induced by cigarette smoke via suppression of ERK-SP1 pathway. Phytotherapy Research 30: 1926-1936.

Podder, B., Kim, Y.S., Zerin, T. and Song, H.Y., 2012. Antioxidant effect of silymarin on paraquat-induced human lung adenocarcinoma A549 cell line. Food and Chemical Toxicology 50: 3206-3214.

Raina, K., Agarwal, C. and Agarwal, R., 2013. Effect of silibinin in human colorectal cancer cells: targeting the activation of NF-κB signaling. Molecular Carcinogenesis 52: 195-206.

Razavi-Azarkhiavi, K., Ali-Omrani, M., Solgi, R., Bagheri, P., Haji-Noormohammadi, M., Amani, N. and Sepand, M.R., 2014. Silymarin alleviates bleomycin-induced pulmonary toxicity and lipid peroxidation in mice. Pharmaceutical Biology 52: 1267-1271.

Ribeiro, V.R., Romao-Veiga, M., Nunes, P.R., de Oliveira, L., Romagnoli, G.G., Peracoli, J.C. and Peracoli, M., 2022. Silibinin downregulates the expression of the Th1 and Th17 profiles by modulation of STATs and transcription factors in pregnant women with preeclampsia. International Immunopharmacology 109: 108807.

Rigby, C.M., Roy, S., Deep, G., Guillermo-Lagae, R., Jain, A.K., Dhar, D., Orlicky, D.J., Agarwal, C. and Agarwal, R., 2017. Role of p53 in silibinin-mediated inhibition of ultraviolet B radiation-induced DNA damage, inflammation and skin carcinogenesis. Carcinogenesis 38: 40-50.

Rigon, C., Marchiori, M., da Silva Jardim, F., Pegoraro, N.S., Chaves, P., Velho, M.C., Beck, R., Ourique, A.F., Sari, M., Oliveira, S.M. and Cruz, L., 2019. Hydrogel containing silibinin nanocapsules presents effective anti-inflammatory action in a model of irritant contact dermatitis in mice. European Journal of Pharmaceutical Sciences 137: 104969.

Robinson, M.W., Harmon, C. and O'Farrelly, C., 2016. Liver immunology and its role in inflammation and homeostasis. Cellular and Molecular Immunology 13: 267-276.

Salamone, F., Galvano, F., Cappello, F., Mangiameli, A., Barbagallo, I. and Li Volti, G., 2012. Silibinin modulates lipid homeostasis and inhibits nuclear factor kappa B activation in experimental nonalcoholic steatohepatitis. Translational Research 59: 477-486.

Saliou, C., Valacchi, G. and Rimbach, G., 2001. Assessing bioflavonoids as regulators of NF-kappa B activity and inflammatory gene expression in mammalian cells. Methods in Enzymology 335: 380-387.

Sarubbo, F., Ramis, M.R., Kienzer, C., Aparicio, S., Esteban, S., Miralles, A. and Moranta, D., 2018. Chronic silymarin, quercetin and naringenin treatments increase monoamines synthesis and hippocampal Sirt1 levels improving cognition in aged rats. Journal of Neuroimmune Pharmacology 13: 24-38.

Saxena, N., Dhaked, R.K. and Nagar, D.P., 2022. Silibinin ameliorates abrin induced hepatotoxicity by attenuating oxidative stress, inflammation and inhibiting Fas pathway. Environmental Toxicology and Pharmacology 93: 103868.

Schümann, J., Prockl, J., Kiemer, A.K., Vollmar, A.M., Bang, R. and Tiegs, G., 2003. Silibinin protects mice from T cell-dependent liver injury. Journal of Hepatology 39: 333-340.

Sharifi, R., Pasalar, P., Kamalinejad, M., Dehpour, A.R., Tavangar, S.M., Paknejad, M., Mehrabani Natanzi, M., Nourbakhsh, M., Ahmadi Ashtiani, H.R., Akbari, M. and Rastegar, H., 2013. The effect of silymarin (*Silybum marianum*) on human skin fibroblasts in an *in vitro* wound healing model. Pharmaceutical Biology 51: 298-303.

Sharifi, R., Rastegar, H., Kamalinejad, M., Dehpour, A.R., Tavangar, S.M., Paknejad, M., Mehrabani Natanzi, M., Ghannadian, N., Akbari, M. and Pasalar, P., 2012. Effect of topical application of silymarin (*Silybum marianum*) on excision wound healing in albino rats. Acta Medica Iranica 50: 583-588.

Shen, H.H., Alex, R., Bellner, L., Raffaele, M., Licari, M., Vanella, L., Stec, D.E. and Abraham, N.G., 2020. Milk thistle seed cold press oil attenuates markers of the metabolic syndrome in a mouse model of dietary-induced obesity. Journal of Food Biochemistry 44: e13522.

Shen, Y., Zhao, H., Wang, Z., Guan, W., Kang, X., Tai, X. and Sun, Y., 2019. Silibinin declines blue light-induced apoptosis and inflammation through MEK/ERK/CREB of retinal ganglion cells. Artificial Cells, Nanomedicine, and Biotechnology 47: 4059-4065.

Shokouhi, G., Kosari-Nasab, M. and Salari, A.A., 2020. Silymarin sex-dependently improves cognitive functions and alters TNF-α, BDNF, and glutamate in the hippocampus of mice with mild traumatic brain injury. Life Sciences 257: 118049.

Sokar, S.S., El-Sayad, M.E., Ghoneim, M.E. and Shebl, A.M., 2017. Combination of Sitagliptin and silymarin ameliorates liver fibrosis induced by carbon tetrachloride in rats. Biomedicine and Pharmacotherapy 89: 98-107.

Soleimani, H., Behfar, M. and Hobbenaghi, R., 2021. Tenogenic effects of silymarin following experimental Achilles tendon transection in rats. Veterinary Research Forum 12: 69-75.

Son, Y., Lee, H.J., Rho, J.K., Chung, S.Y., Lee, C.G., Yang, K., Kim, S.H., Lee, M., Shin, I.S. and Kim, J.S., 2015. The ameliorative effect of silibinin against radiation-induced lung injury: protection of normal tissue without decreasing therapeutic efficacy in lung cancer. BMC Pulmonary Medicine 15: 68.

Song, J.M., Qian, X., Molla, K., Teferi, F., Upadhyaya, P., O Sullivan, G., Luo, X. and Kassie, F., 2015. Combinations of indole-3-carbinol and silibinin suppress inflammation-driven mouse lung tumorigenesis by modulating critical cell cycle regulators. Carcinogenesis 36: 666-675.

Song, J., Pan, W., Sun, Y., Han, J., Shi, W. and Liao, W., 2017. Aspergillus fumigatus-induced early inflammatory response in pulmonary microvascular endothelial cells: Role of p38 MAPK and inhibition by silibinin. International Immunopharmacology 49: 195-202.

Speciale, A., Muscarà, C., Molonia, M.S., Cimino, F., Saija, A. and Giofrè, S.V., 2021. Silibinin as potential tool against SARS-Cov-2: In silico spike receptor-binding domain and main protease molecular docking analysis, and *in vitro* endothelial protective effects. Phytotherapy Research 35: 4616-4625.

Stolf, A.M., Campos Cardoso, C., Morais, H., Alves de Souza, C.E., Lomba, L.A., Brandt, A.P., Agnes, J.P., Collere, F.C., Galindo, C.M., Corso, C.R., Spercoski, K.M., Locatelli Dittrich, R., Zampronio, A.R., Cadena, S. and Acco, A., 2018. Effects of silymarin on angiogenesis and oxidative stress in streptozotocin-induced diabetes in mice. Biomedicine and Pharmacotherapy 108: 232-243.

Surai, P.F., 2015. Silymarin as a natural antioxidant: an overview of the current evidence and perspectives. Antioxidants 4: 204-247.

Surai, P.F., 2020. Vitagene in avian biology and poultry health. Wageningen Academic Publishers, Wageningen, The Netherlands.

Tewari-Singh, N., Jain, A.K., Inturi, S., Agarwal, C., White, C.W. and Agarwal, R., 2012. Silibinin attenuates sulfur mustard analog-induced skin injury by targeting multiple pathways connecting oxidative stress and inflammation. PloS One 7: e46149.

Thibaut, R., Gage, M.C., Pineda-Torra, I., Chabrier, G., Venteclef, N. and Alzaid, F., 2022. Liver macrophages and inflammation in physiology and physiopathology of non-alcoholic fatty liver disease. The FEBS Journal 289: 3024-3057.

Toklu, H.Z., Tunali Akbay, T., Velioglu-Ogunc, A., Ercan, F., Gedik, N., Keyer-Uysal, M. and Sener, G., 2008. Silymarin, the antioxidant component of *Silybum marianum*, prevents sepsis-induced acute lung and brain injury. The Journal of Surgical Research 145: 214-222.

Tong, W.W., Zhang, C., Hong, T., Liu, D.H., Wang, C., Li, J., He, X.K. and Xu, W.D., 2018. Silibinin alleviates inflammation and induces apoptosis in human rheumatoid arthritis fibroblast-like synoviocytes and has a therapeutic effect on arthritis in rats. Scientific Reports 8: 3241.

Toomari, E., Hajian, S., Mojab, F., Omidkhah, T. and Nasiri, M., 2021. Evaluation the effect of *Silybum marianum* ointment on episiotomy wound healing and pain intensity in primiparous women: a randomized triple blind clinical trial. BMC Complementary Medicine and Therapies 21: 253.

Uçmak, F., Ekin, N., İbiloğlu, İ., Arslan, S., Kaplan, İ. and Şenateş, E., 2016. Prophylactic administration of silybin ameliorates L-Arginine-induced acute pancreatitis. Medical Science Monitor 22: 3641-3646.

Vangaveti, S., Das, P. and Kumar, V.L., 2021. Metformin and silymarin afford protection in cyclosporine A induced hepatorenal toxicity in rat by modulating redox status and inflammation. Journal of Biochemical and Molecular Toxicology 35: e22614.

Vargas-Mendoza, N., Ángeles-Valencia, M., Madrigal-Santillán, E.O., Morales-Martínez, M., Tirado-Lule, J.M., Solano-Urrusquieta, A., Madrigal-Bujaidar, E., Álvarez-González, I., Fregoso-Aguilar, T., Morales-González, Á. and Morales-González, J.A., 2020. Effect of silymarin supplementation on physical performance, muscle and myocardium histological changes, bodyweight, and food consumption in rats subjected to regular exercise training. International Journal of Molecular Sciences 21: 7724.

Vargas-Mendoza, N., Angeles-Valencia, M., Morales-González, Á., Morales-Martínez, M., Madrigal-Bujaidar, E., Álvarez-González, I., Fregoso-Aguilar, T., Delgado-Olivares, L., Madrigal-Santillán, E.O. and Morales-González, J.A., 2021. Effect of silymarin supplementation in lung and liver histological modifications during exercise training in a rodent model. Journal of Functional Morphology and Kinesiology 6: 72.

Wang, C., Wang, Z., Zhang, X., Zhang, X., Dong, L., Xing, Y., Li, Y., Liu, Z., Chen, L., Qiao, H., Wang, L. and Zhu, C., 2012. Protection by silibinin against experimental ischemic stroke: up-regulated pAkt, pmTOR, HIF-1α and Bcl-2, down-regulated Bax, NF-κB expression. Neuroscience Letters 529: 45-50.

Wang, L., Huang, Q.H., Li, Y.X., Huang, Y.F., Xie, J.H., Xu, L.Q., Dou, Y.X., Su, Z.R., Zeng, H.F. and Chen, J.N., 2018. Protective effects of silymarin on triptolide-induced acute hepatotoxicity in rats. Molecular Medicine Reports 17: 789-800.

Wu, W.T., Chen, Y.R., Lu, D.H., Senatov, F.S., Yang, K.C. and Wang, C.C., 2021. Silymarin modulates catabolic cytokine expression through Sirt1 and SOX9 in human articular chondrocytes. Journal of Orthopaedic Surgery and Research 16: 147.

Xu, W., Sun, Y., Wang, J., Wang, B., Xu, F., Xie, Z. and Wang, Y., 2022. Controlled release of silibinin in GelMA hydrogels inhibits inflammation by inducing M2-type macrophage polarization and promotes vascularization *in vitro*. RSC Advances 12: 13192-13202.

Yang, H.L. and Shi, X.W., 2021. Silybin alleviates experimental autoimmune encephalomyelitis by suppressing dendritic cell activation and Th17 cell differentiation. Frontiers in Neurology 12: 659678.

Yardım, A., Kucukler, S., Özdemir, S., Çomaklı, S., Caglayan, C., Kandemir, F.M. and Çelik, H., 2021. Silymarin alleviates docetaxel-induced central and peripheral neurotoxicity by reducing oxidative stress, inflammation and apoptosis in rats. Gene 769: 145239.

Yassin, N., AbouZid, S.F., El-Kalaawy, A.M., Ali, T.M., Elesawy, B.H. and Ahmed, O.M., 2021. Tackling of renal carcinogenesis in Wistar rats by *Silybum marianum* total extract, silymarin, and silibinin via modulation of oxidative stress, apoptosis, Nrf2, PPARγ, NF-κB, and PI3K/Akt signaling pathways. Oxidative Medicine and Cellular Longevity 2021: 7665169.

Ye, Z., Zhang, X., Huang, Q., Zhang, W. and Ye, M., 2021. Synergistic hepatoprotective effect of combined administration of Lachnum polysaccharide with silymarin. Bioorganic and Medicinal Chemistry Letters 46: 128159.

Yu, W., Tu, Y., Long, Z., Liu, J., Kong, D., Peng, J., Wu, H., Zheng, G., Zhao, J., Chen, Y., Liu, R., Li, W. and Hai, C., 2022a. Reactive oxygen species bridge the gap between chronic inflammation and tumor development. Oxidative Medicine and Cellular Longevity 2022: 2606928.

Yu, C., Wang, D., Yang, Z. and Wang, T., 2022b. Pharmacological effects of polyphenol phytochemicals on the intestinal inflammation via targeting TLR4/NF-κB signaling pathway. International Journal of Molecular Sciences 23: 6939.

Zarpou, S., Mosavi, H., Bagheri, A., Malekzadeh Shafaroudi, M. and Khonakdar-Tarsi, A., 2021. NF-κB and NLRP3 gene expression changes during warm hepatic ischemia-reperfusion in rats with and without silibinin. Gastroenterology and Hepatology From Bed to Bench 14: 267-275.

Zaulet, M., Kevorkian, S., Dinescu, S., Cotoraci, C., Suciu, M., Herman, H., Buburuzan, L., Badulescu, L., Ardelean, A. and Hermenean, A., 2017. Protective effects of silymarin against bisphenol A-induced hepatotoxicity in mouse liver. Experimental and Therapeutic Medicine 13: 821-828.

Zhang, B., Wang, B., Cao, S., Wang, Y. and Wu, D., 2017. Silybin attenuates LPS-induced lung injury in mice by inhibiting NF-κB signaling and NLRP3 activation. International Journal of Molecular Medicine 39: 1111-1118.

Zhang, B., Xu, D., She, L., Wang, Z., Yang, N., Sun, R., Zhang, Y., Yan, C., Wei, Q., Aa, J., Liu, B., Wang, G. and Xie, Y., 2018. Silybin inhibits NLRP3 inflammasome assembly through the NAD+/SIRT2 pathway in mice with nonalcoholic fatty liver disease. FASEB Journal 32: 757-767.

Zhang, J., Shi, Q., Hu, Y. and Li, X., 2022. Silibinin augments the effect of clopidogrel on atherosclerosis in diabetic ApoE deficiency mice. Clinical Hemorheology and Microcirculation 80: 353-361.

Zhang, R., Xu, D., Zhang, Y., Wang, R., Yang, N., Lou, Y., Zhao, H., Aa, J., Wang, G. and Xie, Y., 2021. Silybin restored CYP3A expression through the Sirtuin 2/Nuclear Factor κ-B pathway in mouse nonalcoholic fatty liver disease. Drug Metabolism and Disposition 49: 770-779.

Zhao, X.A., Chen, G.M., Liu, Y., Chen, Y.X., Wu, H.Y., Chen, J., Xiong, Y.L., Tian, C., Wang, G.Y., Jia, B., Xia, J., Wang, J., Yan, X.M., Zhang, Z.P., Huang, R. and Wu, C., 2017. Inhibitory effect of silymarin on CCl_4-induced liver fibrosis by reducing Ly6C^{hi} monocytes infiltration. International Journal of Clinical and Experimental Pathology 10: 11941-11951.

Zhao, X., Wang, H., Yang, Y., Gou, Y., Wang, Z., Yang, D. and Li, C., 2021. Protective effects of silymarin against D-Gal/LPS-induced organ damage and Inflammation in mice. Drug Design, Development and Therapy 15: 1903-1914.

Zheng, R., Ma, J., Wang, D., Dong, W., Wang, S., Liu, T., Xie, R., Liu, L., Wang, B. and Cao, H., 2018. Chemopreventive effects of silibinin on colitis-associated tumorigenesis by inhibiting IL-6/STAT3 signaling pathway. Mediators of Inflammation 2018: 1562010.

Zheng, W., Feng, Z., Lou, Y., Chen, C., Zhang, C., Tao, Z., Li, H., Cheng, L. and Ying, X., 2017. Silibinin protects against osteoarthritis through inhibiting the inflammatory response and cartilage matrix degradation *in vitro* and *in vivo*. Oncotarget 8: 99649-99665.

Zheng, Y., Chen, J., Wu, X., Zhang, X., Hu, C., Kang, Y., Lin, J., Li, J., Huang, Y., Zhang, X. and Li, C., 2022. Enhanced anti-inflammatory effects of silibinin and capsaicin combination in lipopolysaccharide-induced RAW264.7 cells by inhibiting NF-κB and MAPK activation. Frontiers in Chemistry 10: 934541.

Zhu, Z. and Sun, G., 2018. Silymarin mitigates lung impairments in a rat model of acute respiratory distress syndrome. Inflammopharmacology 26: 747-754.

Chapter 11
Silymarin and gut health

Actions speak louder than words

*Anton Surai[1] and Peter F. Surai[2-7]**
[1]Healthy Food Services, Bristol, UK; [2]Vitagene and Health Research Centre, Bristol, UK; [3]Department of Microbiology and Biochemistry, Faculty of Veterinary Medicine, Trakia University, Stara Zagora, Bulgaria; [4]Department of Animal Nutrition, Faculty of Agricultural and Environmental Sciences, Szent Istvan University, Hungary; [5]Saint-Petersburg State Academy of Veterinary Medicine, St. Petersburg, Russia; [6]Sumy National Agrarian University, Sumy, Ukraine; [7]Odessa National Academy of Food Technologies, Odessa, Ukraine
psurai@feedfood.co.uk

Abstract

Gut health recently has become a fashionable topic of research since it was realised that gut plays a fundamental role in maintaining our health. On the one hand, the intestine is the major place of nutrient absorption and its integrity is of a paramount importance for healthy nutrition. On the other hand, intestinal microbiota is believed to be involved in regulation of the main physiological functions of the body affecting digestive, nervous, muscle and other systems. Furthermore, the gut is a place where food/feed-derived microbes, including pathogens, meet the protective weaponry of the body in the form of gut immune system and therefore human/animal health starts in the gut. A delicate balance between antioxidants and prooxidants (redox balance) in cells is an important determinant of various physiological processes and maintenance of this balance is the main aim of the so-called integrated antioxidant system of the human/animal body. The data presented in this chapter clearly demonstrates protective effects of silymarin (SM) in gut health maintenance. It seems likely, that SM can improve gut health and adaptive ability of human/farm animals and poultry to various stresses by activating Nrf2, suppressing NF-κB and upregulating major vitagenes. However, molecular mechanisms of such regulatory actions of SM in the gut require more research. Taking into account high concentrations of phytochemicals in the gut, it could well be that they play an essential part in maintaining an optimal antioxidant-prooxidant balance in the digestive tract responsible for additional health effects of polyphenolics including SM. In animal nutrition and disease prevention strategy SM alone, or in combination with other hepato-active compounds (carnitine, betaine, taurine, vitamin B12, etc.), could have similar hepatoprotective effects as described in humans with similar mechanisms of protective action.

Keywords: silymarin, gut health, inflammation, NF-κB, Nrf2, vitagenes, redox homeostasis

DOI:10.3920/978-90-8686-944-2_011,

11.1 Introduction

Gut health recently has become a fashionable topic of research since it was realised that gut plays a fundamental role in maintaining our health. On the one hand, the intestine is the major place of nutrient absorption and its integrity is of a paramount importance for healthy nutrition. On the other hand, intestinal microbiota is believed to be involved in regulation of the main physiological functions of the body affecting digestive, nervous, muscle and other systems. Furthermore, the gut is a place where food/feed-derived microbes, including pathogens, meet the protective weaponry of the body in the form of gut immune system and therefore human/animal health starts in the gut. A delicate balance between antioxidants and prooxidants (redox balance) in cells is an important determinant of various physiological processes and maintenance of this balance is the main aim of the so-called integrated antioxidant system of the human/animal body. This system was developed during evolution to provide antioxidant defence and give a chance for human/animals to survive in an oxygenated atmosphere. Recent data suggest that the antioxidant-prooxidant balance starts in the intestine. When food is consumed and appears in the stomach and then in the small intestine, it contains a range of antioxidants but may also contain a range of potentially dangerous substances.

Keeping a balance between antioxidants and prooxidants in the intestine is a very important task in which diet plays a crucial role. In general, the prooxidants or their sources which can be found in the GIT include:

- oxidised poly-unsaturated fatty acids;
- iron ions;
- nitrites and nitrates;
- heavy metals;
- mycotoxins;
- immune cells;
- other sources.

The physicochemical environment of the gastrointestinal tract depends on many factors, with diet, bacterial metabolites and body secretion being major determinants (Sanderson, 1999). There is a delicate balance between the environment of the lumen and epithelial cell functionality, and dietary factors are responsible for gene expression in the intestine and its adaptation. In this regard, oxidative stress could cause changes in this balance affecting the absorption of nutrients. Even if each of those lipid peroxidation promoters is present at a very low concentration, their combination could be much more powerful. For example, lipid hydroperoxides can produce peroxyl radicals in presence of iron or copper ions and once the chain reaction of lipid peroxidation has started many other food-derived PUFAs can be oxidised. It has been calculated that the pH and temperature, as well as presence of oxygen in stomach can be favourable for lipid peroxidation (Kanner and Lapidot, 2001). Recent data indicate that the average human or animal/poultry diet contains a range of various prooxidants. In many cases those contaminants are found in the food/feed in low or very low concentrations, however, their various combinations could be an important source of free radical production in the gut.

It is well appreciated that human/animal gut has a complex antioxidant defence network (McLean *et al.*, 2015; Surai, 2002; Surai, 2018; Surai and Fisinin, 2015; Surai *et al.*, 2004; 2020; Tang *et al.*, 2019). There are some antioxidants, such as antioxidant enzymes, including GPx, SOD, CAT, GSH, Trx and coenzyme Q, which can be synthesised in the body. However, the diet is the major provider of nutrients possessing antioxidant properties directly (vitamin E, carotenoids, ascorbic acid, flavonoids, etc.) or being essential for the synthesis of antioxidant enzymes. For example, selenium (Se) is an essential part of a range of selenoproteins performing antioxidant functions (e.g. GPx, TrxR, MsrB, selenoproteins P and W, etc.); manganese (Mn) is an integral part of mitochondrial SOD2; zinc (Zn) and copper (Cu) are important parts of cytosolic SOD1; iron (Fe) is an integral part of CAT.

Recently the vitagene concept has been developed and special attention has been paid to possible applications of the concept in the development of the effective strategy for preventing negative consequences of commercially relevant stresses in poultry/animal production (Surai, 2020). It is important to emphasise that nutritional modulation of vitagene expression and activities is considered to be a new promising direction in nutritional sciences (Surai, 2020). It is important to note that vitagenes operate in the body in close relationship with various transcription factors, including Nrf2 and NF-κB. Therefore, vitagene activation withing the framework of cell signalling have a great variety of additional applications, including gut health and immunity. Elucidating the cellular factors and signalling pathways that maintain intestinal integrity, epithelial proliferation and differentiation is vital to our understanding of gut adaptation to various stresses (Li *et al.*, 2020a).

This chapter presents recent research data related to possible molecular mechanisms of regulatory roles of vitagenes in gut health maintenance in stressful commercial conditions of industrial poultry/animal production with a specific emphasis to possible protective actions of SM.

11.2 Vitagenes in gut defence

Nutritional modulation of vitagenes described earlier (Surai, 2020) is of great importance for gut health maintenance. Vitagenes are expressed in the gut and defensive antioxidant compounds coded by vitagene represent major protective mechanism in the gut. This is especially important in conditions of prohibition of feed antibiotics, a situation when natural gut protective mechanisms are of paramount importance.

11.2.1 SOD

Protective roles of SOD in poultry and animal husbandry have been recently reviewed (Surai, 2016; 2020), however, data on SOD expression and activity in the intestine are quite limited. Protective roles of SOD in animal/poultry physiology are summarised in Figure 11.1. In this sense, it should be noted that SOD is important vitagene being the main driving force in cell/body adaptation to various stress conditions.

In avian intestine electron microscopy with immunostaining allowed to identify that SOD activity was associated with the apical microvilli and, to a lesser degree, with the terminal web (Davis *et al.*, 1989). The surface epithelia of gastrointestinal tract of rats was shown to have high expression of SOD1 and SOD2 suggesting that they play important protective roles in the gut (Dobashi *et al.*, 1989). Hamster tissues from various organs with an intensive cell renewal, including intestine, showed strong SOD immunostaining in differentiated cells (Oberley *et al.*, 1990).

In the gut indirect immunofluorescent staining and histochemistry showed strong SOD2 immunoreactivity in parietal cells, most intramural nerve cell bodies, the colonic interstitial cells at the submucosa-circular muscle layer interface, and intestinal epithelium cells. At the same time, weak to moderate SOD2 immunoreactivity was detected in small submucosal arteries, smooth muscle cells, esophageal striated muscle, gastric epithelium, esophageal epithelium, and intestinal glands (Fang and

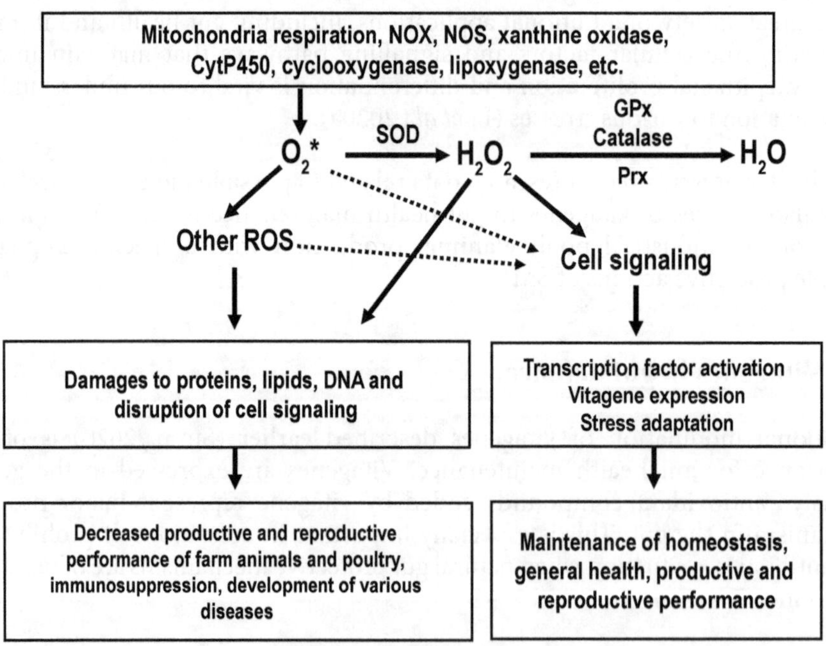

Figure 11.1. Protective roles of SOD in animal/poultry physiology (adapted from Surai, 2020).

Christensen, 1995). In general, SOD in the small intestine and colon of the rat includes both SOD1 and SOD2 with cytosolic form of the enzyme (SOD1) to be characterised by increased expression in comparison to SOD2 (Frederiks and Bosch, 1997; Table 11.1).

In the human gut SOD1 and SOD2 are reported to predominantly expressed in intestinal epithelial cells (Kruidenier *et al.*, 2003).

It is known that SOD can provide significant protection against mucosal damage induced by OH* radicals (Rubinstein *et al.*, 1993). In auto-perfused segments of cat ileum pretreatment with SOD was shown to significantly attenuated the capillary permeability increase induced by regional ischemia (Granger *et al.*, 1981). SOD2 was found to function as a cytokine-regulated acute phase protein involved in cellular protection from free radical-mediated damage. In particular, exposure of intestinal epithelial cell to LPS or pro-inflammatory cytokines (TNF-α) led to a marked increase in SOD2 mRNA. It was proven that de novo transcription but not protein synthesis was required for the LPS- and TNF-α-dependent induction in SOD2 mRNA. Interestingly, treatment with pro-inflammatory IL-1β dramatically increased (12-fold) SOD2 mRNA, however no change was observed due to treatment with IL-6 or IFN-α, immuno-competent molecules which in acute inflammation have anti-inflammatory properties (Valentine and Nick, 1992).

Extracellular H_2O_2 was found to induce damage to cultured gastric mucosal cells and therefore it was suggested that intracellular SOD plays an important role in preventing H_2O_2 damage. Susceptibility to lysis by H_2O_2 was indicated to be inversely related to inhibition of SOD activity (Hiraishi *et al.*, 1994). When SOD is inhibited or overwhelmed, accumulated O_2* would be responsible for reduction of stored Fe^{3+} to Fe^{2+} with following reaction with H_2O_2 and formation of more toxic species, which ultimately would lead to cell damage (Hiraishi *et al.*, 1994). SOD activity in the gastric mucosa was shown to decrease significantly during I/R simultaneously with gastric mucosal injury and it was demonstrated that the decrease in SOD activity in

Table 11.1. Localisation of SOD activity in tissues of 3-month-old male Wistar rats (adapted from Frederiks and Bosch, 1997).[1]

Tissue	SOD activity	SOD1	SOD2
Small intestine			
Enterocytes	+	++	+
Goblet cells	+	++	+
Colon			
Resorptive cells	++	++	+
Goblet cells	+	++	+

[1] + = moderate; ++ = high.

gastric mucosa aggravated mucosal injury by free radicals overproduction and lipid peroxidation (Tanaka and Yuda, 1993). Interestingly, *Lactobacillus* were shown to provide protection to the intestinal barrier and to attenuate oxidative stress in colitis in rats and Crohn's disease in mice by producing bacterial SOD (Han *et al.*, 2006; LeBlanc *et al.*, 2011). In mice exposed to DON, supplementation with fullerene C60 was reported to significantly increase the activities of SOD in the intestine and liver (Liao *et al.*, 2021).

There is a significant difference in total SOD activity between different segments of the chicken gut (Figure 11.2). Based on the SOD activity the laying hen intestinal segments can be placed in the following descending order: duodenum>jejunum= ileum>>ceca>colon. On the one hand, the total SOD activity in the duodenum was significantly (by 40%) higher than that in jejunum or ileum (Surai *et al.*, 2018). On the other hand, the total SOD activity in the ceca was shown to be significantly (by 32%) lower than that in jejunum or ileum, but substantially higher (by 24%) in comparison to that in the colon. Interestingly, lipid peroxidation (MDA) was found to be highest in jejunum and the order of the intestinal segments in accordance with MDA level (jejunum>duodenum>ileum>ceca=colon) is not the same as for SOD, reflecting importance of other protective mechanisms in the intestine (beyond SOD) responsible for antioxidant defences.

There is a need for more detailed evaluation of the antioxidant system of the chicken gut depending on age, nutrition and stress. It would be also particularly important

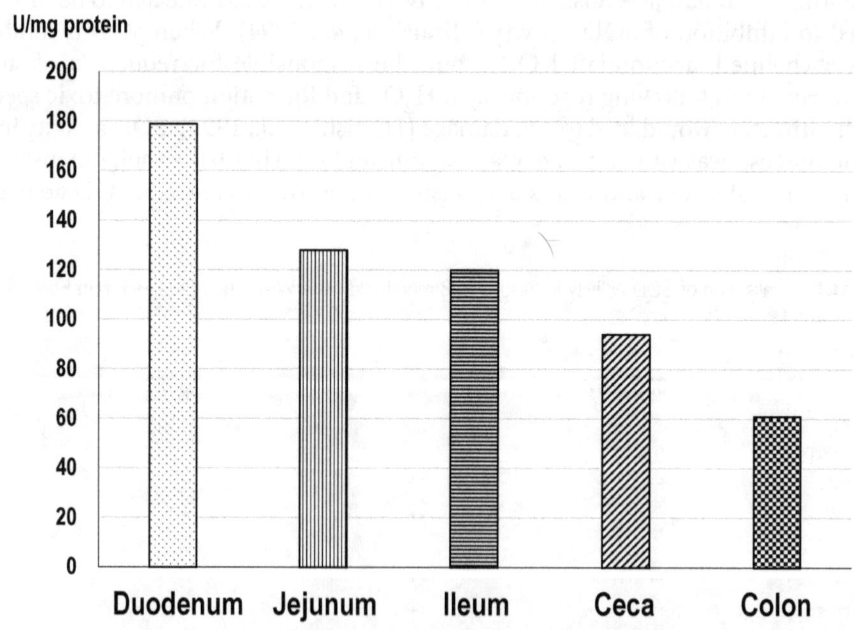

Figure 11.2. Superoxide dismutase activity in chicken gut (adapted from Surai *et al.*, 2018).

to study a relationship between antioxidant defences and microbiota in the chicken gut to understand molecular mechanisms of the maintenance of healthy gut in stress conditions.

A comprehensive study of the antioxidant defence system development in growing chickens conducted by Tang *et al.* (2019) indicates that:

- The heart was characterised by the highest SOD activity in comparison to that of the intestine, liver, and kidney.
- During chicken growth SOD activity in the intestine (duodenum, jejunum, and ileum) was maintained at a comparatively high level.
- SOD activity in the gut is age-dependent: at day 3 the duodenum SOD was the highest and at day 21 the lowest in comparison to its activity in the jejunum and ileum.
- The mucous epithelium was characterised by the highest abundance of SOD1 compared with that in the submucosa and muscular layers.
- SOD1 was highly expressed in mature epithelial cells in comparison to the immature cells located in the crypt.
- A sharp decrease in SOD1, SOD2, and GPx7 mRNA levels was evident at 11 d of age in the entire small intestinal tract.
- Ad day 3 posthatch duodenum, jejunum and ileum have similar level of expression of Nrf2. Furthermore, Nrf2 expression in the duodenum did not depend on bird age, while in the jejunum and ileum, Nrf2 was highly expressed at early age (d3 and d11) and decreased from 3 weeks of age (Tang *et al.*, 2019).

In vitamin-D-replete chicks, SOD1 was shown to be associated with the apical border (microvilli) of the duodenal absorptive cells (Davis *et al.*, 1989). SOD3 expression was found to be decreased in the ileum of laying hens in the late phase of production compared to those at peak production (Wang *et al.*, 2019). Since antioxidant-pro-oxidant balance in the gut plays an important role in chicken health and immunity (Surai and Fisinin, 2015), special emphasis should be given to this area of research.

11.2.1.1 SOD in the gut under various stress conditions

Chronic cyclic heat stress in chickens was shown to downregulate the expression of SOD1 and SOD2 in the duodenum (Dridi *et al.*, 2022). Under cold stress in quails, the SOD expression was reported to be decreased in duodenum, jejunum and ileum of quails. This was associated with a simultaneous increase in the mRNA expression of NF-κB in the same intestinal parts (Fu *et al.*, 2013). Under acute heat stress in chickens, elevated expression of HSP70 (by L-(1)-Glutamine) was indicated to increase the antioxidant capacity of the intestine through improving both enzymatic (including SOD and GPx) and nonenzymatic systems (Gu *et al.*, 2012). High stocking density in laying hens was indicated to significantly decrease SOD activity in the jejunum (Wang *et al.*, 2021). OTA was reported to dramatically decrease SOD activity in chicken caeca while organic Se supplementation was able to partly alleviate that decrease in SOD activity (Yang *et al.*, 2020).

Feeding of DON-contaminated feed (3.5 mg DON/kg) to 4-week-old piglets for 42 days was observed to significantly decrease expression of SOD3, GPx2 and GPx3 (but not GPx4) in the ileum. However, expressions of those antioxidant enzymes were not affected by DON in the jejunum (Lessard *et al.*, 2015). In the caecal tonsil of broilers fed on Met-deficient diet for 40 days SOD activities in cecum tonsil were significantly decreased when compared with the control Met-adequate group (Wu *et al.*, 2018). In a chronic oxidative stress young pig model induced by D-galactose dietary supplementation of α-ketoglutarate (0.5%) for 28 days was shown to increase the SOD and GPx activities including relative mRNA expression in the intestine (Li *et al.*, 2020c).

In piglet colon total superoxide dismutase (T-SOD) and SOD2 activities were increased on day 1 and 3 post-weaning in comparison with day 0 or days 7-14 after weaning. Interestingly, SOD1 activity did not change during the same period (Zhou *et al.*, 2019). Weaning stress in goats was associated with decreased SOD activity in the gut, in particular SOD activity was significantly lower in the lower gut of the young goats at postweaning (age of 11 postnatal weeks) than that in younger pre-weaning goats (at 2 postnatal weeks). Interestingly, a probiotic (*Lactobacillus plantarum*) increased SOD activity in ileum and a plant extract-based prebiotic was able to increase SOD activity in both of ileum and jejunum (Chen *et al.*, 2020). Various avian diseases are shown to negatively affect antioxidant defences including decrease SOD activity in jejunal and ileal parts of the gut challenged with *Salmonella pullorum* (Wang *et al.*, 2012). Broilers fed a diet supplemented with 1×10^9 cfu *Clostridium butyricum*/kg diet had greater SOD activity in the ileal mucosa on d21 and in jejunal mucosa on d42 than those in the other groups fed antibiotic aureomycin or lower doses of the probiotic (Liao *et al.*, 2015).

The mRNA expression of intestinal (ileal) Cu/Zn-superoxide dismutase (*SOD1*) was shown to be significantly upregulated in quercetin-supplemented (200, 400 or 800 mg/kg) broiler chickens (Abdel-Latif *et al.*, 2021). A combination of vitamin E and quercetin fed to aged breeder hens was observed to increase SOD1 expression and SOD activity in duodenum, jejunum and ileum (Amevor *et al.*, 2022). Dietary L-theanine (300 or 600 mg/kg for 14 days) in Chaohu ducks was indicated to increase jejunum SOD activity (Zhang *et al.*, 2019a). In *E. Tenella*-challenged broilers an organic acids mixture was found to increase SOD2 in the caecal tissue (Balta *et al.*, 2021). Dietary magnolol (100-400 mg/kg) was shown to increase expression of SOD in breast muscle, but at the same time it significantly decreased total SOD activity in the muscles. In the same experiment magnolol did not affect SOD activity in broiler jejunum (Xie *et al.*, 2022a).

In earlier study with similar magnolol dosage (100-300 mg/kg) there was an increase in the activity of total SOD in both serum and ileal mucosa on d 42 with increasing magnolol levels (Du *et al.*, 2021). The authors showed that SOD1 expression in the jejunum was linearly up-regulated with increasing magnolol levels. Dietary cottonseed oil (6%) was demonstrated to increase the expression of the SOD and GPx genes in the intestines of 42-day-old broiler (Araujo *et al.*, 2019). Orally administrated *Bacillus coagulans* to newly hatched chicks for 7 days were shown to increase SOD activity in chicken duodenum (Xie *et al.*, 2022b). An *Artemisia argyi* aqueous extract in the broiler diet was shown to increase the T-SOD activity of duodenum and jejunum (Zhao *et al.*, 2016). In weaned piglets dietary probiotics or synbiotics supplementation increased the colonic SOD activity (Wang *et al.*, 2020a).

It could well be that effects of various nutritional and environmental factors on SOD expression and activity could be mediated via Nrf2 modulation. For example, resveratrol (RSV) was observed to mitigate oxidative stress-induced intestinal barrier damages through PI3K/Akt-mediated Nrf2 signalling pathway (Zhuang *et al.*, 2019). Pretreatment of IPEC-J2 cells with RSV improved activities of SOD1, CAT and GPx. Under oxidative stress RSV was reported to upregulate Akt phosphorylation, Nrf2 phosphorylation, and expression levels of such antioxidant genes as HO-1, SOD1, and CAT in a dose-dependent manner and knockdown of Nrf2 was shown to abrogate RSV-mediated protection against oxidative stress and prevented increase in expression of SOD1, CAT, and GPx. Similarly, the PI3K/Akt inhibitor (LY294002) also abrogated protective effect of RSV and suppressed Nrf2 phosphorylation and AO gene expression under oxidative stress conditions (Zhuang *et al.*, 2019).

11.2.2 HSP70

Recently, new mechanisms of adaptive defences of the gastrointestinal mucosa at the intracellular level have been characterised. One of these responses, known as the heat shock response, is considered to be a universal fundamental mechanism necessary for cell survival under a variety of unfavourable conditions (Santoro, 2000). As mentioned above, intestinal cells are challenged with a great variety of potentially toxic compounds and their protection is a vital part of the strategy to maintain animal/poultry health. In mammalian/avian cells, the induction of the heat shock response requires the activation and translocation to the nucleus of one or more heat shock transcription factors, which control the expression of a specific set of genes encoding cytoprotective heat shock proteins (Santoro, 2000). HSPs have a broad range of functions related to their major role in cellular homeostasis and protect cells against apoptosis and cell death. The expression of HSP27, heat shock cognate 70 (HSC 70), HSP70 and HSP90 along the GIT of young pigs and the effect of weaning on this expression were studied (David *et al.*, 2002). It should be mentioned that on the one hand under normal physiological conditions HSP70 proteins function as ATP-dependent molecular chaperones maintaining important cell functions related to proteostasis. On the other hand, under various stress conditions additional synthesis of stress inducible HSP70 increases the ability of stressed cells to deal with increased concentrations of unfolded or denatured proteins (Surai, 2020). Protective functions of HSP70 are summarised in Figure 11.3.

There is a site specificity in HSP expression in the gut. For example, the expression of HSP27 and HSP70 was increased in the stomach and duodenum between 6 and 12 h post-weaning and between 24 and 48 h in the mid-jejunum, ileum and colon. At the same time, their expressions were transiently decreased in the ileum. In normal

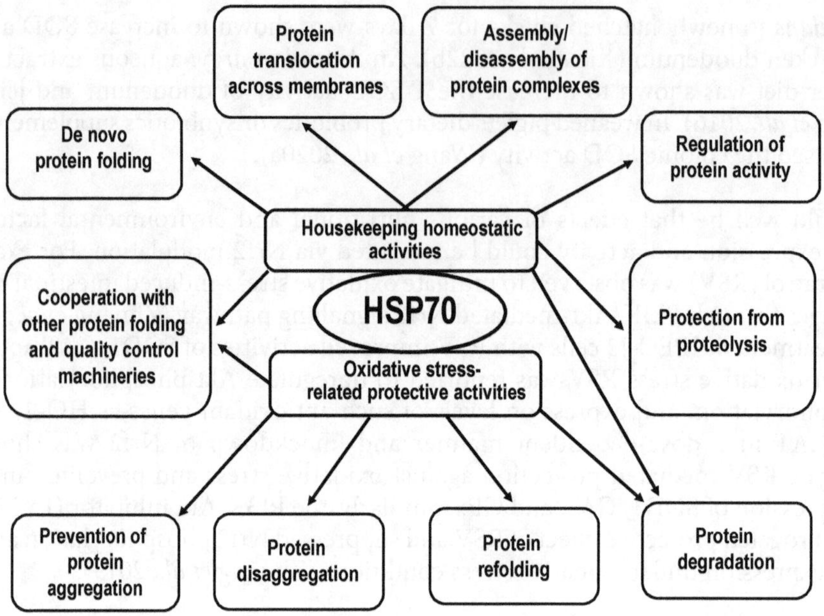

Figure 11.3. Protective functions of HSP70 (adapted from Surai, 2020).

porcine GIT, HSP expression is gut region- and cell type-specific in response to dietary components, microbes, and microbial metabolites to which the mucosa surface is exposed (Liu *et al.*, 2014).

Therefore, HSPs function as molecular chaperones in regulating cellular homeostasis and promoting survival. However, if the stress is too high, a signal that leads to programmed cell death, apoptosis, is activated, thereby providing a finely tuned balance between survival and death (Kopecek *et al.*, 2001). In addition to extracellular stimuli, several non-stressful conditions induce HSPs during normal cellular growth and development. In particular, the HSP family is activated under oxidative stress and provides an important protection against protein denaturation and modifications by capping and refolding or drives damaged proteins into appropriate proteolytic pathways (Yenari, 2002). HSPs have been assigned to multiple subcellular sites and implicated in multiple functions ranging from stress response, intracellular trafficking, antigen processing, control of cell proliferation, differentiation, and tumorigenesis (Wadhwa *et al.*, 2002).

Therefore, in response to environmental or physiological stresses cells increase synthesis of HSP (Tsukimi and Okabe, 2001). ROS-mediated damage has been implicated in the pathophysiology of the gastrointestinal mucosa and HSPs are suggested to play an important role in cytoprotection against oxidative stress-induced injury (Prabhu and Balasubramanian, 2002). For example, the mammalian intestinal epithelial cells respond to heat stress by producing heat shock proteins that provide protection in stress conditions, which would otherwise lead to cell damage or death.

The protective effects of HSPs are seen in heat stress, infection, and inflammation (Malago *et al.*, 2002). The molecular mechanisms of heat shock response-induced cytoprotection involve inhibition of proinflammatory cytokine production and induction of cellular proliferation for restitution of the damaged epithelium (Malago *et al.*, 2002). It is interesting to note that HSP72, the stress-inducible form of HSP70, was detected in samples from rat distal colon, proximal colon, and terminal ileum, but was not found in proximal small bowel or other organs (liver, kidney, spleen, heart, and brain) of unstressed animals (Beck *et al.*, 1995). HSPs play an important role in gastric mucosal defence under conditions of stress. For example, exposure of rats to restraint and water-immersion stress caused rapid HSP70 mRNA expression and HSP70 accumulation in gastric mucosa and the extent of HSP70 induction inversely correlated to the severity of mucosal damage (Rokutan, 1999). Therefore, HSP70 is involved in repair of partially damaged proteins and substantially contributes to protection of the gastrointestinal mucosa against various necrotising factors (Tsukimi and Okabe, 2001). Exposure of mice to thermal stress was shown to result in the rapid induction and expression of HSP70 in the intestine and other organs (the liver, pancreas, heart, lung and adrenal cortex) not constitutively expressing HSP70 (Huang *et al.*, 2001). HSP70 is reported to maintain barrier function as a result of stabilisation of the tight junctions between intestinal epithelial cells (Kojima *et al.*, 2003; Liedel *et al.*, 2011; Musch *et al.*, 1999).

Mother's milk-induced HSP70 expression was indicated to preserve intestinal epithelial barrier function in an immature rat pup model (Liedel *et al.*, 2011). Geranylgeranylacetone, a clinically used antiulcer drug, was reported to increase expression of HSP70 in the small intestine and suppress indomethacin-induced lesions (e.g. inflammation) of the small intestines in wild-type mice (Asano *et al.*, 2009). Intestinal HSP70 was shown to play a protective role as a result of re-establishing the balance between the intestinal post-inflammatory and anti-inflammatory cytokines in a post-infectious irritable bowel syndrome mouse model (Lan *et al.*, 2016).

In patients with inflammatory bowel diseases, HSP70 expression was found to be significantly increased during the active stage of the disease and overexpression of HSP70 was reported to protect against the development of inflammation in the large intestinal mucosa provoked by various damaging factors (Samborski and Grzymisławski, 2015). The authors suggested that microbiota can affect HSP70 expression in the gut and it seems likely that augmentation of HSP70 expression in the gut could be considered as an important strategy to deal with various gut integrity-related problems. Co-localised HSP70 and tight junction protein zona occludens-1 (ZO-1) reported recently, suggest physical interaction of HSP70 and tight junction proteins to protect tight junction function (Rentea *et al.*, 2018).

11.2.3 HO-1

It is accepted that HO-1, known as HSP32, can be induced by various stresses and HO-1 induction and the maintenance of its appropriate activity is critical in protecting the intestinal epithelial cells from oxidative injury (Fujii *et al.*, 2003). Cytoprotective action of HO-1 is summarised in Figure 11.4.

There is a range of stress-related factors which are able to activate HO-1 expression, mainly via Nrf2 pathway and products of HO-1 action on heme are believed to be involved in cytoprotection (Surai, 2020). It is interesting that in the aforementioned experiment HO-1 was markedly induced following LPS treatment in the mucosal epithelial cells in the upper intestine (duodenum and jejunum) but not in the lower intestine (ileum and colon). It seems likely, that there is a delicate interaction between HO-1 and other antioxidant defence mechanisms to maintain mucosal integrity and repair of acute mucosal damage. It was suggested that activation of HO-1 could be an important natural defensive mechanism to alleviate inflammation and tissue injury in the gastrointestinal tract (Guo *et al.*, 2001). Increased expression of HO-1 was shown to be a protective mechanism behind alleviation of the intestinal injury by hydrogen gas in a model of severe sepsis in mice (Li *et al.*, 2015), or due to pharmacological preconditioning with vitamin C after haemorrhagic shock in rats (Zhao *et al.*, 2014), ischemic preconditioning in the late phase of IR injury of the intestine (Mallick *et al.*,

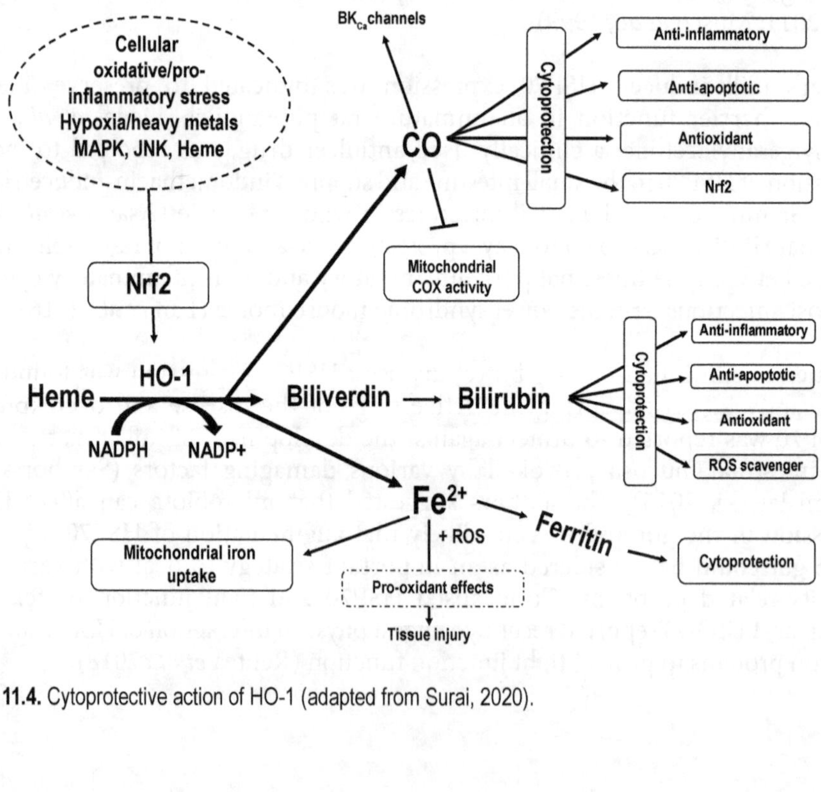

Figure 11.4. Cytoprotective action of HO-1 (adapted from Surai, 2020).

2010), or haemorrhagic shock-induced intestinal tissue injury in rats (Inoue *et al.*, 2008; Umeda *et al.*, 2009).

Induction of HO-1 was suggested to be a mechanism of protective action of hypothermia (Attuwaybi *et al.*, 2003), hemin (Attuwaybi *et al.*, 2004) or a somatostatin analogue, octreotide (Takano *et al.*, 2012) against I/R-induced impairment of intestinal integrity in rats. Similarly, induction of HO-1 was indicated to improve impaired intestinal transit after burn injury in rats (Gan and Chen *et al.*, 2007). The HO-1 system is believed to provide gut cytoprotection and decreasing I/R injury by inhibiting inflammation, oxidation, and apoptosis (Liao *et al.*, 2013).

A great number of publications indicated that HO-1/CO system is characterised by potent antioxidant, antiapoptotic, anti-inflammatory and cytoprotective activities against I/R injury. This was demonstrated by genetic overexpression of HO-1 cDNA or pharmacological induction with drugs/nutrients (Cheng and Rong, 2017). Resveratrol was shown to protect oxidative stress-induced intestinal epithelial barrier dysfunction by upregulating HO-1 and SOD expression. It is of note that protective effects of resveratrol were abolished by the HO-1 inhibition or HO-1 knockdown by siRNA (Wang *et al.*, 2016). Similarly, HO-1 was found to serve as an effector of the anti-inflammatory action of hydrogen sulphide donor (NaHS-PC) in postischemic murine small intestine (Zuidema *et al.*, 2011). Fish oil dietary supplementation was shown to induce HO-1 expression in the mouse intestine associated with increased concentration of 4-Hydroxy hexenal, a product of n-3 PUFAs peroxidation (Nakagawa *et al.*, 2014). Furthermore, in endotoxic shock model, intestinal preconditioning was able to prevent inflammatory responses by modulating HO-1 expression (Tamion *et al.*, 2007). HO-1 is shown to be important player in the anti-inflammatory activities of M-CSF-polarised M2 macrophages (Sierra-Filardi *et al.*, 2010). HO-1 production by intestinal $CX3CR1^+$ macrophages in mouse was found to help resolving gut inflammation (Marelli *et al.*, 2017).

Nutritional modulation of the function of intestinal macrophages to restore the immunological homeostasis associated with upregulated HO-1 activity and rebalance the enteric commensal flora is considered as a promising strategy to deal with gut inflammation (Ju *et al.*, 2018). Furthermore, HO-1 has been considered as an immunomodulator playing a key role in the homeostasis maintenance in the gastrointestinal tract. The protective role of HO-1 in the control of the intestinal inflammation is associated with its connection with the gut microbiota (Marelli and Allavena, 2020).

Low dose of DON was reported to trigger low-grade inflammation in liver and changes in gut microbiota in mice. Interestingly, HO-1 was reported to exert protective effect in DON-induced hepatotoxicity, which was suggested to be associated with microbiota modulation by HO-1 (Peng *et al.*, 2019). Interestingly, a food-grade bacterium genetically modified to deliver bioactive HO-1 *in situ* was reported to possess a protective effect against intestinal mucosal injury in rats with endotoxemia as a result of modulation of the immune system (Pang *et al.*, 2008). The central role of HO-1 in modulating the immune system is associated with decreasing secretion of inflammatory cytokines, such as TNF-α, IL-1β, IL-6 and IL-17 and increased levels of anti-inflammatory mediators such as IL-10 or IL-22 due to increased production of CO (Marelli and Allavena, 2020). In addition, as a result of the low levels of HO-1, the processes of phagocytosis were impaired and the dysbiosis occurred leading to chronic inflammation in the gut (Marelli and Allavena, 2020).

11.2.4 Thioredoxin system

Thioredoxin and TrxR are considered to be also important members of vitagene family playing protective roles in the gut. A summary of thioredoxin system is shown in Figure 11.5, indicating that biological roles of the thioredoxin system are diverse. They include antioxidant defence, gene regulation, modulation of protein phosphorylation, regulation of apoptosis and redox regulation of various cellular functions including cell proliferation, differentiation and maintenance of viability, regulation of the synthesis of DNA and its repair, involvement in hormone action and cytokine function as well as in protein biosynthesis (Surai, 2020).

Interestingly, Takaishi *et al* (2003) identified rat Trx as a growth-promoting factor for intestinal epithelial cells, while Higashikubo *et al.* (1999) showed that cellular oxidative stress caused an increase in the activity of Trx, which is involved in the defence mechanism against oxidative stress. In particular, H_2O_2 was cytotoxic to the small intestine epithelial cell line, IEC-6 and the glutathione S-transferase and TrxR

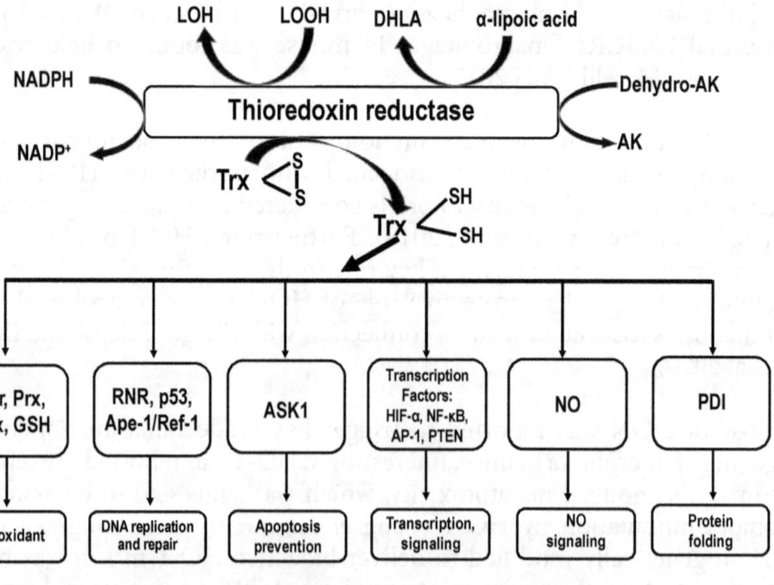

Figure 11.5. Thioredoxin system functions (adapted from Surai, 2020).

activities and SH content decreased dose-dependently with H_2O_2 treatment, while Trx activity increased at low H_2O_2 concentrations. is not clear at present, but clearly, they participate in maintenance of the redox balance in the gut. It is important to note that Trx expression is particularly high in the small intestinal mucosa and colon (Gasdaska *et al.*, 1996), while TrxR expression in small intestine is substantially higher than in colon.

All three thioredoxin reductases are expressed in the intestine at least at the mRNA level, which is relatively unaffected by marginal Se deficiency and in the case of TrxR2 and TrxR3 rather increased when Se becomes limited (Kipp *et al.*, 2009). The presence of a full complement of Trx/TrxR proteins in stomach, duodenum, jejunum, ileum and colon suggesting their function in antioxidant defence and redox regulation in the intestinal tract (Godoy *et al.*, 2011). Furthermore, the selenoproteins GPx2, TrxR2 and TrxR3 in the gut are regulated by the Wnt pathway (Kipp *et al.*, 2012).

It has been also shown that unstimulated lamina propria T lymphocytes exhibited high expression of Trx which involved in the regulation of intracellular redox homeostasis in these cells (Sido *et al.*, 2005). The authors suggested Trx to play a key role in the specialised intestinal microenvironment in amplifying immediate immune responses. Membrane-bound Trx converts human β-defensin 1 to a potent antimicrobial peptide *in vivo* (Jaeger *et al.*, 2013). Recently *Caenorhabditis elegans* Trx-3, the first metazoan thioredoxin with a tissue-specific expression pattern restricted to intestine has been characterised (Jiménez-Hidalgo *et al.*, 2014). Its role in the gut redox balance maintenance and search for avian orthologs await investigation.

11.2.5 Glutathione system

The importance of cellular GSH/GSSG redox pair in modulating cell transitions and their oxidative susceptibility has been clearly demonstrated (Jefferies *et al.*, 2003). Accumulating evidence clearly indicate that Trx- and GSH-systems are two major thiol-dependent redox systems in mammalian/avian cells operating in concert. In particular, Trx system is known to provide electrons to Trx-dependent peroxidases, involved in the repair of oxidised proteins by reducing Msr and regulates the activities of many oxidative-sensitive transcription factors, including NF-κB and Nrf2 and providing optimal conditions for the redox signalling (Surai, 2020). At the same time the GSH is considered to be a backup system responsible for reduction of Trx when the electron transfer pathway from TrxR is interrupted/damaged. A cooperative work inside GSH- and Trx-systems are shown in Figure 11.6.

It was shown that the intestinal epithelium is capable of transporting luminal GSH to augment intracellular peroxide catabolism and suggested that the loss of mucosal redox balance is a driving force in etiology of chronic gut pathologies (Aw, 2005). The gut contains internally-originated antioxidant enzymes SOD, GPx and CAT and they represent an important mechanism of the enterocyte defence from oxidative damage. A specific gastrointestinal GPx2 has been described in 1993 (Chu *et al.*, 1993). GPx2 activity was expressed in both the villus and crypt regions of the rat

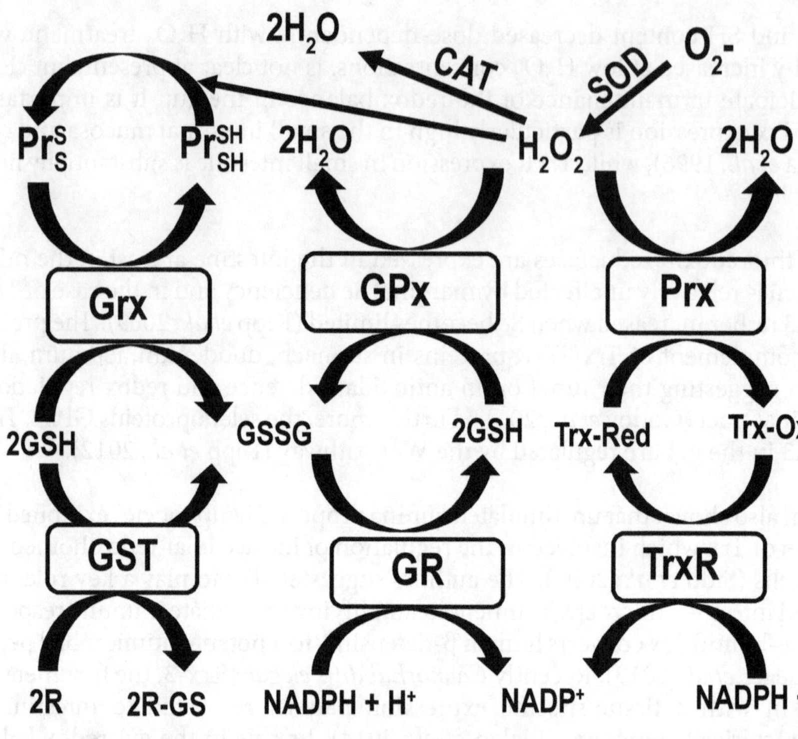

Figure 11.6. Glutathione and thioredoxin systems in mammalian/avian cells (adapted from Surai, 2020).

mucosal epithelium and its activity nearly equalled that of classical GPx throughout the small intestine and colorectal segments (Esworthy *et al.*, 1998). When enzymatic activity in liver, small intestine, cecum, and colon of rats was compared, GPx2 was highest in large bowel (Meinl *et al.*, 2009).

GPx2 was detected in proximal, transverse and distal colon being located in the luminal epithelium and lymphatic tissue of rats (Drew *et al.*, 2005). GPx2 could be considered as a barrier against hydroperoxide resorption (Brigelius-Flohé, 1999; Brigelius-Flohé and Maiorino, 2013). Furthermore, in the gastrointestinal tract there are at least three more selenoproteins, including plasma GPx, selenoprotein P and TrxR (Mörk *et al.*, 1998). GSH and GSH-dependent enzymes contribute significantly towards intestinal antioxidant defences and an important peroxide detoxification pathway in the intestine is based on the GSH redox system (LeGrand and Aw, 1998).

In this system GPx reduces peroxides at the expense of GSH oxidation. Oxidised glutathione is reduced back to the active form by GR utilising reducing potential of NADPH which is produced in the pentose phosphate pathway. Various studies in mouse models of colon cancer and selenoprotein gene deletion studies indicated that selenoproteins play a pivotal role in the maintenance of gut homeostasis. In particular, GPx has been extensively studied for its redox regulation, antioxidant and anti-inflammatory roles in preventing chronic intestinal inflammation (Reeves and Hoffman, 2009; Speckmann and Steinbrenner, 2014). GPx1 is shown to be expressed in all cell types of the gut, whereas GPx2 is predominantly expressed in the epithelial cells, including the paneth cells, of the gastrointestinal mucosa (Brigelius-Flohé *et al.*, 2001; Esworthy *et al.*, 1998; Florian *et al.*, 2001) and GPx4 is found to be expressed in epithelial cells and the lamina propria of the intestine (Speckmann *et al.*, 2011; Takahashi *et al.*, 1987).

Up-regulation by the Nrf2/Keap1 system indicates that GPx2 is an antioxidant and anti-inflammatory enzyme (Brigelius-Flohé and Flohé, 2020). In fact, an increased apoptotic cell proportion in the crypts of the colon was reported as a major pathological observation in gpx2-/- mice under unstressed condition (Florian *et al.*, 2010). However, in a model of inflammation-mediated colon carcinogenesis, inflammatory scores were shown to be increased in gpx2-/- than in WT mice (Krehl *et al.*, 2012). It is of note an existence of a cooperative action of various AO enzymes, including GPx, in the gut. On the one hand, a double knock-out of GPx2 and GPx1 caused ileo-colitis (Esworthy *et al.*, 2001). On the other hand, in the colon of gpx2-/- mice a compensatory dramatic overexpression of gpx1 at the transcriptional and translational level were observed (Florian *et al.*, 2010).

Interestingly, in gpx2-/- mice the total GPx activity in the gut was shown to be significantly increased in comparison to wild type mice (Müller *et al.*, 2013) and unique role of GPx2 in preventing ectopic apoptosis in the intestine awaits further investigation (Brigelius-Flohé and Flohé, 2020). Loss of epithelium specific GPx2 was reported to lead to aberrant cell fate decisions during intestinal differentiation in mice (Lennicke *et al.*, 2017). A significant increase in SOD1, SOD3, Prx6, GPx2, GPx7 expression during I/R-induced damage of the small intestine was observed in rats. Interestingly, injection of exogenous Prx6 prior to induced ischemia showed a significant protective effect in the intestine leading to minimisation of oxidative injury with reducing necrosis and apoptosis simultaneously with normalisation of expression of antioxidant enzymes (Gordeeva *et al.*, 2015).

Importantly, protective effect of *Lactobacillus plantarum* (Wang *et al.*, 2018) and *Bifidobacterium bifidum* (Din *et al.*, 2020) in dextran sodium sulphate-induced colitis in mice was associated with up-regulation of ROS-scavenging enzymes, including GPx2. Similarly, gene expression of SOD2 in jejunum tissue of weaned piglets was increased after oral administration of *Lactobacillus reuteri* in the form of a liquid preparation (Zhang *et al.*, 2017a). When porcine epithelial cells were treated with zearalenone (10 μM for 24 h), microarray results identified 190 genes significantly and differentially expressed, of which 70% were up-regulated, including GPx6, GPx2, GPx1 (Taranu *et al.*, 2015). It seems likely that interactions between various antioxidants withing the antioxidant defence network is of great importance in the animal/chicken gut. For example, vitamin E (200 mg/kg BW) was shown to reduce toxic effect of phoxim (organophosphate pesticides) on intestinal structure, alleviated the oxidative stress in intestinal tissue, decreased the level of proinflammatory TNF-α and increased expression of GPx2 and SOD in rats (Sun *et al.*, 2018).

Gut microbiota was indicated to affect host amino acid and GSH metabolism in mice (Mardinoglu *et al.*, 2015). Under oxidative stress conditions, imposed by peroxidised oil dietary consumption in weaned piglets, jejunal integrity is shown to be dependent on the local and hepatic GSH redox system, which is responsible for the elimination of luminal peroxides, and thereby protecting duodenal barrier function (Degroote *et al.*, 2019). Interestingly, GPx8 is shown to protect against colitis by negatively regulating caspase-4/11 activity and decreasing inflammation and mice lacking GPx8 (the oxidative stress sensor) are characterised by increased susceptibility to colitis and endotoxic shock and disturbed gut microbiome (Hsu *et al.*, 2020).

11.2.6 Sirtuins

It is generally accepted that SIRTs are involved in the intestine protection in stress conditions. For example, mice with an intestinal specific SIRT1 deficiency (Sirt1int-/-) were characterised by dysregulated intestinal cell differentiation with altered gut microbiota (Lo Sasso *et al.*, 2014a). SIRT1 is shown to have anti-inflammatory effects in the intestine via regulating the gut microbiota (Wellman *et al.*, 2017). SIRT1 deficiency in the intestine was reported to elevate the number of secretory cells, including intestinal Paneth and goblet cells (Wellman *et al.*, 2017). SIRT1 was reported to alleviate endoplasmic reticulum stress-mediated apoptosis of intestinal epithelial cells in an ulcerative colitis model system (Ren *et al.*, 2019). Curcumin and resveratrol were shown to exert their protective effects on dextran sulphate sodium (DSS)-induced colitis in mice partially through regulating SIRT1/mTOR signalling leading to suppression of the intestinal inflammation (Zhang *et al.*, 2019b). Resveratrol was shown to have protective effects against radiation-induced intestinal injury at least partly via activation of SIRT1 (Zhang *et al.*, 2017b). In general, defective expression of SIRT1 is believed to contribute to activation of inflammatory pathways in the human gut (Caruso *et al.*, 2014).

Interestingly, other SIRTs are believed to be also involved in gut integrity maintenance. For example, compared to wild type mice, SIRT2 deficient mice showed exaggeration of cellular adhesion with sepsis in the small intestine, while SIRT2 overexpression showed protective effects (Buechler *et al.*, 2017). Interestingly, under basal condition, SIRT2 deficiency did not affect the basal phenotype and intestinal morphology, whereas SIRT2 deficiency (Sirt2-/-) was observed to promote DSS-induced inflammatory responses. Interestingly, anti-inflammatory action of SIRT2 was shown to be associated with regulation of NF-κB acetylation and macrophage polarisation (Lo Sasso *et al.*, 2014b).

SIRT2 was found to be expressed in small intestinal villi and its levels were shown to be dramatically increased in differentiated intestinal cells compared with undifferentiated cells and it was clearly shown that SIRT2 to be essential for maintenance of normal intestinal homeostasis (Li *et al.*, 2020a). Deletion of SIRT2 was reported to result in decreased enterocyte and goblet cell differentiation, whereas SIRT2 deficiency increased the Paneth cell lineage and it seems likely that SIRT2 regulates intestinal cell differentiation through regulation of Wnt/β-catenin signalling (Li *et al.*, 2020a). SIRT3 deficiency was shown to cause an impaired intestinal permeability and inflammation in high fat fed mice, which was attenuated by sodium butyrate (Chen *et al.*, 2019). Furthermore, SIRT3 was reported to be anti-inflammatory factor interacting with the gut microbiota during colon tumorigenesis (Zhang *et al.*, 2018). It is believed that Prx3 is a key protective factor for intestinal I/R injury, and SIRT3-mediated Prx3 deacetylation was indicated to alleviate intestinal I/R-induced mitochondrial oxidative damage and apoptosis (Wang *et al.*, 2020b). Importantly, SIRT6 was found to be predominantly expressed in epithelial cells in intestinal crypts and its expression was decreased in colitis in both mice and humans (Liu *et al.*, 2017).

Protective effects of SIRT6 to intestine was confirmed in a study showing increased susceptibility of the cells to injurious insults after knockdown of SIRT6 expression, while YAMC cells with SIRT6 overexpression were characterised by increased resistance to injurious insult. Intestinal epithelial-specific *Sirt6* ($Sirt6^{IEC\text{-}KO}$) knockout mice were indicated to show increased susceptibility to DSS-induced colitis (Liu *et al.*, 2017). The authors showed that protective effects of SIRT6 on intestinal epithelial cells challenged with inflammatory injury was related to preservation of R-spondin-1 (a critical growth factor for intestinal epithelial cells) levels in the cells. By targeting SIRT6 and MAPK13, microRNA-351-5p was shown to aggravate I/R injury associated with increased intestinal mucosal oxidative stress, inflammation, and apoptosis (Hu *et al.*, 2018).

Redox signalling is proven to play a critical role in the physiology and pathophysiology of gastrointestinal tract (Perez *et al.*, 2017). Progression of gut inflammation is believed to rely on the balance between pro-inflammatory redox-sensitive pathways, such as NLRP3 inflammasome and NF-κB, and the adaptive up-regulation of Nrf2 and vitagenes, including SOD, GPx2 and other protective mechanisms (Perez *et al.*, 2017; Surai, 2020).

Analysis of the literature related to poultry/pig diet showed that on the one hand, there is a range of harmful compounds in the diet, including oxidised PUFAs, traces of mycotoxins, heavy metals and other environmental pollutants. Recently a detrimental role of air pollution, including particulate matter has been linked to redox disbalance in the gut and detrimental changes in microbiota (Feng *et al.*, 2020). Therefore, emissions of harmful agents and dust in poultry/pig production could have detrimental effects on animal gut health by imposing oxidative stress. Furthermore, dietary nitrate can affect gut health via modulation of intestinal microbiota metabolism (Rocha and Laranjinha, 2020).

It is important to mention host-immune, host-microbiota and immune-microbiota crosstalk during physiological conditions and disease processes rely on the redox homeostasis in the gut (Campbell and Colgan, 2019). The authors suggested that redox signals derived from immune cells, parenchymal cells and the gut microbiota, are associated with various redox products produced locally (e.g. GSH, Trx, etc.) and it seems likely that dietary antioxidants and pro-oxidants could also have regulatory effects for gut signalling and adaptation.

On the one hand, a combination of prooxidant compounds could potentially stimulate lipid peroxidation, compromise redox homeostasis and cause DNA and protein damages in the intestine leading to decrease absorption efficacy of various nutrients and deteriorating FCR. On the other hand, the diet contains a range of antioxidant compounds, including vitamin E, ascorbic acid, carnitine, TAU, coenzyme Q, flavonoids, etc., which potentially can deal with those free radicals produced in the digestive tract as a result of aforementioned toxic compounds action (Surai and Fisinin, 2015). Therefore, a balance between antioxidants and prooxidants in the digestive tract can be maintained by optimal dietary supplementation of natural antioxidants and nutrients upregulating antioxidant defences and vitagenes in the gut.

Conceptually, some nutrients which are not well absorbed could have health-promoting properties. For example, it is well known that various flavonoids/polyphenols are not well absorbed in the small intestine (Surai, 2014; 2015). As a result, many of them will be available in the large intestine providing there an important antioxidant protection, preventing lipid peroxidation, damages to DNA and proteins. Since depending on condition those compounds can show antioxidant or prooxidant properties it is highly likely that small amounts of dietary flavonoids could alert antioxidant defence systems in the gut and help stress adaptation (Surai, 2020).

11.3 Gut redox balance and microbiota

It is believed that under physiological conditions, the gut cell can tolerate a certain level of ROS due to its antioxidant capacity, which is critical for intestinal homeostasis (Tian *et al.*, 2017). However, in stress conditions an excessive ROS production can break an existing antioxidant-prooxidant (redox) balance and enhance membrane permeability, alter the inflammatory response, and cause lipid and protein modifications, DNA damage and apoptosis (Tian *et al.*, 2017). The human and animal/avian gastrointestinal tracts harbour trillions of commensal microorganisms, collectively known as the microbiota (Bhat and Kapila, 2017). For example, chicken intestinal tract is composed of duodenum, jejunum, ileum, cecum, and colon, and there are significant differences in microbiota concentration and composition between the aforementioned gut sections (Xiao *et al.*, 2017).

Interestingly, cecum is characterised by the most complex microbial community dominated by the phyla *Firmicutes*, *Bacteroidetes*, *Actinobacteria* and *Proteobacteria* (Sergeant *et al.*, 2014). On the other hand, at the genus level, the major microbial genera across all gut sections were shown to be *Lactobacillus*, *Enterococcus*, *Bacteroides*, and *Corynebacterium* (Xiao *et al.*, 2017). Furthermore, *Bacteroides* was shown to be the dominant group in cecum, while *Lactobacillus* was predominant in the small intestine sections (duodenum, jejunum and ileum; Xiao *et al.*, 2017).

The microbiota's various bacterial members are involved in a physiological network of cooperation and competition within the gut (Stecher *et al.*, 2015). On the one hand, microbiota is shaped by environmental factors. On the other hand, gut environment including redox balance is shaped by microbiota. Redox signalling in the gut regulates many physiological functions, including self-renewal, proliferation, migration and differentiation of epithelial cells (Perez *et al.*, 2017). By modulating NADPH oxidases commensal microbiota substantially contribute to this signalling and normal commensal microbiota is responsible for so called colonisation resistance by creating hostile/unfavourable conditions for colonisation of enteric pathogens (Stecher *et al.*, 2015).

Interestingly, the same nutritional (antibiotics and other drugs) or environmental (changes in diet or disease challenge) factors can affect antioxidant-prooxidant balance (Surai and Fisinin, 2015) and disrupt microbiota in the gut (Stecher *et al.*, 2015). For example, experimental infection with *Cryptosporidium parvum* in immunocompromised Swiss albino mice caused an increase in lipid peroxidation and decrease in GSH, CAT and SOD at the peak of infection in the intestine and liver (Bhagat *et al.*, 2017). An important consequence of redox balance and microbiota disturbances is inflammatory host responses and activation of immune cells resulting in further production of ROS in the gut and deepen the problem. Furthermore, under inflammatory conditions, the microbial community could shift from obligate to facultative anaerobes (Rigottier-Gois, 2013). For example, the gut microbiota is shown to contribute to the control of *Compilobacter jejuni* colonisation and could prevent lesion development (Han *et al*, 2017).

Of note, intestinal microbiota is shown to play an important role in mucosal immunity and dysbiosis is associated with the pathogenesis of inflammatory diseases (Shi *et al.*, 2017). In the complex intestinal ecosystem, there could be a range of microbes able to facilitate oxidation/reduction reactions and maintenance of the redox balance. A redox based response within cells is emerging as an important and conserved element of host cell and symbiotic microbe interaction (Jones and Neish, 2017). It has been suggested that in the gut commensal microflora, in particular *Lactobacillus* species, are able to stimulate rapid, non-pathogenic levels of ROS production which would oxidise reactive cysteine residues within proteins controlling cell signalling pathways. A number of studies revealed that proteins that harbour reactive cysteine residues, for example Keap1 or IκB, could function as redox sensors and transducers of signalling initiated by increased ROS concentrations (Jones and Neish, 2017). It has been shown that ROS production by intestinal epithelial cells is mediated by receptors and enzymatic processes similar to those employed by phagocytic cells to induce microbial death (Neish *et al.*, 2013). Reversible oxidation of cysteine residues is responsible for adaptive response to fluctuating levels of ROS and ROS signalling in the gut is suggested to represent an evolutionary ancient form of host cell and microbe cross-talk (Jones *et al.*, 2012; Neish and Jones, 2014).

Free radical production in the gut due to commensal microbiota could also oxidise Trx and GSH, changing redox balance in the cell and inducing the transcription factors such as the Nrf2 and NF-κB. This could lead to modulation of gut inflammation and other cellular processes. It seems likely that the aforementioned microbiota-host interactions represent a universal mechanism used by bacterial communities to affect a variety of signalling and homeostatic processes in the host (Lee, 2008). Of interest, it was shown that the loss of mucus due to pathogenic bacteria is associated with significantly increased ROS production (Alam *et al.*, 2016) further aggravating disturbances in the redox balance of the gut. Therefore, two important balances in the gut namely antioxidants/prooxidants and commensal/pathogenic microbiota work in synergy. They maintain gut redox balance via transcription factors (e.g. Nrf2 and NF-κB) and vitagene modulation and are main protective mechanisms of the healthy gut (Figure 11.7).

Interestingly, probiotics may modulate the redox status of the gut via their metal ion chelating ability, antioxidant systems modulation, regulating signalling pathways, enzyme producing ROS, and intestinal microbiota (Wang *et al.*, 2017a). However, the authors raised several questions as to efficacy of probiotics in modulation of gut health. For example, incapability of probiotic bacteria to colonise the gut and their elimination shortly after substantially restrict their long-term action. Interestingly, *Bacillus* amyloliquefaciens SC06 was shown to alleviate the oxidative stress of intestinal porcine epithelial cells via modulating Nrf2/Keap1 signalling pathway and decreasing ROS production (Wang *et al.*, 2017b). Clearly there is a need for more detailed elucidation of the microbial population in poultry/animal gut depending on the diet, feed supplements, including pre- and probiotics and vitagene-modulating nutrients. The characterisation of the stress factors leading to intestinal dysbiosis and

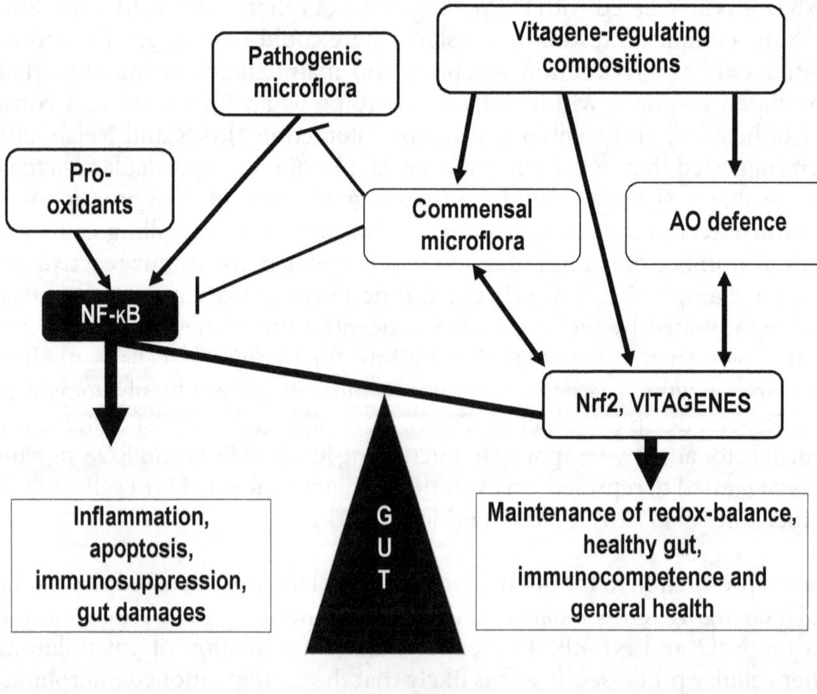

Figure 11.7. Antioxidant-prooxidant balance and microbiota in the gut (adapted from Surai, 2018; 2020).

the identification of the microbial taxa contributing to pathological effects present a new direction of future research to better understand the impact of the microbiota on health and disease (Weiss and Hennet, 2017). Therefore, interactions between RONS, vitagene-regulated antioxidants and microbiota represent an important mechanism of the gut integrity/health maintenance in stressful conditions of commercial poultry production.

11.4 Protective effects of silymarin in the gut

It seems likely that the gut is the major place of antioxidant action of polyphenols (Surai *et al.*, 2003; 2004; Surai and Fisinin, 2015). Reduction of oxidative damage, modulation of colonic flora and variation in gene expression are involved in the modulation of intestinal function by polyphenols. For example, to study the molecular effects of wine polyphenols at the gene level, the microarray technology was used: rats were treated with 50 mg/kg/BW wine polyphenols for 14 days. Global expression analysis of 5,707 genes revealed an extensive down-regulation of genes involved in a wide range of physiological functions, such as metabolism, transport, signal transduction and intercellular signalling (Dolara *et al.*, 2005). It was shown that two major regulatory pathways were downregulated in the colon mucosa in polyphenols treated rats: inflammatory response and steroid metabolism. Since flavonoids are consumed in concentrations usually much higher than other antioxidant compounds, their protective effect during digestion is of great importance. For example, it has been shown that flavonoids not only prevented an accumulation of peroxidised lipids but can also switch prooxidant properties of heme-proteins to antioxidant ones (Kanner and Lapidot, 2001).

Dietary polyphenols can also modulate *in vivo* oxidative damage in the gastrointestinal tract of rodents (Giovannelli *et al.*, 2000) supporting the hypothesis that dietary polyphenols might have both a protective and a therapeutic potential in oxidative damage-related pathologies. Emerging evidence indicates that the antioxidant-prooxidant balance (redox status) in various parts of the intestine depends on the level of antioxidants and pro-oxidants provided by the diet and released by cells themselves, as well as on the level of absorption of both antioxidants and pro-oxidants (Surai, 2018; 2020; Surai and Fisinin, 2015; Surai *et al.*, 2003; 2004). In a model system mimicking stomach conditions, it was shown that both lipid peroxidation and co-oxidation of vitamin E and β-carotene were inhibited at pH 3.0 by red wine polyphenols (Gorelik *et al.*, 2005). In the gut, an interaction between different antioxidants could bring about their maximum synergistic effects. It has been found that consumption of partially oxidised food could increase lipid peroxidation in the stomach and the absorption of cytotoxic lipid peroxidation products into the body.

The addition of red wine polyphenols to the meal may alter these outcomes (Gorelik *et al.*, 2008a), therefore red wine polyphenols exert a beneficial effect by the novel function, inhibition of absorption of the lipid peroxidation products, including MDA (Gorelik *et al.*, 2008b). These findings explain the potentially harmful effects of oxidised fats found in foods/feeds (Surai *et al.*, 2003) and the important benefit of dietary polyphenols in the diet. There are also multiple studies suggesting that locating the biological site of action of polyphenols in the gastrointestinal tract may lead to a revision in our understanding of how flavonoids, including SM/SB, work *in vivo* and may help to elucidate the mechanisms of the health-promoting action of SM/SB and other polyphenols (Kanner *et al.*, 2012).

Redox signalling in gut inflammation is complex and poorly understood. However, it is generally accepted that homeostatic control of the intestinal epithelial redox environment is central for nutrient digestion and absorption, stem cell proliferation, apical enterocyte apoptosis, and immune response (Circu and Aw, 2012). In this context, polyphenols may play a role in intestinal mucosa integrity, inflammation and permeability (Martínes *et al.*, 2013; Surai, 2014; Surai *et al.*, 2004). For example, wine phenolics were able to prevent or delay the progression of intestinal diseases characterised by oxidative stress and inflammation, acting as both free radical scavengers and modulators of specific inflammation-related genes involved in cellular redox signalling (Biasi *et al.*, 2014). They exert their effects by modulating cell signalling pathways, mainly activated in response to oxidative and inflammatory stimuli, and Nrf2 and NF-κB are the principal downstream effectors (Biasi *et al.*, 2011). For example, pigs administered a grape seed and grape marc extract had a lower transactivation of NF-κB and Nrf2 and a lower expression of various target genes of these transcription factors in the duodenal mucosa (but not in the liver and plasma) than control pigs (Gessner *et al.*, 2013).

Furthermore, the ratio of villus height: crypt depth and the gain/feed ratio were higher in the animals fed a gape extract than in control pigs. In mice, the dietary grape seed extract decreased proliferation and enhanced differentiation of epithelial cell and the changes in gut epithelium were associated with the suppression of NF-κB signalling (Yang *et al.*, 2014). Polyphenolic compounds could also affect gut integrity. For example, grape seed extract (0.1%) supplied to rats with drinking water for 21 days significantly increased the expression of gut junction protein occludin in the proximal colon and reduced faecal levels of the neutrophil protein calprotectin, compared with control (Goodrich *et al.*, 2012). It was also reported that a naturally occurring flavonoid procyanidin B2 could modulate cellular redox status and the antioxidant enzyme defence system in colonic cells protecting against oxidative stress and xenobiotics (Rodríguez-Ramiro *et al.*, 2011a,b).

It is possible to suggest that there is a biological reason for some antioxidants not to be absorbed completely and to provide antioxidant protection in lower parts of the intestine (Surai and Fisinin, 2015; Surai *et al.*, 2003; 2004). Comparatively low bioavailability and antioxidant potential of various polyphenolics could be beneficial for humans/animals providing antioxidant protection in various parts of the digestive tract, including the large intestine where levels of other antioxidants would be quite low. The same is true for SM. For example, SB concentration in the gut could reach 800 μM (Köck *et al.*, 2013), a concentration exceeding the requirement for its direct antioxidant activity. However, it is still unclear whether SM has any direct antioxidant effects *in vivo*, although it might be capable of exerting such effects within the gastrointestinal tract, where SM may come into direct contact with cells without having undergone absorption and metabolism (Surai *et al.*, 2004). It has been suggested that gastroprotective effects of SM might be related to the protection of gastric mucosal NO and non-protein sulfhydryl groups and the modulation of capsaicin-sensitive gastric sensory afferents (Shin *et al.*, 2013). Oral administration of SM (20-200 mg/kg) was shown to dose-dependently decrease gastric lesions in ethanol-induced gastritis model in rats. Furthermore, SM was also reported to significantly suppress the development of gastric lesions in other model systems including aspirin- or water immersion-restraint stress-induced gastritis models.

Interestingly, in ethanol-induced gastritis model, gastroprotective effect of SM was demonstrated to be blocked by nitric oxide (NO) synthase inhibitor (l-NAME), SH blocker (N-ethylmaleimide) or transient receptor potential vanilloid 1 antagonist (capsazepine). In the same model, ethanol-induced decrease in gastric mucus and non-protein sulfhydryl groups was reported to be reversed by SM with simultaneous suppression of lipid peroxidation (Shin *et al.*, 2013). The beneficial effects of SM, on a murine model of colitis was also shown (Esmaily *et al.*, 2009). SM effectively reduced colonic damage, lipid peroxidation, neutrophil infiltration and the content of inflammatory cytokines alongside increasing total antioxidant capacity of colonic tissue.

In trinitrobenzene sulfonic acid-induced colitis model, SB treatment significantly reduced several components of inflammatory colitis such as NF-κB activity, levels of IL-1β, TNF-α, TBARS, protein carbonyl, MPO activity, and an improvement in antioxidant capability of the colon tissue (Esmaily *et al.*, 2011). Furthermore, SB (50 mg/kg/BW) was reported to modulate gut microbial enzymes, colonic oxidative stress and Wnt/β-catenin signalling resulting in antiproliferative effect against 1,2-di-methylhydrazine-induced colon carcinogenesis in experimental rats (Sangeetha *et al.*, 2012). Protective effects of SB on *Helicobacter pylori*-induced gastritis were also demonstrated (Cho *et al.*, 2021). *H. pylori* infection-induced elevated translocation and DNA binding of NF-κB and STAT3 were found to be inhibited by SB treatment. Moreover, SB administration substantially mitigated dysplasia and hyperplasia in mouse stomach caused by *H. pylori* infection in combination with high salt diet. Furthermore, pretreatment with SB was able to attenuate the up-regulation of COX-2 and iNOS in *H. pylori*-infected MKN-1 cells and mouse stomach (Cho *et al.*, 2021). Using SM-loaded chitosan-montmorillonite microbeads was shown to be a promising approach for the treatment of gastric ulcer (Sharma *et al.*, 2018).

In a rat model of indomethacin-induced gastric injury SM (50 mg/kg) was reported to have a gastro-protective effect evidenced by attenuation of the severity of gastric mucosal damage. This was mediated via suppression of gastric inflammation by decreasing proinflammatory MPO activity, TNF-α and IL-6 expressions along with reducing NF-κB p65 expression. Furthermore, SM attenuated oxidative stress by increasing the antioxidant and the cyto-protective defence mechanisms including Nrf2 induction (Arafa Keshk *et al.*, 2017).

It is also well known that polyphenols are providing antioxidant protection in the lower intestine and can alter colonic flora (Moco *et al.*, 2012). Polyphenols are usually extensively metabolised by gut bacteria into a complex series of end-products that affect the functional ecology of symbiotic partners that can alter the host physiology (Moco *et al.*, 2012). It has been suggested that the consumption of a diet rich in plant foods with high dietary polyphenol content may enhance the gastrointestinal health of the host through microbiota modulation. For example, grape antioxidant dietary fibre intake stimulates proliferation of *Lactobacillus* and slightly affects the composition of *Bifidobacterium* species in the cecum of rats (Pozuelo *et al.*, 2012). It appears that dietary polyphenols may have the ability to modify the gut microbial balance, but this effect is indirect, i.e. it is mediated by biotransformation products, rather than the original plant compounds (Parkar *et al.*, 2013). It should be mentioned that polyphenol-microbiota interactions are complex and subject to large inter-individual variability, leading to different polyphenol-metabolising phenotypes or 'metabotypes' (Bolca *et al.*, 2013). It seems likely that SM/SB, similar to other polyphenolics, could affect animal/poultry microbiota. Recently it has been shown that SM/SB could alleviate memory impairment of transgenic APP/PS1 mice associated with their regulatory effect on the gut microbiota composition (Shen *et al.*, 2019). Interestingly, SM/SB was shown to decrease the microbiota diversity and affected abundances of several key bacterial species associated with AD development.

In another study, SM demonstrated protective effects against dietary-induced obesity and liver steatosis associated with gut microbiota composition changes. At the phylum level, SM decreased levels of Firmicutes, and the ratio of *Firmicutes-to-Bacteroidetes*, while at the genus level, SM decreased levels of *Lachnoclostridium, Lachnospiraceae_UCG-006, and Mollicutes_RF9* and increased levels of *Blautia, Akkermansia and Bacteroides*. Importantly, SM also demonstrated an inhibitory effect on such beneficial bacteria, as *Alloprevotella* and *Lactobacillus*. Furthermore, the production of acetate, propionate, and butyrate in SM-treated mouse was increased while the generation of formate and conversion of cytotoxic secondary metabolites were shown to be reduced due to SM treatment (Li *et al.*, 2020b). It has been recently shown that the flavonolignans, including SM/SB, are relatively resistant to biotransformation by gut microbiota (Valentová *et al.*, 2020). In the *E. coli*-infected broiler chicks SM dietary supplementation (500 and 1000 mg/kg) resulted in improved growth performance via suppressing the ileal pathogen microbial numbers and enhancing the villi absorptive surface area (Jahanian *et al.*, 2021). Broiler chickens fed a diet containing graded levels of SM were characterised by linearly increased the nutrient digestibility of dry matter and caecal *Lactobacillus* counts and by reduced the methyl mercaptans and acetic acid emission in broilers (Shanmugam *et al.*, 2022). In HFD-fed hamsters, a silybin-2-hydroxypropyl-β-cyclodextrin was demonstrated to modulate gut health by restoring the gut microbiota and intestinal integrity (Ren *et al.*, 2022).

Therefore, it seems likely that reduction of oxidative damage and inflammation, modulation of colonic flora and variation in gene expression are involved in the modulation of intestinal function by polyphenols, including SM.

11.5 Conclusions

The compromised gut health is a common problem in commercial poultry and animal production. The severity of the problem significantly increased as a result of antibiotic withdrawal. For many years growth-promoting properties of feed antibiotics were used by broiler producers to maintain healthy chicken gut, improve FCR and economics of meat production in general. However, common usage of feed antibiotics in poultry and pig industries led to their residues in meat and eggs. Consumption of animal products contaminated with residues of antibiotics was one of the important driving force for antibiotic resistance development in humans. As a result, antibiotic usage as feed additives were prohibited in most countries with developed poultry production and their therapeutic usage was also restricted.

Therefore antibiotic-free poultry and animal production is on the agenda of many leading commercial companies. This increased research efforts to better understand biology of chicken/animal gut health in efforts to find natural alternative to antibiotics. On the one hand, great attention has been given to prebiotics, probiotics, organic acids, essential oils, butyrates, medium-chain fatty acids, polyphenolics, etc. as possible gut health enhancers. On the other hand, redox balance in the gut become a centre of research devoted to elucidation of molecular mechanisms of natural gut protection under various stress conditions via activation of various transcription factors, vitagenes and additional synthesis of a range protective molecules possessing antioxidant properties.

A summary of stress adaptation associated with vitagene activation is shown in Figure 11.8.

First of all, vitagenes are responsible for encoding protective molecules, including SOD, HSP70, HO-1, elements of Trx- and GSH-systems and sirtuins. In response to stress, vitagene activation and additional synthesis of protective molecules provide optimal AO defences, proteostasis, redox balance and gene expression providing effective adaptation to stressful conditions to overcome them with minimal losses. Furthermore, nutritional modulation of vitagenes by using various supplements including carnitine, TAU, betaine, vitamins and minerals emerged as a new approach to deal with commercially-relevant stresses. It seems likely, that SM/SB can also improve adaptive ability of farm animals and poultry to commercially relevant stresses by activating Nrf2 and suppressing NF-κB. However, molecular mechanisms of such regulatory actions of SM/SB require more research.

Furthermore, immunomodulating and anti-inflammatory properties od SM/SB deserve more attention in future research. It could well be that some dietary constituents which are not well absorbed could have health-promoting properties by maintaining redox balance in the large intestine, where concentration of other antioxidants (vitamin E, carotenoids, ascorbate, etc.) could be low, but prooxidants (iron, oxidised PUFAs, etc.) and substrates of oxidation are still present. This protective effect in the large intestine could be responsible, for example, for bowl cancer prevention.

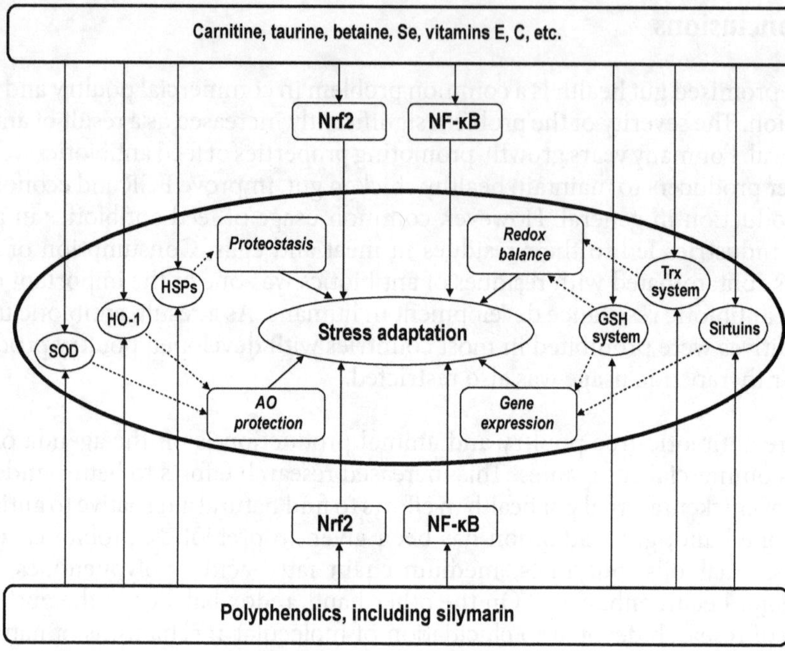

Figure 11.8. Vitagenes in stress adaptation (adapted from Surai, 2020).

Therefore, there could be a biological reason for some diet constituents/nutrients not being absorbed, but still being involved in antioxidant protection in the lower gut. Taking into account high concentrations of phytochemicals in the gut, it could well be that they play an essential part in maintaining an optimal antioxidant-prooxidant balance in the digestive tract responsible for additional health effects of phytochemicals including SM. In animal nutrition and disease prevention strategy SM alone, or in combination with other hepato-active compounds (carnitine, betaine, TAU, vitamin B12, etc.), could have similar hepatoprotective effects as described in humans with similar mechanisms of protective action.

References

Abdel-Latif, M.A., Elbestawy, A.R., El-Far, A.H., Noreldin, A.E., Emam, M., Baty, R.S., Albadrani, G.M., Abdel-Daim, M.M. and Abd El-Hamid, H.S., 2021. Quercetin dietary supplementation advances growth performance, gut microbiota, and intestinal mRNA expression genes in broiler chickens. Animals 11: 2302.

Alam, A., Leoni, G., Quiros, M., Wu, H., Desai, C., Nishio, H., Jones, R.M., Nusrat, A. and Neish, A.S., 2016. The microenvironment of injured murine gut elicits a local pro-restitutive microbiota. Nature Microbiology 1: 15021.

Amevor, F.K., Cui, Z., Du, X., Ning, Z., Deng, X., Xu, D., Shu, G., Wu, Y., Cao, X., Shuo, W., Tian, Y., Li, D., Wang, Y., Zhang, Y., Du, X., Zhu, Q., Han, X. and Zhao, X., 2022. Supplementation of dietary quercetin and vitamin E promotes the intestinal structure and immune barrier integrity in aged breeder hens. Frontiers in Immunology 13: 860889.

Arafa Keshk, W., Zahran, S.M., Katary, M.A. and Abd-Elaziz Ali, D., 2017. Modulatory effect of silymarin on nuclear factor-erythroid-2-related factor 2 regulated redox status, nuclear factor-κB mediated inflammation and apoptosis in experimental gastric ulcer. Chemico-Biological Interactions 273: 266-272.

Araujo, R.S., Oliveira, A.C., Sousa, F., Dourado, L., Guimarães, S., Silva, W., Biagiotti, D., Bayão, G. and Sousa, K., 2019. Effects of cottonseed oil and ferrous sulfate on the performance and expression of antioxidant enzymes in broilers. Poultry Science 98: 3860-3869.

Asano, T., Tanaka, K., Yamakawa, N., Adachi, H., Sobue, G., Goto, H., Takeuchi, K. and Mizushima, T., 2009. HSP70 confers protection against indomethacin-induced lesions of the small intestine. The Journal of Pharmacology and Experimental Therapeutics 330: 458-467.

Attuwaybi, B.O., Hassoun, H.T., Zou, L., Kozar, R.A., Kone, B.C., Weisbrodt, N.W. and Moore, F.A., 2003. Hypothermia protects against gut ischemia/reperfusion-induced impaired intestinal transit by inducing heme oxygenase-1. The Journal of Surgical Research 115: 48-55.

Attuwaybi, B.O., Kozar, R.A., Moore-Olufemi, S.D., Sato, N., Hassoun, H.T., Weisbrodt, N.W. and Moore, F.A., 2004. Heme oxygenase-1 induction by hemin protects against gut ischemia/reperfusion injury. The Journal of Surgical Research 118: 53-57.

Aw, T.Y., 2005. Intestinal glutathione: determinant of mucosal peroxide transport, metabolism, and oxidative susceptibility. Toxicology and Applied Pharmacology 204: 320-328.

Balta, I., Marcu, A., Linton, M., Kelly, C., Stef, L., Pet, I., Ward, P., Pircalabioru, G.G., Chifiriuc, C., Gundogdu, O., Callaway, T. and Corcionivoschi, N., 2021. The *in vitro* and *in vivo* anti-virulent effect of organic acid mixtures against Eimeria tenella and Eimeria bovis. Scientific Reports 11: 16202.

Beck, S.C., Paidas, C.N., Mooney, M.L., Deitch, E.A. and De Maio, A., 1995. Presence of the stress inducible form of hsp-70 (hsp-72) in normal rat colon. Shock 3: 398-402.

Bhagat, M., Sood, S., Yadav, A., Verma, P., Manzoor, N., Chakraborty, D., Katoch, R. and Sangha, N., 2017. Alterations in oxidative stress parameters and its associated correlation with clinical disease on experimental Cryptosporidium parvum infection in Swiss albino mice. Journal of Parasitic Diseases 41: 707-712.

Bhat, M.I. and Kapila, R., 2017. Dietary metabolites derived from gut microbiota: critical modulators of epigenetic changes in mammals. Nutrition Reviews 75: 374-389.

Biasi, F., Astegiano, M., Maina, M., Leonarduzzi, G. and Poli, G., 2011. Polyphenol supplementation as a complementary medicinal approach to treating inflammatory bowel disease. Current Medicinal Chemistry 18: 4851-4865.

Biasi, F., Deiana, M., Guina, T., Gamba, P., Leonarduzzi, G. and Poli, G., 2014. Wine consumption and intestinal redox homeostasis. Redox Biology 2: 795-802.

Bolca, S., Van de Wiele, T. and Possemiers, S., 2013. Gut metabotypes govern health effects of dietary polyphenols. Current opinion in Biotechnology 24: 220-225.

Brigelius-Flohé, R. and Maiorino, M., 2013. Glutathione peroxidases. Biochimica et Biophysica Acta 1830: 3289-3303.

Brigelius-Flohé, R. and Flohé, L., 2020. Regulatory phenomena in the glutathione peroxidase superfamily. Antioxidants and Redox Signaling 33: 498-516.

Brigelius-Flohé, R., 1999. Tissue-specific functions of individual glutathione peroxidases. Free Radical Biology and Medicine 27: 951-965.

Brigelius-Flohé, R., Muller, C., Menard, J., Florian, S., Schmehl, K. and Wingler, K., 2001. Functions of GI-GPx: lessons from selenium-dependent expression and intracellular localization. BioFactors 14: 101-106.

Buechler, N., Wang, X., Yoza, B.K., McCall, C.E. and Vachharajani, V., 2017. Sirtuin 2 regulates microvascular inflammation during sepsis. Journal of Immunology Research 2017: 2648946.

Campbell, E.L. and Colgan, S.P., 2019. Control and dysregulation of redox signalling in the gastrointestinal tract. Nature reviews. Gastroenterology and Hepatology 16: 106-120.

Caruso, R., Marafini, I., Franzè, E., Stolfi, C., Zorzi, F., Monteleone, I., Caprioli, F., Colantoni, A., Sarra, M., Sedda, S., Biancone, L., Sileri, P., Sica, G.S., MacDonald, T.T., Pallone, F. and Monteleone, G., 2014. Defective expression of SIRT1 contributes to sustain inflammatory pathways in the gut. Mucosal Immunology 7: 1467-1479.

Chen, M., Hui, S., Lang, H., Zhou, M., Zhang, Y., Kang, C., Zeng, X., Zhang, Q., Yi, L. and Mi, M., 2019. SIRT3 deficiency promotes high-fat diet-induced nonalcoholic fatty liver disease in correlation with impaired intestinal permeability through gut microbial dysbiosis. Molecular Nutrition and Food Research 63: e1800612.

Chen, K., Liu, Y., Cheng, Y., Yan, Q., Zhou, C., He, Z., Zeng, J., He, J. and Tan, Z., 2020. Supplementation of Lactobacillus plantarum or Macleaya cordata extract alleviates oxidative damage induced by weaning in the lower gut of young goats. Animals 10: 548.

Cheng, Y. and Rong, J., 2017. Therapeutic potential of heme oxygenase-1/carbon monoxide system against ischemia-reperfusion injury. Current Pharmaceutical Design 23: 3884-3898.

Cho, K., Lee, H.G., Piao, J.Y., Kim, S.J., Na, H.K. and Surh, Y.J., 2021. Protective effects of silibinin on Helicobacter pylori-induced gastritis: NF-κB and STAT3 as potential targets. Journal of Cancer Prevention 26: 118-127.

Chu, F.F., Doroshow, J.H. and Esworthy, R.S., 1993. Expression, characterization, and tissue distribution of a new cellular selenium-dependent glutathione peroxidase, GSHPx-GI. Journal of Biological Chemistry 268: 2571-2576.

Circu, M.L. and Aw, T.Y., 2012. Intestinal redox biology and oxidative stress. Seminars in Cell and Developmental Biology 23: 729-737.

David, J.C., Grongnet, J.F. and Lalles, J.P., 2002. Weaning affects the expression of heat shock proteins in different regions of the gastrointestinal tract of piglets. Journal of Nutrition 132: 2551-2561.

Davis, W.L., Matthews, J.L., Shibata, K., Kipnis, M., Farmer, G.R., Cortinas, E., Meiyr, J.C. and Goodman, D.B., 1989. The immunocytochemical localization of superoxide dismutase in the enterocytes of the avian intestine: the effect of vitamin D3. The Histochemical Journal 21: 194-202.

Degroote, J., Wang, W., Vergauwen, H., De Smet, S., Van Ginneken, C. and Michiels, J., 2019. Impact of a dietary challenge with peroxidized oil on the glutathione redox status and integrity of the small intestine in weaned piglets. Animal 13: 1641-1650.

Din, A.U., Hassan, A., Zhu, Y., Zhang, K., Wang, Y., Li, T., Wang, Y. and Wang, G., 2020. Inhibitory effect of Bifidobacterium bifidum ATCC 29521 on colitis and its mechanism. The Journal of Nutritional Biochemistry 79: 108353.

Dobashi, K., Asayama, K., Kato, K., Kobayashi, M. and Kawasi, A., 1989. Immunohistochemical localization of copper-zinc and manganese superoxide dismutases in rat tissues. Acta Histochemica et Cytochemica 22: 351-365.

Dolara, P., Luceri, C., De Filippo, C., Femia, A.P., Giovannelli, L., Caderni, G., Cecchini, C., Silvi, S., Orpianesi, C. and Cresci, A., 2005. Red wine polyphenols influence carcinogenesis, intestinal microflora, oxidative damage and gene expression profiles of colonic mucosa in F344 rats. Mutation Research 591: 237-246.

Drew, J.E., Farquharson, A.J., Arthur, J.R., Morrice, P.C. and Duthie, G.G., 2005. Novel sites of cytosolic glutathione peroxidase expression in colon. FEBS Letters 579: 6135-6139.

Dridi, J.S., Greene, E.S., Maynard, C.W., Brugaletta, G., Ramser, A., Christopher, C.J., Campagna, S.R., Castro, H.F. and Dridi, S., 2022. Duodenal metabolic profile changes in heat-stressed broilers. Animals 12: 1337.

Du, E., Fan, Q., Zhao, N., Zhang, W., Wei, J., Chen, F., Huang, S. and Guo, W., 2021. Supplemental magnolol improves the antioxidant capacity and intestinal health of broiler chickens. Animal Science Journal 92: e13665.

Esmaily, H., Hosseini-Tabatabaei, A., Rahimian, R., Khorasani, R., Baeeri, M., Barazesh-Morgani, A., Yasa, N., Khademi, Y. and Abdollahi, M., 2009. On the benefits of silymarin in murine colitis by improving balance of destructive cytokines and reduction of toxic stress in the bowel cells. Central European Journal of Biology 4: 204-213.

Esmaily, H., Vaziri-Bami, A., Miroliaee, A.E., Baeeri, M. and Abdollahi, M., 2011. The correlation between NF-κB inhibition and disease activity by coadministration of silibinin and ursodeoxycholic acid in experimental colitis. Fundamental and Clinical Pharmacology 25: 723-733.

Esworthy, R.S., Aranda, R., Martín, M.G., Doroshow, J.H., Binder, S.W. and Chu, F.F., 2001. Mice with combined disruption of Gpx1 and Gpx2 genes have colitis. American Journal of Physiology. Gastrointestinal and Liver Physiology 281: G848-G855.

Esworthy, R.S., Swiderek, K.M., Ho, Y.S. and Chu, F.F., 1998. Selenium-dependent glutathione peroxidase-GI is a major glutathione peroxidase activity in the mucosal epithelium of rodent intestine. Biochimica et Biophysica Acta 1381: 213-226.

Fang, S. and Christensen, J., 1995. Manganese superoxide dismutase and reduced nicotinamide adenine dinucleotide diaphorase colocalize in the rat gut. Gastroenterology 109: 1429-1436.

Feng, J., Cavallero, S., Hsiai, T. and Li, R., 2020. Impact of air pollution on intestinal redox lipidome and microbiome. Free Radical Biology and Medicine 151: 99-110.

Florian, S., Krehl, S., Loewinger, M., Kipp, A., Banning, A., Esworthy, S., Chu, F.F. and Brigelius-Flohé, R., 2010. Loss of GPx2 increases apoptosis, mitosis, and GPx1 expression in the intestine of mice. Free radical Biology and Medicine 49: 1694-1702.

Florian, S., Wingler, K., Schmehl, K., Jacobasch, G., Kreuzer, O.J., Meyerhof, W. and Brigelius-Flohé, R., 2001. Cellular and subcellular localization of gastrointestinal glutathione peroxidase in normal and malignant human intestinal tissue. Free Radical Research 35: 655-663.

Frederiks, W.M. and Bosch, K.S., 1997. Localization of superoxide dismutase activity in rat tissues. Free radical Biology and Medicine 22: 241-248.

Fu, J., Liu, C.P., Zhang, Z.W., Xing, M.W. and Xu, S.W., 2013. Influence of inflammatory pathway markers on oxidative stress induced by cold stress in intestine of quails. Research in Veterinary Science 95: 495-501.

Fujii, H., Takahashi, T., Nakahira, K., Uehara, K., Shimizu, H., Matsumi, M., Morita, K., Hirakawa, M., Akagi, R. and Sassa, S., 2003. Protective role of heme oxygenase-1 in the intestinal tissue injury in an experimental model of sepsis. Critical Care Medicine 31: 893-902.

Gan, H.T. and Chen, J.D., 2007. Induction of heme oxygenase-1 improves impaired intestinal transit after burn injury. Surgery 141: 385-393.

Gasdaska, J.R., Gasdaska, P.Y., Gallegos, A. and Powis, G., 1996. Human thioredoxin reductase gene localization to chromosomal position 12q23-q24.1 and mRNA distribution in human tissue. Genomics 37: 257-259.

Gessner, D.K., Fiesel, A., Most, E., Dinges, J., Wen, G., Ringseis, R. and Eder, K., 2013. Supplementation of a grape seed and grape marc meal extract decreases activities of the oxidative stress-responsive transcription factors NF-κB and Nrf2 in the duodenal mucosa of pigs. Acta Veterinaria Scandinavica 55: 18.

Giovannelli, L., Testa, G., De Filippo, C., Cheynier, V., Clifford, M.N. and Dolora, P., 2000. Effect of complex polyphenols and tannins from red wine on DNA oxidative damage of rat colon mucosa *in vivo*. European Journal of Nutrition 39: 207-212.

Godoy, J.R., Funke, M., Ackermann, W., Haunhorst, P., Oesteritz, S., Capani, F., Elsässer, H.P. and Lillig, C.H., 2011. Redox atlas of the mouse. Immunohistochemical detection of glutaredoxin-, peroxiredoxin-, and thioredoxin-family proteins in various tissues of the laboratory mouse. Biochimica et Biophysica Acta 1810: 2-92.

Goodrich, K.M., Fundaro, G., Griffin, L.E., Grant, A., Hulver, M.W., Ponder, M.A. and Neilson, A.P., 2012. Chronic administration of dietary grape seed extract increases colonic expression of gut tight junction protein occludin and reduces fecal calprotectin: a secondary analysis of healthy Wistar Furth rats. Nutrition Research 32: 787-794.

Gordeeva, A.E., Temnov, A.A., Charnagalov, A.A., Sharapov, M.G., Fesenko, E.E. and Novoselov, V.I., 2015. Protective effect of peroxiredoxin 6 in ischemia/reperfusion-induced damage of small intestine. Digestive Diseases and Sciences 60: 3610-3619.

Gorelik, S., Lapidot, T., Shaham, I., Granit, R., Ligumsky, M., Kohen, R. and Kanner, J., 2005. Lipid peroxidation and coupled vitamin oxidation in simulated and human gastric fluid inhibited by dietary polyphenols: health implications. Journal of Agricultural and Food Chemistry 53: 3397-3402.

Gorelik, S., Ligumsky, M., Kohen, R. and Kanner, J., 2008a. The stomach as a 'bioreactor': when red meat meets red wine. Journal of Agricultural and Food Chemistry 56: 5002-5007.

Gorelik, S., Ligumsky, M., Kohen, R. and Kanner, J., 2008b. A novel function of red wine polyphenols in humans: prevention of absorption of cytotoxic lipid peroxidation products. FASEB Journal 22: 41-46.

Granger, D.N., Rutili, G. and McCord, J.M., 1981. Superoxide radicals in feline intestinal ischemia. Gastroenterology 81: 22-29.

Gu, X.H., Hao, Y. and Wang, X.L., 2012. Overexpression of heat shock protein 70 and its relationship to intestine under acute heat stress in broilers: 2. Intestinal oxidative stress. Poultry Science 91: 790-799.

Guo, X., Shin, V.Y. and Cho, C.H., 2001. Modulation of heme oxygenase in tissue injury and its implication in protection against gastrointestinal diseases. Life Sciences 69: 3113-3119.

Han, W., Mercenier, A., Ait-Belgnaoui, A., Pavan, S., Lamine, F., van Swam, I.I., Kleerebezem, M., Salvador-Cartier, C., Hisbergues, M., Bueno, L., Theodorou, V. and Fioramonti, J., 2006. Improvement of an experimental colitis in rats by lactic acid bacteria producing superoxide dismutase. Inflammatory Bowel Diseases 12: 1044-1052.

Han, Z., Willer, T., Li, L., Pielsticker, C., Rychlik, I., Velge, P., Kaspers, B. and Rautenschlein, S., 2017. Influence of the gut microbiota composition on Campylobacter jejuni colonization in chickens. Infection and Immunity 85: e00380-17.

Higashikubo, A., Tanaka, N., Noda, N., Maeda, I., Yagi, K., Mizoguchi, T. and Nanri, H., 1999. Increase in thioredoxin activity of intestinal epithelial cells mediated by oxidative stress. Biological and Pharmaceutical Bulletin 22: 900-903.

Hiraishi, H., Terano, A., Sugimoto, T., Harada, T., Razandi, M. and Ivey, K.J., 1994. Protective role of intracellular superoxide dismutase against extracellular oxidants in cultured rat gastric cells. The Journal of Clinical Investigation 93: 331-338.

Hsu, J.L., Chou, J.W., Chen, T.F., Hsu, J.T., Su, F.Y., Lan, J.L., Wu, P.C., Hu, C.M., Lee, E.Y. and Lee, W.H., 2020. Glutathione peroxidase 8 negatively regulates caspase-4/11 to protect against colitis. EMBO Molecular Medicine 12: e9386.

Hu, Y., Tao, X., Han, X., Xu, L., Yin, L., Sun, H., Qi, Y., Xu, Y. and Peng, J., 2018. MicroRNA-351-5p aggravates intestinal ischaemia/reperfusion injury through the targeting of MAPK13 and Sirtuin-6. British Journal of Pharmacology 175: 3594-3609.

Huang, L., Mivechi, N.F. and Moskophidis, D., 2001. Insights into regulation and function of the major stress-induced hsp70 molecular chaperone *in vivo*: analysis of mice with targeted gene disruption of the hsp70.1 or hsp70.3 gene. Molecular and Cellular Biology 21: 8575-8591.

Inoue, K., Takahashi, T., Uehara, K., Shimuzu, H., Ido, K., Morimatsu, H., Omori, E., Katayama, H., Akagi, R. and Morita, K., 2008. Protective role of heme oxygenase 1 in the intestinal tissue injury in hemorrhagic shock in rats. Shock 29: 252-261.

Jaeger, S.U., Schroeder, B.O., Meyer-Hoffert, U., Courth, L., Fehr, S.N., Gersemann, M., Stange, E.F. and Wehkamp, J., 2013. Cell-mediated reduction of human β-defensin 1: a major role for mucosal thioredoxin. Mucosal Immunology 6: 1179-1190.

Jahanian, E., Mahdavi, A.H. and Jahanian, R., 2021. Silymarin improved the growth performance via modulating the microbiota and mucosal immunity in Escherichia coli-challenged broiler chicks. Livestock Science 249: 104529.

Jefferies, H., Bot, J., Coster, J., Khalil, A., Hall, J.C. and McCauley, R.D., 2003. The role of glutathione in intestinal dysfunction. Journal of Investigative Surgery 16: 315-323.

Jiménez-Hidalgo, M., Kurz, C.L., Pedrajas, J.R., Naranjo-Galindo, F.J., González-Barrios, M., Cabello, J., Sáez, A.G., Lozano, E., Button, E.L., Veal, E.A., Fierro-González, J.C., Swoboda, P. and Miranda-Vizuete, A., 2014. Functional characterization of thioredoxin 3 (TRX-3), a Caenorhabditis elegans intestine-specific thioredoxin. Free Radical Biology & Medicine 68: 205-219.

Jones, R.M., Mercante, J.W. and Neish, A.S., 2012. Reactive oxygen production induced by the gut microbiota: pharmacotherapeutic implications. Current Medicinal Chemistry 19: 1519-1529.

Jones, R.M. and Neish, A.S., 2017. Redox signaling mediated by the gut microbiota. Free Radical Biology & Medicine 105: 41-47.

Ju, S., Ge, Y., Li, P., Tian, X., Wang, H., Zheng, X. and Ju, S., 2018. Dietary quercetin ameliorates experimental colitis in mouse by remodeling the function of colonic macrophages via a heme oxygenase-1-dependent pathway. Cell Cycle 17: 53-63.

Kanner, J. and Lapidot, T., 2001. The stomach as a bioreactor: dietary lipid peroxidation in the gastric fluid and the effects of plant-derived antioxidants. Free Radical Biology & Medicine 31: 1388-1395.

Kanner, J., Gorelik, S., Roman, S. and Kohen, R., 2012. Protection by polyphenols of postprandial human plasma and low-density lipoprotein modification: the stomach as a bioreactor. Journal of Agricultural and Food Chemistry 60: 8790-8796.

Kipp, A., Banning, A., Van Schothorst, E.M., Méplan, C., Schomburg, L., Evelo, C., Coort, S., Gaj, S., Keijer, J., Hesketh, J. and Brigelius-Flohé, R., 2009. Four selenoproteins, protein biosynthesis, and Wnt signalling are particularly sensitive to limited selenium intake in mouse colon. Molecular Nutrition and Food Research 53: 1561-1572.

Kipp, A.P., Müller, M.F., Göken, E.M., Deubel, S. and Brigelius-Flohé, R., 2012. The selenoproteins GPx2, TrxR2 and TrxR3 are regulated by Wnt signalling in the intestinal epithelium. Biochimica et Biophysica Acta 1820: 1588-1596.

Köck, K., Xie, Y., Hawke, R.L., Oberlies, N.H. and Brouwer, K.L., 2013. Interaction of silymarin flavonolignans with organic anion-transporting polypeptides. Drug Metabolism and Disposition 41: 958-965.

Kojima, K., Musch, M.W., Ren, H., Boone, D.L., Hendrickson, B.A., Ma, A. and Chang, E.B., 2003. Enteric flora and lymphocyte-derived cytokines determine expression of heat shock proteins in mouse colonic epithelial cells. Gastroenterology 124: 1395-1407.

Kopecek, P., Altmannova, K. and Weigl, E., 2001. Stress proteins: nomenclature, division and functions. Biomedical Papers of the Medical Faculty of the University Palacky 45: 39-47.

Krehl, S., Loewinger, M., Florian, S., Kipp, A.P., Banning, A., Wessjohann, L.A., Brauer, M.N., Iori, R., Esworthy, R.S., Chu, F.F. and Brigelius-Flohé, R., 2012. Glutathione peroxidase-2 and selenium decreased inflammation and tumors in a mouse model of inflammation-associated carcinogenesis whereas sulforaphane effects differed with selenium supply. Carcinogenesis 33: 620-628.

Kruidenier, L., Kuiper, I., van Duijn, W., Marklund, S.L., van Hogezand, R.A., Lamers, C.B. and Verspaget, H.W., 2003. Differential mucosal expression of three superoxide dismutase isoforms in inflammatory bowel disease. The Journal of Pathology 201: 7-16.

Lan, C., Sun, X.N., Zhou, X.C., Yang, B., Huang, B.L., Deng, T.Z., He, Z.T. and Han, X.Y., 2016. Preinduced intestinal HSP70 improves visceral hypersensitivity and abnormal intestinal motility in PI-IBS mouse model. Asian Pacific Journal of Tropical Medicine 9: 302-305.

LeBlanc, J.G., del Carmen, S., Miyoshi, A., Azevedo, V., Sesma, F., Langella, P., Bermúdez-Humarán, L.G., Watterlot, L., Perdigon, G. and de Moreno de LeBlanc, A., 2011. Use of superoxide dismutase and catalase producing lactic acid bacteria in TNBS induced Crohn's disease in mice. Journal of Biotechnology 151: 287-293.

Lee, W.J., 2008. Bacterial-modulated signaling pathways in gut homeostasis. Science Signaling 1: pe24.

LeGrand, T.S. and Aw, T.Y., 1998. Chronic hypoxia alters glucose utilization during GSH-dependent detoxication in rat small intestine. American Journal of Physiology 274: G376-G384.

Lennicke, C., Rahn, J., Wickenhauser, C., Lichtenfels, R., Müller, A.S., Wessjohann, L.A., Kipp, A.P. and Seliger, B., 2017. Loss of epithelium-specific GPx2 results in aberrant cell fate decisions during intestinal differentiation. Oncotarget 9: 539-552.

Lessard, M., Savard, C., Deschene, K., Lauzon, K., Pinilla, V.A., Gagnon, C.A., Lapointe, J., Guay, F. and Chorfi, Y., 2015. Impact of deoxynivalenol (DON) contaminated feed on intestinal integrity and immune response in swine. Food and Chemical Toxicology 80: 7-16.

Li, Y., Li, Q., Chen, H., Wang, T., Liu, L., Wang, G., Xie, K. and Yu, Y., 2015. Hydrogen gas alleviates the intestinal injury caused by severe sepsis in mice by increasing the expression of heme oxygenase-1. Shock 44: 90-98.

Li, C., Zhou, Y., Rychahou, P., Weiss, H.L., Lee, E.Y., Perry, C.L., Barrett, T.A., Wang, Q. and Evers, B.M., 2020a. SIRT2 contributes to the regulation of intestinal cell proliferation and differentiation. Cellular and Molecular Gastroenterology and Hepatology 10: 43-57.

Li, X., Wang, Y., Xing, Y., Xing, R., Liu, Y. and Xu, Y., 2020b. Changes of gut microbiota during silybin-mediated treatment of high-fat diet-induced non-alcoholic fatty liver disease in mice. Hepatology Research 50: 5-14.

Li, Y., Wang, P., Yin, J., Jin, S., Su, W., Tian, J., Li, T. and Yao, K., 2020c. Effects of ornithine α-ketoglutarate on growth performance and gut microbiota in a chronic oxidative stress pig model induced by d-galactose. Food and Function 11: 472-482.

Liao, Y.F., Zhu, W., Li, D.P. and Zhu, X., 2013. Heme oxygenase-1 and gut ischemia/reperfusion injury: A short review. World journal of Gastroenterology 19: 3555-3561.

Liao, S., Liu, G., Tan, B., Qi, M., Li, J., Li, X., Zhu, C., Huang, J., Yin, Y. and Tang, Y., 2021. Fullerene C60 protects against intestinal injury from deoxynivalenol toxicity by improving antioxidant capacity. Life 11: 491.

Liao, X.D., Ma, G., Cai, J., Fu, Y., Yan, X.Y., Wei, X.B. and Zhang, R.J., 2015. Effects of Clostridium butyricum on growth performance, antioxidation, and immune function of broilers. Poultry Science 94: 662-667.

Liedel, J.L., Guo, Y., Yu, Y., Shiou, S.R., Chen, S., Petrof, E.O., Hu, S., Musch, M.W. and Claud, E.C., 2011. Mother's milk-induced Hsp70 expression preserves intestinal epithelial barrier function in an immature rat pup model. Pediatric Research 69: 395-400.

Liu, F., Bu, H.F., Geng, H., De Plaen, I.G., Gao, C., Wang, P., Wang, X., Kurowski, J.A., Yang, H., Qian, J. and Tan, X.D., 2017. Sirtuin-6 preserves R-spondin-1 expression and increases resistance of intestinal epithelium to injury in mice. Molecular Medicine 23: 272-284.

Liu, H.Y., Dicksved, J., Lundh, T. and Lindberg, J.E., 2014. Expression of heat shock proteins 27 and 72 correlates with specific commensal microbes in different regions of porcine gastrointestinal tract. American Journal of Physiology – Gastrointestinal and Liver Physiology 306: G1033-1041.

Lo Sasso, G., Menzies, K.J., Mottis, A., Piersigilli, A., Perino, A., Yamamoto, H., Schoonjans, K. and Auwerx, J., 2014b. SIRT2 deficiency modulates macrophage polarization and susceptibility to experimental colitis. PloS One 9: e103573.

Lo Sasso, G., Ryu, D., Mouchiroud, L., Fernando, S.C., Anderson, C.L., Katsyuba, E., Piersigilli, A., Hottiger, M.O., Schoonjans, K. and Auwerx, J., 2014a. Loss of Sirt1 function improves intestinal anti-bacterial defense and protects from colitis-induced colorectal cancer. PloS One 9: e102495.

Malago, J.J., Koninkx, J.F. and Van Dijk, J.E., 2002. The heat shock response and cytoprotection of the intestinal epithelium. Cell Stress Chaperones 7: 191-199.

Mallick, I.H., Winslet, M.C. and Seifalian, A.M., 2010. Ischemic preconditioning of small bowel mitigates the late phase of reperfusion injury: heme oxygenase mediates cytoprotection. American Journal of Surgery 199: 223-231.

Mardinoglu, A., Shoaie, S., Bergentall, M., Ghaffari, P., Zhang, C., Larsson, E., Bäckhed, F. and Nielsen, J., 2015. The gut microbiota modulates host amino acid and glutathione metabolism in mice. Molecular Systems Biology 11: 834.

Marelli, G. and Allavena, P., 2020. The good and the bad side of heme-oxygenase-1 in the gut. Antioxidants and Redox Signaling 32: 1071-1079.

Marelli, G., Erreni, M., Anselmo, A., Taverniti, V., Guglielmetti, S., Mantovani, A. and Allavena, P., 2017. Heme-oxygenase-1 production by intestinal CX3CR1$^+$ macrophages helps to resolve inflammation and prevents carcinogenesis. Cancer Research 77: 4472-4485.

Martínez, J.A., Etxeberría, U., Galar, A. and Milagro, F.I., 2013. Role of dietary polyphenols and inflammatory processes on disease progression mediated by the gut microbiota. Rejuvenation Research 16: 435-437.

McLean, J.A., Karadas, F., Surai, P.F., McDevitt, R.M. and Speake, B.K., 2005. Lipid-soluble and water-soluble antioxidant activities of the avian intestinal mucosa at different sites along the intestinal tract. Comparative Biochemistry and Physiology Part B: Biochemistry and Molecular Biology 141: 366-372.

Meinl, W., Sczesny, S., Brigelius-Flohé, R., Blaut, M. and Glatt, H., 2009. Impact of gut microbiota on intestinal and hepatic levels of phase 2 xenobiotic-metabolizing enzymes in the rat. Drug Metabolism and Disposition 37: 1179-1186.

Moco, S., Martin, F.P. and Rezzi, S., 2012. Metabolomics view on gut microbiome modulation by polyphenol-rich foods. Journal of Proteome Research 11: 4781-4790.

Mörk, H., Lex, B., Scheurlen, M., Dreher, I., Schutze, N., Köhrle, J. and Jakob, F., 1998. Expression pattern of gastrointestinal selenoproteins – targets for selenium supplementation. Nutrition and Cancer 32: 64-70.

Müller, M.F., Florian, S., Pommer, S., Osterhoff, M., Esworthy, R.S., Chu, F.F., Brigelius-Flohé, R. and Kipp, A.P., 2013. Deletion of glutathione peroxidase-2 inhibits azoxymethane-induced colon cancer development. PloS One: e72055.

Musch, M.W., Sugi, K., Straus, D. and Chang, E.B., 1999. Heat-shock protein 72 protects against oxidant-induced injury of barrier function of human colonic epithelial Caco2/bbe cells. Gastroenterology 117: 115-122.

Nakagawa, F., Morino, K., Ugi, S., Ishikado, A., Kondo, K., Sato, D., Konno, S., Nemoto, K., Kusunoki, C., Sekine, O., Sunagawa, A., Kawamura, M., Inoue, N., Nishio, Y. and Maegawa, H., 2014. 4-Hydroxy hexenal derived from dietary n-3 polyunsaturated fatty acids induces anti-oxidative enzyme heme oxygenase-1 in multiple organs. Biochemical and Biophysical Research Communications 443: 991-996.

Neish, A.S. and Jones, R.M., 2014. Redox signaling mediates symbiosis between the gut microbiota and the intestine. Gut Microbes 5: 250-253.

Neish, A.S., 2013. Redox signaling mediated by the gut microbiota. Free Radical Research 47: 950-957.

Oberley, T.D., Oberley, L.W., Slattery, A.F., Lauchner, L.J. and Elwell, J.H., 1990. Immunohistochemical localization of antioxidant enzymes in adult Syrian hamster tissues and during kidney development. The American Journal of Pathology 137: 199-214.

Pang, Q., Ji, Y., Li, Y., Bermúdez-Humarán, L.G., Hu, G. and Zeng, Y., 2008. Intragastric administration with recombinant Lactococcus lactis producing heme oxygenase-1 prevents lipopolysaccharide-induced endotoxemia in rats. FEMS Microbiology Letters 283: 62-68.

Parkar, S.G., Trower, T.M. and Stevenson, D.E., 2013. Fecal microbial metabolism of polyphenols and its effects on human gut microbiota. Anaerobe 23: 12-19.

Peng, Z., Liao, Y., Chen, L., Liu, S., Shan, Z., Nüssler, A.K., Yao, P., Yan, H., Liu, L. and Yang, W., 2019. Heme oxygenase-1 attenuates low-dose of deoxynivalenol-induced liver inflammation potentially associating with microbiota. Toxicology and Applied Pharmacology 374: 20-31.

Pérez, S., Taléns-Visconti, R., Rius-Pérez, S., Finamor, I. and Sastre, J., 2017. Redox signaling in the gastrointestinal tract. Free Radical Biology & Medicine 104: 75-103.

Pozuelo, M.J., Agis-Torres, A., Hervert-Hernández, D., Elvira López-Oliva, M., Muñoz-Martínez, E., Rotger, R. and Goñi, I., 2012. Grape antioxidant dietary fiber stimulates Lactobacillus growth in rat cecum. Journal of Food Science 77: H59-H62.

Prabhu, R. and Balasubramanian, K.A., 2002. Heat preconditioning attenuates oxygen free radical mediated alterations in the intestinal brush border membrane induced by surgical manipulation. Journal of Surgical Research 107: 227-233.

Reeves, M.A. and Hoffmann, P.R., 2009. The human selenoproteome: recent insights into functions and regulation. Cellular and Molecular Life Sciences 66: 2457-2478.

Ren, M.T., Gu, M.L., Zhou, X.X., Yu, M.S., Pan, H.H., Ji, F. and Ding, C.Y., 2019. Sirtuin 1 alleviates endoplasmic reticulum stress-mediated apoptosis of intestinal epithelial cells in ulcerative colitis. World Journal of Gastroenterology 25: 5800-5813.

Ren, L., Ma, X.L., Wang, H.L., Li, R., Cui, J.J., Yan, P.J., Wang, Y.N., Yu, X.Y., Du, P., Yu, H.Y., Guo, H.H., Tang, R., Che, Y.S., Zheng, W.S., Jiang, J.D. and Wang, L.L., 2022. Prebiotic-like cyclodextrin assisted silybin on NAFLD through restoring liver and gut homeostasis. Journal of Controlled Release 348: 825-840.

Rentea, R.M., Guo, Y., Zhu, X., Musch, M.W., Chang, E.B., Gourlay, D.M. and Liedel, J.L., 2018. Role of intestinal Hsp70 in barrier maintenance: contribution of milk to the induction of Hsp70.2. Pediatric Surgery International 34: 323-330.

Rigottier-Gois, L., 2013. Dysbiosis in inflammatory bowel diseases: the oxygen hypothesis. The ISME Journal 7: 1256-1261.

Rocha, B.S. and Laranjinha, J., 2020. Nitrate from diet might fuel gut microbiota metabolism: Minding the gap between redox signaling and inter-kingdom communication. Free Radical Biology and Medicine 149: 37-43.

Rodríguez-Ramiro, I., Martín, M.A., Ramos, S., Bravo, L. and Goya, L., 2011a. Comparative effects of dietary flavanols on antioxidant defences and their response to oxidant-induced stress on Caco2 cells. European Journal of Nutrition 50: 313-322.

Rodríguez-Ramiro, I., Ramos, S., Bravo, L., Goya, L. and Martín, M.Á., 2011b. Procyanidin B2 and a cocoa polyphenolic extract inhibit acrylamide-induced apoptosis in human Caco-2 cells by preventing oxidative stress and activation of JNK pathway. The Journal of Nutritional Biochemistry 22: 1186-1194.

Rokutan, K., 1999. Molecular stress response in the stomach. Nippon Yakurigaku Zasshi 114: 265-272.

Rubinstein, A., Kakunda, A. and Kohen, R., 1993. Protection of the rat jejunal mucosa against oxidative injury by cationized superoxide dismutase. Journal of Pharmaceutical Sciences 82: 1285-1287.

Samborski, P. and Grzymisławski, M., 2015. The role of HSP70 heat shock proteins in the pathogenesis and treatment of inflammatory bowel diseases. Advances in Clinical and Experimental Medicine 24: 525-530.

Sanderson, I.R., 1999. The physicochemical environment of the neonatal intestine. American Journal of Clinical Nutrition 69: 1028S-1034S.

Sangeetha, N., Viswanathan, P., Balasubramanian, T. and Nalini, N., 2012. Colon cancer chemopreventive efficacy of silibinin through perturbation of xenobiotic metabolizing enzymes in experimental rats. European Journal of Pharmacology 674: 430-438.

Santoro, M.G., 2000. Heat shock factors and the control of the stress response. Biochemical Pharmacology 59: 55-63.

Sergeant, M.J., Constantinidou, C., Cogan, T.A., Bedford, M.R., Penn, C.W. and Pallen, M.J., 2014. Extensive microbial and functional diversity within the chicken cecal microbiome. PloS One 9: e91941.

Shanmugam, S., Park, J.H., Cho, S. and Kim, I.H., 2022. Silymarin seed extract supplementation enhances the growth performance, meat quality, and nutrients digestibility, and reduces gas emission in broilers. Animal Bioscience 35: 1215-1222.

Sharma, A., Puri, V., Kakkar, V. and Singh, I., 2018. Formulation and evaluation of silymarin-loaded chitosan-montmorilloite microbeads for the potential treatment of gastric ulcers. Journal of Functional Biomaterials 9: 52.

Shen, L., Liu, L., Li, X.Y. and Ji, H.F., 2019. Regulation of gut microbiota in Alzheimer's disease mice by silibinin and silymarin and their pharmacological implications. Applied Microbiology and Biotechnology 103: 7141-7149.

Shi, N., Li, N., Duan, X. and Niu, H., 2017. Interaction between the gut microbiome and mucosal immune system. Military Medical Research 4: 14.

Shin, J.H., Lee, C.W., Oh, S.J., Yun, J., Lee, K., Park, S.K., Kim, H.M., Han, S.B., Kim, Y., Kim, H.C. and Kang, J.S., 2013. Protective effect of silymarin against ethanol-induced gastritis in rats: role of sulfhydryls, nitric oxide and gastric sensory afferents. Food and Chemical Toxicology 55: 353-357.

Sido, B., Giese, T., Autschbach, F., Lasitschka, F., Braunstein, J. and Meuer, S.C., 2005. Potential role of thioredoxin in immune responses in intestinal lamina propria T lymphocytes. European Journal of Immunology 35: 408-417.

Sierra-Filardi, E., Vega, M.A., Sánchez-Mateos, P., Corbí, A.L. and Puig-Kröger, A., 2010. Heme Oxygenase-1 expression in M-CSF-polarized M2 macrophages contributes to LPS-induced IL-10 release. Immunobiology 215: 788-795.

Speckmann, B. and Steinbrenner, H., 2014. Selenium and selenoproteins in inflammatory bowel diseases and experimental colitis. Inflammatory Bowel Disease 20: 1110-1119.

Speckmann, B., Bidmon, H.J., Pinto, A., Anlauf, M., Sies, H. and Steinbrenner, H., 2011. Induction of glutathione peroxidase 4 expression during enterocytic cell differentiation. Journal of Biological Chemistry 286: 10764-10772.

Stecher, B., 2015. The roles of inflammation, nutrient availability and the commensal microbiota in enteric pathogen infection. Microbiology Spectrum 3: 10.1128.

Sun, Y., Zhang, J., Song, W. and Shan, A., 2018. Vitamin E alleviates phoxim-induced toxic effects on intestinal oxidative stress, barrier function, and morphological changes in rats. Environmental Science and Pollution Research International 25: 26682-26692.

Surai, K.P., Surai, P.F., Speake, B.K. and Sparks, N.H., 2003. Antioxidant-prooxidant balance in the intestine: Food for thought. 1. Prooxidants. Nutritional Genomics and Functional Foods 1: 51-70.

Surai, K.P., Surai, P.F., Speake, B.K. and Sparks, N.H., 2004. Antioxidant-prooxidant balance in the intestine: food for thought 2. Antioxidants. Current Topics in Nutraceutical Research 2: 27-46.

Surai, P.F., 2002. Natural antioxidants in avian nutrition and reproduction. Nottingham University Press, Nottingham, UK.

Surai, P.F., 2014. Polyphenol compounds in the chicken/animal diet: from the past to the future. Journal of Animal Physiology and Animal Nutrition 98: 19-31.

Surai, P.F., 2015. Silymarin as a natural antioxidant: an overview of the current evidence and perspectives. Antioxidants 4: 204-247.

Surai, P.F., 2016. Antioxidant systems in poultry biology: superoxide dismutase. Journal of Animal Research and Nutrition 1: 1-8.

Surai, P.F., 2018. Selenium in poultry nutrition and health. Wageningen Academic Publishers, Wageningen, The Netherlands.

Surai, P.F., 2020. Vitagene in avian biology and poultry health. Wageningen Academic Publishers, Wageningen, The Netherlands.

Surai, P.F. and Fisinin, V.I., 2015. Antioxidant-prooxidant balance in the intestine: applications in chick placement and pig weaning. Journal of Veterinary Science and Medicine 3: 16.

Surai, P.F., Kochish, I.I. and Shapovalov, S.O., 2018. Superoxide dismutase activity in chicken gut. British Poultry Abstracts 11-12.

Takahashi, K., Avissar, N., Whitin, J. and Cohen, H., 1987. Purification and characterization of human plasma glutathione peroxidase: a selenoglycoprotein distinct from the known cellular enzyme. Archives of Biochemistry and Biophysics 256: 677-686.

Takaishi, S., Sawada, M., Seno, H., Kayahara, T., Morita-Fujisawa, Y., Fukuzawa, H. and Chiba, T., 2003. Growth promoting effect of thioredoxin on intestinal epithelial cells. Digestive Diseases and Sciences 48: 379-385.

Takano, T., Yonemitsu, Y., Saito, S., Itoh, H., Onohara, T., Fukuda, A., Takai, M. and Maehara, Y., 2012. A somatostatin analogue, octreotide, ameliorates intestinal ischemia-reperfusion injury through the early induction of heme oxygenase-1. The Journal of Surgical Research 175: 350-358.

Tamion, F., Richard, V., Renet, S. and Thuillez, C., 2007. Intestinal preconditioning prevents inflammatory response by modulating heme oxygenase-1 expression in endotoxic shock model. American journal of physiology. Gastrointestinal and Liver Physiology 293: G1308-G1314.

Tanaka, J. and Yuda, Y., 1993. Role of lipid peroxidation in gastric mucosal lesions induced by ischemia-reperfusion in the pylorus-ligated rat. Biological and Pharmaceutical Bulletin 16: 29-32.

Tang, D., Wu, J., Jiao, H., Wang, X., Zhao, J. and Lin, H., 2019. The development of antioxidant system in the intestinal tract of broiler chickens. Poultry Science 98: 664-678.

Taranu, I., Braicu, C., Marin, D.E., Pistol, G.C., Motiu, M., Balacescu, L., Beridan Neagoe, I. and Burlacu, R., 2015. Exposure to zearalenone mycotoxin alters *in vitro* porcine intestinal epithelial cells by differential gene expression. Toxicology Letters 232: 310-325.

Tian, T., Wang, Z. and Zhang, J., 2017. Pathomechanisms of oxidative stress in inflammatory bowel disease and potential antioxidant therapies. Oxidative Medicine and Cellular Longevity 2017: 4535194.

Tsukimi, Y. and Okabe, S., 2001. Recent advances in gastrointestinal pathophysiology: role of heat shock proteins in mucosal defense and ulcer healing. Biological and Pharmaceutical Bulletin 24: 1-9.

Umeda, K., Takahashi, T., Inoue, K., Shimizu, H., Maeda, S., Morimatsu, H., Omori, E., Akagi, R., Katayama, H. and Morita, K., 2009. Prevention of hemorrhagic shock-induced intestinal tissue injury by glutamine via heme oxygenase-1 induction. Shock 31: 40-49.

Valentine, J.F. and Nick, H.S., 1992. Acute-phase induction of manganese superoxide dismutase in intestinal epithelial cell lines. Gastroenterology 103: 905-912.

Valentová, K., Havlík, J., Kosina, P., Papoušková, B., Jaimes, J.D., Káňová, K., Petrásková, L., Ulrichová, J. and Křen, V., 2020. Biotransformation of silymarin flavonolignans by human fecal microbiota. Metabolites 10: 29.

Wadhwa, R., Taira, K. and Kaul, S.C., 2002. An Hsp70 family chaperone, mortalin/mthsp70/PBP74/Grp75: what, when, and where? Cell Stress and Chaperones 7: 309-316.

Wang, N., Han, Q., Wang, G., Ma, W.P., Wang, J., Wu, W.X., Guo, Y., Liu, L., Jiang, X.Y., Xie, X.L. and Jiang, H.Q., 2016. Resveratrol protects oxidative stress-induced intestinal epithelial barrier dysfunction by upregulating heme oxygenase-1 expression. Digestive Diseases and Sciences 61: 2522-2534.

Wang, Y., Guo, Y., Chen, H., Wei, H. and Wan, C., 2018. Potential of Lactobacillus plantarum ZDY2013 and Bifidobacterium bifidum WBIN03 in relieving colitis by gut microbiota, immune, and anti-oxidative stress. Canadian Journal of Microbiology 64: 327-337.

Wang, Y., Wu, Y., Wang, Y., Xu, H., Mei, X., Yu, D., Wang, Y. and Li, W., 2017a. Antioxidant properties of probiotic bacteria. Nutrients 9: 521.

Wang, Y., Wu, Y., Wang, Y., Fu, A., Gong, L., Li, W. and Li, Y., 2017b. Bacillus amyloliquefaciens SC06 alleviates the oxidative stress of IPEC-1 via modulating Nrf2/Keap1 signaling pathway and decreasing ROS production. Applied Microbiology and Biotechnology 101: 3015-3026.

Wang, K., Zhu, Q., Kong, X., Song, M., Azad, M., Xiong, L., Zheng, Y. and He, Q., 2020a. Dietary probiotics or synbiotics supplementation during gestation, lactation, and nursery periods modifies colonic microbiota, antioxidant capacity, and immune function in weaned piglets. Frontiers in Veterinary Science 7: 597832.

Wang, Z., Sun, R., Wang, G., Chen, Z., Li, Y., Zhao, Y., Liu, D., Zhao, H., Zhang, F., Yao, J. and Tian, X., 2020b. SIRT3-mediated deacetylation of PRDX3 alleviates mitochondrial oxidative damage and apoptosis induced by intestinal ischemia/reperfusion injury. Redox Biology 28: 101343.

Wang, J., Zhang, C., Zhang, T., Yan, L., Qiu, L., Yin, H., Ding, X., Bai, S., Zeng, Q., Mao, X., Zhang, K., Wu, C., Xuan, Y. and Shan, Z., 2021. Dietary 25-hydroxyvitamin D improves intestinal health and microbiota of laying hens under high stocking density. Poultry Science 100: 101132.

Wang, L.C., Zhang, T.T., Wen, C., Jiang, Z.Y., Wang, T. and Zhou, Y.M., 2012. Protective effects of zinc-bearing clinoptilolite on broilers challenged with Salmonella pullorum. Poultry Science 91: 1838-1845.

Wang, W.W., Wang, J., Zhang, H.J., Wu, S.G. and Qi, G.H., 2019. Transcriptome analysis reveals mechanism underlying the differential intestinal functionality of laying hens in the late phase and peak phase of production. BMC Genomics 20: 970.

Weiss, G.A. and Hennet, T., 2017. Mechanisms and consequences of intestinal dysbiosis. Cellular and Molecular Life Sciences 74: 2959-2977.

Wellman, A.S., Metukuri, M.R., Kazgan, N., Xu, X., Xu, Q., Ren, N., Czopik, A., Shanahan, M.T., Kang, A., Chen, W., Azcarate-Peril, M.A., Gulati, A.S., Fargo, D.C., Guarente, L. and Li, X., 2017. Intestinal epithelial Sirtuin 1 regulates intestinal inflammation during aging in mice by altering the intestinal microbiota. Gastroenterology 153: 772-786.

Wu, B.Y., Zhu, M., Ruan, T., Li, L.J., Lyu, Y.N. and Wang, H.S., 2018. Oxidative stress, apoptosis and abnormal expression of apoptotic protein and gene and cell cycle arrest in the cecal tonsil of broilers induces by dietary methionine deficiency. Research in Veterinary Science 121: 65-75.

Xiao, Y., Xiang, Y., Zhou, W., Chen, J., Li, K. and Yang, H., 2017. Microbial community mapping in intestinal tract of broiler chicken. Poultry Science 96: 1387-1393.

Xie, Q., Xie, K., Yi, J., Song, Z., Zhang, H. and He, X., 2022a. The effects of magnolol supplementation on growth performance, meat quality, oxidative capacity, and intestinal microbiota in broilers. Poultry Science 101: 101722.

Xie, S., Zhang, H., Matjeke, R.S., Zhao, J. and Yu, Q., 2022b. Bacillus coagulans protect against Salmonella enteritidis-induced intestinal mucosal damage in young chickens by inducing the differentiation of goblet cells. Poultry Science 101: 101639.

Yang, G., Wang, H., Kang, Y. and Zhu, M.J., 2014. Grape seed extract improves epithelial structure and suppresses inflammation in ileum of IL-10-deficient mice. Food and Function 5: 2558-2563.

Yang, S., Li, L., Yu, L., Sun, L., Li, K., Tong, C., Xu, W., Cui, G., Long, M. and Li, P., 2020. Selenium-enriched yeast reduces caecal pathological injuries and intervenes changes of the diversity of caecal microbiota caused by Ochratoxin-A in broilers. Food and Chemical Toxicology 137: 111139.

Yenari, M.A., 2002. Heat shock proteins and neuroprotection. Advances in Experimental Medicine and Biology 513: 281-299.

Zhang, D., Shang, T., Huang, Y., Wang, S., Liu, H., Wang, J., Wang, Y., Ji, H. and Zhang, R., 2017a. Gene expression profile changes in the jejunum of weaned piglets after oral administration of Lactobacillus or an antibiotic. Scientific Reports 7: 15816.

Zhang, H., Yan, H., Zhou, X., Wang, H., Yang, Y., Zhang, J. and Wang, H., 2017b. The protective effects of Resveratrol against radiation-induced intestinal injury. BMC Complementary and Alternative Medicine 17: 410.

Zhang, C., Chen, K.K., Zhao, X.H., Wang, C. and Geng, Z.Y., 2019a. Effect of l-theanine on the growth performance, immune function, and jejunum morphology and antioxidant status of ducks. Animal 13: 1145-1153.

Zhang, L., Xue, H., Zhao, G., Qiao, C., Sun, X., Pang, C. and Zhang, D., 2019b. Curcumin and resveratrol suppress dextran sulfate sodium-induced colitis in mice. Molecular Medicine Reports 19: 3053-3060.

Zhang, Y., Wang, X.L., Zhou, M., Kang, C., Lang, H.D., Chen, M.T., Hui, S.C., Wang, B. and Mi, M.T., 2018. Crosstalk between gut microbiota and Sirtuin-3 in colonic inflammation and tumorigenesis. Experimental and Molecular Medicine 50: 1-11.

Zhao, B., Fei, J., Chen, Y., Ying, Y.L., Ma, L., Song, X.Q., Wang, L., Chen, E.Z. and Mao, E.Q., 2014. Pharmacological preconditioning with vitamin C attenuates intestinal injury via the induction of heme oxygenase-1 after hemorrhagic shock in rats. PloS One 9: e99134.

Zhao, F., Shi, B., Sun, D., Chen, H., Tong, M., Zhang, P., Guo, X. and Yan, S., 2016. Effects of dietary supplementation of Artemisia argyi aqueous extract on antioxidant indexes of small intestine in broilers. Animal Nutrition 2: 198-203.

Zhou, Z., Zhang, J., Zhang, X., Mo, S., Tan, X., Wang, L., Li, J., Li, Y., Ding, X., Liu, X., Ma, X., Yang, H. and Yin, Y., 2019. The production of short chain fatty acid and colonic development in weaning piglets. Journal of Animal Physiology and Animal Nutrition 103: 1530-1537.

Zhuang, Y., Wu, H., Wang, X., He, J., He, S. and Yin, Y., 2019. Resveratrol attenuates oxidative stress-induced intestinal barrier injury through PI3K/Akt-mediated Nrf2 signaling pathway. Oxidative Medicine and Cellular Longevity 2019: 7591840.

Zuidema, M.Y., Peyton, K.J., Fay, W.P., Durante, W. and Korthuis, R.J., 2011. Antecedent hydrogen sulfide elicits an anti-inflammatory phenotype in postischemic murine small intestine: role of heme oxygenase-1. American journal of physiology. Heart and Circulatory Physiology 301: H888-H894.

Part IV.

Practical applications of silymarin in clinical practice

Practice makes perfect

Chapter 12
Hepatoprotective properties of silymarin

Where there's will, there's way.

Anton Surai[1] and Peter F. Surai[2-7]*
[1]Healthy Food Services, Bristol, UK; [2]Vitagene and Health Research Centre, Bristol, UK; [3]Department of Microbiology and Biochemistry, Faculty of Veterinary Medicine, Trakia University, Stara Zagora, Bulgaria; [4]Department of Animal Nutrition, Faculty of Agricultural and Environmental Sciences, Szent Istvan University, Hungary; [5]Saint-Petersburg State Academy of Veterinary Medicine, St. Petersburg, Russia; [6]Sumy National Agrarian University, Sumy, Ukraine; [7]Odessa National Academy of Food Technologies, Odessa, Ukraine
psurai@feedfood.co.uk

Abstract

Among polyphenols silymarin (SM), an extract from a medicinal plant *Silybum Marianum*, also known as milk thistle, has a special place, having been used in human medicine for the management of liver diseases since ancient times. Since redox disbalance and oxidative stress are considered to be important pathological mechanisms underlying major liver disease phenotypes, usage of natural antioxidants in liver disease prevention and management is well justified. Among many different dietary supplements used for liver support/treatment SM received tremendous attention due to its antioxidant, anti-inflammatory and redox-regulating properties. A range of *in vitro* and *in vivo* animal studies clearly proved the point that SM is an important hepatoprotectant which can be used singly or in combinations with other nutrients/drugs to deal with various liver disorders/diseases. However, clinical trials with SM and its combinations with other antioxidants were not always as successful as one could expect. On the one hand, in various clinical trials SM was found to improve liver integrity as evidenced by decreased activity in plasma of liver derived enzymes. On the other hand, the evidence of SM protective effects in clinical trials was comparatively low quality and new well designed clinical trials should be conducted with a bigger number of participants. Since SM is a comparatively safe, non-toxic supplement with low risks of drug interactions it could be effectively used as an additional/adjunct therapy for liver problems singly or in combination with various drugs. It seems likely that new developments in this area of research will put more light on the protective effects of SM in various liver disorders.

Keywords: silymarin, liver diseases, protection, Nrf2, NF-κB, vitagenes, redox homeostasis

DOI:10.3920/978-90-8686-944-2_012,

12.1 Introduction

Liver diseases, including non-alcoholic fatty liver disease, alcoholic liver disease (ALD), chronic viral hepatis, autoimmune hepatitis, hepatic schistosomiasis, liver cirrhosis and hepatocellular carcinoma with a poor long-term clinical prognosis are important risk factors and major causes of illness and death worldwide (Wang *et al.*, 2014). It has been demonstrated that SM has protective effects in major cases of liver damage as a result of three important activities, namely anti-inflammatory, antioxidant and immunomodulatory actions which are responsible for antagonising the progression of hepatitis to cirrhosis and hepatocellular carcinoma (Federico *et al.*, 2017b). Protective effects of SM against liver diseases could be executed via different mechanisms (Camini and Costa, 2020; Tighe *et al.*, 2020):

- AO protection and redox balance maintenance;
- cell membrane stabilisation and permeability regulation;
- promotion of ribosomal RNA synthesis, an important event in hepatic regeneration;
- inhibition of stellate hepatocytes transformation into myofibroblasts preventing fibrosis;
- anti-inflammatory action via suppression of NF-κB and inhibition of the synthesis and release of pro-inflammatory cytokines;
- anti-toxic action;
- anti-cancer action.

In general, SM is reported to have protective effects in metabolic-associated NAFLD, alcoholic liver disease, viral hepatitis, drug-induced liver injury and amanita mushroom poisoning (Kren *et al.*, 2021; Tighe *et al.*, 2020). In particular, a shortcut review on usage of SB to reduce liver transplantation and death after poisoning with amatoxin-containing mushrooms was conducted and included five papers presented substantial evidence to answer the clinical question. It was concluded that, only the limited evidence supports SB efficacy, however, taking into account the lack of alternative treatments and the relatively few adverse effects, SB could be recommended to be used in patients with amatoxin-containing mushrooms poisoning (Lacombe and St-Onge, 2016). However, the SM clinical efficacy needs to be further elucidated (Tighe *et al.*, 2020).

12.2 Silymarin and non-alcoholic fatty liver disease

NAFLD is characterised by excessive fat accumulation (>5% fat in the hepatocytes by histology in the absence of excess alcohol consumption; Yaqub *et al.*, 2021). It should be taking into account that NAFLD is a spectrum of liver conditions, ranging from hepatic steatosis with a low risk of progression; non-alcoholic steatohepatitis (NASH), associated with inflammation and hepatocellular injury to fibrosis and ultimately further advancing to cirrhosis and hepatocellular carcinoma (Kuchay *et al.*, 2021). In general, NAFLD is an acquired metabolic stress-related liver injury closely related to other disorders including type 2 diabetes mellitus (insulin resistance) and obesity. For general populations, the prevalence rate of NAFLD comprises about 20-30%

in Western countries and much less (5-18%) in Asia making it the most common cause of chronic liver disease worldwide (Gruneau *et al.*, 2023; Yaqub *et al.*, 2021) and the prevalence of NAFLD among people with diabetes and in the obese patients can reach 50% and 80% respectively (Majumdar *et al.*, 2021; Yaqub *et al.*, 2021). The prevalence rate of NASH is much lower comprising 1.5-6.5% (Majumdar *et al.*, 2021). Cardiovascular disease is considered to be the main cause of mortality in NAFLD and risk of cancer is almost doubled in NAFLD patients (Majumdar *et al.*, 2021).

The pathogenesis of NAFLD is a multifactorial involving the combination and interaction of genetic, environmental, nutritional, behavioural and other factors (Yaqub *et al.*, 2021) and characterised by hepatic lipid accumulation, insulin resistance, lipotoxicity, gut dysbiosis and inflammation (Tilg *et al.*, 2021). The NAFLD development is closely associated with redox disbalance and oxidative stress leading to modified metabolism, mitochondrial damage, protein misfolding/oxidation. Furthermore, ER stress response and other biochemical changes lead to a persistent chronic systemic inflammation state, associated with disbalance of pro- and anti-inflammatory cytokines expression and synthesis regulated by a range of redox-sensitive transcription factors including NF-κB and Nrf2 (Delli Bovi *et al.*, 2021; Podrini *et al.*, 2013; Yaqub *et al.*, 2021). There is expanding evidence that NAFLD patients often have a compromised antioxidant status, disturbed redox balance and systemic oxidative stress (Arroyave-Ospina *et al.*, 2021).

At present, there are no approved pharmacologic treatments for the disease (Gruneau *et al.*, 2023). Lifestyle modification (healthy diet, exercise and weight loss) remains the main first-line intervention in NAFLD (Majumdar *et al.*, 2021). However, several agents/drugs targeting various mechanisms of the disease, including redox disbalance, oxidative stress and inflammation have been investigated or are currently under investigation in animal models and in clinical trials (Majumdar *et al.*, 2021). In many cases pharmacologic treatments target type 2 diabetes mellitus (improving insulin resistance) and indirectly affecting NASH/NAFLD (Gruneau *et al.*, 2023). Since SM/SB is characterised by antioxidant, anti-toxic and anti-inflammatory properties (Surai, 2015; 2022) it is a good candidate for a complementary therapy of NAFLD and a recent update on this issue is summarised below.

12.2.1 *In vitro* studies

In human adipose tissue derived mesenchymal stem cells, SB (10 μM) was shown to increase UCP expression by stimulation of SIRT1, PPARα, and PGC-1α, improving metabolic parameters and decreasing lipid mass leading to the formation of functional adipocytes (Barbagallo *et al.*, 2016). Furthermore, incubation of steatotic cells with SB (50 μM) was demonstrated to significantly reduce TG accumulation via promoting lipid catabolism and inhibiting lipogenic pathways associated with the restoration of the AO balance (reduction in ROS content, lipid peroxidation and decreased NF-κB expression) which was compromised by excessive lipid accumulation (Vecchione *et al.*, 2016).

An *in vitro* model of the NAFLD progression based on sequential exposure of hepatocytes to high concentrations of fatty acids (FA) and TNF-α was used to assess protective effects of SB. It was shown that the exposure to 50 μM SB reduced fat accumulation and counteracted the FA-induced increased lipid peroxidation and mitochondrial damage as a result of (Vecchione *et al.*, 2017):

- increased the mitochondrial size and improved the mitochondrial cristae organisation;
- induced mitochondrial FA oxidation;
- decreased basal and maximal respiration and ATP production in SH cells;
- stimulated ATP production in SS cells;
- rescued the FA-induced apoptotic signals and oxidative stress in SH cells.

By activating the Caspase 8 and Fas-associated protein with death domain-like apoptosis regulator (CFLAR)-JNK pathway in oleic acid-treated HepG2 cells, SB was shown to regulate its downstream target genes participated in lipid metabolism, including PPARα, sterol regulatory element binding protein-1c (SREBP-1C) and patatin-like phospholipase domain-containing protein 3 (PNPLA3), glucose uptake (PI3K-AKT), oxidative stress (NRF2, CYP2E1, CYP4A) and inflammatory response (NO; Liu *et al.*, 2018).

Autophagy is considered to be involved in NAFLD development. SM was observed to reduce lipid accumulation in HepG2 cells exposed to high-fructose by inducing autophagy via the AMPK/mTOR signalling pathway. Indeed, the protein content of phosphorylated-mTOR was found to be decreased, while phosphorylated-AMPK was increased due to SM treatment (Li *et al.*, 2019). The effect of SB in a well-established *in vitro* coculture model of early-stage NASH based on cell treatment with FFA was studied. It was shown that FFAs imposed a fast redox unbalance in both hepatic satellite cells and hepatocytes leading to an increase in collagen synthesis and deposition. Furthermore, in hepatocytes, FFA caused a reduction in the activity of MMP2-9 contributing to the enhanced extracellular collagen deposition. The aforementioned effects were shown to be ameliorated by the supplementation of SB (5 or 7.5 μM; Anfuso *et al.*, 2019).

SB was suggested to serve as a novel and cost-effective dietary supplement for treatment and/or prevention of hepatic steatosis associated with NAFLD progression. Fructose and fatty acid combination *in vitro* led to reduced cell viability, increased apoptosis, oxidative stress and mitochondrial respiration, major indicators of severe steatosis and liver dysfunction. Hepatic cell abnormalities including mitochondrial dysfunction were shown to be almost completely alleviated by SB treatment (50 μM; Grasselli *et al.*, 2019). In a rat hepatoma cell model of NAFLD progression the beneficial effect of SB was found to involve amelioration of the FA profile of lipid droplets, stimulation of the mitochondrial oxidation, upregulation of miR-122, restoration of the levels of aquaporin-9 and glycerol permeability and reduction of the activation of NF-κB, and autophagy turnover (Baldini *et al.*, 2020). SM was reported to act as a hepatoprotective agent modulating the pro-fibrogenic stimuli of hepatic stellate (LX-2) cells and its effects depended on stress levels in the cellular environment. In particular, 100 μM of SM was shown to reduce the synthesis of actin filaments in activated cells, the synthesis of the protein level of α-SMA, and other pro-fibrotic factors such as CTGF and PFGF and also protected the cells from the negative effects of dimethyl sulfoxide (Silva *et al.*, 2020).

12.2.2 *In vivo* studies

Major molecular mechanisms for the hepatoprotective effect of SB on NAFLD in rats were shown to include (Yao *et al.*, 2011):

- mitochondrial membrane stabilisation;
- improved antioxidant defences;
- oxidative stress inhibition;
- improved insulin resistance.

In an experimental mouse model of NAFLD effects of SB (20 mg/kg, i.p. for 4 weeks) on liver and myocardium injury were investigated. Evidently, SB was shown to markedly improve hepatic and myocardial damage associated with reduction in oxidants (isoprostanes, 8-deoxyguanosine, nitrites/nitrates) and restoration of AO defences in the liver and in the heart of the experimental animals. Furthermore, SB was reported to ameliorate damaged liver mitochondrial respiratory chain and to attenuate increased pro-inflammatory cytokine expression (Salamone *et al.*, 2012). The capacity of SB to limit mitochondrial failure is considered to be a part of its hepatoprotective property (Serviddio *et al.*, 2014). In male C57BL/6 mice fed with HFD to induce obesity and insulin resistance SM treatment (30 and 60 mg/kg for 18 days) was shown to improve diet-induced liver damage and insulin resistance associated with decreasing inflammation (Guo *et al.*, 2016). SB (50 and 100 mg/kg for 8 weeks) was found to improve HFD-induced NAFD in hamsters through reducing de novo lipogenesis and increasing FA oxidation simultaneously with inducing p-AMPKα expression (Cui *et al.*, 2017). High fat and high carbohydrate diet (HFHCD) supplemented with SM (210 mg/kg diet) was shown to significantly improve glycemia, visceral fat, lipid profile, and liver fibrosis. SM also ameliorated HFHCD-induced (both *in vitro* and *in vivo*) ALT, hepatic inflammation, oxidative stress, and apoptosis (Marin *et al.*, 2017). Effects of the combination of SB with lisinopril (MK-521) on renal fibrosis *in vitro* (HK-2 cells) and *in vivo* (HFD-induced renal fibrosis mouse model) were studied. The expressions of collagen I, α-SMA, Smad2 and Smad3 in TGF-β-treated HK-2 cells were shown to be decreased by MK-521 and SB (20-80 μM) further inhibited them. Furthermore, SB (100 mg/kg) also significantly enhanced anti-fibrotic effect of MK-521 on HFD-induced renal fibrosis mice (Ma *et al.*, 2020).

In *in vivo* and *in vitro* models of NAFLD based on C57BL/6 mice fed a HFD or palmitate (PA) treated HepG2 cells, respectively, SB was discovered to abolish oxidative stress, to restore NAD^+ levels and to induce the SIRT1/AMPK pathway (Salomone *et al.*, 2017). Furthermore, SB was reported to improve palmitate-induced insulin resistance in C2C12 myotubes by attenuating IRS-1/PI3K/Akt pathway inhibition (Li *et al.*, 2015). The administration of SM (30 mg/kg body weight/d for 4 weeks) was indicated to significantly ameliorate HFD-induced glucose metabolic disorders, oxidative stress and pathological alterations in the mouse kidney. Furthermore, SM mitigated renal lipid accumulation, fatty acid β-oxidation and mitochondrial biogenesis in HFD mice and PA treated HK2 cells. In addition, SM was found to partly restore mitochondrial membrane potential of PA-treated HK2 cells (Feng *et al.*, 2017).

It was shown that SB can inhibit endoplasmic reticulum stress and prevent NLRP3 inflammasome activation in the NAFLD models including HFD-fed mice and cultured hepatocytes by regulation of the NAD^+/SIRT2 pathway (Zhang *et al.*, 2018). In the *in vivo* study based on male C57BL/6 mice fed with methionine- choline-deficient diet and the *in vitro* study with mouse NCTC-1469 cells pretreated with oleic acid plus palmitic acid, SM was able to alleviate hepatic lipid accumulation and oxidative stress (increased the expression of Nrf2 and the activities of CAT, GPx and HO-1) in mice with non-alcoholic steatohepatitis by regulating CFLAR-JNK pathway (Liu *et al.*, 2019b).

The results of experiments with mice fed HFD or with HepG2 cells treated with palmitic acid indicated that SB intervention was associated with reduced triglyceride content, miR-122 expression and the mRNA and improved lipid metabolism as evidenced by reduced protein expressions of fatty acid synthase and acetyl-CoA carboxylase as well as with increased mRNA and protein expression of carnitine palmitoyl transferase 1A (CPT1A, Yang *et al.*, 2021). The authors concluded that SB could improve hepatic lipid metabolism by reducing the expression of miR-122.

SM (100 and 200 mg/kg) was shown to attenuate fructose-induced NAFLD in mice through the regulation of endoplasmic reticulum stress proteins GRP78 and XBP-1 (Sahin *et al.*, 2020). SB was found to alleviate hepatic lipid accumulation in methionine-choline deficient diet-induced NAFLD in mice via activating PPARα (Cui *et al.*, 2021). SB is considered as a CYP3A (clinically significant group of cytochrome P-450 isoenzymes) inhibitor. In mouse model of NAFLD caused by HFD, SB was reported to restore CYP3A expression and to suppress liver inflammation and to inhibit NF-κB nuclear translocation through elevation of SIRT2 expression and promotion of p65 deacetylation (Zhang *et al.*, 2021).

In mice SM is shown to have beneficial effects on ameliorating NAFLD which was associated with restoration of HFD-induced changes of gut microbiota composition and increasing production of beneficial short-chain fatty acids, including acetate, propionate, and butyrate and decreasing generation of formate and conversion of cytotoxic secondary metabolites such as lithocholic acid and deoxy-cholic acid (Li *et al.*, 2020). In two-year-old dogs, SB (12.75 mg per 10 kg body weight) was shown to improve liver function as indicative by decreased serum ALT, AST and GGT activities (Gogulski *et al.*, 2021).

Interestingly, protective effects of SM were also observed in NASH. For example, in irinotecan-induced NASH, SM hepatoprotective actions seem to involve the inhibition of oxidative stress and protein nitrosylation leading to prevention of activation of hepatic fibrosis mechanisms (Marcolino Assis-Júnior *et al.*, 2017). It has been suggested that anti-inflammatory effect of SB in a mouse model of NASH was mediated by blocking the NF-κB-signalling pathway through the inhibition of O-GlcNAcylation (Lee *et al.*, 2018). SB (105 mg/kg/day for 8 weeks) was also shown to alleviates hepatic steatosis and fibrosis in a NASH mouse model by inhibiting oxidative stress via activation of the Nrf2 pathway and upregulating Nrf2 target genes as well as by suppressing the NF-κB signalling pathway in the NASH liver (Ou *et al.*, 2018).

Protective effects of SM were also shown in various other models. For instance, liposomal SM was demonstrated to have improved *in vitro* and *in vivo* hepatoprotective effects in alcohol-induced hepatotoxicity in Wistar rats as evidenced by improvement in liver function, increased efficacy in combating inflammatory conditions, increased antioxidant defences and reversal of histological changes compared to SM alone (Kumar *et al.*, 2019). SM (300 mg/kg) was observed to decrease NF-κB expression in the liver of CCl_4-treated rats (Yan and Zhang, 2021). In rats with type 2 diabetes hepatoprotective effects of SM (60 mg/kg and 120 mg/kg for 60 days) on liver injury was reported to be mediated by upregulation of irisin (polypeptide, best known as the exercise-induced chemokine) and reduction of oxidative stress (Kheiripour *et al.*, 2019).

SM was shown to have protective effects on hypercholesterolaemic, bile duct ligated and obese animals. For example, in hypercholesterolaemic rats, SB (300 and 600 mg/kg for 60 days) was reported to significantly reduce both serum and hepatic total cholesterol, triglycerides, VLDL-C, LDL-C and to increase HDL-C at both doses (Gobalakrishnan *et al.*, 2016). In experimental obstructive jaundice model (bile ducts ligation) SM was reported to ameliorate oxidative stress and liver histopathology in rats (Onalan *et al.*, 2016). In bile duct ligated female Sprague Dawley rats, treatment with milk thistle extract (600 mg/kg) was shown to attenuate cholestatic liver injury as evidenced by decreased ALT, AST, MDA and MPO activities in serum (Alaca *et al.*, 2017). SM (10 and 100 mg/kg for seven consecutive days) was reported to significantly ameliorate bile duct obstruction-induced compromised antioxidant system and to mitigate cholaemic nephropathy (Ommati *et al.*, 2021).

SB (50 mg/kg, IP twice per week, for 8 weeks) was discovered to attenuate adipose tissue inflammation and to ameliorate obesity and its complications in diet-induced obesity model in mice as evidenced by reversing fatty liver disease, hyperglycaemia, hyperinsulinemia and hypertriglyceridemia and restoring glucose homeostasis (Alsaggar *et al.*, 2020). In obese mice SB (54 mg/kg body weight, intragastrically) was shown to improve glucose metabolism, to decrease the concentration of TC, TG, and LDL-C and to increase the concentration of HDL-C in the serum of mice. In white adipose tissue of HFD-fed mice differentially expressed proteins were related to PPAR, lipolysis of fat cells, metabolism of glycerides and oxidative phosphorylation (Wang *et al.*, 2020). Therefore, HFD was demonstrated to increase the expressions of various proteins implicated in lipid synthesis and transport in the liver leading to disorders of liver lipid metabolism. SM was able to decrease liver lipid deposition and increase insulin sensitivity by regulating the expressions of those proteins including perilipin-2, phosphatidate phosphatase LPIN1, farnesyl pyrophosphate synthase, and glutathione S-transferase A1 (Wang *et al.*, 2022).

A high-fat/high-cholesterol diet was demonstrated to cause abnormal lipid metabolism, polyol metabolism, amino acid metabolism, the urea cycle and the TCA cycle evidenced in the serum and liver of C57BL/6 J mice. In the same experiment SB treatment (50 or 100 mg/kg for 4 weeks) was able to ameliorate hepatic lipid accumulation and to modulate global metabolic pathways in animals (Sun *et al.*, 2020). It seems likely that, SM hepatoprotective role could be associated with upregulation of hepatic Farnesoid-X activated receptors (FXR). In an experiment, obesity, insulin resistance, hyperlipidaemia, and fatty liver were induced in mice by feeding HFD for 3 months. SM (40 mg/100 g for 6 weeks) was shown to enhance FXR transactivity and inhibited NF-κB signalling, ameliorated insulin resistance, dyslipidaemia and inflammation, and reconstituted the bile acid pool in liver of diet-induced obesity (Gu *et al.*, 2016).

In addition, in APAP-induced liver damages in rats, milk thistle extract (MTE, 200 mg/kg/day for 28 days) led to a marked (6.5-fold) upregulation of hepatic FXR expression (Khalili *et al.*, 2021). APAP treatment was recorded to be associated with a significant elevation of liver transaminase along with the architectural injuries in the liver. In contrast, chronic concomitant administration of MTE significantly restored the liver function and structural abnormality. Interestingly, 2-fold increased MTE dose (400 mg/kg/day) was found to have similar protective effect on the liver but was less effective in activation (2.3-fold) of FXR expression (Khalili *et al.*, 2021). Furthermore, TAA-inducted liver cirrhosis was shown to be associated with significant deterioration of liver and renal functions together with increasing expression of hepatic and renal TGF-β1 and decreasing expression of hepatic and renal FXR.

Giving SM (50 mg/kg/day/4 weeks p.o.) to rats was found to induce hepatic and renal improvement which was evidenced biochemically and histologically. Rats fed SM for four weeks were characterised by significant increase of the hepatic and renal expression of FXR compared to control untreated rats. Interestingly, the expression of hepatic and renal FXR in the TAA-treated group showed significantly lower levels of expression compared to the control group and SM significantly increased it (Magdy *et al.*, 2018).

In general, the etiology and pathophysiology of acute and chronic liver diseases are not fully understood and need further elucidation. However, accumulating information clearly indicates that the FXR is involved in regulation of a range of important physiological functions and biochemical processes in the liver, including the bile acid synthesis and haemostasis, glucose and lipid metabolism, cholesterol efflux and transport with a negative correlation between the hepatic FXR gene expression and deterioration of the liver disease (Panzitt and Wagner, 2021). FXR activation is reported to be associated with improvement of endothelial vasodilation, while experiments with FXR-deficient animals further substantiated an important regulatory role of FXR in the liver functioning (Panzitt and Wagner, 2021; Stofan and Guo, 2020).

There are several publications describing combined effects of SM with other antioxidants. For example, a combination of SB (47 mg) and vitamin E (15 mg) complexed with phospholipids administered to rats fed a choline-deprived or HFD, was reported to effectively ameliorate hepatocyte fat deposition, NO derivatives formation, and mitochondrial alterations and improving AO defences including improved GSH and thioredoxin AO activity (Grattagliano *et al.*, 2013). Furthermore, hepatoprotective effects (reducing cytokine-induced PGE2, IL-8 and MCP-1 production, inhibiting NF-κB nuclear translocation and improving AO defences) of a combination of SB with S-adenosylmethionine on canine hepatocytes *in vitro* were shown (Au *et al.*, 2013).

There were also several attempts to use SM with improved bioavailability. For example, combined application of SB and tangeretin (an efflux transporter inhibitor increasing the bioavailability of SB) was shown to attenuate the progression of NASH in mice via modulation of lipid metabolism: inhibiting fatty acid generating and transporting proteins, cholesterol metabolism enzyme (CYP27A1) as well as nuclear transcription factors FXR, PPAR-γ, and LXR (Suguro *et al.*, 2020). Interestingly, SB phytosome (400 mg/kg) was reported to have similar protective effects as α-R-Lipoic Acid (200 mg/kg) in mitigating chronic hepatitis in rats as a result of inhibition of oxidative stress and inflammatory cytokines production (Ali *et al.*, 2016). Chitosan-functionalised lipid-polymer hybrid nanoparticles are shown to enhance efficacy of oral delivery of SM and they demonstrated a desirable lipid-lowering effect in a mouse model of NAFLD (Liang *et al.*, 2018).

It should be mentioned that milk thistle can also be effective in the liver protection. For instance, in an NAFLD mouse model oxidative stress induced by feeding with high energy diet (HED) caused reduction of testosterone level, testicular spermatogenic cell numbers and testicular histopathological damage and decreased semen quality in quail. At the same time feeding milk thistle seed (1%) was shown to ameliorate most HED-induced detrimental changes (Çeribaşı *et al.*, 2020).

There was a range of hepatotoxicity models where SM/SB showed protective effects. In particular, among toxicants imposing hepatotoxicity CCl_4, valproic acid, thioacetamide, fructose, diclofenac, APAP, etc. were tested. In addition, NASH rats, HFD-induced NAFLD, MCD diet-induced NASH, restraint stress-induced acute liver injury, HepG2 cells and HFD-induced liver inflammation were also used (Wadhwa *et al.*, 2022). For more details on anti-toxic effects of SM/SB see Chapter 8. In general, in most toxicity models hepatoprotective effects of SM/SB were clearly shown, including

- improvement of liver integrity (decreased ALT, AST, GGT in plasma/serum);
- decreased expression of NF-κB and pro-inflammatory cytokines and reduced liver inflammation;
- improved Nrf2 expression and enhanced AO defence network mechanisms;
- vitagene activation and improved stress adaptation (Figure 12.1).

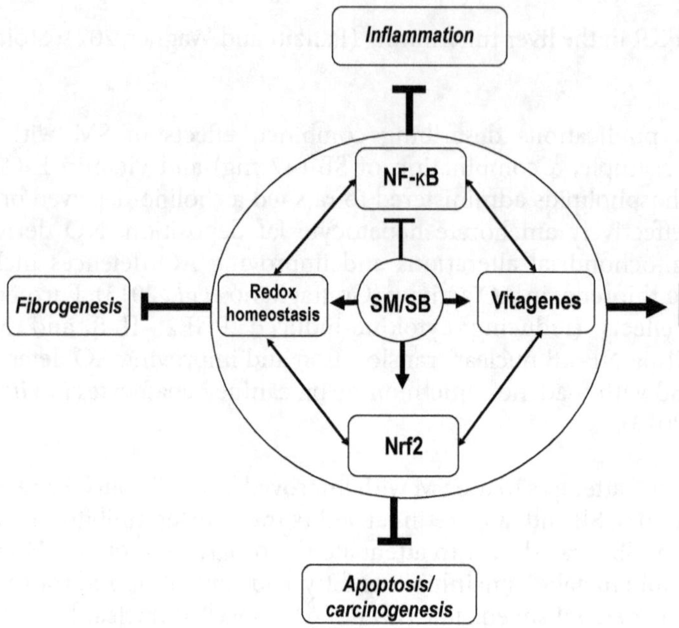

Figure 12.1. Liver protection by SM/SB.

Since redox disbalance and oxidative stress are considered to play crucial roles during the progression of NAFLD and hepatic steatosis (Wadhwa *et al.*, 2022) the aforementioned protective effects of SM/SB are of paramount importance for the development of effective means to protect human liver under various stressful conditions as well as liver of farm animals and poultry under commercially-relevant stresses.

12.2.3 Clinical trials

A meta-analysis of 8 randomised control trials involved 587 patients with NAFLD showed that SM significantly decreased activity of liver's enzymes (AST and ALT) released into blood (serum/plasma) and reflecting improvement of liver integrity (Zhong *et al.*, 2017). There were also attempts to combine SM with other antioxidants to improve liver protection. For example, treatment with SM + vitamin E (210 mg a day of SM formulation containing 60% SM and 30 IU of vitamin E, for 6 months) of patients diagnosed with NAFLD was associated with a decrease in transaminases (AST, ALT and GGT) without an accompanying weight loss (Aller *et al.*, 2018). Similarly, SB in combination with vitamin D and vitamin E (303 mg of silybin-phospholipid complex, 10 mg of vitamin D, and 15 mg of vitamin E twice a day) consumed for 6 months by NAFLD patients (n=60) caused a significant improvement in metabolic markers, oxidative stress and endothelial dysfunction in comparison to not treated nonalcoholic fatty liver disease patients (Federico *et al.*, 2019). In a recent meta-analysis based on four studies (totally 168 participants) that examined the effect of SB-phospholipid-vitamin E complex (SB 94 mg, phosphatidylcholine 194 mg, vitamin E acetate 50% 89.28 mg) intake on liver enzymes among NAFLD or NASH patients it was shown that SB-vitamin E complex intake was associated with a significantly decreased circulating GGT level without any significant effect on serum AST and ALT levels (Derakhshandeh-Rishehri *et al.*, 2020).

Two trials testing SM in NASH have been conducted. In a clinical-trial with 64 NASH patients who were randomly divided as case group (n=33, receiving 210 mg/day SM orally for 8 weeks) and control group (n=31, receiving placebo), SM was indicated to decrease serum AST and ALT reflecting improvement in the liver integrity (Solhi *et al.*, 2014). A long-term (12 months) treatment with SB conjugated with phosphatidylcholine in patients with NASH was shown to induce increased CAT activity in human endothelial cells (Federico *et al.*, 2017a).

There were also several clinical trials showing protective effects of SM against liver damages associated with other clinical conditions/diseases. First of all, in a double-blind clinical trial, 74 patients with acne and taking isotretinoin were randomly assigned into intervention (n=37) and control (n=37) groups. The patients in the intervention group received a 140 mg SM capsule per day for 30 days while the control group patients received a placebo once a day for 30 days. At the end of the study, a significant difference was reported to be observed between the two groups in levels of serum AST and ALT. In this study SM showed a protective effect on the liver as evidenced by preventing liver enzymes from increasing in blood (Mirnezami *et al.*, 2020). Secondly, in a double-blinded clinical trial patients with hypoxia were treated with SM at a dose of 280 mg with orally gavage technique and the control group was treated with a placebo every 8 h for 3 days. In the SM group, liver enzymes (AST, ALT and GGT) in serum were lower than the placebo group on the third day after treatment (Jamalian *et al.*, 2020). Finally, in a one-year, randomised, double-blinded, placebo-controlled clinical trial conducted on 90 trauma patients it was shown that SM supplementation (140 mg, three times daily for 14 days) significantly improved some antioxidant markers (TAC and thiol) and decreased liver enzymes (AST, ALT, ALP) in blood samples of patients with trauma-induced liver injury (Mirzaei *et al.*, 2021).

It is important to mention that usually NAFLD is associated with obesity and metabolic disturbances, however, NAFLD can also occur in non-obese individuals, especially in Asian populations and its major causes can be summarised as follows (Wood, 2010):

- metabolic: insulin resistance and increased visceral adiposity;
- drugs: amiodarone, tamoxifen, diltiazem;
- infectious-Inflammatory disorders: hepatitis C, HIVc, celiac disease, small intestinal bacterial overgrowth;
- genetic disorders: abetalipoproteinemia, lipodystrophies, cholesterol ester storage diseased, Wolman disease, Wilson's disease, PNPLA3 mutation.

Various interventions have been conducted in attempts to find an effective treatment for patients with NAFLD. These include (Lombardi *et al.*, 2017):

- lifestyle modifications such as dietary changes and increased exercise;
- agents that decrease:
  - weight (e.g. orlistat);
  - insulin resistance (insulin-sensitising agents, such as metformin and thiazolidinediones including pioglitazone and rosiglitazone);
  - oxidative stress (e.g. vitamin E, herbal preparations such as SM, and S-adenosylmethionine);
- other agents such as:
  - statins (e.g. simvastatin, atorvastatin);
  - secondary bile acids or analogues, including ursodeoxycholic acid or obeticholic acid;
  - omega-3 fatty acids that play a role in fat metabolism;
  - angiotensin-converting enzyme inhibitors including ramipril or angiotensin II receptor antagonists such as losartan;
- weight reduction surgery (bariatric surgery).

However, it should be mentioned that the optimal pharmacological treatment for patients with NAFLD until now remains uncertain.

Recently the comparative benefits and harms of different interventions in NAFLS have been assessed using standard Cochrane methodology (Lombardi *et al.*, 2017). In particular, the Cochrane Central Register of Controlled Trials (CENTRAL), MEDLINE, Embase, Science Citation Index Expanded, the World Health Organisation International Clinical Trials Registry Platform, and ClinicalTrials.com to August 2016 have been searched. The authors identified 77 trials including 6,287 participants that met the inclusion criteria. Forty-one trials (3,829 participants) provided detailed information for one or more outcomes. The authors concluded that all the evidence was very low quality: 35 trials included only participants with NASH, 5 trials included only participants with diabetes mellitus and 14 trials included only participants without diabetes mellitus. At the same time the follow-up in the trials ranged from 1 month to 24 months. When a comparison between antioxidants (vitamin E or other antioxidants; milk thistle (SM or *Silybum marianum* extract); S-adenosylmethionine) versus no intervention was conducted, it was concluded that (Lombardi *et al.*, 2017):

- there was no mortality in either group;
- none of the participants developed serious adverse events in the trial;
- there was no evidence of difference in the number of serious adverse events between antioxidants and no intervention;
- none of the trials reported health-related quality of life.

Similarly, there was no evidence of beneficial effects of bile acids or thiazolidinediones in NAFLD treatment. The authors concluded that due to the very low-quality evidence they were uncertain about the effectiveness of any pharmacological treatments of NAFLD including patients with steatohepatitis and therefore, further well-designed randomised clinical trials with sufficiently large sample sizes and long follow-up periods are necessary (Lombardi *et al.*, 2017).

Recently through active ingredient screening, PPI network construction, target prediction, KEGG pathway, GO biological process analysis, and experimental verification, *S. marianum's* hepatoprotective mechanism for NAFLD was clarified (Jiang *et al.*, 2022). Indeed, it was confirmed that the active hepatoprotective ingredient of *S. marianum* was silymarin. Based on accumulating evidence the authors indicated that SM can significantly improve major markers of liver health, including

- improvement of the levels of ALT, AST, HDL-C, LDL-C, TC and TG;
- decrease of protein expressions of IL-6, Caspase 3, MAPK1, VEGFA, p53; and
- increase of protein expression of AKT1 (Jiang *et al.*, 2022).

12.3 Antiviral hepatoprotective activity of silymarin

There is a range of papers describing antiviral activities of SM/SB. The most frequent target for SM intervention is shown to be hepatitis C virus (HCV) and clinical trials with SM were conducted in patients with chronic hepatitis C (Liu *et al.*, 2019a). However, dengue virus (DENV), influenza A virus, human immunodeficiency virus, togaviruses – chikungunya virus and mayaro virus, and hepatitis B virus are also important targets for SM (Kren, 2021; Ferraz *et al.*, 2021). For-example, SM clearly showed anti-DENV activity (Low *et al.*, 2021) and was effective against Enterovirus A71 (a major neurovirulent agent causing severe hand, foot and mouth disease associated with neurological complications and death; Lalani *et al.*, 2021).

12.3.1 Inhibition of hepatitis C virus

Hepatitis C is an inflammation of the liver caused by the hepatitis C virus. The virus is known to cause both acute and chronic hepatitis and globally about 58 million people have chronic hepatitis C virus infection with 1.5 million new infections occurring per year and approximately 290,000 people died from hepatitis C complications in 2019 (WHO, 2022). It is estimated that about 118,000 people in the UK had chronic hepatitis C in 2019 (NHS, 2022). Hepatitis C can be treated with medicines that stop the virus multiplying inside the body and until recently, most people would have taken 2 main medicines called pegylated interferon (Peg-IFN) and ribavirin (RBV). Recently new hepatitis C medicines have been developed making treatment more effective, easier to tolerate, with shorter treatment courses (NHS, 2022).

In 2007 SM was shown to inhibit T-cell inflammatory cytokines, hepatocyte NF-κB signalling, and HCV infection (Polyak *et al.*, 2007) probably via the JAK-STAT antiviral signalling pathway leading to inhibition of HCV replication. Multiple effects of SM on the HCV lifecycle were demonstrated including blockage of entry/fusion, replication, and virion production in the host cells associated with attenuating HCV-induced oxidative stress, NF-κB activation and pro-inflammatory cytokines production (Morishima *et al.*, 2010; Wagoner *et al.*, 2010). It seems likely that anti-HCV activity of SM and its constituents could be mediated via (Liu *et al.*, 2019a):

- affecting RNA-dependent RNA polymerase activity;
- inducing anti-inflammatory and anti-proliferative gene expressions;

- blocking clathrin-mediated endocytosis;
- targeting the HCV NS4B protein;
- blocking viral cell-to-cell spread.

Therefore, SM was suggested (Wagoner *et al.*, 2011) to provide hepatoprotection by multiple actions that collectively leading to reduced inflammation by several mechanisms including inhibition of NF-κB signalling, T cell proliferation, inflammatory cytokine production and virus infection. Furthermore, SM antiviral effects are likely executed via blocking virus entry, HCV RNA and protein expression, and virus transmission impacting multiple steps of the virus life cycle (Wagoner *et al.*, 2011). The data on protective effects of SM or its constituents in patients with HCV are not consistent with several unsuccessful attempts to decrease HCV viral load (Fried *et al.*, 2012; Gabbay *et al.*, 2007; Tanamly *et al.*, 2004). However, using SB-vitamin E-phospholipid complex, possessing improved SB solubility and availability and additional AO potential due to vitamin E in two randomised controlled trials with HCV patients was effective in decreasing viral load, reducing liver fibrosis, reducing depression and anxiety and increasing work ability in comparison to patients on a standard treatment with Peg-IFN + RBV (Malaguarnera *et al.*, 2015; 2016).

It is important to note that SM could be a great help as an adjuvant therapy in treating patients which do not respond to a traditional therapy or having adverse effects of it. For example, two weeks intravenous infusion of SM (combined with 7 days of Peg-IFN+RBV treatment) to chronic hepatitis C patients non-responders to a traditional therapy was shown to dose-dependently decrease HCV viral load (Biermer and Berg, 2009; Biermer *et al.*, 2012; Ferenci *et al.*, 2008; Rutter *et al.*, 2011). The authors suggested that SM could block both viral infection and viral production or release in chronic hepatitis C patients (Guedj *et al.*, 2012). Similarly, in hepatitis C patients intolerable to IFN-containing treatments, intravenous infusion of SM in combination with RBV and vitamin D therapy a sustained virological response was achieved (Dahari *et al.*, 2015). It seems likely that newly developed anti-HCV drugs will improve hepatitis C treatment but taking into account information that the current antiviral agents can only abrogate viral replication without displaying any hepatoprotective effects, combining such drugs with SM or its derivatives could be a valuable option to improve the patient conditions (Liu *et al.*, 2019a).

There is also a report suggesting COVID-19 treatment with SB exploring dual targeting of host cytokine storm and virus replication machinery (Bosch-Barrera *et al.*, 2020) and silybin B was identified as a potential anti-COVID drug (Srivastava *et al.*, 2021) and this direction of research requires urgent attention. The mosquito-borne chikungunya virus (CHIKV) is responsible for chikungunya fever, characterised by severe back and small joint pain, and debilitating arthritis associated with crippling pains that persist for a long period of time. SM is reported to exhibit significant antiviral activity against CHIKV, reducing both CHIKV replication efficiency and down-regulating production of viral proteins involved in replication (Lani *et al.*, 2015). Recent *in vitro* analysis demonstrated that SB could exhibit significant dose-dependent anti-CHIKV activity within 12.5-100-μM concentrations with CC_{50} as 50.90 μM confirming that SB is a promising candidate drug against CHIKV infection (Dutta *et al.*, 2022).

In vitro the antiviral activity of SM against Zika virus (ZIKV) infection in Vero cells was investigated. SM showed significant inhibition of ZIKV infection, protecting cells infected with EC_{50} equal to 34.17 μg/ml, and its greatest protective efficiency was achieved at 125 μg/ml, when cell viability did not differ from the control without infection (da Silva *et al.*, 2020). SM was shown to exert direct extracellular virucidal effects against Enterovirus 71 (EV-A71) with IC_{50} of 15.2±3.53 μg/ml with SI of 10.53. Furthermore, SM was reported to block both viral attachment and entry of EV-A71 to inhibit infection in Vero cells (Lalani *et al.*, 2020; 2021). SM and its derivatives are reported to have antiviral activities against liver and non-liver pathogens, and they can be included into broad-spectrum antivirals category of treatments to be used as a complementary approach to improve antiviral therapy (Liu *et al.*, 2019a). A recent comparative evaluation of flavonoids revealed the superiority and promising inhibition activity of SB against SARS-CoV-2 showing significant interference with SARS-CoV-2 entry and replication through multi-targeting activity (Hamdy *et al.*, 2022).

12.4 Conclusions

Based on clinical features and causative agents, liver diseases include non-alcoholic fatty liver disease, alcoholic liver disease, metabolic-associated fatty liver disease and drug-induced liver injury (Aghemo *et al.*, 2022), chronic viral hepatis, autoimmune hepatitis, hepatic schistosomiasis, liver cirrhosis and hepatocellular carcinoma (Wang *et al.*, 2014). Since redox disbalance and oxidative stress are considered to be important pathological mechanisms underlying all liver disease phenotypes, usage of natural antioxidants in liver disease prevention and management is well justified. Among many different dietary supplements used for liver support/treatment SM/SB has received tremendous attention due to its antioxidant, anti-inflammatory and redox-regulating properties. Furthermore, based on pharmacodynamic and pharmacokinetic properties the expert panel reached an agreement on SM as a safe hepatoprotective agent (Aghemo *et al.*, 2022). A range of *in vitro* and *in vivo* animal studies clearly proved the point that SM/SB is an important hepatoprotectant which can be used singly or in combinations with other drugs to deal with various liver diseases. Interestingly, 38.5% of the silymarin flavonolignans down-regulated proteins and 53.8% of the up-regulated proteins were illustrated to be involved in the hepatoprotective activity (Dwivedi *et al.*, 2022).

However, clinical trials with SM and its combinations with other antioxidants were not always as successful as one could expect. On the one hand, in various clinical trials SM was found to improve liver integrity as evidenced by decreased activity in plasma of liver derived ALT, AST, GGT, etc. (de Avelar *et al.*, 2017; Jamalian *et al.*, 2020; Saller *et al.*, 2001; Tao *et al.*, 2019; Zhong *et al.*, 2017). In the most recent meta-analysis of eight randomised clinical trials (up to June 2020) evaluating the efficacy of treatment with SM in individuals with NAFLD compared to placebo,

SM was shown to be effective in reducing transaminase (ALT and AST) levels in individuals with NAFLD (Kalopitas *et al.*, 2021). On the other hand, the evidence of SM protective effects in clinical trials was comparatively low quality (Lombardi *et al.*, 2017) and new well designed clinical trials should be conducted with a bigger number of participants. In particular, the optimised SM phytosomal formulations could significantly improve SM oral bioavailability and increase its therapeutic bio-efficacy (Shriram *et al.*, 2022). Since SM is a comparatively safe, non-toxic supplement with low risks of drug interactions (Tighe *et al.*, 2020) it could be effectively used as an additional/adjunct therapy for liver problems singly or in combination with other drugs. It sems likely that new developments in this area of research will put more light on the protective effects of SM in various liver disorders. Recently, an international expert panel of clinicians concluded that SM has significant roles in prevention and treatment of various liver diseases including alcoholic liver disease, nonalcoholic fatty liver disease/metabolic dysfunction-associated fatty liver disease, drug-induced liver injury, and liver cirrhosis (Gillessen *et al.*, 2022).

References

Aghemo, A., Alekseeva, O.P., Angelico, F., Bakulin, I.G., Bakulina, N.V., Bordin, D., Bueverov, A.O., Drapkina, O.M., Gillessen, A., Kagarmanova, E.M., Korochanskaya, N.V., Kucheryavii, U.A., Lazebnik, L.B., Livzan, M.A., Maev, I.V., Martynov, A.I., Osipenko, M.F., Sas, E.I., Starodubova, A., Uspensky, Y.P. and Yakovlev, A.A., 2022. Role of silymarin as antioxidant in clinical management of chronic liver diseases: a narrative review. Annals of Medicine 54: 1548-1560.

Alaca, N., Özbeyli, D., Uslu, S., Şahin, H.H., Yiğittürk, G., Kurtel, H., Öktem, G. and Çağlayan Yeğen, B., 2017. Treatment with milk thistle extract, *Silybum marianum*, ursodeoxycholic acid, or their combination attenuates cholestatic liver injury in rats: Role of the hepatic stem cells. The Turkish Journal of Gastroenterology 28: 476-484.

Ali, S.O., Darwish, H.A. and Ismail, N.A., 2016. Curcumin, silybin phytosome® and α-R-lipoic acid mitigate chronic hepatitis in rat by inhibiting oxidative stress and inflammatory cytokines production. Basic & Clinical Pharmacology & Toxicology 118: 369-380.

Aller, R., Laserna, C., Rojo, M.Á., Mora, N., García Sánchez, C., Pina, M., Sigüenza, R., Durà, M., Primo, D., Izaola, O. and de Luis, D., 2018. Role of the PNPLA3 polymorphism rs738409 on silymarin + vitamin E response in subjects with non-alcoholic fatty liver disease. Revista Espanola de Enfermedades Digestivas 110: 634-640.

Alsaggar, M., Bdour, S., Ababneh, Q., El-Elimat, T., Qinna, N. and Alzoubi, K.H., 2020. Silibinin attenuates adipose tissue inflammation and reverses obesity and its complications in diet-induced obesity model in mice. BMC Pharmacology & Toxicology 21: 8.

Anfuso, B., Giraudi, P.J., Tiribelli, C. and Rosso, N., 2019. Silybin modulates collagen turnover in an *in vitro* model of NASH. Molecules 24: 1280.

Arroyave-Ospina, J.C., Wu, Z., Geng, Y. and Moshage, H., 2021. Role of oxidative stress in the pathogenesis of non-alcoholic fatty liver disease: Implications for prevention and therapy. Antioxidants 10: 174.

Au, A.Y., Hasenwinkel, J.M. and Frondoza, C.G., 2013. Hepatoprotective effects of S-adenosylmethionine and silybin on canine hepatocytes *in vitro*. Journal of Animal Physiology and Animal Nutrition 97: 331-341.

Baldini, F., Portincasa, P., Grasselli, E., Damonte, G., Salis, A., Bonomo, M., Florio, M., Serale, N., Voci, A., Gena, P., Vergani, L. and Calamita, G., 2020. Aquaporin-9 is involved in the lipid-lowering activity of the nutraceutical silybin on hepatocytes through modulation of autophagy and lipid droplets composition. Biochimica et Biophysica Acta. Molecular and Cell Biology of Lipids 1865: 158586.

Barbagallo, I., Vanella, L., Cambria, M.T., Tibullo, D., Godos, J., Guarnaccia, L., Zappalà, A., Galvano, F. and Li Volti, G., 2016. Silibinin regulates lipid metabolism and differentiation in functional human adipocytes. Frontiers in Pharmacology 6: 309.

Biermer, M. and Berg, T., 2009. Rapid suppression of hepatitis C viremia induced by intravenous silibinin plus ribavirin. Gastroenterology 137: 390-391.

Biermer, M., Schlosser, B., Fülöp, B., van Bömmel, F., Brodzinski, A., Heyne, R., Keller, K., Sarrazin, C. and Berg, T., 2012. High-dose silibinin rescue treatment for HCV-infected patients showing suboptimal virologic response to standard combination therapy. Journal of Viral Hepatitis 19: 547-553.

Bosch-Barrera, J., Martin-Castillo, B., Buxó, M., Brunet, J., Encinar, J.A. and Menendez, J.A., 2020. Silibinin and SARS-CoV-2: Dual targeting of host cytokine storm and virus replication machinery for clinical management of COVID-19 patients. Journal of Clinical Medicine 9: 1770.

Camini, F.C. and Costa, D.C., 2020. Silymarin: not just another antioxidant. Journal of Basic and Clinical Physiology and Pharmacology 31: 4.

Çeribaşı, S., Türk, G., Özçelik, M., Doğan, G., Çeribaşı, A.O., Mutlu, S.İ., Erişir, Z., Güvenç, M., Güngören, G., Acısu, T.C., Akarsu, S.A., Kaya, Ş.Ö., Sönmez, M., Yüce, A., Çiftçi, M., Çambay, Z., Bağcı, E., Azman, M.A. and Şimşek, Ü.G., 2020. Negative effect of feeding with high energy diets on testes and metabolic blood parameters of male Japanese quails, and positive role of milk thistle seed. Theriogenology 144: 74-81.

Cui, C.X., Deng, J.N., Yan, L., Liu, Y., Fan, J.Y., Mu, H.N., Sun, H.Y., Wang, Y.H. and Han, J.Y., 2017. Silibinin capsules improves high fat diet-induced nonalcoholic fatty liver disease in hamsters through modifying hepatic de novo lipogenesis and fatty acid oxidation. Journal of Ethnopharmacology 208: 24-35.

Cui, S., Pan, X.J., Ge, C.L., Guo, Y.T., Zhang, P.F., Yan, T.T., Zhou, J.Y., He, Q.X., Cheng, L.H., Wang, G.J., Hao, H.P. and Wang, H., 2021. Silybin alleviates hepatic lipid accumulation in methionine-choline deficient diet-induced nonalcoholic fatty liver disease in mice via peroxisome proliferator-activated receptor α. Chinese Journal of Natural Medicines 19: 401-411.

da Silva, T.F., Ferraz, A.C., Almeida, L.T., Caetano, C., Camini, F.C., Lima, R., Andrade, A., de Oliveira, D.B., Rocha, K., Silva, B.M., de Magalhães, J.C. and Magalhães, C., 2020. Antiviral effect of silymarin against Zika virus *in vitro*. Acta Tropica 211: 105613.

Dahari, H., Shteingart, S., Gafanovich, I., Cotler, S.J., D'Amato, M., Pohl, R.T., Weiss, G., Ashkenazi, Y.J., Tichler, T., Goldin, E. and Lurie, Y., 2015. Sustained virological response with intravenous silibinin: individualized IFN-free therapy via real-time modelling of HCV kinetics. Liver International 35: 289-294.

de Avelar, C.R., Pereira, E.M., de Farias Costa, P.R., de Jesus, R.P. and de Oliveira, L., 2017. Effect of silymarin on biochemical indicators in patients with liver disease: Systematic review with meta-analysis. World Journal of Gastroenterology 23: 5004-5017.

Delli Bovi, A.P., Marciano, F., Mandato, C., Siano, M.A., Savoia, M. and Vajro, P., 2021. Oxidative stress in non-alcoholic fatty liver disease. An updated mini review. Frontiers in Medicine 8: 595371.

Derakhshandeh-Rishehri, S.M., Heidari-Beni, M. and Eftekhari, M.H., 2020. The effects of Reasil, silibyn-phospholipid-vitamin E complex on liver enzymes in patients with non-alcoholic fatty liver disease, NAFLD or non-alcoholic steato-hepatitis, NASH: A systemic review and meta-analysis of RCTS. Acta Endocrinologica 2005: 223-231.

Dutta, S.K., Sengupta, S. and Tripathi, A., 2022. In silico and *in vitro* evaluation of silibinin: a promising anti-Chikungunya agent. *In vitro* Cellular & Developmental Biology. Animal 58: 255-267.

Dwivedi, P.S.R., Patil, V.S., Khanal, P., Bhandare, V., Gurav, S., Harish, D.R., Patil, B.M. and Roy, S., 2022. System biology-based investigation of Silymarin to trace hepatoprotective effect. Computers in Biology and Medicine 142: 105223.

Federico, A., Conti, V., Russomanno, G., Dallio, M., Masarone, M., Stiuso, P., Tuccillo, C., Caraglia, M., Manzo, V., Persico, M., Filippelli, A. and Loguercio, C., 2017a. A long-term treatment with silybin in patients with non-alcoholic steatohepatitis stimulates catalase activity in human endothelial cells. *In vivo* 31: 609-618.

Federico, A., Dallio, M. and Loguercio, C., 2017b. Silymarin/silybin and chronic liver disease: A marriage of many years. Molecules 22: 191.

Federico, A., Dallio, M., Masarone, M., Gravina, A.G., Di Sarno, R., Tuccillo, C., Cossiga, V., Lama, S., Stiuso, P., Morisco, F., Persico, M. and Loguercio, C., 2019. Evaluation of the effect derived from silybin with vitamin D and vitamin E administration on clinical, metabolic, endothelial dysfunction, oxidative stress parameters, and serological worsening markers in nonalcoholic fatty liver disease patients. Oxidative Medicine and Cellular Longevity 2019: 8742075.

Feng, B., Meng, R., Bin Huang, Bi, Y., Shen, S. and Zhu, D., 2017. Silymarin protects against renal injury through normalization of lipid metabolism and mitochondrial biogenesis in high fat-fed mice. Free Radical Biology & Medicine 110: 240-249.

Ferenci, P., Scherzer, T.M., Kerschner, H., Rutter, K., Beinhardt, S., Hofer, H., Schöniger-Hekele, M., Holzmann, H. and Steindl-Munda, P., 2008. Silibinin is a potent antiviral agent in patients with chronic hepatitis C not responding to pegylated interferon/ribavirin therapy. Gastroenterology 135: 1561-1567.

Ferraz, A.C., Almeida, L.T., da Silva Caetano, C.C., da Silva Menegatto, M.B., Souza Lima, R.L., de Senna, J., de Oliveira Cardoso, J.M., Perucci, L.O., Talvani, A., Geraldo de Lima, W., de Mello Silva, B., Barbosa Reis, A., de Magalhães, J.C. and Lopes de Brito Magalhães, C., 2021. Hepatoprotective, antioxidant, anti-inflammatory, and antiviral activities of silymarin against mayaro virus infection. Antiviral Research 194: 105168.

Fried, M.W., Navarro, V.J., Afdhal, N., Belle, S.H., Wahed, A.S., Hawke, R.L., Doo, E., Meyers, C.M., Reddy, K.R. and Silymarin in NASH and C Hepatitis, SyNCH Study Group, 2012. Effect of silymarin, milk thistle on liver disease in patients with chronic hepatitis C unsuccessfully treated with interferon therapy: a randomized controlled trial. JAMA 308: 274-282.

Gabbay, E., Zigmond, E., Pappo, O., Hemed, N., Rowe, M., Zabrecky, G., Cohen, R. and Ilan, Y., 2007. Antioxidant therapy for chronic hepatitis C after failure of interferon: results of phase II randomized, double-blind placebo controlled clinical trial. World Journal of Gastroenterology 13: 5317-5323.

Gillessen, A., Angelico, F., Chen, J., Lu, L., Lucena, M.I., Fu, Q., Xie, Q., Andrade, R.J., Xie, W., Xu, X., Yu, Y., Mao, Y. and Nan, Y., 2022. Silymarin for Treating Toxic Liver Disease: International Consensus Recommendations. Gastro Hep Advances 1: 882-893.

Gobalakrishnan, S., Asirvatham, S.S. and Janarthanam, V., 2016. Effect of silybin on lipid profile in hypercholesterolaemic rats. Journal of Clinical and Diagnostic Research 10: FF01-FF5.

Gogulski, M., Cieślak, A., Grabska, J., Ardois, M., Pomorska-Mól, M., Kołodziejski, P.A., Libera, K., Strompfová, V. and Szumacher-Strabel, M., 2021. Effects of silybin supplementation on nutrient digestibility, hematological parameters, liver function indices, and liver-specific mi-RNA concentration in dogs. BMC Veterinary Research 17: 228.

Grasselli, E., Baldini, F., Vecchione, G., Oliveira, P.J., Sardão, V.A., Voci, A., Portincasa, P. and Vergani, L., 2019. Excess fructose and fatty acids trigger a model of non-alcoholic fatty liver disease progression *in vitro*: Protective effect of the flavonoid silybin. International Journal of Molecular Medicine 44: 705-712.

Grattagliano, I., Diogo, C.V., Mastrodonato, M., de Bari, O., Persichella, M., Wang, D.Q., Liquori, A., Ferri, D., Carratù, M.R., Oliveira, P.J. and Portincasa, P., 2013. A silybin-phospholipids complex counteracts rat fatty liver degeneration and mitochondrial oxidative changes. World Journal of Gastroenterology 19: 3007-3017.

Gruneau, L., Ekstedt, M., Kechagias, S. and Henriksson, M., 2023. Disease progression modeling for economic evaluation in nonalcoholic fatty liver disease – a systematic review. Clinical Gastroenterology and Hepatology 21: 283-298. S1542-3565.

Gu, M., Zhao, P., Huang, J., Zhao, Y., Wang, Y., Li, Y., Li, Y., Fan, S., Ma, Y.M., Tong, Q., Yang, L., Ji, G. and Huang, C., 2016. Silymarin ameliorates metabolic dysfunction associated with diet-induced obesity via activation of Farnesyl X receptor. Frontiers in Pharmacology 7: 345.

Guedj, J., Dahari, H., Pohl, R.T., Ferenci, P. and Perelson, A.S., 2012. Understanding silibinin's modes of action against HCV using viral kinetic modeling. Journal of Hepatology 56: 1019-1024.

Guo, Y., Wang, S., Wang, Y. and Zhu, T., 2016. Silymarin improved diet-induced liver damage and insulin resistance by decreasing inflammation in mice. Pharmaceutical Biology 54: 2995-3000.

Hamdy, R., Mostafa, A., Abo Shama, N.M., Soliman, S. and Fayed, B., 2022. Comparative evaluation of flavonoids reveals the superiority and promising inhibition activity of silibinin against SARS-CoV-2. Phytotherapy Research 36: 2921-2939.

Jamalian, M., Mahmodiyeh, B., Saveiee, S. and Solhi, H., 2020. Investigating the impact of silymarin on liver oxidative injury. Journal of Family Medicine and Primary Care 9: 1707-1711.

Jiang, G., Sun, C., Wang, X., Mei, J., Li, C., Zhan, H., Liao, Y., Zhu, Y. and Mao, J., 2022. Hepatoprotective mechanism of *Silybum marianum* on nonalcoholic fatty liver disease based on network pharmacology and experimental verification. Bioengineered 13: 5216-5235.

Kalopitas, G., Antza, C., Doundoulakis, I., Siargkas, A., Kouroumalis, E., Germanidis, G., Samara, M. and Chourdakis, M., 2021. Impact of silymarin in individuals with nonalcoholic fatty liver disease: A systematic review and meta-analysis. Nutrition 83: 111092.

Khalili, A., Fallah, P., Hashemi, S.A., Ahmadian-Attari, M.M., Jamshidi, V., Mazloom, R., Beikzadeh, L. and Bayat, G., 2021. New mechanistic insights into hepatoprotective activity of milk thistle and chicory quantified extract: The role of hepatic Farnesoid-X activated receptors. Avicenna Journal of Phytomedicine 11: 367-379.

Kheiripour, N., Karimi, J., Khodadadi, I., Tavilani, H., Taghi Goodarzi, M. and Hashemnia, M., 2019. Hepatoprotective effects of silymarin on liver injury via irisin upregulation and oxidative stress reduction in rats with type 2 diabetes. Iranian Journal of Medical Sciences 44: 108-117.

Křen, V., 2021. Chirality matters: Biological activity of optically pure silybin and Its congeners. International Journal of Molecular Sciences 22: 7885.

Kuchay, M.S., Martínez-Montoro, J.I., Choudhary, N.S., Fernández-García, J.C. and Ramos-Molina, B., 2021. Non-alcoholic fatty liver disease in lean and non-obese individuals: current and future challenges. Biomedicines 9: 1346.

Kumar, N., Rai, A., Reddy, N.D., Shenoy, R.R., Mudgal, J., Bansal, P., Mudgal, P.P., Arumugam, K., Udupa, N., Sharma, N. and Rao, C.M., 2019. Improved *in vitro* and *in vivo* hepatoprotective effects of liposomal silymarin in alcohol-induced hepatotoxicity in Wistar rats. Pharmacological Reports 71: 703-712.

Lacombe, G. and St-Onge, M., 2016. Towards evidence-based emergency medicine: best BETs from the Manchester Royal Infirmary. BET 1: Silibinin in suspected amatoxin-containing mushroom poisoning. Emergency Medicine Journal 33: 76-77.

Lalani, S.S., Anasir, M.I. and Poh, C.L., 2020. Antiviral activity of silymarin in comparison with baicalein against EV-A71. BMC Complementary Medicine and Therapies 20: 97.

Lalani, S., Masomian, M. and Poh, C.L., 2021. Functional insights into silymarin as an antiviral agent against enterovirus A71, EV-A71. International Journal of Molecular Sciences 22: 8757.

Lani, R., Hassandarvish, P., Chiam, C.W., Moghaddam, E., Chu, J.J., Rausalu, K., Merits, A., Higgs, S., Vanlandingham, D., Abu Bakar, S. and Zandi, K., 2015. Antiviral activity of silymarin against chikungunya virus. Scientific Reports 5: 11421.

Lee, S.J., Nam, M.J., Lee, D.E., Park, J.W., Kang, B.S., Lee, D.S., Lee, H.S. and Kwon, O.S., 2018. Silibinin ameliorates O-GlcNAcylation and inflammation in a mouse model of nonalcoholic steatohepatitis. International Journal of Molecular Sciences 19: 2165.

Li, H.B., Yang, Y.R., Mo, Z.J., Ding, Y. and Jiang, W.J., 2015. Silibinin improves palmitate-induced insulin resistance in C2C12 myotubes by attenuating IRS-1/PI3K/Akt pathway inhibition. Brazilian Journal of Medical and Biological Research 48: 440-446.

Li, X., Wang, Y., Xing, Y., Xing, R., Liu, Y. and Xu, Y., 2020. Changes of gut microbiota during silybin-mediated treatment of high-fat diet-induced non-alcoholic fatty liver disease in mice. Hepatology Research 50: 5-14.

Li, Y., Ren, L., Song, G., Zhang, P., Yang, L., Chen, X., Yu, X. and Chen, S., 2019. Silibinin ameliorates fructose-induced lipid accumulation and activates autophagy in HepG2 cells. Endocrine, Metabolic & Immune Disorders Drug Targets 19: 632-642.

Liang, J., Liu, Y., Liu, J., Li, Z., Fan, Q., Jiang, Z., Yan, F., Wang, Z., Huang, P. and Feng, N., 2018. Chitosan-functionalized lipid-polymer hybrid nanoparticles for oral delivery of silymarin and enhanced lipid-lowering effect in NAFLD. Journal of Nanobiotechnology 16: 64.

Liu, C.H., Jassey, A., Hsu, H.Y. and Lin, L.T., 2019a. Antiviral activities of silymarin and derivatives. Molecules 24: 1552.

Liu, Y., Xu, W., Zhai, T., You, J. and Chen, Y., 2019b. Silibinin ameliorates hepatic lipid accumulation and oxidative stress in mice with non-alcoholic steatohepatitis by regulating CFLAR-JNK pathway. Acta Pharmaceutica Sinica. B 9: 745-757.

Liu, Y., Yu, Q. and Chen, Y., 2018. Effect of silibinin on CFLAR-JNK pathway in oleic acid-treated HepG2 cells. Biomedicine & Pharmacotherapy 108: 716-723.

Lombardi, R., Onali, S., Thorburn, D., Davidson, B.R., Gurusamy, K.S. and Tsochatzis, E., 2017. Pharmacological interventions for non-alcohol related fatty liver disease, NAFLD: an attempted network meta-analysis. The Cochrane Database of Systematic Reviews 3: CD011640.

Low, Z.X., OuYong, B.M., Hassandarvish, P., Poh, C.L. and Ramanathan, B., 2021. Antiviral activity of silymarin and baicalein against dengue virus. Scientific Reports 11: 21221.

Ma, Z., Zang, W., Wang, H. and Wei, X., 2020. Silibinin enhances anti-renal fibrosis effect of MK-521 via downregulation of TGF-β signaling pathway. Human Cell 33: 330-336.

Magdy, Y.M., El-Kharashi, O.A., El-Waseef, D., Nabih, E.S. and Abd El Samad, A.A., 2018. Insights into hepatic and renal FXR/DDAH-1/eNOS pathway and its role in the potential benefit of rosuvastatin and silymarin in hepatic nephropathy. Experimental and Molecular Pathology 105: 293-310.

Majumdar, A., Verbeek, J. and Tsochatzis, E.A., 2021. Non-alcoholic fatty liver disease: Current therapeutic options. Current Opinion in Pharmacology 61: 98-105.

Malaguarnera, G., Bertino, G., Chisari, G., Motta, M., Vecchio, M., Vacante, M., Caraci, F., Greco, C., Drago, F., Nunnari, G. and Malaguarnera, M., 2016. Silybin supplementation during HCV therapy with pegylated interferon-α plus ribavirin reduces depression and anxiety and increases work ability. BMC Psychiatry 16: 398.

Malaguarnera, M., Motta, M., Vacante, M., Malaguarnera, G., Caraci, F., Nunnari, G., Gagliano, C., Greco, C., Chisari, G., Drago, F. and Bertino, G., 2015. Silybin-vitamin E-phospholipids complex reduces liver fibrosis in patients with chronic hepatitis C treated with pegylated interferon α and ribavirin. American Journal of Translational Research 7: 2510-2518.

Marcolino Assis-Júnior, E., Melo, A.T., Pereira, V., Wong, D., Sousa, N., Oliveira, C., Malveira, L., Moreira, L.S., Souza, M., Almeida, P. and Lima-Júnior, R., 2017. Dual effect of silymarin on experimental non-alcoholic steatohepatitis induced by irinotecan. Toxicology and Applied Pharmacology 327: 71-79.

Marin, V., Gazzin, S., Gambaro, S.E., Dal Ben, M., Calligaris, S., Anese, M., Raseni, A., Avellini, C., Giraudi, P.J., Tiribelli, C. and Rosso, N., 2017. Effects of oral administration of silymarin in a juvenile murine model of non-alcoholic steatohepatitis. Nutrients 9: 1006.

Mirnezami, M., Jafarimanesh, H., Rezagholizamenjany, M., Alimoradian, A. and Ranjbaran, M., 2020. The effect of silymarin on liver enzymes in patients taking isotretinoin: A randomized clinical trial. Dermatologic Therapy 33: e13236.

Mirzaei, E., Sabetian, G., Masjedi, M., Heidari, R., Mirjalili, M., Dehghanian, A. and Vazin, A., 2021. The effect of silymarin on liver enzymes and antioxidant status in trauma patients in the intensive care unit: a randomized double blinded placebo-controlled clinical trial. Clinical and Experimental Hepatology 7: 149-155.

Morishima, C., Shuhart, M.C., Wang, C.C., Paschal, D.M., Apodaca, M.C., Liu, Y., Sloan, D.D., Graf, T.N., Oberlies, N.H., Lee, D.Y., Jerome, K.R. and Polyak, S.J., 2010. Silymarin inhibits *in vitro* T-cell proliferation and cytokine production in hepatitis C virus infection. Gastroenterology 138: 671-681.e6812.

National Health Service (NHS), 2022. Hepatitis C. NHS, Leeds, UK. Available at: https://tinyurl.com/4hzxzahs.

Ommati, M.M., Farshad, O., Azarpira, N., Ghazanfari, E., Niknahad, H. and Heidari, R., 2021. Silymarin mitigates bile duct obstruction-induced cholemic nephropathy. Naunyn-Schmiedeberg's Archives of Pharmacology 394: 1301-1314.

Onalan, A.K., Tuncal, S., Kilicoglu, S., Celepli, S., Durak, E., Kilicoglu, B., Devrim, E., Barlas, A.M. and Kismet, K., 2016. Effect of silymarin on oxidative stress and liver histopathology in experimental obstructive jaundice model. Acta Cirurgica Brasileira 31: 801-806.

Ou, Q., Weng, Y., Wang, S., Zhao, Y., Zhang, F., Zhou, J. and Wu, X., 2018. Silybin alleviates hepatic steatosis and fibrosis in NASH mice by inhibiting oxidative stress and involvement with the Nf-κB pathway. Digestive Diseases and Sciences 63: 3398-3408.

Panzitt, K. and Wagner, M., 2021. FXR in liver physiology: Multiple faces to regulate liver metabolism. Biochimica et Biophysica acta. Molecular Basis of Disease 1867: 166133.

Podrini, C., Borghesan, M., Greco, A., Pazienza, V., Mazzoccoli, G. and Vinciguerra, M., 2013. Redox homeostasis and epigenetics in non-alcoholic fatty liver disease, NAFLD. Current Pharmaceutical Design 19: 2737-2746.

Polyak, S.J., Morishima, C., Shuhart, M.C., Wang, C.C., Liu, Y. and Lee, D.Y., 2007. Inhibition of T-cell inflammatory cytokines, hepatocyte NF-kappaB signaling, and HCV infection by standardized silymarin. Gastroenterology 132: 1925-1936.

Rutter, K., Scherzer, T.M., Beinhardt, S., Kerschner, H., Stättermayer, A.F., Hofer, H., Popow-Kraupp, T., Steindl-Munda, P. and Ferenci, P., 2011. Intravenous silibinin as 'rescue treatment' for on-treatment non-responders to pegylated interferon/ribavirin combination therapy. Antiviral Therapy 16: 1327-1333.

Sahin, E., Bagci, R., Bektur Aykanat, N.E., Kacar, S. and Sahinturk, V., 2020. Silymarin attenuated nonalcoholic fatty liver disease through the regulation of endoplasmic reticulum stress proteins GRP78 and XBP-1 in mice. Journal of Food Biochemistry 44: e13194.

Salamone, F., Galvano, F., Cappello, F., Mangiameli, A., Barbagallo, I. and Volti, G.L., 2012. Silibinin modulates lipid homeostasis and inhibits nuclear factor kappa B activation in experimental nonalcoholic steatohepatitis. Translational Research 159: 477-486.

Saller, R., Meier, R. and Brignoli, R., 2001. The use of silymarin in the treatment of liver diseases. Drugs 61: 2035-2063.

Salomone, F., Barbagallo, I., Godos, J., Lembo, V., Currenti, W., Cinà, D., Avola, R., D'Orazio, N., Morisco, F., Galvano, F. and Li Volti, G., 2017. Silibinin restores NAD^+levels and induces the SIRT1/AMPK pathway in non-alcoholic fatty liver. Nutrients 9: 1086.

Serviddio, G., Bellanti, F., Stanca, E., Lunetti, P., Blonda, M., Tamborra, R., Siculella, L., Vendemiale, G., Capobianco, L. and Giudetti, A.M., 2014. Silybin exerts antioxidant effects and induces mitochondrial biogenesis in liver of rat with secondary biliary cirrhosis. Free Radical Biology & Medicine 73: 117-126.

Shriram, R.G., Moin, A., Alotaibi, H.F., Khafagy, E.S., Al Saqr, A., Abu Lila, A.S. and Charyulu, R.N., 2022. Phytosomes as a plausible nano-delivery system for enhanced oral bioavailability and improved hepatoprotective activity of silymarin. Pharmaceuticals 15: 790.

Silva, C.M., Ferrari, G.D., Alberici, L.C., Malaspina, O. and Moraes, K., 2020. Cellular and molecular effects of silymarin on the transdifferentiation processes of LX-2 cells and its connection with lipid metabolism. Molecular and Cellular Biochemistry 468: 129-142.

Solhi, H., Ghahremani, R., Kazemifar, A.M. and Hoseini Yazdi, Z., 2014. Silymarin in treatment of non-alcoholic steatohepatitis: A randomized clinical trial. Caspian Journal of Internal Medicine 5: 9-12.

Srivastava, R., Tripathi, S., Unni, S., Hussain, A., Haque, S., Dasgupta, N., Singh, V. and Mishra, B.N., 2021. Silybin B and cianidanol inhibit M^{pro} and spike protein of SARS-CoV-2: Evidence from in silico molecular docking studies. Current Pharmaceutical Design 27: 3476-3489.

Stofan, M. and Guo, G.L., 2020. Bile acids and FXR: Novel targets for liver diseases. Frontiers in Medicine 7: 544.

Suguro, R., Pang, X.C., Yuan, Z.W., Chen, S.Y., Zhu, Y.Z. and Xie, Y., 2020. Combinational application of silybin and tangeretin attenuates the progression of non-alcoholic steatohepatitis, NASH in mice via modulating lipid metabolism. Pharmacological Research 151: 104519.

Sun, R., Xu, D., Wei, Q., Zhang, B., Aa, J., Wang, G. and Xie, Y., 2020. Silybin ameliorates hepatic lipid accumulation and modulates global metabolism in an NAFLD mouse model. Biomedicine & Pharmacotherapy 123: 109721.

Surai, P.F., 2015. Silymarin as a natural antioxidant: an overview of the current evidence and perspectives. Antioxidants 4: 204-247.

Surai, P.F., 2022. Silymarin as a vitagene modulator: effects on mitochondria integrity in stress conditions. In: Ostojik, S.M. (ed) Molecular nutrition and mitochondria. Elsevier, Academic Press, London, UK, pp. 535-559.

Tanamly, M.D., Tadros, F., Labeeb, S., Makld, H., Shehata, M., Mikhail, N., Abdel-Hamid, M., Shehata, M., Abu-Baki, L., Medhat, A., Magder, L.S., Afdhal, N.H. and Strickland, G.T., 2004. Randomised double-blinded trial evaluating silymarin for chronic hepatitis C in an Egyptian village: study description and 12-month results. Digestive and Liver Disease 36: 752-759.

Tao, L., Qu, X., Zhang, Y., Song, Y. and Zhang, S.X., 2019. Prophylactic therapy of silymarin, milk thistle on antituberculosis drug-induced liver injury: A meta-analysis of randomized controlled trials. Canadian Journal of Gastroenterology & Hepatology 2019: 3192351.

Tighe, S.P., Akhtar, D., Iqbal, U. and Ahmed, A., 2020. Chronic liver disease and silymarin: A biochemical and clinical review. Journal of Clinical and Translational Hepatology 8: 454-458.

Tilg, H., Adolph, T.E., Dudek, M. and Knolle, P., 2021. Non-alcoholic fatty liver disease: the interplay between metabolism, microbes and immunity. Nature Metabolism 3: 1596-1607.

Vecchione, G., Grasselli, E., Cioffi, F., Baldini, F., Oliveira, P.J., Sardão, V.A., Cortese, K., Lanni, A., Voci, A., Portincasa, P. and Vergani, L., 2017. The nutraceutic Silybin counteracts excess lipid accumulation and ongoing oxidative stress in an *in vitro* model of non-alcoholic fatty liver disease progression. Frontiers in Nutrition 4: 42.

Vecchione, G., Grasselli, E., Voci, A., Baldini, F., Grattagliano, I., Wang, D.Q., Portincasa, P. and Vergani, L., 2016. Silybin counteracts lipid excess and oxidative stress in cultured steatotic hepatic cells. World Journal of Gastroenterology 22: 6016-6026.

Wadhwa, K., Pahwa, R., Kumar, M., Kumar, S., Sharma, P.C., Singh, G., Verma, R., Mittal, V., Singh, I., Kaushik, D. and Jeandet, P., 2022. Mechanistic insights into the pharmacological significance of silymarin. Molecules 27: 5327.

Wagoner, J., Morishima, C., Graf, T.N., Oberlies, N.H., Teissier, E., Pécheur, E.I., Tavis, J.E. and Polyak, S.J., 2011. Differential *in vitro* effects of intravenous versus oral formulations of silibinin on the HCV life cycle and inflammation. PloS One 6: e16464.

Wagoner, J., Negash, A., Kane, O.J., Martinez, L.E., Nahmias, Y., Bourne, N., Owen, D.M., Grove, J., Brimacombe, C., McKeating, J.A., Pécheur, E.I., Graf, T.N., Oberlies, N.H., Lohmann, V., Cao, F., Tavis, J.E. and Polyak, S.J., 2010. Multiple effects of silymarin on the hepatitis C virus lifecycle. Hepatology 51: 1912-1921.

Wang, F.S., Fan, J.G., Zhang, Z., Gao, B. and Wang, H.Y., 2014. The global burden of liver disease: the major impact of China. Hepatology 60: 2099-2108.

Wang, F., Chen, S., Ren, L., Wang, Y., Li, Z., Song, T., Zhang, H. and Yang, Q., 2020. The effect of silibinin on protein expression profile in white adipose tissue of obese mice. Frontiers in Pharmacology 11: 55.

Wang, Y., Zhao, H., Yang, L., Zhang, H., Yu, X., Fei, W., Zhen, Y., Gao, Z., Chen, S. and Ren, L., 2022. Quantitative proteomics analysis based on tandem mass tag labeling coupled with labeling coupled with liquid chromatography-tandem mass spectrometry discovers the effect of silibinin on non-alcoholic fatty liver disease in mice. Bioengineered 13: 6750-6766.

Wood, N.J., 2010. Liver: Nonobese individuals in the developing world are at risk of nonalcoholic fatty liver and liver disease. Nature Reviews. Gastroenterology & Hepatology 7: 357.

World Health Organization (WHO), 2022. Hepatitis C. WHO, Geneva, Switzerland. Available at: https://www.tinyurl.com/6yzfakb8.

Yan, B. and Zhang, C., 2021. Liver protection mechanism and absorption promotion technology of silybin based on intelligent medical analysis. Journal of Healthcare Engineering 2021: 9968016.

Yang, L., Liu, Q., Zhang, H., Wang, Y., Li, Y., Chen, S., Song, G. and Ren, L., 2021. Silibinin improves nonalcoholic fatty liver by regulating the expression of miR-122: An *in vitro* and *in vivo* study. Molecular Medicine Reports 23: 335.

Yao, J., Zhi, M. and Minhu, C., 2011. Effect of silybin on high-fat-induced fatty liver in rats. Brazilian Journal of Medical and Biological Research 44: 652-659.

Yaqub, S., Ananias, P., Shah, A., Luenam, K., Jose, A.M., Melo, J.P., Turkistani, A. and Mohammed, L., 2021. Decoding the pathophysiology of non-alcoholic fatty liver disease progressing to non-alcoholic steatohepatitis: A systematic review. Cureus 13: e18201.

Zhang, B., Xu, D., She, L., Wang, Z., Yang, N., Sun, R., Zhang, Y., Yan, C., Wei, Q., Aa, J., Liu, B., Wang, G. and Xie, Y., 2018. Silybin inhibits NLRP3 inflammasome assembly through the NAD^+/SIRT2 pathway in mice with nonalcoholic fatty liver disease. FASEB Journal 32: 757-767.

Zhang, R., Xu, D., Zhang, Y., Wang, R., Yang, N., Lou, Y., Zhao, H., Aa, J., Wang, G. and Xie, Y., 2021. Silybin restored CYP3A expression through the Sirtuin 2/Nuclear Factor κ-B pathway in mouse nonalcoholic fatty liver disease. Drug Metabolism and Disposition 49: 770-779.

Zhong, S., Fan, Y., Yan, Q., Fan, X., Wu, B., Han, Y., Zhang, Y., Chen, Y., Zhang, H. and Niu, J., 2017. The therapeutic effect of silymarin in the treatment of nonalcoholic fatty disease: A meta-analysis, PRISMA of randomized control trials. Medicine 96: e9061.

Chapter 13
Neuroprotective properties of silymarin

Laughter is the best medicine

Peter F. Surai[1-6] and Anton Surai[7]*
[1]Vitagene and Health Research Centre, Bristol, UK; [2]Department of Microbiology and Biochemistry, Faculty of Veterinary Medicine, Trakia University, Stara Zagora, Bulgaria; [3]Department of Animal Nutrition, Faculty of Agricultural and Environmental Sciences, Szent Istvan University, Hungary; [4]Saint-Petersburg State Academy of Veterinary Medicine, St. Petersburg, Russia; [5]Sumy National Agrarian University, Sumy, Ukraine; [6]Odessa National Academy of Food Technologies, Odessa, Ukraine; [7]Healthy Food Services, Bristol, UK
psurai@feedfood.co.uk

Abstract

Protective effects of SM in neurodegeneration shown in various animal models are associated with activation of Nrf2 and vitagenes leading to improvement of antioxidant defences and reduction of oxidative stress, prevention/reduction of inflammation and apoptosis by inhibiting NF-κB, inhibition of microglia activation, upregulation of neurotrophic factors and attenuation of autophagy, etc. This chapter presents recent data on protective effects of SM against Alzheimer (AD) and Parkinson diseases (PD). On one hand, it was demonstrated in various model systems that protective actions of SM in Alzheimer's disease are associated with improvement of various important cellular events including redox homeostasis, Ca^{2+}-homeostasis, neurogenesis, oestrogen receptor activities, insulin signalling, gut microbiota composition and autophagy. On the other hand, beneficial effects of SM in Alzheimer's disease are related to ameliorating oxidative stress and preventing mitochondria disfunction, Tau phosphorylation, microglia activation, neuroinflammation and apoptosis. Similarly, protective effects of SM in Parkinson's disease were also demonstrated in model systems and there are quite a few similarities in molecular mechanisms of protective effects of SM against PD and AD with prevention of oxidative stress and maintaining redox balance in the brain and neurones to play a crucial role in such protective actions of SM. Oxidative stress and redox disbalance are common hallmarks of several neurodegenerative diseases including Parkinson's and Alzheimer's diseases. Furthermore, it seems likely that regulatory actions of SM on Nrf2, NF-κB, MAPK and JNK are of paramount importance in their protective actions in neurogenerative diseases including Parkinson's and Alzheimer's diseases. Clearly, more research is warrant in this exciting area.

Keywords: silymarin, neurodegeneration, Alzheimer's disease, Parkinson's disease, mechanisms

DOI:10.3920/978-90-8686-944-2_013,

13.1 Introduction

Neurodegenerative diseases include a group of human disorders where the progressive and irreversible damage and loss of specific neuronal networks lead to the clinical manifestation of the disease with the most common being Alzheimer's disease (AD), Parkinson's disease (PD), amyotrophic lateral sclerosis (ALS) and multiple sclerosis (MS; Pardillo-Díaz *et al.*, 2022). Clinical manifestations of neurodegenerative diseases include cognitive and behavioural disorders associated with movement disorders (Dugger and Dickson, 2017). Based on experimental results with rodent and primate models at least four well defined mechanisms of such changes in CNS were defined including:

- oxidative stress, calcium (Ca^{2+}) imbalance and mitochondrial dysfunction;
- neuroinflammation;
- cell death, including apoptosis;
- proteotoxic stress, associated with abnormalities in the lysosomal/autophagosomal and ubiquitin proteasomal systems, disruption of autophagy and the accumulation of α-synuclein.

Oxidative stress is a common hallmark of several neurodegenerative diseases. SM has been recently shown to have neuroprotective activities against neurodegenerative diseases such as Parkinson's and Alzheimer's diseases. Anti-Parkinson's potential of SM has been recently analysed in detail (Ullah and Khan, 2018). Recently, protective effects of SM on neurodegeneration in various animal models have been also reviewed (Amato *et al.*, 2019) and its protective mechanisms include:

- improvement of antioxidant defences and reduction of oxidative stress;
- prevention/reduction of inflammation and apoptosis by inhibiting NF-κB;
- inhibition of microglia activation;
- upregulation of neurotrophic factors and attenuation of autophagy;
- downregulation of AChE activity, Aβ aggregation, attenuation of amyloid β plaque burden;
- increase of the brain-derived neurotrophic factor BDNF levels;
- the oestrogen-like activity through selective activation of Erβ;
- increase of brain energy metabolism and cholinergic functions;
- regulation of relative abundance of several key bacterial species involved in AD development.

Recent data on protective effects of SM against Alzheimer and Parkinson diseases are analysed below.

13.2 Silymarin and Alzheimer's disease

Alzheimer's disease (AD) is the most common form of dementia (the loss of cognitive functioning), a group of symptoms associated with declining of brain functions affecting memory, thinking skills and other mental abilities accounting for 60-80% of dementia cases. AD was first described by German physician Dr Alois Alzheimer in 1906. AD is most common in elderly (>65-year-old) people with increasing risk of the disease with age, affecting about 1 in 14 people over the age of 65 and 1 in every 6 people over the age of 80. It is estimated that more than 520,000 people in the UK have dementia associated with Alzheimer's disease (Alzheimer.org.uk, 2022). In general, estimates vary, but many experts suggest that more than 6 million Americans may have dementia caused by Alzheimer's and AD is currently ranked as the sixth leading cause of death in the United States and may rank third for older people in Europe, North and South America (Jeremic *et al.*, 2021; NIA, 2022).

In India, more than 4 million people are suffering from Alzheimer's disease and other types of dementia (Dhapola *et al.*, 2021). There are approximately 50 million people worldwide with dementia (Lichtenthaler *et al.*, 2022) and up to 70% of them are estimated to have Alzheimer's disease (Mayoclinic.org, 2022). The first sign of AD is believed to be short term memory loss. At the next stage of the further disease development more severe memory problems, disorientation, confusion, difficulty planning or making decisions, low mood or anxiety, personality changes (becoming aggressive, demanding and suspicious) and problems with language and speech appear (NHS, 2022a).

AD development represents a very complex neurodegenerative process and the two most widely accepted points of view on AD etiology in the scientific medical community are the hypothesis of the amyloid cascade formation and the phosphorylation of the tau protein (Jeremic *et al.*, 2021). It seems likely that abnormal proteins build up in the brain, including amyloid-β (a fragment of a larger protein, which proteolytically derives from the amyloid precursor protein; APP) deposits known as 'plaques' (around/between brain cells), and tau 'tangles' (twisted fibres called intracellular neurofibrillary tangles (NFT) built up inside brain cells) are responsible for damages to brain cells and a loss of connections between them (Princiotta Cariddi *et al.*, 2022) being the fundamental neuropathological pillars of the disease.

Amyloid beta (Aβ) is shown to be the major component of the senile plaques, whereas tau protein is the main component of neurofibrillary tangles found in the brain of AD patients being key players in neuronal degeneration (Walia *et al.*, 2022). Senile plaques are the aggregated forms of Aβ peptides that are formed as a result of sequential cleavage of the APP by specific enzymes called β- and γ-secretases. Furthermore, intraneuronal NFTs are associated with hyperphosphorylated tau protein deeply participating in synaptic loss and cognitive impairment and it seems likely that defective clearance of Aβ and tau protein could be the main contributor to AD (Li *et al.*, 2021a).

Therefore, previously healthy neurons in the brain are believed to stop properly functioning, lose connections with other neurons, and eventually die. It seems likely that 'plaques' and 'tangles' are responsible for blocking communication among nerve cells and disrupting their functions and survival. The alterations/damages initially can be seen in the hippocampus and the entorhinal cortex, in the regions of the brain that controls memory, but at later stages of the disease other parts of the brain are affected leading to appearance of a range AD symptoms (NIA, 2022). Aβ plaques and hyperphosphorylated tau protein aggregates leading to cognitive deficits and behavioural problems, are considered to be the hallmarks of the AD (Johri, 2021). There is a range of genes involved in this disease including APP gene, presenilin genes (PS1 & PS2), ApoE gene, and α-macroglobulin gene (Dhapola *et al.*, 2021) and there are more than 40 genetic variants which are related to risk factors that enhance the susceptibility to the development of the late-onset AD (Jeremic *et al.*, 2021).

The exact cause of AD is not yet fully understood and changes in the brain may begin many years before symptoms appear. It is believed that a combination of genetic (a family history of the condition), environmental (air pollution), and lifestyle factors that affect the brain over time are responsible for the development of AD. It should be emphasised that a number of lifestyle risk factors for AD can be modified including high dietary fat, low physical activity, hypertension, diabetes mellitus, increased homocysteine and cholesterol, etc. (Jeremic *et al.*, 2021).

There's currently no cure for Alzheimer's disease and it is impossible to stop the disease process in the brain, but medicines are available that can help relieve/improve some of the symptoms by removing amyloid from the brain or temporarily slow down the worsening/progression of dementia symptoms and improve quality of life. Therapy could consist of drugs that prevent oxidative stress and mitochondria dysfunction restoring redox balance in the brain cells, modulate immune inflammatory response, restore insulin tolerance, etc. Therefore, disease-modifying therapy presents a range of significant challenges for AD clinical practice (Jeremic *et al.*, 2021). Changes in life style (stopping smoking and cutting down on alcohol), diet (eating a healthy, balanced diet and maintaining a healthy weight) and physical activity are believed to reduce risk or delay the onset of dementia (NHS, 2022a).

Considering molecular mechanisms of AD neuropathology development, several plausible pathophysiological events have been identified in the AD brain (Johri, 2021) including

- oxidative stress;
- mitochondrial dysfunction;
- disruption of Ca^{2+} homeostasis;
- inflammation;
- apoptosis; and
- deficient glucose metabolism.

The etiology of AD is still puzzling, but it has been suggested that oxidative stress plays a key role in the pathogenesis of AD (Walia *et al.*, 2022). Interestingly, oxidative stress is interconnected practically with all the aforementioned pathological events and mitochondrial dysfunction leads to increased ROS production and decreased AO defences. Ca^{2+} homeostasis is of great importance in maintaining general cellular homeostasis and the disruption of Ca^{2+} homeostasis confers mitochondrial damage inevitably leading to excess ROS production and oxidative stress. Cell redox balance regulates inflammatory reactions and oxidative stress could induce inflammatory pathways, a fundamental process in disease development and progression. The same is true for apoptosis, excessive oxidative stress and mitochondria dysfunction are key events in apoptosis initiation. Finally, carbohydrate metabolism provides key regulatory intermediates participating in AO defences and alteration of glucose metabolism could also affect ROS production and the antioxidant defence network.

The chronic stress (environmental, emotional, nutritional, etc.) can lead to oxidative stress (OS) in the parts of the brain associated with suppressed cell proliferation and reduced neurogenesis and involved in pathogenesis of depression and AD (Juszczyk *et al.*, 2021). In this context, OS is reported to facilitates the expression of APP and beta-secretase (BACE1) participated in the increased generation of Aβ and OS also restricts Aβ clearance and favours its accumulation in the brain (Walia *et al.*, 2022). Of note, secretases are a group of proteases processing the AD-linked neuronal APP and also controlling microglial functions (Lichtenthaler *et al.*, 2022).

The oxidative stress caused by Aβ is considered to be associated with formation of complexes between Aβ and redox active metals, including Cu, Zn and Fe. Therefore, the metal-amyloid complexes are responsible for ROS formation leading to excitotoxicity, membrane depolarisation and impairment of mitochondrial function (Ionescu-Tucker and Cotman, 2021). Involvement of innate and adaptive immunity abnormalities in AD development and a systemic failure of cell-mediated Aβ clearance as an important factor of AD progression (Li *et al.*, 2021a) deserve more attention. Interestingly, on the one hand, microglia (the resident macrophage cells located throughout the brain and spinal cord) are able to phagocytose Aβ and, thus, reducing its abundance. On the other hand, microglia are also believed to contribute to Aβ aggregation and excessive neuroinflammation (Lichtenthaler *et al.*, 2022).

The neuroinflammation (persistent microglial activation) associated with the glial activation and release of proinflammatory mediators including NO, IL-1β, Il-18, TNF-α, prostaglandins, and chemokines (fractalkine, MIP-1α, IP10, MCP-1, etc.) substantially contribute to neuronal death in AD patients (de Oliveira *et al.*, 2021). Growing evidence supports a central role for vitagenes (Calabrese *et al.*, 2007), including sirtuins (Fernando and Wijayasinghe, 2021) in the regulation of neuroinflammation and AD development.

It should be also noted that brain is the organ that is most susceptible to the ROS-induced damage due to high levels of PUFAs, low levels of antioxidants, low repair capacity, and non-replicating natures of neurons (Ionescu-Tucker and Cotman, 2021; Walia *et al.*, 2022). It is logical to suggest that by prevention of oxidative stress and controlling optimal redox balance it is possible to ameliorate at least some oxidative-stress-induced events in AD brain. Therefore, the antioxidant therapy may provide benefits and slow down the progress of AD to advance stages by ameliorating neuronal degeneration. However, the findings from the clinical studies of preventive action of antioxidants in AD showed inconsistent results (Walia *et al.*, 2022). The authors suggested that inconsistent outcome of the clinical trials could be a result of poor study design, selection of the wrong antioxidant, inability of the molecule to cross the blood-brain barrier, treatment in the advanced state of disease, etc. It has been shown that mouse models cannot recapitulate the full phenotype of human AD and somatic mutation models have not been available (Li *et al.*, 2021b) limiting progress in the area of AD research.

There is a range of AD models based on invertebrates including insects (Drosophila melanogaster) and common round worms (*Coenorhabditis elaegans*), mammalian models including mice, rats, dogs or non-human primates (Balmus *et al.*, 2015). Furthermore, neuropsychiatric symptoms resembling AD behaviour in human can be induced in animals by various chemicals including scopolamine, atropine, okadaic acid, STZ, aluminium chloride, ferrous sulphate heptahydrate, L-Buthionine-(S,R)-sulphoximine, amyloid peptide mix, etc. (Balmus *et al.*, 2015). There are also AD models based on transgenic animals, but most of the transgenic AD models were shown to rely on the familial AD forms which account only for about 5% of all the AD cases (Balmus *et al.*, 2015). Furthermore, beyond AD features transgenic animals may also manifest other deficits and in experiments are mainly used genetically modified young animals, while AD is characteristic for elderly patients. Among the non-genetically manipulated neuroinflammation models for AD, LPS-induced animal model is commonly used (Zakaria *et al.*, 2017).

The Senescence Accelerated Mouse-Prone 8 (SAMP8) is a naturally occurring mouse line that displays a phenotype of accelerated aging. Therefore, SAMPS8 is considered to be an ideal model to study AD, characterised by important features of pathogenesis of AD, including oxidative stress, inflammation, amyloid-β (Aβ) deposits, tau protein hyperphosphorylation, endoplasmic reticulum stress, abnormal autophagy activity, etc. (Liu *et al.*, 2020a). Therefore, many Alzheimer's disease animal models have been developed and actively used to study molecular mechanisms of AD development, aetiology elucidation or therapeutic compounds testing. However, it should be borne in mind that an animal model is not exactly the disease, but only a close resemblance of it in an animal organism and cannot reflect all the complex features of AD (Balmus *et al.*, 2015). Therefore, no perfect animal model (mimicking the entire AD features of the human AD) has been designed yet.

SM and SB used in various animal models of AD showed promising results. For example, in mesencephalic mixed neuron-glia cultures SM was indicated to protect dopaminergic neurons against LPS-induced neurotoxicity by inhibiting microglia activation mediated through the inhibition of NF-κB activation (Wang *et al.*, 2002). In an Alzheimer's disease mouse model SM was reported to attenuate the amyloid β plaque burden and improved behavioural abnormalities (Murata *et al.*, 2010). SB was discovered to be an inhibitor of Aβ aggregation and therefore could be considered as a therapeutic agent for the treatment of AD (Yin *et al.*, 2011). It was shown that (+)-taxifolin, isolated from SM is an inhibitor of aggregation of the 42-residue amyloid β-protein (Sato *et al.*, 2013).

SB was found to inhibit AChE activity and amyloid β peptide aggregation. In particular, SB interacted with Aβ and AChE to form various stable complexes leading to downregulation of AChE activity and Aβ aggregations, and to decrease the quantity of AChE. Furthermore, SB-treated APP/PS1 transgenic mice had greater scores in the Morris Water Maze with SB having an ability to increase the number of newly generated microglia, astrocytes, neurons, and neuronal precursor cells (Duan *et al.*, 2015). SB (100 or 200 mg/kg for 8 weeks) was observed to reverse learning and suppress memory impairments in APP/PS1 transgenic mice via prevention/inhibition of oxidative stress (MDA, GSH and SOD) and amelioration of apoptosis as evidenced by suppression of the activation of caspase-3. Furthermore, increased levels of synaptophysin and PSD95 in experimental mice were observed as a result of SB treatment (Bai *et al.*, 2017).

Oral administration of SB (100 or 200 mg/kg once per day by gavage for 2 months from 6 to 8 months of age) to APP/PS1 mice was shown to significantly attenuate the cognitive deficits in the Y-maze test, novel object recognition test, and Morris water maze test. Furthermore, SB reduced Aβ deposition and the levels of soluble Aβ1-40/1-42 in the hippocampus due to downregulation of APP and BACE1 and upregulation of the zinc-metalloprotease neprilysin in APP/PS1 mice. In addition, SB ameliorated oxidative stress as evidenced by decreased MDA content and increased activities of the antioxidant enzymes (CAT and SOD; Bai *et al.*, 2019). Protective effects of SM and SB (by gavage at a dosage of 100 mg/kg once a day for 15 days) administration on transgenic APP/PS1 mice having important mutations associated with early-onset Alzheimer's disease were investigated. It was shown that compared to control animals, SM and SB administration were associated with alleviation of memory deficits and reduction of the amyloid plaque burden in the brain of APP/PS1 mice and tended to decrease the microbiota diversity regulating abundances of several key bacterial species associated with AD development (Shen *et al.*, 2019).

In addition, in an Alzheimer's disease model, SB was found to significantly attenuate memory impairment, simultaneously with attenuation of ERs, mitogen-activated protein kinases and PI3K-Akt pathways in the hippocampus of amyloid β (Aβ1-42)-injected rats (Song *et al.*, 2018). The effect of SM on the passive avoidance learning in a rat model of AD induced by the intracerebroventricular injection of Aβ peptide (Aβ1-42) in Wistar rats was evaluated. SM was used at 70 and 140 mg/kg once a day, for 4 weeks leading to memory function improvement, decreased brain amyloid plaques and suppressed APP expression (Yaghmaei *et al.*, 2014).

It seems likely that underlying neuroprotective mechanism of SM is associated with its capacity to inhibit oxidative stress in the brain, it also shows additional advantages by influencing various pathways, including (Borah *et al.*, 2013):

- β-amyloid aggregation;
- inflammatory mechanisms;
- cellular apoptotic machinery; and
- oestrogenic receptor mediation.

The potential of SM to slow the progression of neurodegenerative disorder such as Alzheimer's disease by using CL4176 *C. elegans* model for AD was evaluated. *C. elegans* CL4176 transgenic animal is known to induce expression of amyloid beta-protein

(Aβ1-42) in muscle tissues in the case of subjection to temperature of 23 °C and above leading to worm paralysis. Therefore, CL4176 animals treated with SM (25 μM or 50 μM) was reported to show delayed paralysis via enhancing resistance to oxidative stress (Kumar *et al.*, 2015). In *Caenorhabditis elegans* Alzheimer's model SM was shown to extend lifespan and reduced proteotoxicity (Xu *et al.*, 2019).

Protective effects of SB on the β-amyloid peptide such as amyloid β-protein (Aβ) and insulin amyloid fibrillation have been reported (Katebi *et al.*, 2018; Liu *et al.*, 2020b; Sciacca *et al.*, 2017; Yin *et al.*, 2011; Zeng *et al.*, 2016). As reported, SB reduced the cerebral plaque burden and brain microglial activation associated with an improvement of the behavioural abnormalities induced by AD pathology (Amato *et al.*, 2019; Yin *et al.*, 2011). In the mouse Alzheimer's disease model, SB encapsulated in macrophage-derived exosomes (Exo-SB) was illustrated to induce dual inhibition of Aβ aggregation and astrocyte activation to alleviate inflammation-mediated neuronal damage and cognitive impairment through its effects on the NF-κB pathway (Huo *et al.*, 2021). In an experiment with SH-SY5Y cells SB (224 and 448 μM) was shown to have an inhibitory effect on lysozyme amyloid fibrillation process (Chen *et al.*, 2021).

SM (20-80 μM) was found to protect glial cells against peroxide-induced ROS formation, ATP depletion, and cell damage and NF-κB or/and PKC signalling pathways were involved in the process. SM also is shown to reduce LPS-induced injures in spinal neuronal/glial cell cultures. *In vivo*, intrathecal administration of SM immediately after eliciting contusive spinal cord injury was able to improve hindlimb locomotor behaviour in the rats (Tsai *et al.*, 2010). SM in the form of encapsulated nano-liquid crystals was observed to have improved activity against beta amyloid induced cytotoxicity (Singh *et al.*, 2020).

In a mice model of HFD-induced experimental dementia SM (200 mg/kg/day, p.o. for 15 days) significantly reversed cognitive deficits and the biochemical changes, including TBARS, GSH and MPO activity (Neha Kumar *et al.*, 2014). Streptozotocin, a glucosamine-nitrosourea derivative, is often used for the induction of AD-like pathology in experimental animals. Protective effects of SB against STZ-induced memory impairment were shown to be associated with improvement of brain energy metabolism and cholinergic functions (Tota *et al.*, 2011). In STZ-induced diabetic rats SM supplementation (200 mg/kg/day for 35 days) was shown to ameliorate cognitive impairment and to improve anxiety-related behaviour and learning and memory by increasing the brain-derived neurotrophic factor levels (Yön *et al.*, 2019).

Intracerebroventricular injection of STZ to rats was indicated to cause memory damage, to sharply reduce the number of nissl bodies and to destroy morphological structure of hippocampal neuronal cells, while SB (25, 50 and 100 mg/kg) was able to ameliorate the damages. In addition, SB was illustrated to significantly decrease STZ-induced tau protein hyperphosphorylation (ser404) in hippocampus and cerebral cortex, to inhibit apoptosis of neurons induced by STZ, and to up-regulate insulin signal transduction pathway (Liu *et al.*, 2020b).

SB was reported to enhance antioxidant defences to show neuroprotective actions in LPS-induced neuroinflammatory injuries and Aβ-induced Alzheimer's disease model in rats (Song *et al.*, 2016; 2017b). SB (50 and 100 mg/ kg for 4 weeks) was reported to ameliorate $A\beta_{25-35}$-induced memory deficits in rats by modulating autophagy and preventing neuroinflammation associated with oxidative stress (Song *et al.*, 2017a). Furthermore, protective effect of SB on learning and memory impairment in LPS-treated rats was shown to be mediated via ROS-BDNF-TrkB pathway (Song *et al.*, 2016). To increase its pharmacological effects, SB was encapsulated into human serum albumin (HSA) nanoparticles and protective effects of SB-HSA nanoparticles on LPS-induced oxidative stress in neuron-like cells (SH-SY5Y) were evaluated *in vitro*. It was reported that co-incubation of LPS-treated cells with SB (50 µg/ml) or SB-HSA nanoparticles was associated with the recovery of cell viability, activation of SOD and CAT, increase of GSH content, and reduction of ROS level, Caspase-3 activity and fragmentation of DNA. In such a model system the neuroprotective and antioxidant activities of SB-HAS nanoparticles were higher in comparison to free SB (Pan *et al.*, 2021). Earlier, similar results were reported with SM. In particular, it was shown that SM-HSA noncomplex possessed increased activity in reducing LPS-induced oxidative stress by restoring cell viability and elevation of SOD and CAT activity *in vitro* and *in vivo* (Sohrabi *et al.*, 2019).

Recent review on silymarin's inhibition and treatment effects for Alzheimer's Disease (Guo *et al.*, 2019) reported that SM has great potential for the treatment of AD by
- inhibiting the formation and development of Aβ;
- enhancing cholinergic energy;
- providing oxidative stress protection; and
- promoting inhibition of neuroinflammation.

An important mechanism associated with AD development is mitochondrial dysfunction. Interestingly, SM showed strong protective effects on mitochondria by rescuing MMP and ATP levels from sodium nitroprusside-induced mitochondrial damage (Esselun *et al.*, 2021). SM also showed neuroprotective effect against aluminium chloride-promoted Alzheimer's-like disease in rats (Aboelwafa *et al.*, 2020) and mice (Makhdoomi *et al.*, 2022). Oral administration of SB for three weeks significantly attenuated the cognitive deficits of formaldehyde-induced mice in a *Y*-maze test and Morris water maze test. SB was shown to inhibit the expression of GSK-3*β* in model mice causing a reduction of the phosphorylation of tau proteins ser396 and ser404 mediated by GSK3*β* (Wei *et al.*, 2022). Protective effects of SM/SB in Alzheimer's disease were summarised in Figure 13.1.

Recently in a clinical trial conducted in Iraq 85 subjects with memory impairment were randomly assigned to one of two groups: placebo (n=43) or experimental (n=42) supplied with 250 mg SM twice daily for 16 weeks. The results indicate that SM consumption was associated with improvement of overall cognitive function, including verbal learning and memory function (Hussain *et al.*, 2022).

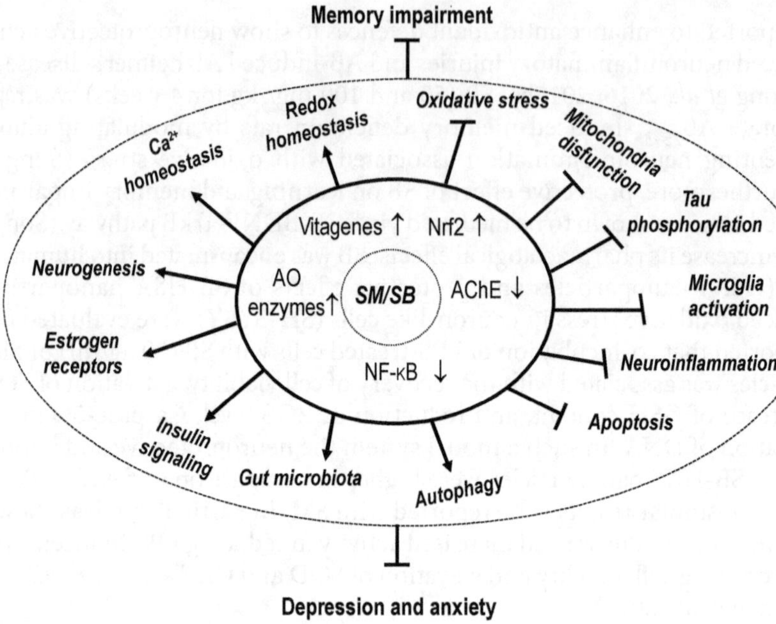

Figure 13.1. Protective effects of SM/SB in Alzheimer disease.

13.3 Silymarin and Parkinson's disease

Parkinson's disease (PD), first described by James Parkinson in 1817, is the second most common neurodegenerative disorder (after Alzheimer's disease) affecting >1% of the population over the age of 60. In 2016 there were about 6.1 million people with PD, a number which more than doubled since 1990 (Dorsey *et al.*, 2018). Currently, more than 10 million people worldwide are living with PD. Importantly, about 60,000 Americans are diagnosed with PD each year with the total number of people with PD in the USA to be about one million. This leads to the combined direct and indirect cost of Parkinson's in the USA of nearly $52 billion per year (Parkinson.org, 2022). There were around 145,000 people with a Parkinson's diagnosis in the UK in 2020 with prediction to increase to around 172,000 people by 2030. (parkinsons.org.uk). The 3 main symptoms of Parkinson's disease are accepted to include involuntary shaking of particular parts of the body (tremor), slow movement and stiff and inflexible muscles. Furthermore, PD patients can also experience depression and anxiety, balance problems, anosmia (loss of sense of smell), insomnia (problems sleeping), memory problems, etc. (NHS, 2022b).

The disease is caused by dopaminergic neuronal damage and loss (>60-80%) of the dopamine-producing cells in the substantia nigra leading to decreased dopamine concentration, (a dopamine-deficiency disorder), abnormal nerve firing patterns within the brain causing impaired movement. The hallmark of PD is presence in the affected brain cells of deposits of the protein alpha-synuclein known as Lewy bodies.

However, exact Lewy bodies functions are still not known. It seems likely, that due to failure of the cell's protein disposal system, including lysosomal/autophagosomal and ubiquitin-proteasomal systems, excessive accumulation of modified proteins can cause neuronal death. The exact pathogenesis of PD is not yet completely understood, but oxidative stress, mitochondrial dysfunction, synaptic dysfunction, neuroinflammation, lysosomal and proteasomal dysfunction (proteotoxic stress), perturbation of calcium and iron metabolism and apoptosis play a critical role in the PD development (Goldman, 2014). Current evidence suggests that oxidative damage and the mitochondrial dysfunction in neurons are major contributors to PD pathogenesis.

Genetic predispositions (several genetic mutations are associated with PD), as well as environmental risk factors (exposure to pesticides, herbicides, heavy metals and other toxic chemicals) are believed to contribute to progression of PD. Unfortunately, today there is no cure available for PD, but medications can improve the motor symptoms presenting a symptomatic treatment for PD. There are three major categories of drugs prescribed for PD patients including drugs that increase the level of dopamine in the brain, drugs that affect other neurotransmitters in the body and medications that help control the non-motor symptoms of the disease. Complementary and supportive therapies for PD include healthy diet, exercise and various alternative approaches (NINDS, 2022), including usage of SM.

It should be mentioned that there is no spontaneous occurrence of parkinsonism in animals but using various toxic chemicals several experimental animal models of PD have been developed. In particular, various neurotoxins can damage the nigrostriatal dopaminergic (DA) system leading to clinical signs of PD. Therefore, MPTP and 6-OHDA are the most frequently used neurotoxins in animal models of PD. MPTP is widely used to create the symptomatology of PD in monkeys and other animals, while 6-OHDA is a neurotoxin of choice in a rodent model of PD (Mokrý, 1995). For example, in the hemi-parkinsonian rat model, behaviour deficit (rotation test) reflecting changes in spontaneous locomotor activity due to dopamine imbalance caused by neurotoxins is registered. To assess locomotor activity of treated animals, T-maze, treadmill running test or sensorimotor tests are employed (Mokrý, 1995). Interestingly, PQ or 1, 1′-dimethyl-4, 4′-bipyridinium ion is an herbicide with a redox property, having the chemical structure analogous to MPP+ and possessing ability to impose oxidative stress and damage the dopaminergic neurons. Therefore, PQ can also be used as a neurotoxicant in PD models (Thirugnanam and Santhakumar, 2022).

SM has been recently shown to have neuroprotective activities against neurodegenerative diseases such as Parkinson's and Alzheimer's diseases. Anti-Parkinson's Potential of SM has been recently analysed in detail (Ullah and Khan, 2018). In maneb (MB)- and PQ-induced mouse model of PD, SM (40 mg/kg for 9 weeks) was reported to significantly improve MB- and PQ-mediated reductions in locomotor activities, dopamine content, TH immunoreactivity, VMAT 2 mRNA expression and the expression of p53 protein. Furthermore, SM was found to attenuate the increases in lipid peroxidation, number of degenerating neurons, nitrite content, mRNA expressions and catalytic activities of cytochrome P-450 2E1 and GST and P-p53, Bax and caspase 9 protein expressions (Singhal *et al.*, 2011). In MB- and PQ-induced Parkinsonism mouse model, SM (40 mg/kg for 9 weeks) significantly resisted the changes in the expression of a few genes related to apoptosis, inflammation, cell cycle, cell-signalling, etc. (Singhal *et al.*, 2013).

Pre-treatment with SM (100, 200 and 300 mg/kg for 5 consecutive days) was demonstrated to reduce brain MPO activity and inflammatory cytokines in 6-OHDA hemi-parkinsonian rats (Haddadi *et al.*, 2013). SM in the same doses ameliorated 6-OHDA-induced motor imbalance by attenuating brain oxidative stress as well as cerebrospinal fluid levels of inflammatory cytokine IL-1β in the rats (Haddadi *et al.*, 2014). Neuroprotective effect of SM was also demonstrated in a MPTP mouse model of Parkinson's disease with MPTP (30 mg/kg) and SM administered to mice intraperitoneally once daily for five consecutive days. Therefore, SM (50 and 100 mg/kg) was shown to preserve dopamine levels which were compromised due to MPTP intoxication. In addition, SM (100 mg/kg) was found to significantly decrease the number of apoptotic cells and preserved dopaminergic neurons in the substantia nigra of MPTP-treated mice (Pérez-H *et al.*, 2014). SB (50 and 100 mg/kg) was reported to ameliorate 1-methyl-4-phenylpyridinium (MPP^+)-induced neurotoxicity in the substantia nigra *in vivo* (Jung *et al.*, 2014).

Furthermore, SB (100 and 200 mg/kg) was reported to protect against a range of MPP(+)-induced detrimental changes including dopamine depletion in striatum, decrease in transfer latency, motor deficits, mitochondrial dysfunction, loss of integrity, oxidative stress and to show anti-apoptotic (inhibiting caspase-3) and anti-inflammatory (decreasing NF-κB expression) effects (Geed *et al.*, 2014). In an experimental rat model of PD induced by unilateral infusion of (6-OHDA; 8 μg/2 μl/rat) into the central region of the substantia nigra pars compacta, short-term treatment with SM (100, 200 and 300 mg/kg, i.p. for 5 days) was shown to improve 6-OHDA-induced catalepsy and motor imbalance in animals. The authors suggested SM to be used in adjunctive therapy along with commonly used anti-parkinsonian drugs (Haddadi *et al.*, 2015).

In a mouse model of MPTP-induced PD, it was observed that SB had an ameliorative effect on motor dysfunction and a protective effect on the dopaminergic neurons associated with mitochondrial stabilisation (Lee *et al.*, 2015a,b). It should be mentioned that mitochondrial dysfunction can increase oxidative stress in PD associated with impaired balance of mitochondrial dynamics and disrupted the integrity of mitochondrial structures (Chandra *et al.*, 2019; Jayaraj *et al.*, 2019). SM (10, 30 and 100 mg/kg) was reported to recover 6-OHDA-induced motor deficits in mice (de Freitas *et al.*, 2018). Pre-treatment of 6-OHDA-intoxicated rats with SM (100, 200 or 300 mg/kg for 5 days) was shown to reduce SNc neuronal apoptosis through inhibition of TLR4 over expression (Haddadi *et al.*, 2018). On the one hand, *in vitro* studies of neuroprotective actions of SM in various PD models have shown (Ullah and Khan, 2018) that:

- antioxidant and anti-inflammatory properties of SM are responsible for its neuroprotection;
- SM can protect dopaminergic neurons from LPS-induced neurotoxicity as a result of inhibiting activation of microglia (anti-inflammatory actions);
- SM is shown to reduce free radicals (superoxide) and pro-inflammatory cytokines (TNF-α) production and inhibits inducible NO synthase;
- SM is reported to regulate NF-κB 100 times better than aspirin;
- SM is found to inhibit several kinases (MAPK and JNK) involved in regulation of NF-κB, without posing any threat to the cell. Notably, SB was reported to suppresses astroglial activation in a mouse model of acute PD by modulating the ERK and JNK signalling pathways (Lee *et al.*, 2015).

On the other hand, *in vivo* studies using various PD models indicated (Ullah and Khan, 2018) that:

- SM is responsible for preservation of dopaminergic neurons (by diminishing apoptosis in the SN) leading to maintenance of striatal dopaminergic levels;
- SM can normalise gene expression of upregulated NF-κB1 and caspase-9;
- the binding affinity of SM for ERβ in CNS regions has also been shown.

In a rat model of PD, male Wistar rats received neurotoxin (6-OHDA; 8 μg/rat) and after 3 weeks (recovery period), the animals were injected (i.p.) with SM (100, 200, or 300 mg/kg for 15 days). The 6-OHDA significantly decreased motor function and compromised antioxidant defences (AO enzymes activity, GSH level, and GSH/GSSG ratio, lipid peroxidation), reduced the population of neurons and tyrosine hydroxylase expression. SM chronic treatment was shown to restore the brain's antioxidant capacity (GSH, GSSG level, and GSH/GSSG ratio) and protected neurons from oxidative stress-induced neurodegeneration and dose-dependently increased the total number of surviving neurons in the SNc. Furthermore, the SM treatment could also improve motor function in parkinsonian animals by increasing tyrosine hydroxylase expression (Haddadi *et al.*, 2020a). SM (40 mg/kg, IP, for 2 weeks) provides protection against MPTP-induced changes in autophagy leading to Parkinsonism (Tripathi *et al.*, 2020).

In a recent study, the cognitive improvement and neuroprotective effect of SB in a mouse model of PD have been studied. SB administration (70, 180 and 240 mg/kg) was observed to significantly attenuate a MPTP-induced cognitive impairment in behavioural tests. In particular, MPTP injection was reported to induce oxidative stress (increased MDA and decreased SOD) which was alleviated by SB treatment. SB administration also restored these mitochondrial disorders including the decline of mitochondrial membrane potential accompanying increased mitochondrial fission and decreased fusion (Liu *et al.*, 2021b). SB (70, 140, or 280 mg/kg in 0.5% sodium carboxymethyl cellulose) was also shown to ameliorate depression/anxiety-like behaviours of PD mouse model and this protective action was associated with attenuated STING-IRF3-IFN-β pathway activation and decreased neuroinflammation (Liu *et al.*, 2021a). SB (280 mg/kg) was shown to attenuate motor dysfunction in a mouse model of Parkinson's disease by suppression of oxidative stress and neuroinflammation along with promotion of mitophagy (Liu *et al.*, 2021b).

There is also a range of publications using other model systems which could be related to PD. For example, in a focal cerebral ischemia rat model SM is shown to be able to slow down the progression of neurodegeneration by protecting neurons from oxidative stress associated damages (Raza *et al.*, 2011). In the cerebral global ischemic rat model SM (50, 100 and/200 mg/kg) was demonstrated to lead to amelioration of cognitive, motor and endogenous defence functions (Muley *et al.*, 2013). Increased iron supplementation in ageing rats was indicated to cause neurochemical and behavioural deficits and SB (25 and 50 mg/kg body weight) treatment significantly and dose-dependently attenuated depletion of striatal dopamine provides dopaminergic neuroprotection by maintaining redox balance in the brain (Chen *et al.*, 2015). SB was reported to rescue learning and memory deficits in novel object recognition test and Morris water maze test as a result of attenuation of microglia activation and preventions of neuroinflammatory reactions in senescence-accelerated mice (Jin *et al.*, 2016).

SM treatment (200 mg/kg) 30 mins post intracerebral haemorrhages (ICH) injury was shown to ameliorate increase in oxidative stress markers and to up-regulate ICH-induced compromised AO system (SOD, GSH, CAT and GST). SM also down regulated the inflammatory responses as evidenced by suppression of NF-κB-p65, caspase-1 and pro-inflammatory cytokine expressions post ICH injury. At the same time SM upregulated Nrf-2/HO-1 pathway leading to improvement of cytoprotection (Yuan *et al.*, 2017). SB (25, 50 and 100 mg/kg) is reported to ameliorate anxiety/depression-like behaviours in amyloid β-treated rats by upregulating BDNF/TrkB pathway and attenuating autophagy in hippocampus (Song *et al.*, 2017b).

SM administration was also associated with improvement in brain derived neurotrophic factor expression, serotonin, dopamine and norepinephrine levels, restoration of AO defences (CAT and GSH) and to reduction in expression of pro-inflammatory cytokines (IL-6, and TNF-α) in cerebral cortex and hippocampus (Thakare *et al.*, 2017). SB is found to exert antidepressant effects by improving neurogenesis through BDNF/TrkB pathway (Li *et al.*, 2018). Furthermore, SM (50 mg/kg for 20 days) was indicated to significantly reduce anxiety- and depression-like symptoms, and neuroinflammation after mild traumatic brain injury in mice (Kosari-Nasab *et al.*, 2018) and this protective effect of SM was suggested to be mediated at least in part through NO leading to increase NO tune (Khoshnoodi *et al.*, 2015).

SB was shown to have protective effects against prothrombin kringle-2-induced neurotoxicity in the nigrostriatal dopaminergic system *in vivo* thus, may be applicable for PD therapy (Leem *et al.*, 2019). SM is found to prevents memory impairments, depressive-like symptoms and anxiety in rats suffering from post-traumatic stress disorder (El-Elimat *et al.*, 2019). SM (50 mg/kg/day) was reported to sex-dependently improve cognitive functions altering TNF-α, BDNF, and glutamate in the hippocampus of mice with mild traumatic brain injury (Shokouhi *et al.*, 2020). The cirrhotic rats consuming SM (50 mg/kg/d SM by food) + Lactulose (LAC; 2 g/kg/d in drinking water) for 8 weeks were characterised by restoration of memory disturbance and improvement of irritated mood (Ghobadi Pour *et al.*, 2020). The rats received SM

(25, 50, and 100 mg/kg) for 14 days following exposure to a model of single prolonged stress (SPS).

Administration of SM was reported to significantly improve anxiety-like behaviours, depression-like behaviours, and freezing behaviour in various tests. Interestingly, SM was able to increase levels of serotonin in the hippocampus (Hipp) and amygdala, and enhanced expression of tryptophan hydroxylase-1 mRNA in the Hipp. SM also suppressed SPS-induced decreases dopamine levels and increased norepinephrine levels in the Hipp (Lee *et al.*, 2020). Interestingly, chitosan-silymarin nanoparticles were shown to be effective in improvement of peripheral nerve regeneration (Ebrahimi-Zadehlou *et al.*, 2021).

Protective effects of SM/SB in Parkinson's disease are summarised in Figure 13.2 and there are quite a few similarities in molecular mechanisms of protective effects of SM/SB against PD and AD with prevention of oxidative stress and maintaining redox balance in the brain and neurones to play a crucial role in such protective actions of SM/SB.

13.4 Conclusions

Oxidative stress and redox disbalance are common hallmarks of several neurodegenerative diseases including Parkinson's and Alzheimer's diseases.

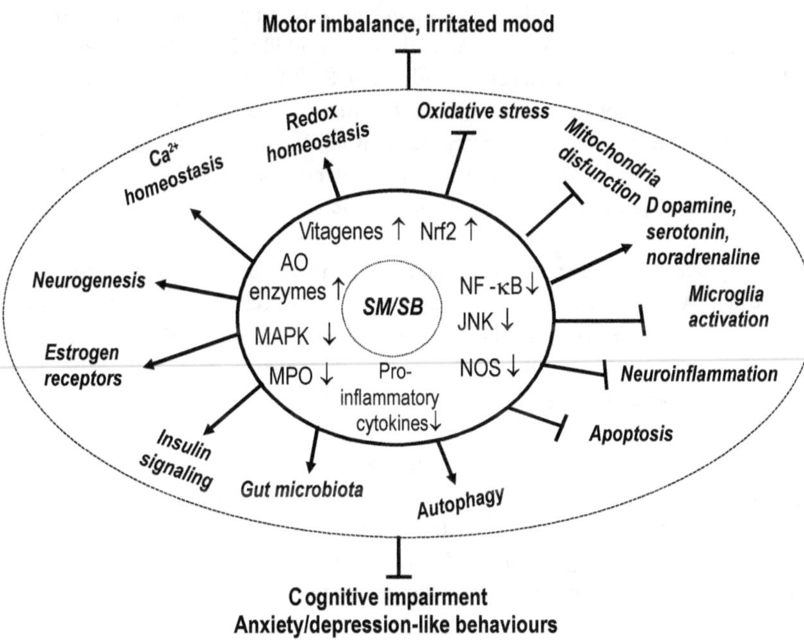

Figure 13.2. Protective effects of SM/SB in Parkinson's disease.

Therefore, the aforementioned data clearly indicate that SM/SB can decrease clinical manifestations of these diseases, including memory impairment, depression and anxiety, motor imbalance, irritated mood, etc. (Haddadi *et al.*, 2020b). Those improvements were clearly associated with improvement of antioxidant defences, redox balance, anti-inflammation and other beneficial changes on the molecular level. Furthermore, it seems likely that regulatory actions of SM/SB on Nrf2, NF-κB, MAPK and JNK are of paramount importance in their protective actions in neurogenerative diseases including Parkinson's and Alzheimer's diseases. Clearly, more research is warrant in this exciting area.

References

Aboelwafa, H.R., El-Kott, A.F., Abd-Ella, E.M. and Yousef, H.N., 2020. The possible neuroprotective effect of silymarin against aluminum chloride-prompted Alzheimer's-like disease in rats. Brain Sciences 10: 628.

Alzheimer's Society (Alzheimer.org.uk), 2022. Alzheimer's disease. Alzheimer's Society, Plymouth, UK. Available at: https://www.tinyurl.com/6yzfakb8.

Amato, A., Terzo, S. and Mulè, F., 2019. Natural compounds as beneficial antioxidant agents in neurodegenerative disorders: A focus on Alzheimer's disease. Antioxidants 8: 608.

Bai, D., Jin, G., Yin, S., Zou, D., Zhu, Q., Yang, Z., Liu, X., Ren, L., Sun, Y. and Gan, S., 2017. Antioxidative and anti-apoptotic roles of silibinin in reversing learning and memory deficits in APP/PS1 mice. Neurochemical Research 42: 3439-3445.

Bai, D., Jin, G., Zhang, D., Zhao, L., Wang, M., Zhu, Q., Zhu, L., Sun, Y., Liu, X., Chen, X., Zhang, L., Li, W. and Cui, Y., 2019. Natural silibinin modulates amyloid precursor protein processing and amyloid-β protein clearance in APP/PS1 mice. The Journal of Physiological Sciences 69: 643-652.

Balmus, I.M., Ciobica, A., Negura, A., Negura, L. and Anton, E., 2015. Basic aspects in selecting a suitable transgenic rodent model for Alzheimer's disease. Psychiatria Danubina 27: 338-345.

Borah, A., Paul, R., Choudhury, S., Choudhury, A., Bhuyan, B., Das Talukdar, A., Dutta Choudhury, M. and Mohanakumar, K.P., 2013. Neuroprotective potential of silymarin against CNS disorders: insight into the pathways and molecular mechanisms of action. CNS Neuroscience & Therapeutics 19: 847-853.

Calabrese, V., Guagliano, E., Sapienza, M., Panebianco, M., Calafato, S., Puleo, E., Pennisi, G., Mancuso, C., Butterfield, D.A. and Stella, A.G., 2007. Redox regulation of cellular stress response in aging and neurodegenerative disorders: role of vitagenes. Neurochemical Research 32: 757-773.

Chandra, G., Shenoi, R.A., Anand, R., Rajamma, U. and Mohanakumar, K.P., 2019. Reinforcing mitochondrial functions in aging brain: An insight into Parkinson's disease therapeutics. Journal of Chemical Neuroanatomy 95: 29-42.

Chen, H., Wang, X., Wang, M., Yang, L., Yan, Z., Zhang, Y. and Liu, Z., 2015. Behavioral and neurochemical deficits in aging rats with increased neonatal Iron intake: Silibinin's neuroprotection by maintaining redox balance. Frontiers in Aging Neuroscience 7: 206.

Chen, X., Deng, X., Han, X., Liang, Y., Meng, Z., Liu, R., Su, W., Zhu, H. and Fu, T., 2021. Inhibition of lysozyme amyloid fibrillation by silybin diastereoisomers: The effects of stereochemistry. ACS Omega 6: 3307-3318.

de Freitas, C.M., Krum, B.N., Chiapinotto Ceretta, A.P., Schaffer, L.F., de Moraes Reis, E., Schwerz, J.P., Barbosa, C.P., Soares, F. and Fachinetto, R., 2018. Silymarin recovers 6-hydroxydopamine-induced motor deficits in mice. Food and Chemical Toxicology 118: 549-556.

de Oliveira, J., Kucharska, E., Garcez, M.L., Rodrigues, M.S., Quevedo, J., Moreno-Gonzalez, I. and Budni, J., 2021. Inflammatory cascade in Alzheimer's disease pathogenesis: A review of experimental findings. Cells 10: 2581.

Dhapola, R., Hota, S.S., Sarma, P., Bhattacharyya, A., Medhi, B. and Reddy, D.H., 2021. Recent advances in molecular pathways and therapeutic implications targeting neuroinflammation for Alzheimer's disease. Inflammopharmacology 29: 1669-1681.

Dorsey, E.R., Sherer, T., Okun, M.S. and Bloem, B.R., 2018. The emerging evidence of the Parkinson pandemic. Journal of Parkinson's Disease 8: S3-S8.

Duan, S., Guan, X., Lin, R., Liu, X., Yan, Y., Lin, R., Zhang, T., Chen, X., Huang, J., Sun, X., Li, Q., Fang, S., Xu, J., Yao, Z. and Gu, H., 2015. Silibinin inhibits acetylcholinesterase activity and amyloid β peptide aggregation: a dual-target drug for the treatment of Alzheimer's disease. Neurobiology of Aging 36: 1792-1807.

Dugger, B.N. and Dickson, D.W., 2017. Pathology of neurodegenerative diseases. Cold Spring Harbor Perspectives in Biology 9: a028035.

Ebrahimi-Zadehlou, P., Najafpour, A. and Mohammadi, R., 2021. Assessments of regenerative potential of silymarin nanoparticles loaded into chitosan conduit on peripheral nerve regeneration: a transected sciatic nerve model in rat. Neurological Research 43: 148-156.

El-Elimat, T., Alzoubi, K.H., AbuAlSamen, M.M., Al Subeh, Z.Y., Graf, T.N. and Oberlies, N.H., 2019. Silymarin prevents memory impairments, anxiety, and depressive-like symptoms in a rat model of post-traumatic stress disorder. Planta Medica 85: 32-40.

Esselun, C., Bruns, B., Hagl, S., Grewal, R. and Eckert, G.P., 2021. Impact of silibinin A on bioenergetics in $PC12APP_{sw}$ cells and mitochondrial membrane properties in murine brain mitochondria. Antioxidants 10: 1520.

Fernando, K. and Wijayasinghe, Y.S., 2021. Sirtuins as potential therapeutic targets for mitigating neuroinflammation associated with Alzheimer's disease. Frontiers in Cellular Neuroscience 15: 746631.

Geed, M., Garabadu, D., Ahmad, A. and Krishnamurthy, S., 2014. Silibinin pretreatment attenuates biochemical and behavioral changes induced by intrastriatal MPP+ injection in rats. Pharmacology, Biochemistry, and Behavior 117: 92-103.

Ghobadi Pour, M., Mirazi, N., Alaei, H., Radahmadi, M., Rajaei, Z. and Monsef Esfahani, A., 2020. The effects of concurrent treatment of silymarin and lactulose on memory changes in cirrhotic male rats. BioImpacts 10: 177-186.

Goldman, S.M., 2014. Environmental toxins and Parkinson's disease. Annual Review of Pharmacology and Toxicology 54: 141-164.

Guo, H., Cao, H., Cui, X., Zheng, W., Wang, S., Yu, J. and Chen, Z., 2019. Silymarin's inhibition and treatment effects for Alzheimer's disease. Molecules 24: 1748.

Haddadi, R., Eyvari Brooshghalan, S., Farajniya, S., Mohajjel Nayebi, A. and Sharifi, H., 2015. Short-term treatment with silymarin improved 6-OHDA-induced catalepsy and motor imbalance in hemi-parkinsonian rats. Advanced Pharmaceutical Bulletin 5: 463-469.

Haddadi, R., Eyvari-Brooshghalan, S., Nayebi, A.M., Sabahi, M. and Ahmadi, S.A., 2020a. Neuronal degeneration and oxidative stress in the SNc of 6-OHDA intoxicated rats; improving role of silymarin long-term treatment. Naunyn-Schmiedeberg's Archives of Pharmacology 393: 2427-2437.

Haddadi, R., Mohajjel Nayebi, A. and Brooshghalan, S.E., 2013. Pre-treatment with silymarin reduces brain myeloperoxidase activity and inflammatory cytokines in 6-OHDA hemi-parkinsonian rats. Neuroscience Letters 555: 106-111.

Haddadi, R., Nayebi, A.M. and Eyvari Brooshghalan, S., 2018. Silymarin prevents apoptosis through inhibiting the Bax/caspase-3 expression and suppresses toll like receptor-4 pathway in the SNc of 6-OHDA intoxicated rats. Biomedicine & Pharmacotherapy 104: 127-136.

Haddadi, R., Nayebi, A.M., Farajniya, S., Brooshghalan, S.E. and Sharifi, H., 2014. Silymarin improved 6-OHDA-induced motor impairment in hemi-parkinsonian rats: behavioral and molecular study. Daru 22: 38.

Haddadi, R., Shahidi, Z. and Eyvari-Brooshghalan, S., 2020b. Silymarin and neurodegenerative diseases: Therapeutic potential and basic molecular mechanisms. Phytomedicine 79: 153320.

Huo, Q., Shi, Y., Qi, Y., Huang, L., Sui, H. and Zhao, L., 2021. Biomimetic silibinin-loaded macrophage-derived exosomes induce dual inhibition of Aβ aggregation and astrocyte activation to alleviate cognitive impairment in a model of Alzheimer's disease. Materials Science & Engineering. C, Materials for Biological Applications 129: 112365.

Hussain, S.A., Abdulrahman, Z.S. and Mustafa, W.W., 2022. Silibinin Improves the Clinical Scores of Memory Function in Patients with Mild Cognitive Impairment: A Double-Blind, Placebo-Controlled Pilot Study. Biomedical and Pharmacology Journal 1: 83-90.

Ionescu-Tucker, A. and Cotman, C.W., 2021. Emerging roles of oxidative stress in brain aging and Alzheimer's disease. Neurobiology of Aging 107: 86-95.

Jayaraj, R.L., Beiram, R., Azimullah, S., Meeran, M., Ojha, S.K., Adem, A. and Jalal, F.Y., 2019. Lycopodium attenuates loss of dopaminergic neurons by suppressing oxidative stress and neuroinflammation in a rat model of Parkinson's disease. Molecules 24: 2182.

Jeremic, D., Jiménez-Díaz, L. and Navarro-López, J.D., 2021. Past, present and future of therapeutic strategies against amyloid-β peptides in Alzheimer's disease: a systematic review. Ageing Research Reviews 72: 101496.

Jin, G., Bai, D., Yin, S., Yang, Z., Zou, D., Zhang, Z., Li, X., Sun, Y. and Zhu, Q., 2016. Silibinin rescues learning and memory deficits by attenuating microglia activation and preventing neuroinflammatory reactions in SAMP8 mice. Neuroscience Letters 629: 256-261.

Johri, A., 2021. Disentangling mitochondria in Alzheimer's disease. International Journal of Molecular Sciences 22: 11520.

Jung, U.J., Jeon, M.T., Choi, M.S. and Kim, S.R., 2014. Silibinin attenuates MPP^+-induced neurotoxicity in the substantia nigra *in vivo*. Journal of Medicinal Food 17: 599-605.

Juszczyk, G., Mikulska, J., Kasperek, K., Pietrzak, D., Mrozek, W. and Herbet, M., 2021. Chronic stress and oxidative stress as common factors of the pathogenesis of depression and Alzheimer's disease: The role of antioxidants in prevention and treatment. Antioxidants 10: 1439.

Katebi, B., Mahdavimehr, M., Meratan, A.A., Ghasemi, A. and Nemat-Gorgani, M., 2018. Protective effects of silibinin on insulin amyloid fibrillation, cytotoxicity and mitochondrial membrane damage. Archives of Biochemistry and Biophysics 659: 22-32.

Khoshnoodi, M., Fakhraei, N. and Dehpour, A.R., 2015. Possible involvement of nitric oxide in antidepressant-like effect of silymarin in male mice. Pharmaceutical Biology 53: 739-745.

Kosari-Nasab, M., Shokouhi, G., Ghorbanihaghjo, A., Abbasi, M.M. and Salari, A.A., 2018. Anxiolytic- and antidepressant-like effects of Silymarin compared to diazepam and fluoxetine in a mouse model of mild traumatic brain injury. Toxicology and Applied Pharmacology 338: 159-173.

Kumar, J., Park, K.C., Awasthi, A. and Prasad, B., 2015. Silymarin extends lifespan and reduces proteotoxicity in C. elegans Alzheimer's model. CNS & Neurological Disorders Drug Targets 14: 295-302.

Lee, Y., Chun, H.J., Lee, K.M., Jung, Y.S. and Lee, J., 2015a. Silibinin suppresses astroglial activation in a mouse model of acute Parkinson's disease by modulating the ERK and JNK signaling pathways. Brain Research 1627: 233-242.

Lee, Y., Park, H.R., Chun, H.J. and Lee, J., 2015b. Silibinin prevents dopaminergic neuronal loss in a mouse model of Parkinson's disease via mitochondrial stabilization. Journal of Neuroscience Research 93: 755-765.

Lee, B., Choi, G.M. and Sur, B., 2020. Silibinin prevents depression-like behaviors in a single prolonged stress rat model: the possible role of serotonin. BMC Complementary Medicine and Therapies 20: 70.

Leem, E., Oh, Y.S., Shin, W.H., Jin, B.K., Jeong, J.Y., Shin, M., Kim, D.W., Jang, J.H., Kim, H.J., Ha, C.M., Jung, U.J., Moon, G.J. and Kim, S.R., 2019. Effects of silibinin against prothrombin Kringle-2-induced neurotoxicity in the nigrostriatal dopaminergic system *in vivo*. Journal of Medicinal Food 22: 277-285.

Li, Y., Laws, S.M., Miles, L.A., Wiley, J.S., Huang, X., Masters, C.L. and Gu, B.J., 2021a. Genomics of Alzheimer's disease implicates the innate and adaptive immune systems. Cellular and Molecular Life Sciences 78: 7397-7426.

Li, S., Wang, C., Wang, W. and Tan, J., 2021b. Trait anxiety, a personality risk factor associated with Alzheimer's disease. Progress in Neuro-Psychopharmacology & Biological Psychiatry 105: 110124.

Li, Y.J., Li, Y.J., Yang, L.D., Zhang, K., Zheng, K.Y., Wei, X.M., Yang, Q., Niu, W.M., Zhao, M.G. and Wu, Y.M., 2018. Silibinin exerts antidepressant effects by improving neurogenesis through BDNF/TrkB pathway. Behavioural Brain Research 348: 184-191.

Lichtenthaler, S.F., Tschirner, S.K. and Steiner, H., 2022. Secretases in Alzheimer's disease: Novel insights into proteolysis of APP and TREM2. Current Opinion in Neurobiology 72: 101-110.

Liu, B., Liu, J. and Shi, J.S., 2020a. SAMP8 mice as a model of age-related cognition decline with underlying mechanisms in Alzheimer's disease. Journal of Alzheimer's Disease 75: 385-395.

Liu, P., Cui, L., Liu, B., Liu, W., Hayashi, T., Mizuno, K., Hattori, S., Ushiki-Kaku, Y., Onodera, S. and Ikejima, T., 2020b. Silibinin ameliorates STZ-induced impairment of memory and learning by up-regulating insulin signaling pathway and attenuating apoptosis. Physiology & Behavior 213: 112689.

Liu, X., Liu, W., Wang, C., Chen, Y., Liu, P., Hayashi, T., Mizuno, K., Hattori, S., Fujisaki, H. and Ikejima, T., 2021a. Silibinin attenuates motor dysfunction in a mouse model of Parkinson's disease by suppression of oxidative stress and neuroinflammation along with promotion of mitophagy. Physiology & Behavior 239: 113510.

Liu, X., Wang, C., Liu, W., Song, S., Fu, J., Hayashi, T., Mizuno, K., Hattori, S., Fujisaki, H. and Ikejima, T., 2021b. Oral administration of silibinin ameliorates cognitive deficits of Parkinson's disease mouse model by restoring mitochondrial disorders in hippocampus. Neurochemical Research 46: 2317-2332.

Makhdoomi, S., Mahboobian, M.M., Haddadi, R., Komaki, A. and Mohammadi, M., 2022. Silibinin-loaded nanostructured lipid carriers (NLCs) ameliorated cognitive deficits and oxidative damages in aluminum chloride-induced neurotoxicity in male mice. Toxicology 477: 153260.

Mayo Clinic (Mayoclinic.org), 2022. Alzheimer's disease. Mayo Clinic, Scottsdale, AZ, USA. Available at: https://www.tinyurl.com/499cp6jt.

Mokrý, J., 1995. Experimental models and behavioural tests used in the study of Parkinson's disease. Physiological Research 44: 143-150.

Muley, M.M., Thakare, V.N., Patil, R.R., Bafna, P.A. and Naik, S.R., 2013. Amelioration of cognitive, motor and endogenous defense functions with silymarin, piracetam and protocatechuic acid in the cerebral global ischemic rat model. Life Sciences 93: 51-57.

Murata, N., Murakami, K., Ozawa, Y., Kinoshita, N., Irie, K., Shirasawa, T. and Shimizu, T., 2010. Silymarin attenuated the amyloid β plaque burden and improved behavioral abnormalities in an Alzheimer's disease mouse model. Bioscience, Biotechnology, and Biochemistry 74: 2299-2306.

Neha Kumar, A., Jaggi, A.S., Sodhi, R.K. and Singh, N., 2014. Silymarin ameliorates memory deficits and neuropathological changes in mouse model of high-fat-diet-induced experimental dementia. Naunyn-Schmiedeberg's Archives of Pharmacology 387: 777-787.

National Health Service (NHS), 2022a. Alzheimer's disease. NHS, Leeds, UK. Available at: https://www.tinyurl.com/mu5e7w9e.

National Health Service (NHS), 2022b. Parkinson's disease. NHS, Leeds, UK. Available at: https://www.tinyurl.com/3tm7myvz.

National Institute of Aging (NIA), 2022. Alzheimer's disease & Related Dementias. NIA, Bethesda, MD USA. Available at: https://www.tinyurl.com/y6df8uab.

National Institute of Neurological Disorders and Stroke (NINDS), 2022. Parkinson's disease: Challenges, Progress, and Promise. NINDS, Bethesda, MD USA. Available at: https://www.tinyurl.com/4twuvhkv.

Pan, Q., Ban, Y. and Xu, L., 2021. Silibinin-albumin nanoparticles: Characterization and biological evaluation against oxidative stress-stimulated neurotoxicity associated with Alzheimer's disease. Journal of Biomedical Nanotechnology 17: 1123-1130.

Pardillo-Díaz, R., Pérez-García, P., Castro, C., Nunez-Abades, P. and Carrascal, L., 2022. Oxidative stress as a potential mechanism underlying membrane hyperexcitability in neurodegenerative diseases. Antioxidants 11: 1511.

Parkinson's Foundation (Parkinson.org), 2022. Statistics. Parkinson's Foundation, New York, NY, USA. Available at: https://www.tinyurl.com/yck68rs7.

Pérez-H.J., Carrillo, S.C., García, E., Ruiz-Mar, G., Pérez-Tamayo, R. and Chavarría, A., 2014. Neuroprotective effect of silymarin in a MPTP mouse model of Parkinson's disease. Toxicology 319: 38-43.

Princiotta Cariddi, L., Mauri, M., Cosentino, M., Versino, M. and Marino, F., 2022. Alzheimer's disease: From immune homeostasis to neuroinflammatory condition. International Journal of Molecular Sciences 23: 13008.

Raza, S.S., Khan, M.M., Ashafaq, M., Ahmad, A., Khuwaja, G., Khan, A., Siddiqui, M.S., Safhi, M.M. and Islam, F., 2011. Silymarin protects neurons from oxidative stress associated damages in focal cerebral ischemia: a behavioral, biochemical and immunohistological study in Wistar rats. Journal of the Neurological Sciences 309: 45-54.

Sato, M., Murakami, K., Uno, M., Ikubo, H., Nakagawa, Y., Katayama, S., Akagi, K. and Irie, K., 2013. Structure-activity relationship for (+)-taxifolin isolated from silymarin as an inhibitor of amyloid β aggregation. Bioscience, Biotechnology, and Biochemistry 77: 1100-1103.

Sciacca, M., Romanucci, V., Zarrelli, A., Monaco, I., Lolicato, F., Spinella, N., Galati, C., Grasso, G., D'Urso, L., Romeo, M., Diomede, L., Salmona, M., Bongiorno, C., Di Fabio, G., La Rosa, C. and Milardi, D., 2017. Inhibition of Aβ amyloid growth and toxicity by silybins: The crucial role of stereochemistry. ACS Chemical Neuroscience 8: 1767-1778.

Shen, L., Liu, L., Li, X.Y. and Ji, H.F., 2019. Regulation of gut microbiota in Alzheimer's disease mice by silibinin and silymarin and their pharmacological implications. Applied Microbiology and Biotechnology 103: 7141-7149.

Shokouhi, G., Kosari-Nasab, M. and Salari, A.A., 2020. Silymarin sex-dependently improves cognitive functions and alters TNF-α, BDNF, and glutamate in the hippocampus of mice with mild traumatic brain injury. Life Sciences 257: 118049.

Singh, A., Kumar, A., Verma, R.K. and Shukla, R., 2020. Silymarin encapsulated nanoliquid crystals for improved activity against beta amyloid induced cytotoxicity. International Journal of Biological Macromolecules 149: 1198-1206.

Singhal, N.K., Chauhan, A.K., Jain, S.K., Shanker, R., Singh, C. and Singh, M.P., 2013. Silymarin- and melatonin-mediated changes in the expression of selected genes in pesticides-induced Parkinsonism. Molecular and Cellular Biochemistry 384: 47-58.

Singhal, N.K., Srivastava, G., Patel, D.K., Jain, S.K. and Singh, M.P., 2011. Melatonin or silymarin reduces maneb- and paraquat-induced Parkinson's disease phenotype in the mouse. Journal of Pineal Research 50: 97-109.

Sohrabi, M.J., Dehpour, A.R., Attar, F., Hasan, A., Mohammad-Sadeghi, N., Meratan, A.A., Aziz, F.M., Salihi, A., Shekha, M.S., Akhtari, K., Shahpasand, K., Hojjati, S., Sharifi, M., Saboury, A.A., Rezayat, S.M., Mousavi, S.E. and Falahati, M., 2019. Silymarin-albumin nanoplex: Preparation and its potential application as an antioxidant in nervous system *in vitro* and *in vivo*. International Journal of Pharmaceutics 572: 118824.

Song, X., Zhou, B., Cui, L., Lei, D., Zhang, P., Yao, G., Xia, M., Hayashi, T., Hattori, S., Ushiki-Kaku, Y., Tashiro, S.I., Onodera, S. and Ikejima, T., 2017a. Silibinin ameliorates $A\beta_{25-35}$-induced memory deficits in rats by modulating autophagy and attenuating neuroinflammation as well as oxidative stress. Neurochemical Research 42: 1073-1083.

Song, X., Liu, B., Cui, L., Zhou, B., Liu, W., Xu, F., Hayashi, T., Hattori, S., Ushiki-Kaku, Y., Tashiro, S.I. and Ikejima, T., 2017b. Silibinin ameliorates anxiety/depression-like behaviors in amyloid β-treated rats by upregulating BDNF/TrkB pathway and attenuating autophagy in hippocampus. Physiology & Behavior 179: 487-493.

Song, X., Zhou, B., Zhang, P., Lei, D., Wang, Y., Yao, G., Hayashi, T., Xia, M., Tashiro, S., Onodera, S. and Ikejima, T., 2016. Protective effect of silibinin on learning and memory impairment in LPS-treated rats via ROS-BDNF-TrkB pathway. Neurochemical Research 41: 1662-1672.

Song, X., Liu, B., Cui, L., Zhou, B., Liu, L., Liu, W., Yao, G., Xia, M., Hayashi, T., Hattori, S., Ushiki-Kaku, Y., Tashiro, S.I. and Ikejima, T., 2018. Estrogen receptors are involved in the neuroprotective effect of silibinin in $A\beta_{1-42}$-treated rats. Neurochemical Research 43: 796-805.

Thakare, V.N., Aswar, M.K., Kulkarni, Y.P., Patil, R.R. and Patel, B.M., 2017. Silymarin ameliorates experimentally induced depressive like behavior in rats: Involvement of hippocampal BDNF signaling, inflammatory cytokines and oxidative stress response. Physiology & Behavior 179: 401-410.

Thirugnanam, T. and Santhakumar, K., 2022. Chemically induced models of Parkinson's disease. Comparative biochemistry and physiology. Toxicology & Pharmacology 252: 109213.

Tota, S., Kamat, P.K., Shukla, R. and Nath, C., 2011. Improvement of brain energy metabolism and cholinergic functions contributes to the beneficial effects of silibinin against streptozotocin induced memory impairment. Behavioural Brain Research 221: 207-215.

Tripathi, M.K., Rasheed, M., Mishra, A.K., Patel, D.K. and Singh, M.P., 2020. Silymarin protects against impaired autophagy associated with 1-Methyl-4-phenyl-1,2,3,6-tetrahydropyridine-induced parkinsonism. Journal of Molecular Neuroscience 70: 276-283.

Tsai, M.J., Liao, J.F., Lin, D.Y., Huang, M.C., Liou, D.Y., Yang, H.C., Lee, H.J., Chen, Y.T., Chi, C.W., Huang, W.C. and Cheng, H., 2010. Silymarin protects spinal cord and cortical cells against oxidative stress and lipopolysaccharide stimulation. Neurochemistry International 57: 867-875.

Ullah, H. and Khan, H., 2018. Anti-Parkinson potential of silymarin: Mechanistic insight and therapeutic standing. Frontiers in Pharmacology 9: 422.

Walia, V., Kaushik, D., Mittal, V., Kumar, K., Verma, R., Parashar, J., Akter, R., Rahman, M.H., Bhatia, S., Al-Harrasi, A., Karthika, C., Bhattacharya, T., Chopra, H. and Ashraf, G.M., 2022. Delineation of neuroprotective effects and possible benefits of antioxidants therapy for the treatment of Alzheimer's diseases by targeting mitochondrial-derived reactive oxygen species: Bench to bedside. Molecular Neurobiology 59: 657-680.

Wang, M.J., Lin, W.W., Chen, H.L., Chang, Y.H., Ou, H.C., Kuo, J.S., Hong, J.S. and Jeng, K.C., 2002. Silymarin protects dopaminergic neurons against lipopolysaccharide-induced neurotoxicity by inhibiting microglia activation. The European Journal of Neuroscience 16: 2103-2112.

Wei, P., Li, X., Wang, S., Dong, Y., Yin, H., Gu, Z., Na, X., Wei, X., Yuan, J., Cao, J., Gao, H., Su, Y., Chen, Y.X. and Jin, G., 2022. Silibinin ameliorates formaldehyde-induced cognitive impairment by inhibiting oxidative stress. Oxidative Medicine and Cellular Longevity 2022: 5981353.

Xu, J., Yuan, Y., Zhang, R., Song, Y., Sui, T., Wang, J., Wang, C., Chen, Y., Guan, S. and Wang, L., 2019. A deuterohemin peptide protects a transgenic Caenorhabditis elegans model of Alzheimer's disease by inhibiting $A\beta_{1-42}$ aggregation. Bioorganic Chemistry 82: 332-339.

Yaghmaei, P., Azarfar, K., Dezfulian, M. and Ebrahim-Habibi, A., 2014. Silymarin effect on amyloid-β plaque accumulation and gene expression of APP in an Alzheimer's disease rat model. Daru 22: 24.

Yin, F., Liu, J., Ji, X., Wang, Y., Zidichouski, J. and Zhang, J., 2011. Silibinin: a novel inhibitor of Aβ aggregation. Neurochemistry International 58: 399-403.

Yön, B., Belviranlı, M. and Okudan, N., 2019. The effect of silymarin supplementation on cognitive impairment induced by diabetes in rats. Journal of Basic and Clinical Physiology and Pharmacology 30: 20180109.

Yuan, R., Fan, H., Cheng, S., Gao, W., Xu, X., Lv, S., Ye, M., Wu, M., Zhu, X. and Zhang, Y., 2017. Silymarin prevents NLRP3 inflammasome activation and protects against intracerebral hemorrhage. Biomedicine & Pharmacotherapy 93: 308-315.

Zakaria, R., Wan Yaacob, W.M., Othman, Z., Long, I., Ahmad, A.H. and Al-Rahbi, B., 2017. Lipopolysaccharide-induced memory impairment in rats: a model of Alzheimer's disease. Physiological Research 66: 553-565.

Zeng, H.J., Miao, M., Yang, R. and Qu, L.B., 2017. Effect of silybin on the fibrillation of hen egg-white lysozyme. Journal of Molecular Recognition 30: https://doi.org/10.1002/jmr.2566.

Chapter 14
Anti-diabetic properties of silymarin

Peter F. Surai[1-6] and Anton Surai[7]*
[1]Vitagene and Health Research Centre, Bristol, UK; [2]Department of Microbiology and Biochemistry, Faculty of Veterinary Medicine, Trakia University, Stara Zagora, Bulgaria; [3]Department of Animal Nutrition, Faculty of Agricultural and Environmental Sciences, Szent Istvan University, Hungary; [4]Saint-Petersburg State Academy of Veterinary Medicine, St. Petersburg, Russia; [5]Sumy National Agrarian University, Sumy, Ukraine; [6]Odessa National Academy of Food Technologies, Odessa, Ukraine; [7]Healthy Food Services, Bristol, UK
psurai@feedfood.co.uk

Abstract

The number of people with diabetes worldwide was reported to rise almost 4-fold for the last 30 years and diabetes is considered to be a major public health concern due to its life-threatening complications, including blindness, kidney failure, heart attacks, stroke and lower limb amputation. The accumulating evidence from the recent research studies indicates that redox disbalance and oxidative stress are key factors in developing various metabolic and neurodegenerative disorders including diabetes. Therefore, antioxidant activities of silymarin (SM) and its regulating effects on the redox balance could be of great importance in prevention and complementary treatments/support of diabetes patients. The data presented in this chapter clearly indicate that in various diabetes-related model systems *in vitro* and *in vivo* SM supplementation provided protective effects related to decreased oxidative stress and re-establishment of the redox balance in various tissues of experimental animals. Furthermore, effects of SM on glucose metabolism and insulin action (production and resistance) in addition to regulatory effects on lipid metabolism, make SM a supplement of choice for complimentary support of diabetic patients. Protective effects of SM in diabetes patients were confirmed in clinical trials and there is a need for new well-designed clinical trials to further substantiate beneficial effects of SM. Molecular mechanisms of protective effects of SM are diverse, but maintenance of redox homeostasis and prevention of oxidative stress are proven to be key points in SM beneficial effects in diabetes.

Keywords: silymarin, diabetes, oxidative stress, redox homeostasis

14.1 Introduction

Diabetes mellitus is a lifelong condition associated with high levels of blood sugar. Two types of diabetes are distinguished including type 1 diabetes, an autoimmune condition leading to the body's immune system attacks and destruction of the insulin-producing pancreatic β-cells and type 2 diabetes (T2D), a disease associated with a lack of production of insulin or low sensitivity (a resistance) to insulin. It should

DOI:10.3920/978-90-8686-944-2_014,

be mentioned that the majority (87%-91%) of the diabetes cases are related to T2D. The number of people with diabetes worldwide was reported to rise almost 4-fold for the last 30 years: from 108 million in 1980 to 422 million in 2014. Diabetes is considered to be a major public health concern due to its life-threatening complications, including blindness, kidney failure, heart attacks, stroke and lower limb amputation. In 2019 diabetes was reported to be the ninth leading cause of death with an estimated 1.5 million deaths (WHO, 2022). More than 4.9 million people in the UK have diabetes and this figure is predicted to rise up to 5.5 million people by 2030. Furthermore, 13.6 million people are considered to be at increased risk of T2D in the UK, and it was reported that the NHS spends at least £10 billion a year on diabetes (about 10% of its entire budget; Diabetes.org, 2022).

Although the exact aetiologies of T2D are not well defined, it seems likely that immunological, genetic, and environmental factors are among major contributors to the development of T2D that is characterised by alterations in

- antioxidant defences;
- lipid metabolism;
- insulin resistance; and
- pancreatic β-cell dysfunction.

Compromised antioxidant defences and oxidative stress are thought to play a major role in developing and progressing T2D. Recently, a total of 22 case-control studies with 2,853 subjects (1,667 diabetic patients and 1,186 healthy controls) were included in a meta-analysis. The pooled results of the meta-analysis showed a significant difference in the levels of some important indexes of OS, including MDA, NO, GSH and total antioxidant status between the diabetic patients and healthy subjects (Banik and Ghosh, 2021). However, oxidative-stress related changes and adaptive strategy in T2D need further elucidation since no significant difference was observed in the SOD and GPx activities in the aforementioned study.

14.2 Silymarin and diabetes

In various animal models natural compounds are shown to have anti-diabetic activities via several mechanisms including (Salazar-García and Corona, 2021):

- regulation of hyperglycaemia;
- upregulation of AO enzymes, decrease of oxidative stress, and neuronal injury;
- increased insulin secretion;
- improved mitochondrial function, learning, memory, and lipid metabolism.

Major results on protective effects of SM in T2D came from *in vitro* and *in vivo* animal model studies as well as from clinical investigations and they can be summarised as follows.

14.2.1 *In vitro* studies

Chronic hyperglycaemia, a typical situation of T2D, leads to damages in organs and tissues, associated with diabetic complications and glucotoxicity, the condition characterised by increased intracellular accumulation of reactive dicarbonyls, such as methylglyoxal (MGO), glyoxal, and 3-deoxyglucosone. Of note, MGO is considered to be the powerful glycating agent, causing the endogenous non-enzymatic glycoxidation of proteins, lipids, and nucleic acids leading to the formation of advanced glycation end products (Maessen *et al.*, 2015).

There are several publications showing protective effect of SM/SB against glucotoxicity *in vitro*. For example, SB is shown to ameliorate high glucose-induced oxidative stress and podocyte injury *in vitro* and *in vivo* (Khazim *et al.*, 2013). It should be taken into account that podocyte injury is considered as an important contributor to the pathogenesis of diabetic nephropathy associated with the excessive ROS generation. It is also well known that glucotoxicity can cause pancreatic β cell dysfunction including cell apoptosis, impaired glucose-stimulated insulin secretion and intracellular lipid accumulation.

Lipid and carbohydrate metabolism are controlled by a range of transcription factors. Furthermore, insulin induced gene-1 (Insig-1) is known to be an important upstream regulatory factor of SREBP-1c. Some evidence suggests that SB (30.0 μM) could protect β-cells from glucotoxicity and improving cell viability through regulation of the Insig-1/SREBP-1c pathway (Chen *et al.*, 2014). SM was shown to preserve the proliferation of pancreatic β-cells in a pancreatectomy model (Soto *et al.*, 2014). Therefore, SB may be an important therapeutic agent for prevention/treatment of β cell dysfunction. SM (5-25 μg/ml) is shown to protect endothelial cells against high glucose-induced oxidative damage by improving AO defences as evidenced by modulation of antioxidant enzyme activity, GSH concentration and protein carbonyl levels (Palomino *et al.*, 2017). SM was reported to ameliorate diabetes-induced proangiogenic response in brain endothelial cells through a GSK-3*β* inhibition-induced reduction of VEGF release (Alhusban *et al.*, 2017).

Antioxidant-related protective effects of SM could be related to NO production and metabolisms. For instance, SM is reported to inhibit cytokine mixture (TNF-α, IFN-γ, and IL-1β)-induced production of NO in the pancreatic beta cell line MIN6N8a and to suppress iNOS gene expression in a dose-dependent manner. Furthermore, SM was also shown to inhibit extracellular signal-regulated protein kinase-1 and 2 (ERK1/2) phosphorylation (Kim *et al.*, 2014). SB is suggested to protect HUVECs from high glucose induced-damage by activation of autophagy pathway (Rezabakhsh *et al.*, 2018). In a model system based on human serum albumin incubated with glucose, SB (50-200 μg) demonstrated concentration-dependent anti-glycation activity associated with (Neelofar *et al.*, 2019):

- inhibiting glucose-induced glycation at an early stage;
- reducing fructosamine formation;

- restoring α-helicity in albumin;
- reducing carbonyl contents with concomitant increase in free thiol, lysine and arginine residues.

Therefore, SB by preventing the glycation-induced changes in proteins, can ameliorate glycation-mediated pathologies in diabetic individuals. The effect of SM on disruption of inner blood retinal barrier, the primary cause of diabetic macular oedema, was studied in human retinal endothelial cells cultured under diabetogenic conditions. SM (4 μg/ml) was shown to cause a significant decrease in vascular endothelial growth factor-induced permeability indicating that SM could prevent diabetes-induced hyperpermeability in human retinal endothelial cells (García-Ramírez *et al.*, 2018). Anti-diabetic actions of SM could be also related to its effects on insulin secretion. In particular, in HIT-T15 cells, SM (25-100 μM) was found to stimulate insulin secretion in a glucose-dependent manner without lowering intracellular peroxides (Meng *et al.*, 2016).

14.2.2 *In vivo* studies

Most animal models of diabetes are based on usage of toxic chemicals targeting the pancreatic β-cells. The discovery (in 1943) that alloxan (ALX) was able to cause diabetes-like changes via fragmentation of the β-cells was an important step in the development of effective animal models of diabetes development. However, there are some complications caused by ALX, including kidney toxicity, which restrict application of this model. In 1963 another chemical causing diabetes called streptozotocin (STZ) was introduced into the area of medical research. In particular, low-doses of STZ was found to cause mild impairment in insulin secretion, a characteristic change in the later stages of T2D. Again, this treatment does not address the insulin resistance issue commonly seen in patients with T2D. Therefore, later it was suggested to combine HFD (a cause of insulin resistance) with STZ treatment to optimise an animal model of T2D (Gheibi *et al.* 2017).

In a rat model of STZ-nicotinamide-induced type 2 diabetic nephropathy SM treatment (60 mg/kg and 120 mg/kg of SM for 60 days) was associated with significantly decreased levels of blood glucose, glycosylated haemoglobin, urine volume, serum creatinine, serum uric acid, and urine albumin in comparison to the diabetic control group. Results of histopathological studies confirmed the protective action of SM (Sheela *et al*, 2013). In a rat model of STZ plus high-fat diet-induced diabetes SB treatment (15 and 30 mg/kg) was found to significantly ameliorate the development of obliterated retinal capillaries in diabetic rats, in comparison to vehicle treatment. Furthermore, leukostasis and level of the retinal ICAM-1 were reported to decrease in SB-treated diabetic rats (Zhang *et al.*, 2014). In STZ-induced diabetic rats, SM (50 mg/kg) was indicated to mitigate the compromised antioxidant status (total antioxidant capacity in the liver and serum) and to restore the cells of Langerhans islets and to prevent diabetes-induced cellular vacuolation and cell depletion in rats (Amniattalab *et al.*, 2016). In a STZ-induced diabetes rat model, SB (100 and

200 mg/kg for 4 weeks) was indicated to provide protective effects against DNA damage (Toğay *et al.*, 2018).

It seems likely that SB can decrease hepatic glucose production through the activation of gut-brain-liver axis in diabetic rats. In HFD/STZ-induced diabetic Sprague-Dawley (SD) rats it was shown that SB (100 and 300 mg/kg for 4 weeks) significantly inhibited fasting blood glucose. Furthermore, the expression of glucagon-like peptide 1 (GLP-1) receptor in the duodenum and the activation of neurons in the nucleus tractus solitarius were shown to be increased, whereas hepatic glucose production was reported to be decreased due to SB treatment (Xu *et al.*, 2018). Of note, the GLP-1 system affects various physiological processes, including potentiation of glucose-stimulated insulin secretion, gut motility, satiety, and hepatic glucose production. GLP-1 signalling via its receptor (GLP-1R) on target tissues has been extensively studied and GLP-1 receptor agonists are now widely used for the treatment of type 2 diabetes (Rosario *et al.*, 2015).

It should be also mentioned that palmitate exposure increased ROS levels and decreased the GLP-1 content in L-cell line GLUTag cells, while Silychristin A, a constituent of SM, activated vitagene (Nrf2-HO-1/SOD2) pathway to reduce apoptosis and improve GLP-1 production through upregulation of oestrogen receptor α (ERα) in GLUTag cells (Wang *et al.*, 2020; 2022). Furthermore, ERα is considered to be a key regulator of energy homeostasis and glucose metabolism and mediates the protective effects of oestrogens against type 2 diabetes (Guillaume *et al.*, 2017). 17β-oestradiol (E2) acting via ER at physiological concentrations is shown to increase insulin production and protect the pancreatic β-cells against major injuries under diabetic conditions including lipotoxicity, hIAPP, oxidative stress and apoptosis (Mauvais-Jarvis, 2011). Furthermore, regulatory roles of ERs in glucose metabolism and diabetes prevention are well described and include (Wang *et al.*, 2022):

- promotion of insulin synthesis by ERα and enhancement of insulin secretion from pancreatic β-cells by ERβ;
- activation of ERα in the liver leads to modulation of insulin sensitivity and further regulate glucose homeostasis;
- increased ERα expression is also associated with improved glucose homeostasis via elevation of insulin-stimulated glucose transporter (GLUT4) expression in skeletal muscle.

ERα is shown to mediate attenuating effect of SB on palmitic acid-induced apoptosis and mitochondrial dysfunction in pancreatic β-cells (Sun *et al.*, 2019). In rats SM (100 mg/kg) was shown to ameliorate STZ-induced diabetic cardiomyopathy, a leading cause of morbidity and mortality in diabetes mellitus patients. This was associated with the inhibition of TGF-β1/Smad signalling: levels of TGF-β1 and p-Smad2/3 were shown to be decreased, whereas Smad7 was increased as a result of SM administration (Meng *et al.*, 2019). SM (25 mg/kg) was found to ameliorate aspartame-induced variation in mouse behaviour, cerebrocortical morphology and oxidative stress markers (Onaolapo *et al.*, 2017). SM supplementation was indicated to improve anxiety-related behaviour and learning and memory in diabetic rats by increasing the brain-derived neurotrophic factor levels (Yön *et al.*, 2019).

SM was reported to prevent lipid accumulation in the liver of rats with type 2 diabetes via SIRT1 and SREBP-1c (Kheiripour *et al.*, 2018). Therefore, SM can ameliorate the disordered glucose metabolism of mice with diet-induced obesity by activating the hepatic SIRT1 pathway. SM was reported to ameliorate the dyslipidemia, hepatic steatosis, and insulin resistance of the HFD-fed mice. SM also increased the phosphorylation of AKT and FOXO1 and reduced the level of FOXO1 acetylation in insulin-resistant cells. However, SIRT1 knockdown was shown to reduce the aforementioned effects of SM (Feng *et al.*, 2021). The authors suggested the possibility that SM directly binds to SIRT1 and increase its enzymatic activity. It should be mentioned that increased ROS production is associated with a reduction in insulin content in pancreatic β-cells (Chu *et al.*, 2020) and excessive ROS levels are believed to be responsible for insulin resistance in its target tissues (Paglialunga *et al.*, 2015; Quan *et al.*, 2020).

Interestingly, a newly developed SM nano-formulation with enhanced bioavailability (SM-loaded pluronic nanomicelles) was reported to be an effective antidiabetic agent in STZ-induced diabetic rats (El-Far *et al.*, 2016). Peroxisome proliferator-activated receptor gamma (PPARγ) is believed to be a key regulator of glucose and lipid metabolism. Agonists (drugs or naturally occurring substances that can activate physiologic receptors) of PPARγ are used in the treatment of various metabolic diseases including T2D and nonalcoholic fatty liver disease. Interestingly, a component of SM namely isosilybin A was identified as an agonist of PPARγ (Pferschy-Wenzig *et al.*, 2014).

Insulin resistance (IR) is considered to be the driving factor leading to T2D, gestational diabetes and prediabetes.

Furthermore, it seems likely that reduced IR was one of the important mechanisms of the protective effects of SB on NAFLD. In rats fed high-fat diet for 6 weeks SB (0.5 mg/kg) was reported to significantly protect liver function, to down-regulate serum fat, and to improve IR. At the same time, SB was able to ameliorate visceral obesity, enhance lipolysis and inhibit gluconeogenesis in NAFLD rats (Yao *et al.*, 2013). Similarly, SM was demonstrated to attenuate fructose-induced insulin resistance syndrome by reducing de novo hepatic lipogenesis in the rat (Prakash *et al.*, 2014). SB can activate the Nrf2-antioxidant pathways in pancreatic β-cells through regulation of ERα expression. On the one hand, *in vitro* SB (10 μM) was shown to elevate viability, insulin biosynthesis, and insulin secretion of high glucose/palmitate-treated INS-1 cells associated with increased expression of ERα, Nrf2, and HO-1 as well as decreased ROS production.

Furthermore, treatment of INS-1 cells with an ERα antagonist or silencing ERα expression in INS-1 and NIT-1 cells were demonstrated to abolish the protective effects of SB. On the other hand, *in vivo* in high-fat diet/STZ-induced type 2 diabetic rats, SB (100 mg/kg/day for 4 weeks) was indicated to decrease fasting blood glucose with a concurrent increase in levels of serum insulin and to increase expression of ERα, Nrf2 and HO-1 in pancreatic β-cells in pancreatic islets (Chu *et al.*, 2020). A conclusion from the recent review related to effect of SM on insulin indicates that the use of SM improves metabolic and insulin resistance parameters (MacDonald-Ramos *et al.*, 2021).

A hypoglycaemic effect of SM has been shown in several animal experiments where SM:

- Mitigated the pancreatic and hepatic damage by oxidative stress (Feng *et al.*, 2016) as a result of increasing the AO defences in diabetic rats. In fact, after SM and SB treatment of STZ-induced diabetic rats, a significant improvement of glucose level, insulin level, lipid profile, SOD activity, GSH content and decreased MDA were observed (El-Far *et al.*, 2014).
- Had a metabolic regulating effects by reducing the glucagon-induced activation of both gluconeogenesis and glycogenolysis (Colturatto *et al.*, 2012).
- Prevented the activation of the hepatic NF-κB signalling pathway and inhibited inflammasome-mediated IL-1β secretion by macrophages contributing to its beneficial effects on hyperglycaemia and obesity-related insulin resistance (Lu *et al.*, 2018).
- Inhibited protein tyrosine phosphatase 1B (PTP1B), T-cell protein tyrosine phosphatase, and vaccinia H1-related phosphatase (Qin *et al.*, 2018). Of note, inhibition of PTP1B could increase insulin sensitivity, improves glucose tolerance and resistance to fat-induced weight gain (Kren, 2021).

Therefore, these SM activities could be relevant to antidiabetic properties of this preparation.

Diabetes development is very often associated with other metabolic changes and a combination of diabetes, high blood pressure (hypertension) and obesity is called metabolic syndrome. Importantly, in the gerbil *Psammomys obesus*, a unique model of nutritional diabetes resembling the disease in humans, SB (100 mg/kg for 7 weeks) was observed to ameliorate the progression of metabolic syndrome (hyperinsulinemia, hyperglycaemia, dyslipidemia, etc.), oxidative stress (GSH and lipid peroxidation), and liver steatosis (Bouderba *et al.*, 2014).

In 2004 SM was demonstrated to have protective effect against alloxan-induced damage in rat pancreas (Soto *et al.*, 2004). Similarly, in a rat model of alloxan-induced type 2 diabetes SM administration (60 and 120 mg/kg for 2 months) was shown to significantly reduce the fasting blood sugar level and to increase the concentration of insulin. Furthermore, SM was responsible for prevention of diabetes-induced weight loss, attenuation of oxidative stress (MDA, NO, and total thiol molecules content) and significant modulation of serum lipid profile with reduction of the expression of urotensin II and its receptor in the heart leading to improvement of histopathological changes in the heart tissues (Rahimi *et al.*, 2018). It should be mentioned that oxidative stress-induced apoptosis in T2D is an important pathological factor and SM (120 mg/kg for 10 days) is reported to have cytoprotective effect against diabetes-induced cardiomyocyte apoptosis in diabetic rats (Tuorkey *et al.*, 2015).

14.2.3 Clinical investigations

The results of a range of clinical trials have led to SM being recognised as a potential therapy for diabetes. In cirrhotic diabetic-patients SM was found to reduce hyperinsulinemia, lipid peroxidation and daily insulin need (Velussi *et al.*, 1993). Furthermore, long-term (12 months) treatment with SM was effective in controlling hyperinsulinemia (significant reduction of the fasting and mean daily glucose concentrations and HbA1c level), exogenous insulin requirement and lipid peroxidation in cirrhotic diabetic patients (Velussi *et al.*, 1997). Later, it was confirmed that SM has protective effect in the restoration of liver function and in controlling blood glucose level in diabetes patients with liver diseases (Jose *et al.*, 2011).

Furthermore, there are randomised controlled trials which have shown that SM administration was associated with significant reductions in fasting and postprandial blood glucose and HbA1c levels in T2D patients without liver disease (Ebrahimpour-Koujan *et al.*, 2018; Huseini *et al.*, 2006; Hussain, 2007). A 4-month randomised double-blind clinical trial was conducted in 51 type II diabetic patients in two well-matched groups. The first group (n=25) received a SM (200 mg) tablet 3 times a day plus conventional therapy. The second group (n=26) received the same therapy with a placebo tablet instead of SM. The results indicated that compared with placebo or with values at the beginning of the study, a significant reduction in HbA(1)c, FBS, total cholesterol, LDL, triglyceride, AST and GPT levels were observed in SM-treated patients (Huseini *et al.*, 2006).

In a randomised, double-blind, placebo-controlled trial 59 T2D patients with poor glycaemic control were divided into three groups: the first two groups were treated with either 200 mg/day SM or placebo as adjuncts to glibenclamide, and the third group was maintained on glibenclamide alone for 120 days. Compared with placebo, SM treatment was shown to significantly reduce both fasting and postprandial plasma glucose concentrations and significantly reduced HbA(1c) levels (Hussain, 2007). Furthermore, SM supplementation (140 mg, thrice daily) was found to improve some antioxidant indices (SOD, GPX and TAC) and to decrease high sensitivity CRP levels in patients with T2D (Ebrahimpour Koujan *et al.*, 2015). Furthermore, in a paralleled, randomised, triple-blinded, placebo-controlled clinical trial involved 40 T2D patients, SM administration (140 mg, thrice daily for 45 days) was associated with significant reduction in fasting blood sugar, serum insulin, serum triglyceride and triglyceride to high-density lipoprotein cholesterol ratio as compared to the placebo group by 11, 14, 25, 24 and 28% respectively.

Forty T2D patients (twenty males and twenty females) were recruited for the paralleled, randomised, triple-blinded, placebo-controlled clinical trial. The participants were randomly assigned to the SM or placebo groups, receiving either 140 mg of SM, thrice daily (n=20) or placebo (n=20) for 45 days. In comparison to the placebo, SM supplementation was found to lead to:

- significant reduction in fasting blood sugar, serum insulin, homeostatic model assessment for insulin resistance, serum triglyceride and triglyceride to high-density lipoprotein cholesterol ratio;
- significant increase in high-density lipoprotein cholesterol levels and quantitative insulin sensitivity check;
- significantly decrease in total cholesterol and low-density lipoprotein cholesterol concentrations (Ebrahimpour-Koujan *et al.*, 2018).

Based on meta-analysis of eight eligible publications from seven trials it was concluded that SM supplementation was able to decrease fasting blood sugar, haemoglobin A1C, insulin, LDL cholesterol and MDA and increase HDL cholesterol levels. At the same time, SM did not affect total cholesterol or triglyceride concentrations (Hadi *et al.*, 2018). Finally, a meta-analysis of the therapeutic effects of SM for patients with glucose/lipid metabolic dysfunction based on 6 studies involving 1,358 patients have been recently conducted. It has been shown that compared with control, SM reduced levels of fasting blood glucose, homeostatic model assessment for insulin resistance, haemoglobin A1c, total cholesterol, triglyceride, LDL-cholesterol, C-reactive protein and increased HDL-cholesterol. However, SM had no impacts on function indicators of liver and kidney (ALT, AST, creatinine phosphokinase and creatinine) and the complication rate (Xiao *et al.*, 2020). The authors concluded that SM supplementation might be effective and safe way of the management of diabetes mellitus and hyperlipidaemia.

14.3 Silymarin and diabetic complications

SM/SB was shown to be effective in controlling various diabetic complications in several organs including neuropathy, retinopathy, impaired healing, hepatopathy, cardiomyopathy, nephropathy, and osteoporosis (Chu *et al.*, 2018; Stolf *et al.*, 2017). Nephropathy is known to be the primary cause of end-stage renal failure worldwide. In animal models of diabetes protective effect of SM on kidney was associated with preservation of the tubular epithelium and a reduction of inter-tubular haemorrhage, improvement of antioxidant defences and attenuating oxidative stress in renal tissue. The involvement of renal metabolic alterations, organelle dysfunction, and cellular stress responses, especially oxidative stress, in the pathogenesis of diabetic kidney disease have been recently reviewed (Sakashita *et al.*, 2021).

Positive effects of SM on kidney integrity were confirmed in T2D with persistent macroalbuminuria (Stolf *et al.* 2017). Administration of SB (15 and 30 mg/kg/day for 10 weeks) to db/db mice was indicated to improve diabetic condition, as evidenced by the decrease of body weight, HbAc1level and serum insulin level. Furthermore, SB was able to prevent kidney injury and to attenuate oxidative stress and activate AKT signalling pathway and decreasing the levels of p-GSK-3β, Bax and cleaved caspase-3

(Liu *et al.*, 2019b). SM (60 and 120 mg/kg/day) was shown to ameliorate engulfment and cell motility protein 1 (ELMO-1) and kidney injury molecule 1 (KIM1) expression and oxidative stress in the kidney of rats with T2D (Goli *et al.*, 2019).

SB (50 and 100 mg/kg) was reported to ameliorate high-fat diet-induced renal fibrosis of diabetic nephropathy decreasing HFD-induced the upregulation of kidney weight/body weight, microalbuminuria, and fibrotic area. Furthermore, 100 mg/kg SB also markedly reduced collagen I, fibronectin, and p65 expressions in mice renal tissues. Interestingly, protective effects of SB (50 μM) were also demonstrated *in vitro* in human renal glomerular endothelial cells (Liu *et al.*, 2019a).

SB can increase anti-fibrosis effect of valsartan *in vitro* (30 μM) and *in vivo* via inhibition of TGF-β1 signalling pathway and therefore in combination with valsartan it may be used to treat renal fibrosis caused by diabetic nephropathy (Liu *et al.*, 2020). Furthermore, in an *in vitro* study with MPC-5 cells SM (16, 32 and 64 μg/ml) was reported to significantly improve the high-glucose induced up-regulation of podoxin and nephrin, as well as decreased the expression of inflammatory cytokines IL-6, ICAM-1 and TNF-α, and the cell survival rates were also significantly increased in a dose-dependent manner (Chen *et al.*, 2021). SM (100, 300 and 900 mg/kg) nanoliposomes were shown to ameliorate STZ-induced kidney injury by decreasing oxidative stress, renal fibrosis, and co-inhibiting JAK2/STAT3/SOCS1 and TGF-β/Smad signalling pathways in diabetic rats (Chen *et al.*, 2021).

There are several reports showing reno-protective effects of SM under various stress conditions. For example, it was suggested that SM (140 mg every 8 hours for 2 months) could be used as a complementary therapy for end-stage renal disease patients undergoing peritoneal dialysis (Firuzi *et al.*, 2016). In an experimental mouse model of contrast-induced nephropathy SM (50, 200 and 300 mg/kg) was demonstrated to preserve renal function (preventing renal glomerular and tubular injuries) and to decrease systemic and renal oxidative damage in a dose-dependent manner (de Souza Santos *et al.*, 2020). SM (100 mg/kg/day, for seven days) was reported to ameliorate colistin-induced acute nephrotoxicity in rats as evidenced by improved antioxidant defences (SOD and GPx) and some improvements in tubular necrosis (Dumludag *et al.*, 2022).

SM (400 mg/kg) was indicated to ameliorate vancomycin induced nephrotoxicity by downregulating apoptosis in mice. Similar protective effects of SM (400 μg/ml) were reported in Vero cells *in vitro* (Malkani *et al.*, 2020). Interestingly, SM (100 mg/kg) was shown to be more effective than metformin in treating diabetic-induced infertility (Pourheydar *et al.*, 2022) and as hepatoprotective agents in mice fibrotic model caused by carbon tetrachloride (Omar *et al.*, 2022).

Thus, natural compounds, including SM/SB, could contribute to expanding the therapeutic options for treating or reducing the complications associated with T2D (Salazar-García and Corona, 2021). However, only a few clinical studies tested SM as a protectant against T2D or its complications. Hence, there is a need for further research devoted to protective ability of SM in T2D before it can be widely used as dietary supplement to improve the management, decrease antidiabetic drug's side effects or help in treatment of T2D. Molecular mechanisms of protective action of SM/SB in diabetes are summarised in Table 14.1.

14.4 Conclusions

The accumulating evidence from the recent research studies indicates that redox disbalance and oxidative stress are key factors in developing various metabolic and neurodegenerative disorders including T2D (Bhatti *et al.*, 2022). Therefore, antioxidant activities of SM/SB and its regulating effects on the redox balance could be of great importance in prevention and complementary treatments/support of diabetes patients. The aforementioned data clearly indicate that in various model systems *in vitro* and *in vivo* SM/SB supplementation was indicated to provide protective effects related to decreased oxidative stress and re-establishment of the redox balance in

Table 14.1. Molecular mechanisms of protective effects of SM/SB in diabetes.

N	Effects	References
1	Antioxidant action	Surai, 2015; see Chapter 4
2	Vitagene activation	Surai, 2020; see Chapter 7
3	Nrf2 stimulation and increased synthesis of AO enzymes	Surai, 2020; Surai *et al.*, 2019; see Chapter 5
4	Inhibition of NF-κB and suppression of proinflammatory cytokine expression	Surai *et al.*, 2021; see Chapter 6
5	Decreasing insulin concentration and insulin resistance	Federico *et al.*, 2019; Guo *et al.*, 2016; Li *et al.*, 2015; MacDonald-Ramos *et al.*, 2021; Prakash *et al.*, 2014
6	Decreasing blood glucose	Baluchnejadmojarad *et al.*, 2009; Soleymani *et al.*, 2022
7	Restoration of cellular function in the islets of Langerhans (β-cells)	Amniattalab *et al.*, 2016; Gad and El-Maddawy, 2014; Oh *et al.*, 2015
8	Reduction of the AGE formation	Borymska *et al.*, 2022; İnceören *et al.*, 2022; Shin *et al.*, 2015; Wu *et al.*, 2011
9	Hypo-lipidemic and anti-hyperglycaemic effects	Alkuraishy *et al.*,2012; Baluchnejadmojarad *et al.*, 2009; Suh *et al.*, 2015; Vaughu *et al.*, 2006
10	Suppression of cholesterol synthesis, esterification and absorption	Škottová and Krečman, 1998; Sobolová *et al.*, 2006; Vaughu *et al.*, 2006
11	Amelioration of increase in liver content of triglycerides, decreasing VLDL synthesis, and their secretion in the intestine)	Alkuraishy *et al.*, 2012; Lirussi *et al.*, 2002; Soleymani *et al.*, 2022
12	Modulation of adipogenic factors (PPARγ, PPARα, C/EBPα, and FABP4) leading to reduced lipid accumulation and blood lipids normalisation	Barbagallo, *et al.*, 2016; Chou *et al.*, 2012; Mohamed Kamel *et al.*, 2022; Pferschy-Wenzig *et al.*, 2014; Suh *et al.*, 2015; Xiao *et al.*, 2017; Yassin *et al.*, 2021

various tissues of experimental animals. Furthermore, effects of SM/SB on glucose metabolism and insulin action (production and resistance) in addition to regulatory effects on lipid metabolism, make SM/SB a supplement of choice for complimentary support of diabetic patients. Protective effects of SM/SB in diabetes patients were confirmed in clinical trials and there is a need for new well-designed clinical trials to further substantiate beneficial effects of SM/SB. Molecular mechanisms of protective effects of SM/SB (Table 14.1) are diverse, but maintenance of redox homeostasis and prevention of oxidative stress are proven to be key points in SM/SB beneficial effects in diabetes.

References

Alhusban, A., Alkhazaleh, E. and El-Elimat, T., 2017. Silymarin ameliorates diabetes-induced proangiogenic response in brain endothelial cells through a GSK-3β inhibition-induced reduction of VEGF release. Journal of Diabetes Research 2017: 2537216.

Alkuraishy, H.M. and Alwindy, S., 2012. Beneficial effects of Silymarin on lipid profile in hyperlipidemic patients: Placebo controlled clinical trail. WebmedCentral Pharmacology 3: WMC002966.

Amniattalab, A., Malekinejad, H., Rezabakhsh, A., Rokhsartalab-Azar, S. and Alizade-Fanalou, S., 2016. Silymarin: A novel natural agent to restore defective pancreatic β cells in Streptozotocin (STZ)-induced diabetic rats. Iranian Journal of Pharmaceutical Research 15: 493-500.

Baluchnejadmojarad, T.O., Roghani, M.E., Homayounfar, H.O. and Khaste Khodaie, Z., 2009. Protective effects of chronic administration of silymarin on blood glucose and lipids and oxidative stress in diabetic rats. Koomesh 10: 143-150.

Banik, S. and Ghosh, A., 2021. The association of oxidative stress biomarkers with type 2 diabetes mellitus: A systematic review and meta-analysis. Health Science Reports 4: e389.

Barbagallo, I., Vanella, L., Cambria, M.T., Tibullo, D., Godos, J., Guarnaccia, L., Zappalà, A., Galvano, F. and Li Volti, G., 2016. Silibinin regulates lipid metabolism and differentiation in functional human adipocytes. Frontiers in Pharmacology 6: 309.

Bhatti, J.S., Sehrawat, A., Mishra, J., Sidhu, I.S., Navik, U., Khullar, N., Kumar, S., Bhatti, G.K. and Reddy, P.H., 2022. Oxidative stress in the pathophysiology of type 2 diabetes and related complications: Current therapeutics strategies and future perspectives. Free Radical Biology & Medicine 184: 114-134.

Borymska, W., Zych, M., Dudek, S. and Kaczmarczyk-Sedlak, I., 2022. Silymarin from milk thistle fruits counteracts selected pathological changes in the lenses of type 1 diabetic rats. Nutrients 14: 1450.

Bouderba, S., Sanchez-Martin, C., Villanueva, G.R., Detaille, D. and Koceïr, E.A., 2014. Beneficial effects of silibinin against the progression of metabolic syndrome, increased oxidative stress, and liver steatosis in Psammomys obesus, a relevant animal model of human obesity and diabetes. Journal of Diabetes 6: 184-192.

Chen, K., Zhao, L., He, H., Wan, X., Wang, F. and Mo, Z., 2014. Silibinin protects β cells from glucotoxicity through regulation of the Insig-1/SREBP-1c pathway. International Journal of Molecular Medicine 34: 1073-1080.

Chen, Y., Chen, L. and Yang, T., 2021. Silymarin nanoliposomes attenuate renal injury on diabetic nephropathy rats via co-suppressing TGF-β/Smad and JAK2/STAT3/SOCS1 pathway. Life Sciences 271: 119197.

Chou, C.H., Chen, Y.C., Hsu, M.C., Tsai, W.L., Chang, C.Y. and Chiu, C.H., 2012. Effect of silymarin on lipid and alcohol metabolism in mice following long-term alcohol consumption. Journal of Food Biochemistry 36: 369-377.

Chu, C., Gao, X., Li, X., Zhang, X., Ma, R., Jia, Y., Li, D., Wang, D. and Xu, F., 2020. Involvement of estrogen receptor-α in the activation of Nrf2-antioxidative signaling pathways by silibinin in pancreatic β-Cells. Biomolecules & Therapeutics 28: 163-171.

Chu, C., Li, D., Zhang, S., Ikejima, T., Jia, Y., Wang, D. and Xu, F., 2018. Role of silibinin in the management of diabetes mellitus and its complications. Archives of Pharmacal Research 41: 785-796.

Colturato, C.P., Constantin, R.P., Maeda, A.S., Jr, Constantin, R.P., Yamamoto, N.S., Bracht, A., Ishii-Iwamoto, E.L. and Constantin, J., 2012. Metabolic effects of silibinin in the rat liver. Chemico-Biological Interactions 195: 119-132.

de Souza Santos, V., Peters, B., Côco, L.Z., Alves, G.M., de Assis, A., Nogueira, B.V., Meyrelles, S.S., Porto, M.L., Vasquez, E.C., Campagnaro, B.P. and Pereira, T., 2019. Silymarin protects against radiocontrast-induced nephropathy in mice. Life Sciences 228: 305-315.

Diabetes UK (Diabetes.org), 2022. Diabetes statistics. Diabetes UK, London, UK. Available at: https://www.tinyurl.com/5b48mpsh.

Dumludag, B., Derici, M.K., Sutcuoglu, O., Ogut, B., Pasaoglu, O.T., Gonul, I.I. and Derici, U., 2022. Role of silymarin (*Silybum marianum*) in the prevention of colistin-induced acute nephrotoxicity in rats. Drug and Chemical Toxicology 45: 568-575.

Ebrahimpour Koujan, S., Gargari, B.P., Mobasseri, M., Valizadeh, H. and Asghari-Jafarabadi, M., 2015. Effects of *Silybum marianum* (L.) Gaertn. (silymarin) extract supplementation on antioxidant status and hs-CRP in patients with type 2 diabetes mellitus: a randomized, triple-blind, placebo-controlled clinical trial. Phytomedicine 22: 290-296.

Ebrahimpour-Koujan, S., Gargari, B.P., Mobasseri, M., Valizadeh, H. and Asghari-Jafarabadi, M., 2018. Lower glycemic indices and lipid profile among type 2 diabetes mellitus patients who received novel dose of *Silybum marianum* (L) Gaertn. (silymarin) extract supplement: A Triple-blinded randomized controlled clinical trial. Phytomedicine 44: 39-44.

El-Far, M., Negm, A. and Wahdan, M., 2014. Promising biopharmaceutical use of silymarin and silibinin as antidiabetic natural agents in streptozotocin-induced diabetic rats: first comparative assessment. World Journal of Pharmacy and Pharmaceutical Sciences 4: 7-28.

El-Far, Y.M., Zakaria, M.M., Gabr, M.M., El Gayar, A.M., El-Sherbiny, I.M. and Eissa, L.A., 2016. A newly developed silymarin nanoformulation as a potential antidiabetic agent in experimental diabetes. Nanomedicine 11: 2581-2602.

Federico, A., Dallio, M., Masarone, M., Gravina, A.G., Di Sarno, R., Tuccillo, C., Cossiga, V., Lama, S., Stiuso, P., Morisco, F., Persico, M. and Loguercio, C., 2019. Evaluation of the effect derived from silybin with vitamin D and vitamin E administration on clinical, metabolic, endothelial dysfunction, oxidative stress parameters, and serological worsening markers in nonalcoholic fatty liver disease patients. Oxidative Medicine and Cellular Longevity 2019: 8742075.

Feng, B., Huang, B., Jing, Y., Shen, S., Feng, W., Wang, W., Meng, R. and Zhu, D., 2021. Silymarin ameliorates the disordered glucose metabolism of mice with diet-induced obesity by activating the hepatic SIRT1 pathway. Cellular Signalling 84: 110023.

Feng, B., Meng, R., Huang, B., Shen, S., Bi, Y. and Zhu, D., 2016. Silymarin alleviates hepatic oxidative stress and protects against metabolic disorders in high-fat diet-fed mice. Free Radical Research, 50: 314-327.

Firuzi, O., Khajehrezaei, S., Ezzatzadegan, S., Nejati, M., Jahanshahi, K.A. and Roozbeh, J., 2016. Effects of silymarin on biochemical and oxidative stress markers in end-stage renal disease patients undergoing peritoneal dialysis. Hemodialysis International. International Symposium on Home Hemodialysis 20: 558-563.

Gad, S.B. and El-Maddawy, Z.K., 2014. Silymarin improves pancreatic endocrine function in rats. Pakistan Veterinary Journal 34: 214-218.

García-Ramírez, M., Turch, M., Simó-Servat, O., Hernández, C. and Simó, R., 2018. Silymarin prevents diabetes-induced hyperpermeability in human retinal endothelial cells. Endocrinologia, Diabetes y Nutricion 65: 200-205.

Gheibi, S., Kashfi, K. and Ghasemi, A., 2017. A practical guide for induction of type-2 diabetes in rat: Incorporating a high-fat diet and streptozotocin. Biomedicine & Pharmacotherapy 95: 605-613.

Goli, F., Karimi, J., Khodadadi, I., Tayebinia, H., Kheiripour, N., Hashemnia, M. and Rahimi, R., 2019. Silymarin attenuates ELMO-1 and KIM-1 expression and oxidative stress in the kidney of rats with type 2 diabetes. Indian Journal of Clinical Biochemistry 34: 172-179.

Guillaume, M., Montagner, A., Fontaine, C., Lenfant, F., Arnal, J.F. and Gourdy, P., 2017. Nuclear and membrane actions of estrogen receptor alpha: Contribution to the regulation of energy and glucose homeostasis. Advances in Experimental Medicine and Biology 1043: 401-426.

Guo, Y., Wang, S., Wang, Y. and Zhu, T., 2016. Silymarin improved diet-induced liver damage and insulin resistance by decreasing inflammation in mice. Pharmaceutical Biology 54: 2995-3000.

Hadi, A., Pourmasoumi, M., Mohammadi, H., Symonds, M. and Miraghajani, M., 2018. The effects of silymarin supplementation on metabolic status and oxidative stress in patients with type 2 diabetes mellitus: A systematic review and meta-analysis of clinical trials. Complementary Therapies in Medicine 41: 311-319.

Huseini, H.F., Larijani, B., Heshmat, R., Fakhrzadeh, H., Radjabipour, B., Toliat, T. and Raza, M., 2006. The efficacy of *Silybum marianum* (L.) Gaertn. (silymarin) in the treatment of type II diabetes: a randomized, double-blind, placebo-controlled, clinical trial. Phytotherapy Research 20: 1036-1039.

Hussain, S.A., 2007. Silymarin as an adjunct to glibenclamide therapy improves long-term and postprandial glycemic control and body mass index in type 2 diabetes. Journal of Medicinal Food 10: 543-547.

İnceören, N., Emen, S., Toptancı, B.Ç., Kızıl, G. and Kızıl, M., 2022. *In vitro* inhibition of advanced glycation end product formation by ethanol extract of milk thistle (*Silybum marianum* L.) seed. South African Journal of Botany 149: 682-692.

Jose, M.A., Abraham, A. and Narmadha, M.P., 2011. Effect of silymarin in diabetes mellitus patients with liver diseases. Journal of Pharmacology & Pharmacotherapeutics 2: 287-289.

Khazim, K., Gorin, Y., Cavaglieri, R.C., Abboud, H.E. and Fanti, P., 2013. The antioxidant silybin prevents high glucose-induced oxidative stress and podocyte injury *in vitro* and *in vivo*. American journal of physiology. Renal Physiology 305: F691-F700.

Kheiripour, N., Karimi, J., Khodadadi, I., Tavilani, H., Goodarzi, M.T. and Hashemnia, M., 2018. Silymarin prevents lipid accumulation in the liver of rats with type 2 diabetes via sirtuin1 and SREBP-1c. Journal of Basic and Clinical Physiology and Pharmacology 29: 301-308.

Kim, E.J., Kim, J., Lee, M.Y., Sudhanva, M.S., Devakumar, S. and Jeon, Y.J., 2014. Silymarin inhibits cytokine-stimulated pancreatic beta cells by blocking the ERK1/2 pathway. Biomolecules & Therapeutics 22: 282-287.

Křen, V., 2021. Chirality matters: Biological activity of optically pure silybin and Its congeners. International Journal of Molecular Sciences 22: 7885.

Li, H.B., Yang, Y.R.Y., Mo, Z.J., Ding, Y. and Jiang, W.J., 2015. Silibinin improves palmitate-induced insulin resistance in C2C12 myotubes by attenuating IRS-1/PI3K/Akt pathway inhibition. Brazilian Journal of Medical and Biological Research 48: 440-446.

Lirussi, F., Beccarello, A., Zanette, G., De Monte, A., Donadon, V., Velussi, M. and Crepaldi, G., 2002. Silybin-beta-cyclodextrin in the treatment of patients with diabetes mellitus and alcoholic liver disease. Efficacy study of a new preparation of an anti-oxidant agent. Diabetes, Nutrition & Metabolism 15: 222-231.

Liu, K., Zhou, S., Liu, J., Wang, Y., Zhu, F. and Liu, M., 2019a. Silibinin attenuates high-fat diet-induced renal fibrosis of diabetic nephropathy. Drug Design, Development and Therapy 13: 3117.

Liu, R., Wang, Q., Ding, Z., Zhang, X., Li, Y., Zang, Y. and Zhang, G., 2020. Silibinin augments the antifibrotic effect of valsartan through inactivation of TGF-β1 signaling in kidney. Drug Design, Development and Therapy 14: 603-611.

Liu, Y., Ye, J., Cao, Y., Zhang, R., Wang, Y., Zhang, S., Dai, W. and Ye, S., 2019b. Silibinin ameliorates diabetic nephropathy via improving diabetic condition in the mice. European Journal of Pharmacology 845: 24-31.

Lu, C.P., Huang, C.Y., Wang, S.H., Chiu, C.H., Li, L.H., Hua, K.F. and Wu, T.H., 2018. Improvement of hyperglycemia in a murine model of insulin resistance and high glucose- and inflammasome-mediated IL-1β expressions in macrophages by silymarin. Chemico-Biological Interactions 290: 12-18.

MacDonald-Ramos, K., Michán, L., Martínez-Ibarra, A. and Cerbón, M., 2021. Silymarin is an ally against insulin resistance: A review. Annals of Hepatology 23: 100255.

Maessen, D.E., Stehouwer, C.D. and Schalkwijk, C.G., 2015. The role of methylglyoxal and the glyoxalase system in diabetes and other age-related diseases. Clinical Science 128: 839-861.

Malkani, N., Naeem, A., Ijaz, F., Mumtaz, S., Ashraf, S. and Sohail, M.I., 2020. *Silybum marianum* (milk thistle) improves vancomycin induced nephrotoxicity by downregulating apoptosis. Molecular Biology Reports 47: 5451-5459.

Mauvais-Jarvis, F., 2011. Estrogen and androgen receptors: regulators of fuel homeostasis and emerging targets for diabetes and obesity. Trends in Endocrinology & Metabolism 22: 24-33.

Meng, R., Mahadevan, J., Oseid, E., Vallerie, S. and Robertson, R.P., 2016. Silymarin activates c-AMP phosphodiesterase and stimulates insulin secretion in a glucose-dependent manner in HIT-T15 cells. Antioxidants 5: 47.

Meng, S., Yang, F., Wang, Y., Qin, Y., Xian, H., Che, H. and Wang, L., 2019. Silymarin ameliorates diabetic cardiomyopathy via inhibiting TGF-β1/Smad signaling. Cell Biology International 43: 65-72.

Mohamed Kamel, G.A., Harahsheh, E. and Hussein, S., 2022. Mechanisms underlying the hepatoprotective effect of silymarin on fluoxetine-induced liver injury in rats: the implication of peroxisome proliferator-activated receptor-gamma, PPAR-γ. Comparative Clinical Pathology 31: 689-698.

Neelofar, K., Arif, Z., Ahmad, J. and Alam, K., 2019. Inhibitory effect of silibinin on Amadori-albumin in diabetes mellitus: A multi-spectroscopic and biochemical approach. Spectrochimica Acta. Part A, Molecular and Biomolecular Spectroscopy 209: 217-222.

Oh, Y.S., 2015. Plant-derived compounds targeting pancreatic beta cells for the treatment of diabetes. Evidence-Based Complementary and Alternative Medicine 2015: 629863.

Omar, Z., Ahmed, A.A., El-Bakry, M.H., Ahmed, M.A. and Hasan, A., 2022. Metformin versus silymarin as hepatoprotective agents in mice fibrotic model caused by carbon tetrachloride. Annales Pharmaceutiques Francaises 80: 659-668.

Onaolapo, A.Y., Abdusalam, S.Z. and Onaolapo, O.J., 2017. Silymarin attenuates aspartame-induced variation in mouse behaviour, cerebrocortical morphology and oxidative stress markers. Pathophysiology 24: 51-62.

Paglialunga, S., Ludzki, A., Root-McCaig, J. and Holloway, G.P., 2015. In adipose tissue, increased mitochondrial emission of reactive oxygen species is important for short-term high-fat diet-induced insulin resistance in mice. Diabetologia 58: 1071-1080.

Palomino, O.M., Gouveia, N.M., Ramos, S., Martín, M.A. and Goya, L., 2017. Protective effect of *Silybum marianum* and silibinin on endothelial cells submitted to high glucose concentration. Planta Medica 83: 97-103.

Pferschy-Wenzig, E.M., Atanasov, A.G., Malainer, C., Noha, S.M., Kunert, O., Schuster, D., Heiss, E.H., Oberlies, N.H., Wagner, H., Bauer, R. and Dirsch, V.M., 2014. Identification of isosilybin a from milk thistle seeds as an agonist of peroxisome proliferator-activated receptor gamma. Journal of Natural Products 77: 842-847.

Pourheydar, B., Azarm, F., Farjah, G., Karimipour, M. and Pourheydar, M., 2022. Effect of silymarin and metformin on the sperm parameters and histopathological changes of testes in diabetic rats: An experimental study. International Journal of Reproductive Biomedicine 19: 1091-1104.

Prakash, P., Singh, V., Jain, M., Rana, M., Khanna, V., Barthwal, M.K. and Dikshit, M., 2014. Silymarin ameliorates fructose induced insulin resistance syndrome by reducing de novo hepatic lipogenesis in the rat. European Journal of Pharmacology 727: 15-28.

Qin, N., Sasaki, T., Li, W., Wang, J., Zhang, X., Li, D., Li, Z., Cheng, M., Hua, H. and Koike, K., 2018. Identification of flavonolignans from *Silybum marianum* seeds as allosteric protein tyrosine phosphatase 1B inhibitors. Journal of Enzyme Inhibition and Medicinal Chemistry 33: 1283-1291.

Quan, Y., Hua, S., Li, W., Zhan, M., Li, Y. and Lu, L., 2020. Resveratrol bidirectionally regulates insulin effects in skeletal muscle through alternation of intracellular redox homeostasis. Life Sciences 242: 117188.

Rahimi, R., Karimi, J., Khodadadi, I., Tayebinia, H., Kheiripour, N., Hashemnia, M. and Goli, F., 2018. Silymarin ameliorates expression of urotensin II (U-II) and its receptor (UTR) and attenuates toxic oxidative stress in the heart of rats with type 2 diabetes. Biomedicine & Pharmacotherapy 101: 244-250.

Rezabakhsh, A., Fathi, F., Bagheri, H.S., Malekinejad, H., Montaseri, A., Rahbarghazi, R. and Garjani, A., 2018. Silibinin protects human endothelial cells from high glucose-induced injury by enhancing autophagic response. Journal of Cellular Biochemistry 119: 8084-8094.

Rosario, W. and D'Alessio, D., 2015. An innate disposition for a healthier gut: Glp-1r signaling in intestinal epithelial lymphocytes. Diabetes 64: 2329-2331.

Sakashita, M., Tanaka, T. and Inagi, R., 2021. Metabolic changes and oxidative stress in diabetic kidney disease. Antioxidants 10: 1143.

Salazar-García, M. and Corona, J.C., 2021. The use of natural compounds as a strategy to counteract oxidative stress in animal models of diabetes mellitus. International Journal of Molecular Sciences 22: 7009.

Sheela, N., Jose, M.A., Sathyamurthy, D. and Kumar, B.N., 2013. Effect of silymarin on streptozotocin-nicotinamide-induced type 2 diabetic nephropathy in rats. Iranian Journal of Kidney Diseases 7: 117-123.

Shin, S., Lee, J.A., Kim, M., Kum, H., Jung, E. and Park, D., 2015. Anti-glycation activities of phenolic constituents from *Silybum marianum* (milk thistle) flower *in vitro* and on human explants. Molecules 20: 3549-3564.

Skottová, N. and Krecman, V., 1998. Silymarin as a potential hypocholesterolaemic drug. Physiological Research 47: 1-7.

Sobolová, L., Škottová, N., Večeřa, R. and Urbánek, K., 2006. Effect of silymarin and its polyphenolic fraction on cholesterol absorption in rats. Pharmacological Research 53: 104-112.

Soleymani, S., Ayati, M.H., Mansourzadeh, M.J., Namazi, N. and Zargaran, A., 2022. The effects of silymarin on the features of cardiometabolic syndrome in adults: A systematic review and meta-analysis. Phytotherapy Research 36: 842-856.

Soto, C., Mena, R., Luna, J., Cerbón, M., Larrieta, E., Vital, P., Uría, E., Sánchez, M., Recoba, R., Barrón, H., Favari, L. and Lara, A., 2004. Silymarin induces recovery of pancreatic function after alloxan damage in rats. Life Sciences 75: 2167-2180.

Soto, C., Raya, L., Juárez, J., Pérez, J. and González, I., 2014. Effect of silymarin in Pdx-1 expression and the proliferation of pancreatic β-cells in a pancreatectomy model. Phytomedicine 21: 233-239.

Stolf, A.M., Cardoso, C.C. and Acco, A., 2017. Effects of silymarin on diabetes mellitus complications: A review. Phytotherapy Research 31: 366-374.

Sun, Y., Yang, J., Liu, W., Yao, G., Xu, F., Hayashi, T., Onodera, S. and Ikejima, T., 2019. Attenuating effect of silibinin on palmitic acid-induced apoptosis and mitochondrial dysfunction in pancreatic β-cells is mediated by estrogen receptor alpha. Molecular and Cellular Biochemistry 460: 81-92.

Surai, P.F., 2015. Silymarin as a natural antioxidant: an overview of the current evidence and perspectives. Antioxidants 4: 204-247.

Surai, P.F., 2020. Vitagene in avian biology and poultry health. Wageningen Academic Publishers, Wageningen, The Netherlands.

Surai, P.F., Kochish, I.I., Fisinin, V.I. and Kidd, M.T., 2019. Antioxidant defence systems and oxidative stress in poultry biology: An update. Antioxidants 8; 235.

Surai, P.F., Kochish, I.I. and Kidd, M.T., 2021. Redox homeostasis in poultry: Regulatory roles of NF-κB. Antioxidants 10: 186.

Toğay, V.A., Sevimli, T.S., Sevimli, M., Çelik, D.A. and Özçelik, N., 2018. DNA damage in rats with streptozotocin-induced diabetes; protective effect of silibinin. Mutation research. Genetic Toxicology and Environmental Mutagenesis 825: 15-18.

Tuorkey, M.J., El-Desouki, N.I. and Kamel, R.A., 2015. Cytoprotective effect of silymarin against diabetes-induced cardiomyocyte apoptosis in diabetic rats. Biomedical and Environmental Sciences 28: 36-43.

Vaughu, C., Gotto, A.J. and Basson, C.T., 2006. The evolving role of silymarin in management of atherosclerosis. Journal of the American College of Cardiology 36: 1-5.

Velussi, M., Cernigoi, A.M., De Monte, A., Dapas, F., Caffau, C. and Zilli, M., 1997. Long-term (12 months) treatment with an anti-oxidant drug (silymarin) is effective on hyperinsulinemia, exogenous insulin need and malondialdehyde levels in cirrhotic diabetic patients. Journal of Hepatology 26: 871-879.

Velussi, M., Cernigoi, A.M., Viezzoli, L., Dapas, F., Caffau, C. and Zilli, M., 1993. Silymarin reduces hyperinsulinemia, malondialdehyde levels, and daily insulin need in cirrhotic diabetic patients. Current Therapeutic Research 53: 533-545.

Wang, J., Zhang, X., Zhang, L., Yan, T., Wu, B., Xu, F. and Jia, Y., 2020. Silychristin A activates Nrf2-HO-1/SOD2 pathway to reduce apoptosis and improve GLP-1 production through upregulation of estrogen receptor α in GLUTag cells. European Journal of Pharmacology 881: 173236.

Wang, J., Zhang, L., Cao, H., Shi, X., Zhang, X., Gao, Z., Ikeda, K., Yan, T., Jia, Y. and Xu, F., 2022. Silibinin improves L-cell mass and function through an estrogen receptor-mediated antioxidative mechanism. Phytomedicine 99: 154022.

World Health Organization (WHO), 2022. Diabetes. WHO, Geneva, Switzerland. Available at: https://www.tinyurl.com/2nk8ns5c.

Wu, C.H., Huang, S.M. and Yen, G.C., 2011. Silymarin: a novel antioxidant with antiglycation and anti-inflammatory properties *in vitro* and *in vivo*. Antioxidants & Redox Signaling 14: 353-366.

Xiao, F., Gao, F., Zhou, S. and Wang, L., 2020. The therapeutic effects of silymarin for patients with glucose/lipid metabolic dysfunction: A meta-analysis. Medicine 99: e22249.

Xiao, P., Yang, Z., Sun, J., Tian, J., Chang, Z., Li, X., Zhang, B., Ye, Y., Ji, H., Yu, E. and Xie, J., 2017. Silymarin inhibits adipogenesis in the adipocytes in grass carp Ctenopharyngodon idellus *in vitro* and *in vivo*. Fish physiology and Biochemistry 43: 1487-1500.

Xu, F., Yang, J., Negishi, H., Sun, Y., Li, D., Zhang, X., Hayashi, T., Gao, M., Ikeda, K., and Ikejima, T., 2018. Silibinin decreases hepatic glucose production through the activation of gut-brain-liver axis in diabetic rats. Food & Function 9: 4926-4935.

Yao, J., Zhi, M., Gao, X., Hu, P., Li, C. and Yang, X., 2013. Effect and the probable mechanisms of silibinin in regulating insulin resistance in the liver of rats with non-alcoholic fatty liver. Brazilian Journal of Medical and Biological Research 46: 270-277.

Yassin, N., AbouZid, S.F., El-Kalaawy, A.M., Ali, T.M., Elesawy, B.H. and Ahmed, O.M., 2021. Tackling of renal carcinogenesis in Wistar rats by *Silybum marianum* total extract, silymarin, and silibinin via modulation of oxidative stress, apoptosis, Nrf2, PPARγ, NF-κB, and PI3K/Akt signaling pathways. Oxidative Medicine and Cellular Longevity 2021: 7665169.

Yön, B., Belviranlı, M. and Okudan, N., 2019. The effect of silymarin supplementation on cognitive impairment induced by diabetes in rats. Journal of Basic and Clinical Physiology and Pharmacology 30: https://doi.org/10.1515/jbcpp-2018-0109.

Zhang, H.T., Shi, K., Baskota, A., Zhou, F.L., Chen, Y.X. and Tian, H.M., 2014. Silybin reduces obliterated retinal capillaries in experimental diabetic retinopathy in rats. European Journal of Pharmacology 740: 233-239.

Chapter 15

Protective actions of silymarin in arthritis and cardiovascular diseases

Health is not valued till sickness comes

Peter F. Surai[1-6] and Anton Surai[7]*

[1]Vitagene and Health Research Centre, Bristol, UK; [2]Department of Microbiology and Biochemistry, Faculty of Veterinary Medicine, Trakia University, Stara Zagora, Bulgaria; [3]Department of Animal Nutrition, Faculty of Agricultural and Environmental Sciences, Szent Istvan University, Hungary; [4]Saint-Petersburg State Academy of Veterinary Medicine, St. Petersburg, Russia; [5]Sumy National Agrarian University, Sumy, Ukraine; [6]Odessa National Academy of Food Technologies, Odessa, Ukraine; [7]Healthy Food Services, Bristol, UK

psurai@feedfood.co.uk

Abstract

The data presented in this chapter show protective effects of SM in arthritis and cardio-vascular diseases (CVD). Antioxidant, anti-inflammatory, anti-apoptotic and anti-toxic activities of SM are of great importance in prevention/treatment of the diseases, since redox disbalance and oxidative stress are driving forces of the disease development. Protective effects of SM in maintaining redox homeostasis and prevention of oxidative stress in arthritis and CVD are related to AO activities (prevention of LDL oxidation, control of vascular tone and endothelial integrity, etc.); up-regulation of Nrf2 and vitagenes, including sirtuins and HO-1 (adaptation to various stresses); decreasing expression of NF-κB and pro-inflammatory cytokines and prevention of over-inflammation (prevention of inflammatory reactions in vessels as an important mechanism of plaque formation); mitochondrial stabilisation (prevention of ROS overproduction); anti-toxic effects (prevention of cardiotoxicity of various drugs); regulatory actions on lipid/cholesterol metabolism (amelioration of plaque formation); immune-modulating actions (decreased inflammation and control of macrophage participation in plaque formation including preventing cholesterol accumulation in macrophages through the suppression of lipoproteins oxidation and regulation of cholesterol uptake and efflux); protective effects against other diseases (e.g. diabetes) which are important risk factors of CVD; other relevant mechanisms (e.g. regulatory effects on steroid receptors, microbiota, gut health, etc.). In various *in vitro* and *in vivo* animal model studies SM showed very promising results. However, in clinical trials the results are not always consistent due to various factors. In some cases, SM can be used directly for disease prevention/treatment, but it seems likely that use SM as complimentary therapy is of paramount importance in many diseases, due to the ability of SM to decrease toxic effects of a range of drugs. New, well designed clinical trials are needed to further substantiate protective effects of SM in arthritis and CVD.

DOI:10.3920/978-90-8686-944-2_015, © Wageningen Academic Publishers, 2023

Keywords: silymarin, arthritis, CVD, oxidative stress, redox homeostasis

15.1 Introduction

In previous chapters protective effects of SM/SB in fatty liver disease, neurodegenerative diseases and diabetes were described. However, redox disbalance and oxidative stress are considered to be major players in a wide range of other diseases including arthritis (Wruck *et al.*, 2011), atherosclerosis, chronic obstructive pulmonary disease, idiopathic pulmonary fibrosis, hypertension, systemic inflammatory response syndrome, ischaemia-reperfusion injury, cancer, etc. (Forman and Zhang *et al.*, 2021). Molecular mechanisms of protective effects of SM/SB in oxidative-stress-related diseases have been reviewed (Surai, 2015; 2022). Main points related to protective effects of SM/SB in arthritis and CVD are presented below.

15.2 Silymarin and arthritis

Arthritis is a term used to describe disorders that affect joints (joint inflammation) and currently there are many types of arthritis with the most common forms being osteoarthritis (OA; degenerative joint disease affecting 9.6% of men and 18% of women over 60 years of age) and rheumatoid arthritis (RA; affecting about 1% of the world population being more common in women; Abdel-Aziz *et al.*, 2021; NIAMS, 2022; Wu *et al.*, 2022).

OA is a multifactorial disease affecting synovial joints (knee, hip, spine and hand joints) with the joint of the knee being the most often affected site with observed pain, swelling, stiffness and joint instability. Multiple risk factors are reported to contribute to the disease development including age, body weight, mechanical stress, joint injury, genetics, etc. with the inflammation being central to the disease development (Abdel-Aziz *et al.*, 2021). The disease is a result of the interplay between systemic and local (or joint) factors. The systemic factors include age, gender, genetics, bone density, nutrition and obesity, while local ones are related to joint deformity, acute joint injury, joint laxity, muscle weakness, physical activity and occupational factors (Abdel-Aziz *et al.*, 2021). Furthermore, cell senescence, synovial inflammation and epigenetic alterations are believed to be closely involved in OA development (Zhang *et al.*, 2021).

It seems likely that redox disbalance and oxidative stress are among major factors affecting OA development (Lepetsos *et al.*, 2019) and disbalance in cytokine production and excess of pro-inflammatory cytokines lead to inflammation (Molnar *et al.*, 2021). Mono-iodoacetate (MIA) is known to be an inhibitor of glyceraldehyde-3-phosphate dehydrogenase leading to osteoarthritis (OA) signs including chondrocyte death, cartilage degeneration, osteophyte, and measurable changes in animal behaviour. Therefore, MIA-induced rodent model of OA is widely used in research and applications (Xu *et al.*, 2020). Several natural products and dietary supplements showed a potential activity for OA treatment (Abdel-Aziz *et al.*, 2021). The anti-inflammatory properties of SM can help dealing with OA. For example, in a MIA-induced OA model in rat SM was reported to exert anti-inflammatory effect and also to potentiate the anti-inflammatory effect of Celecoxib associated with regulation of the proinflammatory mediators at translational and transcriptional level (Ashkavand *et al.*, 2012). Furthermore, SB protects against OA *in vitro* (1, 10 and 50 μM) by inhibition of IL-1β-induced inflammation as well as PI3K/Akt phosphorylation and NF-κB activation in human OA chondrocytes. Furthermore, SB (200 mg/kg for 8 weeks) showed protective effects against cartilage matrix degradation in surgically induced OA by destabilisation of the medial meniscus in mice (Zheng *et al.*, 2017).

Rheumatoid arthritis (RA) is a typical, chronic, systemic autoimmune disease primarily damaging the joints by affecting the proliferation of joint synovial tissue, the formation of pannus and the destruction of cartilage (Wu *et al.*, 2021). It seems likely that cytokine-mediated pathways are involved in the pathogenesis of RA and at the affected joint, infiltrating immune cells can release a variety of cytokines, regulating immune response, including inflammation and immune pathology (Kondo *et al.*, 2021). Furthermore, it is proven that redox disbalance and oxidative stress are deeply involved in RA development (da Fonseca *et al.*, 2019).

Therefore, anti-inflammatory properties of SM are of great importance in RA prevention and treatment. It seems likely that inhibiting migration and activation of neutrophils in the articulations could be responsible for anti-inflammatory action of SM in RA (Mayer *et al.*, 2005). In particular, SB was shown to alleviate inflammation and induce apoptosis in human rheumatoid arthritis fibroblast-like synoviocytes *in vitro* and having a therapeutic effect on collagen-induced arthritis in rats *in vivo*. This anti-inflammatory SB action was a result of NF-κB suppression and SIRT1 regulation (Tong *et al.*, 2018). SB is considered to be the natural agonist of ERβ and a potential therapeutic tool to decrease inflammation in the treatment of autoimmune diseases, including RA. In T lymphocytes from healthy donors and patients with active RA, SB is reported to upregulate ERβ expression, to induce apoptosis, to inhibit proliferation, and to reduce expression of the pro-inflammatory cytokines IL-17 and TNF-α, through ERβ binding (Dupuis *et al.*, 2018). Among the developed animal models of rheumatoid arthritis (RA), adjuvant-induced arthritis (AIA) model reflecting a number of clinical characteristics of RA in humans, including inflammatory reactions and cartilage damages, is successfully applied in preclinical research. Therefore, in AIA rat model, SB was shown to ameliorate experimental RA and abnormal lipid metabolism by suppression of up-regulated liver X receptor controlling transcriptional programs involved in lipid homeostasis and inflammation with simultaneous reduction of the nuclear translocation of NF-κB (Xie *et al.*, 2021).

SM can also decrease various side effects and improve efficacy of RA drugs. For example, methotrexate (MTX) has been used as RA drug since 1980s and now it is the most commonly used disease modifying anti-rheumatic drug. It is usually used in combination with other RA drugs (Jiang *et al.*, 2021). However, MTX has a number of side effects and a search for drugs/nutrients helping avoid/decrease those side effects continues and SM could be one of those. For example, SM (100 mg/kg/day for 10 days, i.p.) was reported to attenuate MTX-induced pulmonary injury (AST and ALT in plasma, histopathological damage parameters in the rat pulmonary tissue samples) by targeting oxidative stress as evidenced by restoration of GPx and SOD activities in plasma (Kalemci *et al.*, 2015). SB (50, 100, or 150 mg/kg for 5 days) was reported to be also able to ameliorate some of the toxic effects of MTX in testicular tissue of mice (Oufi *et al.*, 2014).

MTX injection to rats caused renal damage exhibited in the form of inflammatory cell infiltration, glomerular and peritubular vascular congestion and swelling of renal tubular epithelium cells and SM showed protective effects. Indeed, SM treatment (300 mg/kg per day, i.p. for five consecutive days) led to statistically significant amelioration in the histological alterations and reduced the number of TUNEL-positive cells as compared with the MTX treated rats. In conclusion, SM treatment leads to a reduction on MTX-induced renal damage in rats (Dabak and Kocaman, 2015). Of note, SB (120 mg twice daily combined with their regular MTX regimen) was shown to improve the effects of MTX in patients with active RA as evidenced by significantly decreased IL-8, IL-6 and TNF-α levels. Significantly elevated Hb, IL-10, and IL-2 levels were also observed in the patients due to SM treatment (Hussain *et al.*, 2016).

15.3 Silymarin and cardiovascular diseases

Cardiovascular diseases (CVDs) are known to be the leading cause of death globally with 17.9 million people died from CVDs in 2019, representing 32% of all global deaths and one third of these deaths takes place in people under 70 years of age. From 1993 to 2019, the global prevalence of CVD nearly doubled and continue increasing (Goldsborough *et al.*, 2022). CVDs are a group of disorders of the heart and blood vessels including (WHO, 2022a):

- coronary heart disease;
- cerebrovascular disease;
- rheumatic heart disease;
- peripheral arterial disease;
- other conditions, including congenital heart disease, deep vein thrombosis and pulmonary embolism.

Four major behavioural risk factors of CVD are unhealthy diet, lack of physical inactivity, tobacco use and harmful use of alcohol. In addition, important CVD risk factors include raised blood pressure, raised blood glucose, raised blood lipids, increased blood cholesterol, especially LDL cholesterol, overweight and obesity, diabetes, metabolic syndrome, chronic inflammatory conditions, family history of CVD, ethnic background, age, gender and stress (NHS, 2022). Therefore, diet optimisation with increased fruit, vegetables and fibre consumption and decreased saturated fat, sugar and salt in the diet, regular physical activity, avoidance of alcohol excess and cessation of smoking are among major health style modifications which can help reducing risks of CVD development (WHO, 2022b).

It is known that heart is working hard in human body: it beats about 100,000 times a day using about 6 kg ATP (more than any other organ) and pumps approximately 10 tons of blood through the body (Neubauer, 2007). In this regard, mitochondria are known to be responsible for maintaining cellular health and their dysfunction involves energy deficits, excessive ROS generation, increased autophagy and apoptosis leading to metabolic abnormalities associated with the development of CVD. Cardiovascular pathologies including ischemic heart disease, heart failure, arterial hypertension, and cardiac arrhythmias are proven to be characterised by mitochondrial dysfunction (Stamerra *et al.*, 2022). CVD is associated with altered mitochondrial biogenesis and clearance leading to decreased ATP production and enhanced ROS formation (Chistiakov *et al.*, 2018). Abnormalities in cardiac energy metabolism are considered to be vital determinant of heart failure (Li *et al.*, 2020). Therefore, it is generally accepted that redox disbalance and oxidative stress are implicated in several forms of CVD including subjects with diabetes, hypertension and other metabolic disturbances. For example, patients with diabetes are shown to have increased blood sugar levels and their blood vessels are prone to damages and they are more likely to develop cardiovascular disease (Li *et al.*, 2020). Excessive ROS generation and a reduction in endogenous antioxidant/redox status are reported to be associated with CVD, including mitochondrial dysfunction, dyslipidaemia, and genetic predisposition (Kong *et al.*, 2022).

In general, abnormalities of lipid, glucose, salt, energy, and ROS metabolism are considered to be major drivers of atherosclerosis, the important pathogenic process underlying CVD associated with the atherosclerotic plaque formation within the arterial wall, obstructing the vessel lumen leading to consequent ischemia of the downstream tissues (Zullo *et al.*, 2022). Most classically successful therapies for CVD display antioxidant, anti-inflammatory and vasoprotective effects. However, only a few 'redox drugs' are in clinical use and many antioxidant strategies and antioxidant supplements have not met expectations (Daiber and Chlopicki, 2020).

Cardio-protective properties of SM/SB presented in a recent review (Taleb *et al.*, 2018) indicate that

- In 9 studies with rats SM/SB improved pulmonary vascular dysfunction, restored endothelial function and vascular tone, reduced blood pressure and heart rate, protected abdominal aorta I/R injury, reduced cerebral ischemic/reperfusion, normalise parameters and reduce cardiotoxicity, anticholesterolemic effects, decreased plasma lipids and increased HDL.
- In 2 studies with mice SM improved endothelial dysfunction, attenuated cardiac hypertrophy and decreased pro-inflammatory NF-κB.
- In 4 studies with rabbits SM protected abdominal aorta I/R injury, decreased cholesterol, reduced triglyceride and increased HDL.
- In 3 human studies SM showed cardioprotection for coronary artery bypass, reduced plasma lipids, increased HDL, reduced cholesterol and triglycerides.
- In 2 *in vitro* studies with HUVECs SM protected ECs, increased nitric oxide content, showed anti-atherosclerotic activity and decreased pro-inflammatory TNF-α.

In various *in vitro* and *in vivo* animal models SM/SB showed protective effects against cardiotoxicity of anti-cancer drugs, including doxorubicin and CS (Razavi and Karimi, 2016) and other cardiotoxic drugs (See Chapter 8). Treatment of hypercholesterolaemic rats with SB was shown to significantly decrease both serum and hepatic total cholesterol, triglycerides, VLDL-C, LDL-C and increased HDL-C (Gobalakrishnan *et al.*, 2016; Wang *et al.*, 2020). It was concluded that SB can increase energy consumption, reduce lipid synthesis, and improve lipid metabolism in mice *in vivo* (Wang *et al.*, 2020). SB treatment showed ameliorative effect against zidovudine + isoniazid-induced hepatotoxicity and hyperlipidaemia in rats (Ramanathan and Sivanesan, 2017). In hypercholesterolemia, SM/SB inhibits 3-hydroxy-3-methylglutaryl coenzyme A (HMG-CoA) reductase, reducing cholesterol synthesis (Sharma *et al.*, 2001). Therefore, SM was reported to have not only antioxidant, but also lipid-lowering, antihypertensive, antidiabetic, antiatherosclerotic, anti-obesity, and hepatoprotective effects (Tajmohammadi *et al.*, 2018).

Vascular dysfunction is believed to be a key initiator in atherosclerosis in the postmenopausal period. Interestingly, SB treatment (50 mg/kg/day) was reported to significantly ameliorate the adverse changes ovariectomised rats, including improved lipid profile and reduced oxidative stress, increased eNOS expression and diminished inflammatory status (Maleki *et al.*, 2022). SM treatment was reported to attenuate cirrhosis- and diabetes-associated cardiac remodelling and reduced cardiac mechanical dysfunctions via mitigation of

- ischemia/reperfusion injury (Rao and Viswanath, 2007);
- chemical-induced cardiotoxicity (Razavi and Karimi, 2016);
- cardiomyopathy (Meng *et al.*, 2019);
- cardiac hypertrophy (Ai *et al.*, 2010).

SM was found to ameliorate diabetic cardiomyopathy via inhibiting TGF-β1/Smad signalling (Meng *et al.*, 2019). SM administration was shown to mitigate cirrhotic-induced cardiac abnormality in the rats (Bayat *et al.*, 2022). Proteomics study on the effect of SB on cardiomyopathy in obese mice showed that TPM1, MYL2 and MYH11 proteins (involved in myocardial contraction) were down-regulated in high-fat diet fed mice and SB demonstrated clear ameliorative effect by up-regulating them (Wang *et al.*, 2021). SM administration as dietary supplements (1% for 4 weeks) to hereditary hypertriglyceridemic rats (a model of metabolic syndrome) was reported to significantly decrease the plasma levels of triglycerides, total cholesterol and markedly increased HDL cholesterol level (Poruba *et al.*, 2015).

Recent analyses of cardioprotective effects of SM in human (Kadoglou *et al.*, 2022) identified 4 major meta-analyses which included:

1. 5 randomised controlled trials (RCTs, 270 patients with T2D): improved glycaemic control, by reducing fasting blood glucose (FBG) and Glycated haemoglobin (HbA1c; Voroneanu *et al.*, 2016);
2. 7 RCTs (370 patients with T2D): improved FBG, HbA1c, Insulin, LDL-Cholesterol, MDA and HDL-Cholesterol levels (Hadi *et al.*, 2018);

3. 10 RCTs (620 adults with dyslipidaemia): improvement of all lipid parameters (Mohammadi *et al.*, 2019);
4. 16 published clinical trials (1,358 patients with glucose/metabolic dysfunction): reduced levels of FBG, insulin resistance, haemoglobin A1c, total cholesterol, triglyceride, LDL-cholesterol, C-reactive protein and increased HDL-cholesterol (Xiao *et al.*, 2020).

The authors indicated a modest improvement in glycaemic and lipid profile, but also noted important limitations of the clinical studies (Kadoglou *et al.*, 2022) including

- small sample size;
- inhomogeneous studies;
- a great variety in dosage, duration of treatment and patients characteristics;
- studies targeted mainly biomarkers and not clinical outcomes.

This led to variable/inconsistent results. The authors also mentioned 5 more randomised, double or triple-blinded, placebo-controlled clinical trials with results published in 2006-2018 with SM or SB usage alone or in combination with vitamins (D, E) and other herbal compounds confirming improved glycaemic indices, insulin sensitivity and lipid profile in T2D patients as a result SM/SB supplementation (Kadoglou *et al.*, 2022). A systematic review of literature and meta-analysis of the available randomised, double-blind, placebo-controlled clinical trials included five eligible trials, with 497 subjects, showed that SM and berberine combination treatment had an advantageous improvement in lipid and glucose profile, exerted a positive effect on TC, TG, HDL-C, LDL-C and fasting plasma glucose (Fogacci *et al.*, 2019).

SB is shown to improve the metabolic aspect and vascular damage in hypertensive patients with normal glucose tolerance patients who are at higher metabolic and cardiovascular risk suggesting that SB might strengthen the effect of antihypertensive drugs giving further cardiovascular protection (Sciacqua *et al.*, 2019). Recently data of 11 clinical trials have been analysed and the results indicated that SM significantly reduced the levels of fasting blood glucose, haemoglobin A1C, total cholesterol, triglyceride, low-density lipoprotein-cholesterol and increased high-density lipoprotein- cholesterol compared to placebo (Soleymani *et al.*, 2022).

Taking into account protective effects of SM/SB in maintaining redox homeostasis and prevention of oxidative stress described in previous chapters it is important to note that they are very relevant to prevention and treatment of CVD (Figure 15.1) including:

- antioxidant activities (prevention of LDL oxidation, control of vascular tone and endothelial integrity, etc.);
- up-regulation of Nrf2 and vitagenes, including sirtuins and HO-1 (adaptation to various stresses);
- decreasing expression of NF-κB and pro-inflammatory cytokines and prevention of over-inflammation (prevention of inflammatory reactions in vessels as an important mechanism of plaque formation);

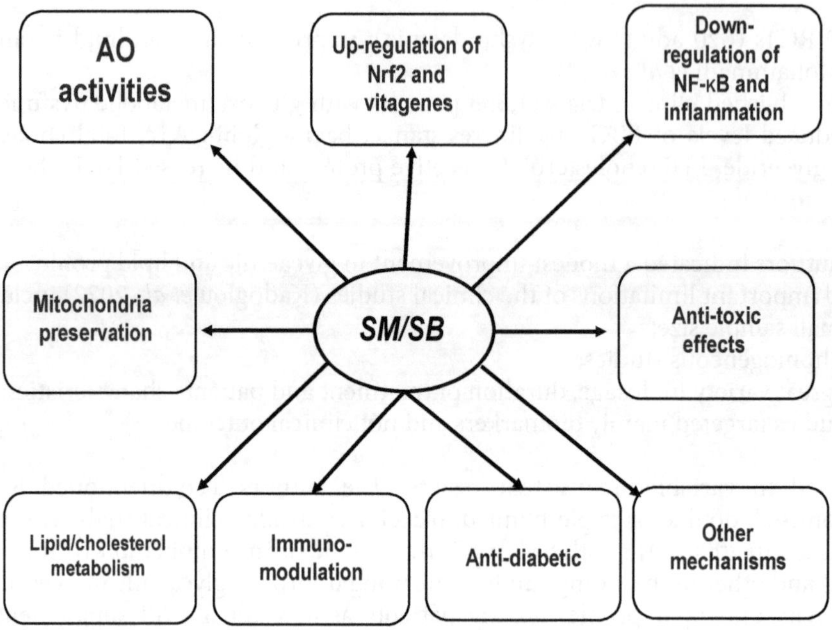

Figure 15.1. Cardioprotective mechanisms of SM/SB.

- mitochondrial stabilisation (prevention of ROS overproduction);
- anti-toxic effects (prevention of cardiotoxicity of various drugs);
- regulatory actions on lipid/cholesterol metabolism (amelioration of plaque formation);
- immune-modulating actions (decreased inflammation and control of macrophage participation in plaque formation including preventing cholesterol accumulation in macrophages through the suppression of lipoproteins oxidation and regulation of cholesterol uptake and efflux);
- protective effects against other diseases (e.g. diabetes) which are important risk factors of CVD;
- other relevant mechanisms (e.g. regulatory effects on steroid receptors, microbiota, gut health, etc.).

15.4 Anticancer activities of silymarin

Recently anti-cancer effects of SM/SB have received tremendous attention and was well covered in comprehensive reviews (Binienda *et al.*, 2020; Delmas *et al.*, 2020; Fallah *et al.*, 2021; Koltai and Fliegel, 2022; Prasad *et al.*, 2020; Tuli *et al.*, 2021; Verdura *et al.*, 2021; Wadhwa *et al.*, 2022). Recent patents related to the anticancer effects of *S. marianum* and silymarin have also been reviewed (Emadi *et al.*, 2022) with a conclusion that SM could be beneficial to oncology patients, including prevention of various side effects of anticancer chemotherapeutics. Because of lack of space in this book, we will not be able to address these issues and interested readers are advised to read the aforementioned review papers.

In general, anti-cancer protective activities of SM/SB are based on similar molecular mechanisms as we described for other diseases including antioxidant, anti-inflammatory, vitagene-activating, immune-modulatory and other activities. As a natural ERβ agonist, SB *in vitro* was demonstrated to induce apoptosis and autophagy, and blocked tumour cell proliferation. It also protected AC16 cardiomyocytes from doxorubicin-induced toxicity. Furthermore, *in vivo* SB was able to induce cell death and autophagy, and reduced tumour volume (Ortona *et al.*, 2022). SB-induced nuclear translocation of apoptosis-inducing factor in human breast cancer MCF-7 cells was also shown to be associated with ER activity (Liu *et al.*, 2020). SM at high doses was reported to provide anticancer effects via various mechanisms, including apoptosis induction, arrest of cell growth due to interruption of the MAPK cascade, downregulation of cyclin-dependent kinases, suppression of vascular endothelial growth factor and its receptor, inhibition of TGF-α and downregulation of protein kinase B and tumour fibrosis (Křen and Valentová, 2022).

It seems likely that wide distribution and easy accessibility of SM compounds with over-the-counter availability as a nutraceutical (not a drug), as well as some controversial issues related to its low bioavailability, has created a sceptical point of view in medical professionals on SM/SB anticancer effects (Koltai and Fliegel, 2022). Therefore, more research efforts in this area are expected in future.

Other protective actions of SM/SB are related to metabolic syndrome (Tajmohammadi *et al.*, 2018; Vahabzadeh *et al.*, 2018), thalassemia (Darvishi Khezri *et al.*, 2016; Moayedi Esfahani *et al.*, 2015; Zou *et al.*, 2017) and photoprotection (Couteau *et al.*, 2012; Kim *et al.*, 2019; Rajnochová Svobodová *et al.*, 2018; Vaid and Katiyar, 2010). Oral SM treatment is considered to be an effective complimentary procedure to improve phototherapy efficacy in patients with vitiligo (Jowkar *et al.*, 2020). Furthermore, SM is used for various skin disorders including melasma, anti-aging, sunscreen, acne, rosacea, psoriasis, skin cancer, photoprotection, cosmeceuticals, etc. (Dorjay *et al.*, 2018).

15.5 Conclusions

The aforementioned data clearly indicate protective effects of SM/SB in arthritis, CVD and cancer. Antioxidant, anti-inflammatory, anti-apoptotic and anti-toxic activities of SM/SB are of great importance in prevention/treatment of the diseases, since redox disbalance and oxidative stress are driving forces of the disease development. In various *in vitro* and *in vivo* animal model studies SM/SB showed very promising results. However, in clinical trials the results are not always consistent due to various factors. In some cases, SM/SB can be used directly for disease prevention/treatment, but it seems likely that use SM/SB as complimentary therapy is of paramount importance in many diseases, due to the ability of SM/SB to decrease toxic effects of a range of drugs. New, well designed clinical trials are needed to further substantiate protective effects of SM/SB in arthritis and CVD.

References

Abdel-Aziz, M.A., Ahmed, H., El-Nekeety, A.A. and Abdel-Wahhab, M.A., 2021. Osteoarthritis complications and the recent therapeutic approaches. Inflammopharmacology 29: 1653-1667.

Ai, W., Zhang, Y., Tang, Q.Z., Yan, L., Bian, Z.Y., Liu, C., Huang, H., Bai, X., Yin, L. and Li, H., 2010. Silibinin attenuates cardiac hypertrophy and fibrosis through blocking EGFR-dependent signaling. Journal of Cellular Biochemistry 110: 1111-1122.

Ashkavand, Z., Malekinejad, H., Amniattalab, A., Rezaei-Golmisheh, A. and Vishwanath, B.S., 2012. Silymarin potentiates the anti-inflammatory effects of Celecoxib on chemically induced osteoarthritis in rats. Phytomedicine 19: 1200-1205.

Bayat, G., Mazloom, R., Hashemi, S.A., Pourkhalili, K., Fallah, P., Shams, A., Esmaeili, P. and Khalili, A., 2022. Silymarin administration attenuates cirrhotic-induced cardiac abnormality in the rats: A possible role of β_1-adrenergic receptors and L-type voltage-dependent calcium channels. Iranian Journal of Medical Sciences 47: 367-378.

Binienda, A., Ziolkowska, S. and Pluciennik, E., 2020. The anticancer properties of silibinin: Its molecular mechanism and therapeutic effect in breast cancer. Anti-Cancer Agents in Medicinal Chemistry 20: 1787-1796.

Chistiakov, D.A., Shkurat, T.P., Melnichenko, A.A., Grechko, A.V. and Orekhov, A.N., 2018. The role of mitochondrial dysfunction in cardiovascular disease: a brief review. Annals of Medicine 50: 121-127.

Couteau, C., Cheignon, C., Paparis, E. and Coiffard, L.J., 2012. Silymarin, a molecule of interest for topical photoprotection. Natural Product Research 26: 2211-2214.

da Fonseca, L., Nunes-Souza, V., Goulart, M. and Rabelo, L.A., 2019. Oxidative stress in rheumatoid arthritis: What the future might hold regarding novel biomarkers and add-on therapies. Oxidative Medicine and Cellular Longevity 2019: 7536805.

Dabak, D.O. and Kocaman, N., 2015. Effects of silymarin on methotrexate-induced nephrotoxicity in rats. Renal Failure 37: 734-739.

Daiber, A. and Chlopicki, S., 2020. Revisiting pharmacology of oxidative stress and endothelial dysfunction in cardiovascular disease: Evidence for redox-based therapies. Free Radical Biology & Medicine 157: 15-37.

Darvishi Khezri, H., Salehifar, E., Kosaryan, M., Aliasgharian, A., Jalali, H. and Hadian Amree, A., 2016. Potential effects of silymarin and its flavonolignan components in patients with β-Thalassemia Major: A comprehensive review in 2015. Advances in Pharmacological Sciences 2016: 3046373.

Delmas, D., Xiao, J., Vejux, A. and Aires, V., 2020. Silymarin and cancer: A dual strategy in both in chemoprevention and chemosensitivity. Molecules 25: 2009.

Dorjay, K., Arif, T. and Adil, M., 2018. Silymarin: An interesting modality in dermatological therapeutics. Indian Journal of Dermatology, Venereology and Leprology 84: 238-243.

Dupuis, M.L., Conti, F., Maselli, A., Pagano, M.T., Ruggieri, A., Anticoli, S., Fragale, A., Gabriele, L., Gagliardi, M.C., Sanchez, M., Ceccarelli, F., Alessandri, C., Valesini, G., Ortona, E. and Pierdominici, M., 2018. The natural agonist of estrogen receptor β silibinin plays an immunosuppressive role representing a potential therapeutic tool in Rheumatoid Arthritis. Frontiers in Immunology 9: 1903.

Emadi, S.A., Ghasemzadeh Rahbardar, M., Mehri, S. and Hosseinzadeh, H., 2022. A review of therapeutic potentials of milk thistle (*Silybum marianum* L.) and its main constituent, silymarin, on cancer, and their related patents. Iranian Journal of Basic Medical Sciences 25: 1166-1176.

Fallah, M., Davoodvandi, A., Nikmanzar, S., Aghili, S., Mirazimi, S., Aschner, M., Rashidian, A., Hamblin, M.R., Chamanara, M., Naghsh, N. and Mirzaei, H., 2021. Silymarin (milk thistle extract) as a therapeutic agent in gastrointestinal cancer. Biomedicine & Pharmacotherapy 142: 112024.

Fogacci, F., Grassi, D., Rizzo, M. and Cicero, A., 2019. Metabolic effect of berberine-silymarin association: A meta-analysis of randomized, double-blind, placebo-controlled clinical trials. Phytotherapy Research 33: 862-870.

Forman, H.J. and Zhang, H., 2021. Targeting oxidative stress in disease: promise and limitations of antioxidant therapy. Nature Reviews. Drug Discovery 20: 689-709.

Gobalakrishnan, S., Asirvatham, S.S. and Janarthanam, V., 2016. Effect of silybin on lipid profile in hypercholesterolaemic rats. Journal of Clinical and Diagnostic Research 10: FF01-FF5.

Goldsborough, E., 3rd, Osuji, N. and Blaha, M.J., 2022. Assessment of cardiovascular disease risk: a 2022 update. Endocrinology and Metabolism Clinics of North America 51: 483-509.

Hadi, A., Pourmasoumi, M., Mohammadi, H., Symonds, M. and Miraghajani, M., 2018. The effects of silymarin supplementation on metabolic status and oxidative stress in patients with type 2 diabetes mellitus: A systematic review and meta-analysis of clinical trials. Complementary Therapies in Medicine 41: 311-319.

Hussain, S.A., Mortada, A.H., Jasim, N.A. and Gorial, F.I., 2016. Silibinin improves the effects of methotrexate in patients with active rheumatoid arthritis: Pilot clinical study. Oman Medical Journal 31: 263.

Jiang, X., Zeng, J., Chen, F. and Li, J., 2021. Systematic review and meta-analysis on the efficacy of methotrexate in rheumatoid arthritis. Annals of Palliative Medicine 10: 10652-10660.

Jowkar, F., Godarzi, H. and Parvizi, M.M., 2020. Can we consider silymarin as a treatment option for vitiligo? A double-blind controlled randomized clinical trial of phototherapy plus oral *Silybum marianum* product versus phototherapy alone. The Journal of Dermatological Treatment 31: 256-260.

Kadoglou, N., Panayiotou, C., Vardas, M., Balaskas, N., Kostomitsopoulos, N.G., Tsaroucha, A.K. and Valsami, G., 2022. A comprehensive review of the cardiovascular protective properties of silibinin/silymarin: A new kid on the block. Pharmaceuticals 15: 538.

Kalemci, S., Topal, Y., Celik, S.Y., Yilmaz, N., Beydilli, H., Kosar, M.I., Dirican, N. and Altuntas, I., 2015. Silibinin attenuates methotrexate-induced pulmonary injury by targeting oxidative stress. Experimental and Therapeutic Medicine 10: 503-507.

Kim, D., Bae, W.R., Kim, Y.S., Shin, D.W., Park, S.G. and Kang, N.G., 2019. Photoprotective effects of *Silybum marianum* extract. Journal of the Society of Cosmetic Scientists of Korea 45: 209-216.

Koltai, T. and Fliegel, L., 2022. Role of silymarin in cancer treatment: Facts, hypotheses, and questions. Journal of Evidence-Based Integrative Medicine 27: 2515690X211068826.

Kondo, N., Kuroda, T. and Kobayashi, D., 2021. Cytokine networks in the pathogenesis of rheumatoid arthritis. International Journal of Molecular Sciences 22: 10922.

Kong, A.S., Lai, K.S., Hee, C.W., Loh, J.Y., Lim, S. and Sathiya, M., 2022. Oxidative stress parameters as biomarkers of cardiovascular disease towards the development and progression. Antioxidants 11: 1175.

Křen, V. and Valentová, K., 2022. Silybin and its congeners: from traditional medicine to molecular effects. Natural Product Reports 39: 1264-1281.

Lepetsos, P., Papavassiliou, K.A. and Papavassiliou, A.G., 2019. Redox and NF-κB signaling in osteoarthritis. Free Radical Biology & Medicine 132: 90-100.

Li, A., Gao, M., Jiang, W., Qin, Y. and Gong, G., 2020. Mitochondrial dynamics in adult cardiomyocytes and heart diseases. Frontiers in Cell and Developmental Biology 8: 584800.

Liu, W., Ji, Y., Sun, Y., Si, L., Fu, J., Hayashi, T., Onodera, S. and Ikejima, T., 2020. Estrogen receptors participate in silibinin-caused nuclear translocation of apoptosis-inducing factor in human breast cancer MCF-7 cells. Archives of Biochemistry and Biophysics 689: 108458.

Maleki, N., Khosh Ravesh, R., Salehiyeh, S., Faisal Faiz, A., Ebrahimi, M., Sharbati, A., Panji, M., Ajami Khiyavi, H., Safizadeh, F., Abbasi, M., Abazari, O., Norbakhsh, R. and Eskandari, Y., 2022. Comparative effects of estrogen and silibinin on cardiovascular risk biomarkers in ovariectomized rats. Gene 823: 146365.

Mayer, K.E., Myers, R.P. and Lee, S.S., 2005. Silymarin treatment of viral hepatitis: a systematic review. Journal of Viral Hepatitis 12: 559-567.

Meng, S., Yang, F., Wang, Y., Qin, Y., Xian, H., Che, H. and Wang, L., 2019. Silymarin ameliorates diabetic cardiomyopathy via inhibiting TGF-β1/Smad signaling. Cell Biology International 43: 65-72.

Moayedi Esfahani, B.A., Reisi, N. and Mirmoghtadaei, M., 2015. Evaluating the safety and efficacy of silymarin in β-thalassemia patients: a review. Hemoglobin 39: 75-80.

Mohammadi, H., Hadi, A., Arab, A., Moradi, S. and Rouhani, M.H., 2019. Effects of silymarin supplementation on blood lipids: A systematic review and meta-analysis of clinical trials. Phytotherapy Research 33: 871-880.

Molnar, V., Matišić, V., Kodvanj, I., Bjelica, R., Jeleč, Ž., Hudetz, D., Rod, E., Čukelj, F., Vrdoljak, T., Vidović, D., Starešinić, M., Sabalić, S., Dobričić, B., Petrović, T., Antičević, D., Borić, I., Košir, R., Zmrzljak, U.P. and Primorac, D., 2021. Cytokines and chemokines involved in osteoarthritis pathogenesis. International Journal of Molecular Sciences 22: 9208.

Neubauer, S., 2007. The failing heart-an engine out of fuel. The New England Journal of Medicine 356: 1140-1151.

National Health Service (NHS), 2022. Cardiovascular disease. NHS, Leeds, UK. Available at: https://www.tinyurl.com/3ux6eu7u.

National Institute of Arthritis and Musculoskeletal and Skin Diseases (NIAMS), 2022. Arthritis and rheumatic diseases. NIAMS, Bethesda, MD, USA. Available at: https://tinyurl.com/hh8jpznj.

Ortona, E., Locatelli, S.L., Pagano, M.T., Ascione, B., Careddu, G., Dupuis, M.L., Marconi, M., Carlo-Stella, C., Malorni, W., Matarrese, P. and Pierdominici, M., 2022. The natural estrogen receptor beta agonist silibinin as a promising therapeutic tool in diffuse large B-cell lymphoma. Anticancer Research 42: 767-779.

Oufi, H.G. and Al-Shawi, N.N., 2014. The effects of different doses of silibinin in combination with methotrexate on testicular tissue of mice. European Journal of Pharmacology 730: 36-40.

Poruba, M., Kazdová, L., Oliyarnyk, O., Malinská, H., Matusková, Z., Tozzi di Angelo, I., Skop, V. and Vecera, R., 2015. Improvement bioavailability of silymarin ameliorates severe dyslipidemia associated with metabolic syndrome. Xenobiotica 45: 751-756.

Prasad, R.R., Paudel, S., Raina, K. and Agarwal, R., 2020. Silibinin and non-melanoma skin cancers. Journal of Traditional and Complementary Medicine 10: 236-244.

Rajnochová Svobodová, A., Gabrielová, E., Michaelides, L., Kosina, P., Ryšavá, A., Ulrichová, J., Zálešák, B. and Vostálová, J., 2018. UVA-photoprotective potential of silymarin and silybin. Archives of Dermatological Research 310: 413-424.

Ramanathan, R. and Sivanesan, K., 2017. Evaluation of ameliorative ability of silibinin against zidovudine and isoniazid-induced hepatotoxicity and hyperlipidaemia in rats: Role of silibinin in phase I and II drug metabolism. Chemico-Biological Interactions 273: 142-153.

Rao, P.R. and Viswanath, R.K., 2007. Cardioprotective activity of silymarin in ischemia-reperfusion-induced myocardial infarction in albino rats. Experimental and Clinical Cardiology 12: 179-187.

Razavi, B.M. and Karimi, G., 2016. Protective effect of silymarin against chemical-induced cardiotoxicity. Iranian Journal of Basic Medical Sciences 19: 916-923.

Sciacqua, A., Perticone, M., Tripepi, G., Addesi, D., Cassano, V., Maio, R., Sesti, G. and Perticone, F., 2019. Metabolic and vascular effects of silybin in hypertensive patients with high 1-h post-load plasma glucose. Internal and Emergency Medicine 14: 77-84.

Sharma, Y., Agarwal, C., Singh, A.K. and Agarwal, R., 2001. Inhibitory effect of silibinin on ligand binding to erbB1 and associated mitogenic signaling, growth, and DNA synthesis in advanced human prostate carcinoma cells. Molecular Carcinogenesis 30: 224-236.

Soleymani, S., Ayati, M.H., Mansourzadeh, M.J., Namazi, N. and Zargaran, A., 2022. The effects of silymarin on the features of cardiometabolic syndrome in adults: A systematic review and meta-analysis. Phytotherapy Research 36: 842-856.

Stamerra, C.A., Di Giosia, P., Giorgini, P., Ferri, C., Sukhorukov, V.N. and Sahebkar, A., 2022. Mitochondrial dysfunction and cardiovascular disease: Pathophysiology and emerging therapies. Oxidative Medicine and Cellular Longevity 2022: 9530007.

Surai, P.F., 2015. Silymarin as a natural antioxidant: an overview of the current evidence and perspectives. Antioxidants 4: 204-247.

Surai, P.F., 2022. Silymarin as a vitagene modulator: effects on mitochondria integrity in stress conditions. In: Ostojik, S.M. (ed) Molecular nutrition and mitochondria. Elsevier, Academic Press, London, UK, pp. 535-559.

Tajmohammadi, A., Razavi, B.M. and Hosseinzadeh, H., 2018. *Silybum marianum* (milk thistle) and its main constituent, silymarin, as a potential therapeutic plant in metabolic syndrome: A review. Phytotherapy Research 32: 1933-1949.

Taleb, A., Ahmad, K.A., Ihsan, A.U., Qu, J., Lin, N., Hezam, K., Koju, N., Hui, L. and Qilong, D., 2018. Antioxidant effects and mechanism of silymarin in oxidative stress induced cardiovascular diseases. Biomedicine & Pharmacotherapy 102: 689-698.

Tong, W.W., Zhang, C., Hong, T., Liu, D.H., Wang, C., Li, J., He, X.K. and Xu, W.D., 2018. Silibinin alleviates inflammation and induces apoptosis in human rheumatoid arthritis fibroblast-like synoviocytes and has a therapeutic effect on arthritis in rats. Scientific Reports 8: 3241.

Tuli, H.S., Mittal, S., Aggarwal, D., Parashar, G., Parashar, N.C., Upadhyay, S.K., Barwal, T.S., Jain, A., Kaur, G., Savla, R., Sak, K., Kumar, M., Varol, M., Iqubal, A. and Sharma, A.K., 2021. Path of silibinin from diet to medicine: A dietary polyphenolic flavonoid having potential anti-cancer therapeutic significance. Seminars in Cancer Biology 73: 196-218.

Vahabzadeh, M., Amiri, N. and Karimi, G., 2018. Effects of silymarin on metabolic syndrome: a review. Journal of the Science of Food and Agriculture 98: 4816-4823.

Vaid, M. and Katiyar, S.K., 2010. Molecular mechanisms of inhibition of photocarcinogenesis by silymarin, a phytochemical from milk thistle, *Silybum marianum* L. Gaertn. International Journal of Oncology 36: 1053-1060.

Verdura, S., Cuyàs, E., Ruiz-Torres, V., Micol, V., Joven, J., Bosch-Barrera, J. and Menendez, J.A., 2021. Lung cancer management with silibinin: A historical and translational perspective. Pharmaceuticals 14: 559.

Voroneanu, L., Nistor, I., Dumea, R., Apetrii, M. and Covic, A., 2016. Silymarin in type 2 diabetes mellitus: A systematic review and meta-analysis of randomized controlled trials. Journal of Diabetes Research 2016: 5147468.

Wadhwa, K., Pahwa, R., Kumar, M., Kumar, S., Sharma, P.C., Singh, G., Verma, R., Mittal, V., Singh, I., Kaushik, D. and Jeandet, P., 2022. Mechanistic insights into the pharmacological significance of silymarin. Molecules 27: 5327.

Wang, F., Chen, S., Ren, L., Wang, Y., Li, Z., Song, T., Zhang, H. and Yang, Q., 2020. The Effect of silibinin on protein expression profile in white adipose tissue of obese mice. Frontiers in Pharmacology 11: 55.

Wang, F., Li, Z., Song, T., Jia, Y., Qi, L., Ren, L. and Chen, S., 2021. Proteomics study on the effect of silybin on cardiomyopathy in obese mice. Scientific Reports 11: 7136.

World Health Organization (WHO), 2022a. Cardiovascular diseases. WHO, Geneva, Switzerland. Available at: https://tinyurl.com/mv9pjxh3.

World Health Organization (WHO), 2022b. Cardiovascular diseases (CVDs). WHO, Geneva, Switzerland. Available at: https://www.tinyurl.com/56era46d.

Wruck, C.J., Fragoulis, A., Gurzynski, A., Brandenburg, L.O., Kan, Y.W., Chan, K., Hassenpflug, J., Freitag-Wolf, S., Varoga, D., Lippross, S. and Pufe, T., 2011. Role of oxidative stress in rheumatoid arthritis: insights from the Nrf2-knockout mice. Annals of the Rheumatic Diseases 70: 844-850.

Wu, Q., Zhao, J. and Guo, W., 2022. Efficacy of massage therapy in improving outcomes in knee osteoarthritis: A systematic review and meta-analysis. Complementary Therapies in Clinical Practice 46: 101522.

Wu, Z., Ma, D., Yang, H., Gao, J., Zhang, G., Xu, K. and Zhang, L., 2021. Fibroblast-like synoviocytes in rheumatoid arthritis: surface markers and phenotypes. International Immunopharmacology 93: 107392.

Xiao, F., Gao, F., Zhou, S. and Wang, L., 2020. The therapeutic effects of silymarin for patients with glucose/lipid metabolic dysfunction: A meta-analysis. Medicine 99: e22249.

Xie, Y., Feng, S.L., Mai, C.T., Zheng, Y.F., Wang, H., Liu, Z.Q., Zhou, H. and Liu, L., 2021. Suppression of up-regulated LXRα by silybin ameliorates experimental rheumatoid arthritis and abnormal lipid metabolism. Phytomedicine 80: 153339.

Xu, J., Yan, L., Yan, B., Zhou, L., Tong, P. and Shan, L., 2020. Osteoarthritis pain model induced by intra-articular injection of mono-iodoacetate in rats. Journal of Visualized Experiments 159: e60649.

Zhang, X.X., He, S.H., Liang, X., Li, W., Li, T.F. and Li, D.F., 2021. Aging, cell senescence, the pathogenesis and targeted therapies of osteoarthritis. Frontiers in Pharmacology 12: 728100.

Zheng, W., Feng, Z., Lou, Y., Chen, C., Zhang, C., Tao, Z., Li, H., Cheng, L. and Ying, X., 2017. Silibinin protects against osteoarthritis through inhibiting the inflammatory response and cartilage matrix degradation *in vitro* and *in vivo*. Oncotarget 8: 99649-99665.

Zou, H., Zhu, X.X., Zhang, G.B., Ma, Y., Wu, Y. and Huang, D.S., 2017. Silibinin: an old drug for hematological disorders. Oncotarget 8: 89307-89314.

Zullo, A., Guida, R., Sciarrillo, R. and Mancini, F.P., 2022. Redox homeostasis in cardiovascular disease: The role of mitochondrial sirtuins. Frontiers in Endocrinology 13: 858330.

Chapter 16
Other beneficial effects of silymarin

A stich in time saves nine

Anton Surai[1] and Peter F. Surai[2-7]*
[1]Healthy Food Services, Bristol, UK; [2]Vitagene and Health Research Centre, Bristol, UK; [3]Department of Microbiology and Biochemistry, Faculty of Veterinary Medicine, Trakia University, Stara Zagora, Bulgaria; [4]Department of Animal Nutrition, Faculty of Agricultural and Environmental Sciences, Szent Istvan University, Hungary; [5]Saint-Petersburg State Academy of Veterinary Medicine, St. Petersburg, Russia; [6]Sumy National Agrarian University, Sumy, Ukraine; [7]Odessa National Academy of Food Technologies, Odessa, Ukraine
psurai@feedfood.co.uk

Abstract

In this chapter additional protective effects of silymarin (SM) are described including amatoxin-containing mushrooms poisoning, burn recovery, anti-aging effects, effects on multidrug resistance, combined protective effects of SM and other antioxidants and SM-drug interactions. Taking into account the lack of alternative effective treatments and the relatively few adverse effects, SM could be an important part of chemotherapy of patients with amatoxin-containing mushrooms poisoning. SM was shown promising results in burn recovery and wound healing. Since taurine and carnitine also possess hepatoprotective properties their combination with SM could be an important addition to the existing hepatoprotectors. Furthermore, various combinations of SM with organic Se deserve more attention. The multidrug resistance (MDR) phenomenon is a serious medical problem creating a major challenge to the treatment of infectious diseases and cancer and various components of SM were shown to modulate MDR by the direct inhibition of P-gp or by downregulating the expression of the dominant transmembrane efflux pumps. Some of SM components were able to completely reverse antibiotic resistance at comparatively low concentrations. This is of great importance for clinical practise and veterinary applications. SM also demonstrated anti-aging effects and decreased detrimental consequences of various stresses, including over-exercising. It seems likely that SM could be an important supplement in sport medicine. Furthermore, various protective effects of SM in stress conditions are a background for its inclusion into anti-stress supplements. SM-drug interactions are of great importance for clinical practice. In general, there are some cases where SM showed inhibition of activities of enzymes and transporters associated with the pharmacokinetics of therapeutic drugs, but SM bioavailability is comparatively low and its concentrations achievable within the human body are usually too low to impose significant inhibition and such effects are unlikely to manifest in clinical settings.

Keywords: silymarin, multidrug resistance, amatoxin, drugs, anti-ageing, anti-stress

DOI:10.3920/978-90-8686-944-2_016,

16.1 Introduction

In previous chapters protective effects of SM/SB in liver diseases, neurological disorders, diabetes, arthritis and CVD were described. However, there is a range of other medical conditions (e.g. amatoxin-containing mushrooms poisoning, multidrug resistance, burn recovery, various stress conditions, etc.) where SM/SB clearly showed protective effects and they will be considered in this chapter.

16.2 SM and amatoxin-containing mushrooms poisoning

The amatoxins include at least 9 different toxins with α-amatoxin being the most hepatotoxic one with the estimated median lethal dose for adults to be about 7-8 mg of toxin. The amatoxins are thermally stable and are not inactivated by cooking. They are found mainly in 3 genera of mushrooms including *Amanita, Lepiota and Galerina.* It is known that the amatoxins are selective inhibitors of RNA polymerases, which are critical enzymes required for the synthesis of messenger RNA and microRNAs, essential elements for protein synthesis and liver homeostasis (Diaz *et al.*, 2018). Therefore, the ingestion of amatoxin-containing mushrooms is known to result in hyperacute liver damage (Gillessen and Schmidt, 2020) and has a bad prognosis due to the high risk of liver failure (Garcia *et al.*, 2015). Of note, amatoxin poisoning is difficult to diagnose due to delayed onset of symptoms. The optimal management of the poisoning is still not determined and therapeutic options usually include various detoxication procedures, chemotherapies and liver transplant and more research work needs to be conducted to improve therapeutic efficacy against amatoxins intoxication (Garcia *et al.*, 2015).

There are some old references for protective effects of SM in mice and dogs poisoned with *A. phallaides* extracts presented by Enjalbert *et al.* (2002) but more importantly is to consider usage of SM in treatment of patients consumed amatoxin-containing mushrooms. Among the amatoxin poisoning cases found in the literature for 20 years, 2,108 amatoxin poisoning cases were adequately documented by hospital reports with detailed therapeutic information and they were analysed in detail by Enjalbert *et al.* (2002). In particular SB was given to 38.2% of patients and the chemotherapies with the lowest mortality rates were shown to include SB as mono-chemotherapy and SB plus benzylpenicillin without and with other drugs. Eight years later additional statistical analysis of the same data confirmed importance of SM in treatment of amatoxin poisoning (Poucheret *et al.*, 2010). Two cases of amatoxin poisoning as a result of *Amanita* mushroom ingestion in the north-eastern United States successfully treated with N-acetylcysteine, high-dose penicillin, cimetidine, and SM, as part of their treatment regimen were described (Ward *et al.*, 2013). It seems likely that parenteral use of a SB-based formulation may be considered as the treatment of choice in amatoxin-containing mushrooms poisoning (Broussard *et al.*, 2001; Mengs *et al.*, 2012). Importantly, there are no antidotes or specific effective treatments for amatoxin-containing mushroom poisonings (Diaz, 2018). Based on animal studies and limited human data, Garcia *et al.* (2015) concluded that SB is the most promising chemical to prevent liver damages and decrease toxicological symptomatology after amatoxin intoxications. A shortcut review on usage of SB to reduce liver transplantation and death after poisoning with amatoxin-containing mushrooms was conducted by Lacombe and St-Onge (2016) based on five papers presented substantial evidence to answer the clinical question. The authors concluded that, only the limited evidence supported SB efficacy.

However, taking into account the lack of alternative effective treatments and the relatively few adverse effects, the authors recommended SB to be used in patients with amatoxin-containing mushrooms poisoning (Lacombe and St-Onge, 2016). Interestingly, in amatoxin poisoning, Portuguese Poisoning Information Center and the National Poisons Center of New Zealand recommend to administrate SM intravenously at a dose of 20-50 mg/kg/day and continued for 48-96 h (Ye and Liu, 2018).

16.3 Silymarin in exercising and stress

SM administration (50 mg/kg) was shown to ameliorate exercise-induced gluconeogenesis and β-oxidation through the regulation of PPARγ, phosphoenol pyruvate carboxykinase and pyruvate dehydrogenase kinase 4 (Choi *et al.*, 2016). Therefore, the authors suggested that intake of SM during exercise might improve endurance. Later anti-fatigue activity of SM was confirmed (Jia and Zhao, 2022). The SM was used orally (50, 100, and 200 mg/kg for 4 weeks). The fatigue level and exercise performance of mice were evaluated. It was shown that SM treatment decreased the blood lactic acid and serum urea nitrogen levels while increased the liver glycogen and muscle glycogen levels. The mouse skeletal muscle integrity after exercising was improved by SM treatment (Jia and Zhao, 2022).

In addition, silymarin decreased plasma lactate and ammonia levels and CK activity after swimming test, this is related to the mechanism that increases energy storage (as glycogen) and release (as blood glucose), and decreases plasma levels of lactate, ammonia, and CK. The observation of the skeletal muscle structures of mice also confirmed that skeletal muscles became more damaged in the control group compared with the silymarin-treated mice after prolonged endurance exercise. Therefore, it is reasonable to infer that silymarin may bear potential pharmacological effects in combating fatigue.

Simultaneous aerobic training and SM (140 mg/kg daily) was found to have interactive effects on reducing glycaemic indices and liver enzymes in men with type 2 diabetes (Ghalandari *et al.*, 2023). In rats subjected to regular exercise training, SM (100 mg/kg, 30-40 min prior to the training session) was reported to improve muscle recovery, to ameliorate inflammation and to promote hypertrophy, vascularisation, and muscle fibre shape/appearance and SM was shown to be more effective than vitamin C (Vargas-Mendoza *et al.*, 2020). SM administration (100 mg) to rats subjected to an 8-week exercise training was found to increase alveolar and bronchial muscle size, improve vascularisation, reduce tissue inflammation and to promote the reduction of lipid content in the liver (Vargas-Mendoza *et al.*, 2021). SB (25, 50 and 100 mg/kg by oral gavage daily prior to physical exercise) was reported to prevent impairment of learning and memory caused by excessive physical exercise in rats, accompanied by reduced apoptosis and senescence in hippocampus cells (Liu *et al.*, 2019). Therefore, it seems likely that SM/SB has protective effects under various stress conditions, including over-exercising.

There is a range of stresses in human life and animal production, including environmental, technological (for animals), nutritional, psychological and internal stresses (Surai, 2020). At the molecular level major stresses disturb redox homeostasis and impose oxidative stress leading to the development of various diseases. Therefore, SM/SB possessing strong antioxidant potential (Chapter 4) can substantially decrease detrimental consequences of various stresses. For instance, SM was reported to significantly suppress the development of gastric lesions in aspirin- or water immersion-restraint stress-induced gastritis models (Shin *et al.*, 2013).

After 5 consecutive weeks of chronic unpredictable mild stress (CUMS), the mice were treated with SB (100, 200 and 400 mg/kg by oral gavage) for 3 consecutive weeks. SB administration was shown to significantly ameliorate the CUMS-induced depressive-like behaviour and improving neuroplasticity and neurotransmission. In particular, SB treatment was indicated to enhance the levels of brain-derived neurotrophic factor (BDNF), serotonin (5-HT) and norepinephrine (NE) in the prefrontal cortex and hippocampus (Yan *et al.*, 2015). Mice subjected to CUMS was found to demonstrate increased immobility time without affecting general locomotion of the animals, reduced BDNF, 5-HT, NE, and DA level, increased serum corticosterone, IL-6 and TNF-α as well as compromised AO defences in the hippocampus and cerebral cortex. SM (100 mg/kg and 200 mg/kg for 3 weeks) was reported to significantly reversed the CUMS-induced changes in the hippocampus and cerebral cortex in mice (Thakare *et al.*, 2018). Interestingly SM was found to activate stress and repair responses that culminate in an anti-inflammatory cellular phenotype (Lovelace *et al.*, 2015). SM was reported to ameliorate restraint stress-induced acute liver injury as a result of mitigation of oxidative stress and reducing inflammatory response associated with blocking JNK activation and subsequently apoptotic signalling (Kim *et al.*, 2016).

SM showed antidepressant-like activity in the acute restraint stress in mice as a result of modulation of corticosterone and oxidative stress response in cerebral cortex and hippocampus (Thakare *et al.*, 2016) with involvement of hippocampal BDNF signalling, inflammatory cytokines and oxidative stress response (Thakare *et al.*, 2017). Intraperitoneal administration of SM protects end organs from multivisceral I/R injury in a rat model. Multivisceral I/R stress in rats damaging end organs was ameliorated by intraperitoneal administration of SM (Koçarslan *et al.*, 2016). For more details on protective effects of SM/SB in I/R-associated stress see Chapter 8. SM was indicated to mitigate lung impairments in a rat model of acute respiratory distress syndrome (Zhu and Sun, 2018). Chronic treatment with SB (1 mg/kg for 40 days) was shown to significantly ameliorate the unpredictable chronic stress-induced behavioural (memory function), biochemical changes (GSH and SOD), and inflammation indexes (serum TNF-α and IL-1β) in stressed mice (Garikapati *et al.*, 2018).

SM was able to prevents memory impairments, depressive-like symptoms and anxiety in a rat model of post-traumatic stress disorder (El-Elimat *et al.*, 2019). SM showed protective effects against chronic unpredictable mild stress induced depressive-like behaviour in mice (Ashraf *et al.*, 2019). SB was reported to prevent depression-like behaviours in a single prolonged stress rat model (Lee *et al.*, 2020). SB was shown to mitigate acute stress-induced anxiety, owing to its anxiolytic properties in the zebrafish model (Nachammai *et al.*, 2021). For protective effects of SM/SB in chemically-induced oxidative stress, see Chapter 8.

As described in Chapter 3, there are at least 8 stress-response pathways responsible for stress sensing and development of the adequate response including nutritional stress response, energy stress response, inflammation stress response, heat shock response, unfolded protein response, hypoxia-induced stress response and DNA damage response. During adaptation to stress various vitagenes (Chapter 7) and transcription factors (Chapter 3, 5 and 6) play important roles. For example, in experimental chemically-induced gastric ulcer SM was found to improve redox status and upregulated Nrf2 with simultaneous reduction in expression of NF-κB and pro-inflammatory markers in gastric tissue (Keshk *et al.*, 2017). Furthermore, SM was shown to regulate the metabolism of sulphur-containing amino acids to maintain the GSH pool through increased cysteine availability in the liver (Kwon *et al.*, 2013).

16.4 Silymarin and burn recovery

Topical application of SM was found to improve the morphological, biochemical and biomechanical properties of experimentally-induced wound defects in rats as evidenced by a significant increase observed in the amount of glycosaminoglycans and collagen present on days 10, 20 and 30 after SM application (Oryan *et al.*, 2012). The 4-week adjuvant treatment with oral SM (140 mg/day) was shown to improve wound recovery in patients with second degree-burn (Mahmoodi-Nesheli *et al.*, 2018). In a model of skin wound healing SB was proven to regulate matrix metalloproteinase 3 (stromelysine1) gene expression as well as extracellular matrix constituents including glycosaminoglycans and collagen production (Tabandeh *et al.*, 2013). It was indicated that 0.2% SB hydrogel possesses potent wound healing activity in incision and excision wound models in mice (Samanta *et al.*, 2016).

16.5 Anti-aging effects of silymarin

It is generally accepted that ageing is associated with redox disbalance, oxidative stress and over-inflammation and therefore it is logical to test anti-aging effects of SM/SB. For example, in mice SB was shown to have protective action against D-galactose-induced senescence associated with inhibiting NF-κB activation and AO system upregulation (Wang *et al.*, 2011). SB was demonstrated to markedly improve endothelial dysfunction in db/db mice by reducing circulating and vascular asymmetric dimethylarginine levels (Li Volti *et al.*, 2011). It is believed that aging-dependent changes including oestrogen depletion could lead to endothelial dysfunction, an important factor in cardiovascular disease development. Interestingly, in aged ovariectomised rats SM treatment was reported to restore the endothelial function and vascular tone and SM action was more effective than oestrogen replacement (Demirci *et al.*, 2014b). The authors suggested that the nitric oxide pathway, oxidative stress prevention and calcium antagonistic features of SM are responsible for its protective effects (Demirci *et al.*, 2014a).

SB (25 and 50 mg/kg body weight) was shown to dose-dependently ameliorate depletion of striatal dopamine and reduced abnormality of behaviour in the aging rats with the neonatal iron supplementation. This was associated with a significant restoration of the redox homeostasis in the substantia nigra of the aging rats (Chen *et al.*, 2015a). SM was demonstrated to extend lifespan and reduce proteotoxicity in *C. elegans* Alzheimer's model (Kumar *et al.*, 2015). It seems likely that anti-elastase effect of SM can be used in various mixtures to gain the anti-aging effects (Pientaweeratch *et al.*, 2016).

In an experiment with old male rats chronic SM treatments (20 mg/kg for 4 weeks) showed restorative effects on cognition and motor coordination associated with reversing the age-induced deficits in monoaminergic neurotransmitters (serotonin, noradrenaline, and dopamine), increasing tryptophan hydroxylase and tyrosine hydroxylase activity and SIRT1 levels and decreasing NF-κB levels in hippocampus (Sarubbo *et al.*, 2018). SM (100 mg/kg) is shown to improve cognitive ability in aged LDLR (+/−) golden Syrian hamsters via mechanisms involving maintaining blood-brain barrier integrity (Gu *et al.*, 2018). The anti-aging properties of SB were studied in rat embryonic fibroblast cells treated with H_2O_2 and protective effect of SM was associated with its antioxidant (decreased ROS production, increased FRAP and rise in the activity of mitochondrial complexes I, II, and IV) and anti-inflammatory (decreased expression of NF-κB and pro-inflammatory cytokines) properties (Baeeri *et al.*, 2018).

In a D-Galactose-induced aging rat model, SM (100 and 200 mg/kg/day) was shown to slow down the progression of age-related hearing loss (Tavanai *et al.*, 2019). SM was reported to be an effective agent for skin protection against the harmful effects of solar radiation including slowing down skin photoaging (Vostálová *et al.*, 2019).

16.6 Silymarin and multidrug resistance

Multidrug resistance (MDR) is an acquired resistance of microorganisms and cancer cells to various drugs of different chemical structures and with different mechanisms of action. An important resistance mechanism is related to drug depletion in cells by membrane efflux proteins. MDR is associated with the overexpression of a variety of proteins (drug transporters) that pump drugs out of the cell, lowering their concentration below the effective levels. The MDR phenomenon is a serious medical problem creating a major challenge to the treatment of infectious diseases with bacterial resistance to tetracyclines, erythromycin, and fluoroquinolones and resistance to cancer therapy. There are 48 human ABC transporter genes and among them, the ability to confer MDR *in vitro* is best characterised for P-glycoprotein (P-gp, also known as ABCB1 or MDR1 P-gp), ABCG2 (also known as breast cancer resistance protein; BCRP), and multidrug resistance-associated protein 1 (MRP1, also known as ABCC1; Hanssen *et al.*, 2021). The ABC transporters families, expressed in various tissues including the liver, intestine, kidney, and brain and many of those transporters are involved in MDR development and P-glycoprotein, Ca^{2+}-dependent efflux pump, is a major player in this process (Catalano *et al.*, 2022).

The phenomenon of antibiotic resistance among bacteria is attributed to misuse and overuse of antimicrobial agents and also associated with various bacterial resistance factors (Rozwadowski and Gawel, 2022). Several plant-derived phytochemicals were shown to be able to modulate various signal transduction pathways and reversing P-gp mediated MDR in tumour cells and therefore modulating the cell signalling pathways by phytochemicals is an important approach in attempts to overcome MDR (Ganesan *et al.*, 2021). Various polyphenols were reported to ameliorate both antineoplastic and bacterial multidrug resistance by inhibiting Adenosine triphosphate Binding Cassette (ABC)-transporters including human P-glycoprotein, breast cancer resistance protein, multidrug resistance-associated protein MRP-1 and bacterial ABC transporters, as well as other bacterial drug efflux pumps (Chambers *et al.*, 2020).

Silychristin A and its 2,3-dehydro-derivative were shown to modulate multidrug resistance by the direct inhibition of P-gp. Interestingly, this action of SM constituents was different from anhydrosilychristin and isosilychristin which modulated multidrug resistance by downregulating the expression of the dominant transmembrane efflux pumps (Viktorová *et al.*, 2019). Furthermore, SB and 2,3-dehydrosilybin showed strong dose-dependent inhibition of P-glycoprotein pump and silybin B was acting directly upon P-glycoprotein *in vitro* and also downregulating the expression of respective multidrug resistance genes altered the expression of P-gp, MRP1 and BCRP (Dobiasová *et al.*, 2020).

Eleven SM flavonolignans have been recently tested for their ability to reverse the multidrug resistance phenotype of *Staphylococcus aureus* and reduce its virulence (Holasová *et al.*, 2022). Importantly, silybin A, 2,3-dehydrosilybin B, and 2,3-dehydrosilybin AB were shown to completely reverse antibiotic resistance at concentrations of 20 μM or less. Furthermore, both 2,3-dehydrosilybin B and AB were reported to decrease the antibiotic-induced gene expression of representative efflux pumps and most of the tested flavonolignans reduced virulence factors, namely bacterial cell to cell communication and cell adhesion to the surface showing great potential as adjunct therapeutics in the control of multidrug-resistant *S. aureus* infections (Holasová *et al.*, 2022). The authors also indicated that the aforementioned properties of SM components possessing antiadhesion effects are closely related to the prevention of biofilm formation as it was noticed earlier with strain of *S. epidermidis* (Evren, and Yurtcu, 2015) and *S. aureus* (Vimberg *et al.*, 2015). Interestingly, SB was shown to restore the sensitivity of CS and taxol in drug-resistant human ovarian cancer cells and reduce drug-induced hepatotoxicity in cell level (Yang *et al.*, 2019).

16.7 Combined protective effects of silymarin and other antioxidants

Taking into account a similarity of hepatoprotective actions of SM (Surai, 2015a; 2020; 2022), TAU (Surai, 2020; Surai *et al.*, 2020; 2021) and carnitine (Surai, 2015b,c,d; 2020) as well as new findings in protective actions of organic Se (Surai, 2018; 2021; Surai *et al.*, 2018) it is reasonable to expect synergistic effects of those nutrients in various stress models. The therapeutic protective effects of SM (300 mg/kg/day for 2 weeks) and TAU (500 mg/kg/day for 2 weeks) against APAP-induced neuro-and hepato-toxicity in adult male albino rats (liver integrity: AST, ALT; liver and brain AO defences: GSH, GSSG, NO, MDA; Liver and brain DNA fragmentation) were comparable (Radwan and Shehata, 2016).

In the model of APAP-induced hepatic toxicity a combination of SM and TAU (22 mg/kg and 100 mg/kg, respectively, twice daily for 7 days) was shown to be more effective than single TAU usage (Omar *et al.*, 2006). In a model of nonalcoholic fatty liver disease associated with metabolic syndrome in rats a combined treatment with SM and TAU showed maximal protective effects (serum liver and cytokine profile) in comparison to results of their single usage (Mi, 2015). In a model of CCl_4-induced rat liver damage the combination therapy (SM+TAU) was more effective than single applications in reducing lipid peroxidation (TBARS levels), NO production, hydroxyproline content in fibrotic liver as well as the activity of serum GGT (Abdel-Moneim *et al.*, 2015). In the cell line CHSE-214 of *Oncorhynchus tshawytscha* treated with H_2O_2 a synergistic protective effects of SM and TAU combination were shown to be concentration-dependent (Olivares-Ferretti *et al.*, 2020). The effects were dose dependent: the TAU treatment showed the highest protective effect on cells at a dose of 100 mg/kg. Combining TAU (100 mg/kg) with SM (10 or 100 mg/kg) showed substantial increase in protective action. However, when the treatment with both molecules was increased to 500 mg/kg of TAU, the protective effect was blocked (Olivares-Ferretti *et al.*, 2020).

Both L-Carnitine and SM were shown to have protective effects against the negative effect of paracetamol through increasing the body weight gain and antioxidant activity (GSH, SOD, MDA) ameliorating liver enzymes, cholesterol and triglycerides (Aziz *et al.*, 2019). Simultaneous administration of SM and L-Carnitine was shown to have protective effects on liver tissue by reducing Diazinon-induced liver injury in rats (Masoumi *et al.*, 2020). The co-administration of L-carnitine or SM with anthracycline chemotherapy was indicated to represents a new therapeutic strategy for better control of anthracycline-induced cardiotoxicity (Zalat *et al.*, 2020a,b).

A treatment of NAFLD patients with a mixture containing vitamin E (200 IU), SM (750 mg) and L-carnitine (1 gram) for 18 weeks was observed to significantly reduce serum glucose and insulin. The authors concluded that the supplement could be useful in the treatment/prevention of nonalcoholic fatty liver disease, diabetes, and the metabolic syndrome due to its ability to reduce markers of liver inflammation, glucose, insulin, and triglycerides (Poulos *et al.*, 2022). In placebo-controlled double-blind clinical trial in men after radical prostatectomy a combination of SM (570 mg) and selenium (240 μg as SeMet) consumed for 6 months was shown to significantly reduce important markers of lipid metabolism known to be associated with prostate cancer progression, namely LDL and total cholesterol in the blood (Vidlar *et al.*, 2010).

The effects of a combination of Se and SM in men with lower urinary tract symptoms, benign prostatic hyperplasia and a prostate specific antigen (PSA) ≤2.5 ng/ml were studies in double-blind, placebo controlled clinical trial. The volunteers were randomly divided into two groups: the first one (n=26) obtained 240 μg selenium (in the form of Se-yeast) plus 570 mg SM daily for 6 months and the second one (n=29) received placebo. The results showed significant beneficial differences between treatment and control groups for the following parameters: International Prostate Symptom Score, urodynamic parameters: maximal rate of urine flow, average flow, bladder volume and ultrasound estimated postvoid residual urine volume, total PSA value and serum selenium levels (Vostalova *et al.*, 2013).

16.8 Silymarin-drug interactions

It is well known that enzymatic drug metabolism and drug transport are important metabolic processes for absorption, disposition, metabolism and elimination of drugs within the body (Iversen *et al.*, 2022). Drug metabolism is reported to be divided into phase I and phase II processes. On the one hand, phase I processes include oxidation, reduction, hydrolysis and hydration, leading to the formation of such functional groups as OH, SH, NH_2 or COOH associated with increased metabolite polarity. On the other hand, phase II processes are associated with drug sulfation, methylation, acetylation, glutathione conjugation, fatty acid conjugation and glucuronidation (Wu *et al.*, 2009).

Drug transporters are known to be involved in the transport of more than half of the most prescribed drugs and are important players in pharmacotherapy. In a recent review the 100 most prescribed drugs in five European countries and Australia were identified. It was shown that 89 of the 100 drugs are metabolised either by Phase I metabolism or Phase II metabolism or are known to be substrates for drug transporters (Iversen *et al.*, 2022). It was also indicated that 67 of the 100 drugs undergo Phase I metabolism with CYP3A4/5 being the predominant metabolising enzyme followed by CYP2D6, CYP2C9, CYP2C19, CYP1A2 and CYP2C8. Among phase II enzymes responsible for metabolism of 17 of the 100 drugs uridine glucuronyl transferases (UGTs) were shown to be the dominant clearance mechanism, while P-glycoprotein pump is the main transporter responsible for the transport of 30 of the 100 drugs (Iversen *et al.*, 2022).

Data on SM/SB involvement in drug-drug interactions (DDI) are diverse and sometime controversial. For example, there was no influence of SM (7 days pretreatment with thrice daily dose of 140 mg) on the pharmacokinetics of ranitidine, a drug reducing the amount of acid the stomach makes (Rao *et al.*, 2007). Co-administration of SM (140 mg, three times daily for 14 days) was reported to significantly increase the plasma concentration of talinolol (the cardioselective beta-receptor antagonist) in healthy volunteers (Han *et al.*, 2009). Pretreatment with an extremely high dose of 1.0 g/kg SM was shown to significantly affect trazodone's (a serotonin modulator used for depression treatment) pharmacokinetics including decrease area under concentration curve (AUC), distribution half-life (t(1/2,alpha)), elimination half-life (t(1/2,beta)), and mean residence time (MRT) in rats (Chang *et al.*, 2009).

Co-administration of SB does not have significant effect on the pharmacokinetics of nifedipine (a calcium channel blocker; Wu *et al.*, 2009). Oral bioavailability of paclitaxel (a chemotherapy drug) was significantly enhanced in the combination with SM (10 and 20 mg/kg; Park *et al.*, 2012). The effects of single and repeated administrations of SM (40 mg/kg) on pharmacokinetics of a P-gp substrate, risperidone (a drug used to treat certain mental/mood disorders), and its major metabolite, 9-hydroxyrisperidone in rats were investigated. The C_{max} of 9-hydroxyrisperidone was significantly increased (1.3-fold) while the other pharmacokinetic parameters were not affected. However, in comparison to single administration of SM, the repeated exposures of SM (5 days) were reported to increase oral bioavailability and affected the pharmacokinetics of risperidone and 9-hydroxyrisperidone (Lee *et al.*, 2013).

The inhibitory effects of milk thistle extracts and isolated constituents on midazolam 1'-hydroxylation were studied using human liver and intestinal microsomes. SM and its constituents silybin A, isosilybin A, isosilybin B, and silychristin at 100 μM were reported to show inhibition (>50%) of CYP3A activity. The highest inhibitory activity calculated as IC_{50} were shown for isosilybin B and silychristin: ~60 and 90 μM, respectively, whereas other constituents were less active with LD50 exceeding 100 μM (Brantley *et al.*, 2013).

In model systems based on the everted sac and non-everted sac SM pretreatment was shown to increase domperidone transport from the duodenum, jejunum, ileum, and colon indicating that SM can increase the bioavailability of domperidone (an anti-sickness medicine). This was confirmed in healthy human volunteers by a significant difference in the pharmacokinetic parameters of domperidone including C_{max}, $T_{1/2}$, AUC0-∞, and AUC0-24 (Yamsani and Yamsani, 2014). Inhibitory effects of SB on pharmacokinetics of imatinib (an oral chemotherapy medication) *in vivo* and *in vitro* were observed. SB (50 mg/kg) was found to significantly decrease the area under the curve of imatinib and to increase the half-life of imatinib (Wang *et al.*, 2014).

SB coadministration in rabbits had no significant effect on pharmacokinetics of nitrendipine in comparison to control group. However, in SB pretreated group of animals an 1.6-1.9-fold increase in area under the concentration-time curve and peak plasma concentration (C_{max}), were observed (Voruganti *et al.*, 2014). SM was reported to affect the pharmacokinetics (a significant reduction of V_{max} and recovery of diabetes-reduced values of AUC and C_{max}) of atorvastatin (a lipid-lowering drug) in diabetic rats (Malekinejad *et al.*, 2014). SB and SM were shown to inhibit raloxifene (a medication used to prevent and treat osteoporosis in postmenopausal women) intestinal glucuronidation and these nutraceuticals were predicted to increase raloxifene systemic exposure by 4- to 5-fold, suggesting high interaction risk (Gufford *et al.*, 2015). SB is shown to inhibit enzyme activities of multiple drug-metabolising enzymes (CYP1A2, CYP2C, CYP3A11, UGT1A1) and to confer significant drug-drug interaction with PPARα agonists via the repression of PPARα activation in a competitive mode (Wang *et al.*, 2015). In rats SB (30 mg/kg) was shown to affect the pharmacokinetics of ivabradine (a medication used to treat heart failure) as evidenced by increased drug plasma concentration (Chen *et al.*, 2015b).

The co-administration of SM (40 mg/kg) and ribavirin (an antiviral medication) was associated with a significantly decreased area under the plasma concentration-time curve and the peak plasma concentration of ribavirin by 31.2-44.5% and 48.9-50.0%, respectively (Liao *et al.*, 2016). The co-administration of SM and simvastatin (SV, a lipid-lowering medication) was reported to significantly increase the C_{max} and AUC_{0-12h} of SV active metabolite simvastatin acid compared with SV alone, while there was no significant difference with regards to T_{max} and $t_{1/2}$. Interestingly, SV pharmacokinetic parameters were not affected by SM pretreatment (Li *et al.*, 2019). SB (25 mg/kg or 50 mg/kg for 2 weeks) was shown to increase blood concentration of brexpiprazole (a serotonin-dopamine activity modulator) in rat by downregulating its main metabolic enzyme CYP3A4 (Yu *et al.*, 2020).

Organic anion-transporting polypeptides (OATPs) belonging to a superfamily of transporters are known to mediate the sodium-independent transport of a wide range of amphiphilic organic compounds, including many various drugs such as statins, angiotensin II receptor blockers, angiotensin converting enzyme inhibitors, chemotherapeutic agents, and anti-diabetic agents (Lynch *et al.*, 2021). Therefore, OATPs mediating the uptake of endogenous compounds and xenobiotics in tissues, are considered to regulate drug absorption and elimination and the ability of SM/SB to impose DDI has been studied. The seven major flavonolignans from SM were demonstrated to be substrates for OATP1B1, OATP1B3, and OATP2B1 (Lynch *et al.*, 2021).

It was demonstrated that SM-drug interactions depend on OATP isoform specificity and concentrations of SM constituents at the site of drug transport. In *in vitro* experiments, OATP1B1- and OATP1B3-mediated oestradiol-17β-glucuronide uptake and OATP2B1-mediated estrone-3-sulphate uptake were shown to be significantly suppressed by the SM flavonolignans. The authors suggested that high SM doses or formulations with improved bioavailability potentially could increase the risk of flavonolignan interactions with OATP substrates in patients (Köck *et al.*, 2013).

It is well known that certain ligand molecules can bind to human serum albumin (HAS) with high affinity, forming stable ligand-HSA complexes and occupying the major drug binding sites. This would affect drug pharmacokinetics in terms of drug tissue distribution and the elimination half-life. The high concentrations of SM components/metabolites were shown to be able to disrupt the albumin binding of warfarin (a blood thinner) and/or other site I ligands in the circulation (Faisal *et al.*, 2021). The authors also showed that some SM components can inhibit CYP2C9, 2C19, and/or 3A4 enzymes at nanomolar or low micromolar concentrations. Silybin A was shown to interact with losartan (an angiotensin receptor blocker) in a genotype-dependent manner: the pharmacokinetic interactions between them were shown to be minor when concomitantly administered at normal doses in genotypes CYP2C9*1/*1 and CYP2C9*1/*3, but moderate interaction was described in CYP2C9*1/*2 genotype (Tanveer *et al.*, 2022).

The clinical degree of SM/SB-drug interaction is believed to depend on many factors including SM/SB concentration, dosage, drug, etc. (Wu *et al.*, 2009). In general, SB is proven to inhibit CYP enzymes, with 2C9 and 3A4 being the most sensitive, but rarely at clinically achievable concentrations. Therefore, it seems likely that CYP-mediated DDI for SB is not a major clinical problem, however sensitive drugs including warfarin, opioids, and anti-arrhythmic agents need more attention (Xie *et al.*, 2019).

As mentioned above accumulating evidence from *in vitro* and *in vivo* studies with various model systems indicated existence of some DDI, but in most cases they are observed in SB concentrations not achievable in human tissues. Furthermore, the clinical relevance of these DDI has not been confirmed in human trials (Tvrdý *et al.*, 2021). In a recent review paper a list of published clinical trials on SB-related DDI included 18 clinical trials with 12 trials did not show such interactions with various drugs including aminopyrine, caffeine, chlorzoxazone, debrisoquine, dextromethorphan, digoxin, indinavir, irinotecan, midazolam, nifedipine, phenylbutazone, ranitidine, rosuvastatin and tolbutamide (Xie *et al.*, 2019).

The most affected drugs included metronidazole (an antibiotic), talinolol (a cardioselective beta-receptor antagonist), domperidone (a dopamine antagonist) and to lesser extent darunavir-ritonavir (protease inhibitor) and losartan (an anti-hypertension drug). The main conclusion from the review of the aforementioned trials is that SM does not pose a clinically relevant risk of drug-drug interaction. The authors mentioned that there are some cases where SM showed inhibition of activities of enzymes and transporters associated with the pharmacokinetics of therapeutic drugs, but SM concentrations achievable within the human body are usually too low to impose significant inhibition and such effects are unlikely to manifest in clinical settings (Xie *et al.*, 2019).

Furthermore, the authors also presented pharmacokinetic studies showing significant effects of SM on talinolol, domperidone, indinavir and metronidazole metabolism and availability. In general, inconsistency of results on risks of DDI with some medications observed in animal models and different clinical trials warrants further clinical studies to address the aforementioned concerns.

16.9 Conclusions

SM-drug interactions are of great importance for clinical practice. In general, there are some cases where SM showed inhibition of activities of enzymes and transporters associated with the pharmacokinetics of therapeutic drugs, but SM bioavailability is comparatively low and its concentrations achievable within the human body are usually too low to impose significant inhibition and such effects are unlikely to manifest in clinical settings. The multidrug resistance (MDR) phenomenon is a serious medical problem creating a major challenge to the treatment of infectious diseases and cancer.

Various components of SM were shown to modulate multidrug resistance by the direct inhibition of P-gp or by downregulating the expression of the dominant transmembrane efflux pumps. Some of SM components were able to completely reverse antibiotic resistance at concentrations of 20 μM or less. This finding is of great importance for clinical practise and veterinary applications. SM also demonstrated anti-aging effects and decreased detrimental consequences of various stresses, including over-exercising. It seems likely that SM could be an important supplement in sport medicine. Furthermore, various protective effects of SM in stress conditions are a background for its inclusion into anti-stress supplements. SM was shown promising results in burn recovery and wound healing.

Furthermore, taking into account the lack of alternative effective treatments and the relatively few adverse effects, SB could be an important part of chemotherapy of patients with amatoxin-containing mushrooms poisoning. Since TAU and carnitine also possess hepatoprotective properties their combination with SM could be an important addition to the existing hepatoprotectors. Furthermore, various combinations of SM with organic Se deserve more attention.

References

Abdel-Moneim, A.M., Al-Kahtani, M.A., El-Kersh, M.A. and Al-Omair, M.A., 2015. Free radical-scavenging, anti-inflammatory/anti-fibrotic and hepatoprotective actions of taurine and silymarin against CCl4 induced rat liver damage. PLoS One 10: e0144509.

Ashraf, A., Mahmoud, P.A., Reda, H., Mansour, S., Helal, M.H., Michel, H.E. and Nasr, M., 2019. Silymarin and silymarin nanoparticles guard against chronic unpredictable mild stress induced depressive-like behavior in mice: involvement of neurogenesis and NLRP3 inflammasome. Journal of Psychopharmacology 33: 615-631.

Aziz, M.A., Zahra, A.E.A., Kheder, Z.A. and Fikry, H.M., 2019. The role of L. methionine, L. carnitine, choline and/or silymarin in hepatoprotection against paracetamol intoxication and oxidative stress in broilers. Slovenian Veterinary Research 56: 717-723.

Baeeri, M., Mohammadi-Nejad, S., Rahimifard, M., Navaei-Nigjeh, M., Moeini-Nodeh, S., Khorasani, R. and Abdollahi, M., 2018. Molecular and biochemical evidence on the protective role of ellagic acid and silybin against oxidative stress-induced cellular aging. Molecular and Cellular Biochemistry 441: 21-33.

Brantley, S.J., Graf, T.N., Oberlies, N.H. and Paine, M.F., 2013. A systematic approach to evaluate herb-drug interaction mechanisms: investigation of milk thistle extracts and eight isolated constituents as CYP3A inhibitors. Drug Metabolism and Disposition 41: 1662-1670.

Broussard, C.N., Aggarwal, A., Lacey, S.R., Post, A.B., Gramlich, T., Henderson, J.M. and Younossi, Z.M., 2001. Mushroom poisoning – from diarrhea to liver transplantation. The American Journal of Gastroenterology 96: 3195-3198.

Catalano, A., Iacopetta, D., Ceramella, J., Scumaci, D., Giuzio, F., Saturnino, C., Aquaro, S., Rosano, C. and Sinicropi, M.S., 2022. Multidrug resistance (MDR): A widespread phenomenon in pharmacological therapies. Molecules 27: 616.

Chambers, C.S., Viktorová, J., Řehořová, K., Biedermann, D., Turková, L., Macek, T., Křen, V. and Valentová, K., 2020. Defying multidrug resistance! Modulation of related transporters by flavonoids and flavonolignans. Journal of Agricultural and Food Chemistry 68: 1763-1779.

Chang, J.C., Wu, Y.T., Lee, W.C., Lin, L.C. and Tsai, T.H., 2009. Herb-drug interaction of silymarin or silibinin on the pharmacokinetics of trazodone in rats. Chemico-Biological Interactions 182: 227-232.

Chen, H., Wang, X., Wang, M., Yang, L., Yan, Z., Zhang, Y. and Liu, Z., 2015a. Behavioral and neurochemical deficits in aging rats with increased neonatal iron intake: Silibinin's neuroprotection by maintaining redox balance. Frontiers in Aging Neuroscience 7: 206.

Chen, X.P., Zheng, H.T., Cai, W.W., Li, M.K., Zhang, J.W. and Hu, J., 2015b. The effect of silibinin on the pharmacokinetics of Ivabradine and N-Desmethylivabradine in rats. Pharmacology 96: 107-111.

Choi, E.J., Kim, E.K., Jeoung, N.H. and Kim, S.H., 2016. Effect of silymarin on gluconeogenesis and lactate production in exercising rats. Food Science and Biotechnology 25: 119-124.

Demirci, B., Demir, O., Dost, T. and Birincioglu, M., 2014a. Treated effect of silymarin on vascular function of aged rats: Dependant on nitric oxide pathway. Pharmaceutical Biology 52: 453-457.

Demirci, B., Dost, T., Gokalp, F. and Birincioglu, M., 2014b. Silymarin improves vascular function of aged ovariectomized rats. Phytotherapy Research 28: 868-872.

Diaz, J.H., 2018. Amatoxin-containing mushroom poisonings: species, toxidromes, treatments, and outcomes. Wilderness & Environmental Medicine 29: 111-118.

Dobiasová, S., Řehořová, K., Kučerová, D., Biedermann, D., Káňová, K., Petrásková, L., Koucká, K., Václavíková, R., Valentová, K., Ruml, T., Macek, T., Křen, V. and Viktorová, J., 2020. Multidrug resistance modulation activity of silybin derivatives and their anti-inflammatory potential. Antioxidants 9: 455.

El-Elimat, T., Alzoubi, K.H., AbuAlSamen, M.M., Al Subeh, Z.Y., Graf, T.N. and Oberlies, N.H., 2019. Silymarin prevents memory impairments, anxiety, and depressive-like symptoms in a rat model of post-traumatic stress disorder. Planta Medica 85: 32-40.

Enjalbert, F., Rapior, S., Nouguier-Soulé, J., Guillon, S., Amouroux, N. and Cabot, C., 2002. Treatment of amatoxin poisoning: 20-year retrospective analysis. Journal of Toxicology. Clinical Toxicology 40: 715-757.

Evren, E. and Yurtcu, E., 2015. *In vitro* effects on biofilm viability and antibacterial and antiadherent activities of silymarin. Folia Microbiologica 60: 351-356.

Faisal, Z., Mohos, V., Fliszár-Nyúl, E., Valentová, K., Káňová, K., Lemli, B., Kunsági-Máté, S. and Poór, M., 2021. Interaction of silymarin components and their sulfate metabolites with human serum albumin and cytochrome P450 (2C9, 2C19, 2D6, and 3A4) enzymes. Biomedicine & Pharmacotherapy 138: 111459.

Ganesan, M., Kanimozhi, G., Pradhapsingh, B., Khan, H.A., Alhomida, A.S., Ekhzaimy, A., Brindha, G.R. and Prasad, N.R., 2021. Phytochemicals reverse P-glycoprotein mediated multidrug resistance via signal transduction pathways. Biomedicine & Pharmacotherapy 139: 111632.

Garcia, J., Costa, V.M., Carvalho, A., Baptista, P., de Pinho, P.G., de Lourdes Bastos, M. and Carvalho, F., 2015. Amanita phalloides poisoning: Mechanisms of toxicity and treatment. Food and Chemical Toxicology 86: 41-55.

Garikapati, D.R., Shaik, P.B. and Penchalaiah, H., 2018. Evaluate neuroprotective effect of silibinin using chronic unpredictable stress (cus) model. International Journal of Physiology, Pathophysiology and Pharmacology 10: 184-191.

Ghalandari, K., Shabani, M., Khajehlandi, A. and Mohammadi, A., 2023. Effect of aerobic training with silymarin consumption on glycemic indices and liver enzymes in men with type 2 diabetes. Archives of Physiology and Biochemistry 129: 76-81. https://doi.org/10.1080/13813455.2020.1797104.

Gillessen, A. and Schmidt, H.H.J., 2020. Silymarin as supportive treatment in liver diseases: A narrative review. Advances in Therapy 37: 1279-1301.

Gu, Y.Y., Huang, P., Li, Q., Liu, Y.Y., Liu, G., Wang, Y.H., Yi, M., Yan, L., Wei, X.H., Yang, L., Hu, B.H., Zhao, X.R., Chang, X., Sun, K., Pan, C.S., Cui, Y.C., Chen, Q.F., Wang, C.S., Fan, J.Y., Ma, Z.Z. and Han, J.Y., 2018. YangXue QingNao Wan and silibinin capsules, the two Chinese medicines, attenuate cognitive impairment in aged LDLR (+/-) golden Syrian hamsters Involving Protection of Blood Brain Barrier. Frontiers in Physiology 9: 658.

Gufford, B.T., Chen, G., Vergara, A.G., Lazarus, P., Oberlies, N.H. and Paine, M.F., 2015. Milk thistle constituents inhibit raloxifene intestinal glucuronidation: A potential clinically relevant natural product-drug interaction. Drug Metabolism and Disposition 43: 1353-1359.

Han, Y., Guo, D., Chen, Y., Tan, Z.R. and Zhou, H.H., 2009. Effect of continuous silymarin administration on oral talinolol pharmacokinetics in healthy volunteers. Xenobiotica 39: 694-699.

Hanssen, K.M., Haber, M. and Fletcher, J.I., 2021. Targeting multidrug resistance-associated protein 1 (MRP1)-expressing cancers: Beyond pharmacological inhibition. Drug Resistance Updates 59: 100795.

Holasová, K., Křížkovská, B., Hoang, L., Dobiasová, S., Lipov, J., Macek, T., Křen, V., Valentová, K., Ruml, T. and Viktorová, J., 2022. Flavonolignans from silymarin modulate antibiotic resistance and virulence in Staphylococcus aureus. Biomedicine & Pharmacotherapy 149: 112806.

Iversen, D.B., Andersen, N.E., Dunvald, A.C.D., Pottegård, A. and Stage, T.B., 2022. Drug metabolism and drug transport of the 100 most prescribed oral drugs. Basic & Clinical Pharmacology & Toxicology 131: 311-324.

Jia, L. and Zhao, F., 2022. Evaluation of silymarin extract from *Silybum marianum* in mice: anti-fatigue activity. Food Science and Human Wellness 11: 914-921.

Keshk, W.A., Zahran, S.M., Katary, M.A. and Ali, D.A.E., 2017. Modulatory effect of silymarin on nuclear factor-erythroid-2-related factor 2 regulated redox status, nuclear factor-κB mediated inflammation and apoptosis in experimental gastric ulcer. Chemico-Biological Interactions 273: 266-272.

Kim, S.H., Oh, D.S., Oh, J.Y., Son, T.G., Yuk, D.Y. and Jung, Y.S., 2016. Silymarin prevents restraint stress-induced acute liver injury by ameliorating oxidative stress and reducing inflammatory response. Molecules 21: 443.

Koçarslan, A., Koçarslan, S., Aydin, M.S., Gunay, Ş., Karahan, M.A., Taşkın, A., Üstunel, M. and Aksoy, N., 2016. Intraperitoneal administration of silymarin protects end organs from multivisceral ischemia/reperfusion injury in a rat model. Brazilian Journal of Cardiovascular Surgery 31: 434-439.

Köck, K., Xie, Y., Hawke, R.L., Oberlies, N.H. and Brouwer, K.L., 2013. Interaction of silymarin flavonolignans with organic anion-transporting polypeptides. Drug Metabolism and Disposition 41: 958-965.

Kumar, J., Park, K.C., Awasthi, A. and Prasad, B., 2015. Silymarin extends lifespan and reduces proteotoxicity in C. elegans Alzheimer's model. CNS & Neurological Disorders Drug Targets 14: 295-302.

Kwon, D.Y., Jung, Y.S., Kim, S.J., Kim, Y.S., Choi, D.W. and Kim, Y.C., 2013. Alterations in sulfur amino acid metabolism in mice treated with silymarin: a novel mechanism of its action involved in enhancement of the antioxidant defense in liver. Planta Medica 79: 997-1002.

Lacombe, G. and St-Onge, M., 2016. Towards evidence-based emergency medicine: best BETs from the Manchester Royal Infirmary. BET 1: Silibinin in suspected amatoxin-containing mushroom poisoning. Emergency Medicine Journal 33: 76-77.

Lee, B., Choi, G.M. and Sur, B., 2020. Silibinin prevents depression-like behaviors in a single prolonged stress rat model: the possible role of serotonin. BMC Complementary Medicine and Therapies 20: 70.

Lee, K.S., Chae, S.W., Park, J.H., Park, J.H., Choi, J.M., Rhie, S.J. and Lee, H.J., 2013. Effects of single or repeated silymarin administration on pharmacokinetics of risperidone and its major metabolite, 9-hydroxyrisperidone in rats. Xenobiotica 43: 303-310.

Li Volti, G., Salomone, S., Sorrenti, V., Mangiameli, A., Urso, V., Siarkos, I., Galvano, F. and Salamone, F., 2011. Effect of silibinin on endothelial dysfunction and ADMA levels in obese diabetic mice. Cardiovascular Diabetology 10: 62.

Li, Y., Wu, Y., Li, Y.J., Meng, L., Ding, C.Y. and Dong, Z.J., 2019. Effects of silymarin on the *in vivo* pharmacokinetics of simvastatin and its active metabolite in rats. Molecules 24: 1666.

Liao, S., Jin, X., Li, J., Zhang, T., Zhang, W., Shi, W., Fan, S., Wang, X., Wang, J., Zhong, B. and Zhang, Z., 2016. Effects of silymarin, glycyrrhizin, and oxymatrine on the pharmacokinetics of Ribavirin and its major metabolite in rats. Phytotherapy Research 30: 618-626.

Liu, B., Liu, W., Liu, P., Liu, X., Song, X., Hayashi, T., Onodera, S. and Ikejima, T., 2019. Silibinin alleviates the learning and memory defects in overtrained rats accompanying reduced neuronal apoptosis and senescence. Neurochemical Research 44: 1818-1829.

Lovelace, E.S., Wagoner, J., MacDonald, J., Bammler, T., Bruckner, J., Brownell, J., Beyer, R.P., Zink, E.M., Kim, Y.M., Kyle, J.E., Webb-Robertson, B.J., Waters, K.M., Metz, T.O., Farin, F., Oberlies, N.H. and Polyak, S.J., 2015. Silymarin suppresses cellular inflammation by inducing reparative stress signaling. Journal of Natural Products 78: 1990-2000.

Lynch, K.D., Montonye, M.L., Tian, D.D., Arman, T., Oyanna, V.O., Bechtold, B.J., Graf, T.N., Oberlies, N.H., Paine, M.F. and Clarke, J.D., 2021. Hepatic organic anion transporting polypeptides mediate disposition of milk thistle flavonolignans and pharmacokinetic silymarin-drug interactions. Phytotherapy Research 35: 3286-3297.

Mahmoodi-Nesheli, M., Alizadeh, S., Solhi, H., Mohseni, J. and Mahmoodi-Nesheli, M., 2018. Adjuvant effect of oral silymarin on patients' wound healing process caused by thermal injuries. Caspian Journal of Internal Medicine 9: 341-346.

Malekinejad, H., Rokhsartalab-Azar, S., Hassani-Dizaj, S., Alizadeh-Fanalou, S., Rezabakhsh, A. and Amniattalab, A., 2014. Effects of silymarin on the pharmacokinetics of atorvastatin in diabetic rats. European Journal of Drug Metabolism and Pharmacokinetics 39: 311-320.

Masoumi, F., Shariati, M. and Mokhtari, M., 2020. Effects of *Silybum marianum* aqueous extract and L-carnitine on stereological changes in diazinon-treated rat liver. Journal Ilmu Ternak dan Veteriner 25: 91.

Mengs, U., Pohl, R.T. and Mitchell, T., 2012. Legalon® SIL: the antidote of choice in patients with acute hepatotoxicity from amatoxin poisoning. Current Pharmaceutical Biotechnology 13: 1964-1970.

Mi, H, 2015. Therapeutic roles of silymarin or/and Taurine on nonalcoholic fatty liver disease associated with metabolic syndrome in rats. Journal of Scientific Research in Science 32: 283-310.

Nachammai, V., Jeyabalan, S. and Muthusamy, S., 2021. Anxiolytic effects of silibinin and naringenin on zebrafish model: A preclinical study. Indian Journal of Pharmacology 53: 457-464.

Olivares-Ferretti, P., Sánchez, R., Ochoa de la Paz, L. and Parodi, J., 2020. A synergy of the nutritional additives taurine and silymarin in salmon farming: evaluation with the CHSE-214 cellular model. Fish Physiology and Biochemistry 46: 945-952.

Omar, A.S., Salwa, N. and Neermen, E.S., 2006. Effect of taurine alone or in combination with either silymarin or melatonin on acute hepatic damage caused by administration of acetaminophen in rats. Bulletin of the National Research Centre 31: 575-591.

Oryan, A., Tabatabaei Naeini, A., Moshiri, A., Mohammadalipour, A. and Tabandeh, M.R., 2012. Modulation of cutaneous wound healing by silymarin in rats. Journal of Wound Care 21: 457-464.

Park, J.H., Park, J.H., Hur, H.J., Woo, J.S. and Lee, H.J., 2012. Effects of silymarin and formulation on the oral bioavailability of paclitaxel in rats. European Journal of Pharmaceutical Sciences 45: 296-301.

Pientaweeratch, S., Panapisal, V. and Tansirikongkol, A, 2016. Antioxidant, anti-collagenase and anti-elastase activities of Phyllanthus emblica, Manilkara zapota and silymarin: an *in vitro* comparative study for anti-aging applications. Pharmaceutical Biology 54: 1865-1872.

Poucheret, P., Fons, F., Doré, J.C., Michelot, D. and Rapior, S., 2010. Amatoxin poisoning treatment decision-making: pharmaco-therapeutic clinical strategy assessment using multidimensional multivariate statistic analysis. Toxicon 55: 1338-1345.

Poulos, J.E., Kalogerinis, P.T., Milanov, V., Kalogerinis, C.T. and Poulos, E.J., 2022. The effects of vitamin E, silymarin and carnitine on the metabolic abnormalities associated with nonalcoholic liver disease. Journal of Dietary Supplements 19: 287-302.

Radwan, O.K. and Shehata, A.M, 2016. Comparison of the therapeutic actions of taurine, methylsulfonylmethane and silymarin against acetaminophen-induced neuro-and hepato-toxicity in adult male albino rats. Journal of Biomedical and Pharmaceutical Research 5: 10-17.

Rao, B.N., Srinivas, M., Kumar, Y.S. and Rao, Y.M., 2007. Effect of silymarin on the oral bioavailability of ranitidine in healthy human volunteers. Drug Metabolism and Drug Interactions 22: 175-185.

Rozwadowski, M. and Gawel, D., 2022. Molecular factors and mechanisms driving multidrug resistance in uropathogenic Escherichia coli-An update. Genes 13: 1397.

Samanta, R., Pattnaik, A.K., Pradhan, K.K., Mehta, B.K., Pattanayak, S.P. and Banerjee, S., 2016. Wound healing activity of silibinin in mice. Pharmacognosy Research 8: 298-302.

Sarubbo, F., Ramis, M.R., Kienzer, C., Aparicio, S., Esteban, S., Miralles, A. and Moranta, D., 2018. Chronic silymarin, quercetin and naringenin treatments increase monoamines synthesis and hippocampal Sirt1 levels improving cognition in aged rats. Journal of Neuroimmune Pharmacology 13: 24-38.

Shin, J.H., Lee, C.W., Oh, S.J., Yun, J., Lee, K., Park, S.K., Kim, H.M., Han, S.B., Kim, Y., Kim, H.C. and Kang, J.S., 2013. Protective effect of silymarin against ethanol-induced gastritis in rats: role of sulfhydryls, nitric oxide and gastric sensory afferents. Food and Chemical Toxicology 55: 353-357.

Surai, P.F., 2015a. Silymarin as a natural antioxidant: An overview of the current evidence and perspectives. Antioxidants 4: 204-247.

Surai, P.F., 2015b. Antioxidant action of carnitine: molecular mechanisms and practical applications. EC Veterinary Science 2: 66-84.

Surai, P.F., 2015c. Carnitine enigma: from antioxidant action to vitagene regulation. Part 1. Absorption, metabolism and antioxidant activities. Journal of Veterinary Science & Medicine 3, 2: 14.

Surai, P.F., 2015d. Carnitine enigma: from antioxidant action to vitagene regulation. Part 2. Transcription factors and practical applications. Journal of Veterinary Science & Medicine 3, 2: 17.

Surai, P.F., 2018. Selenium in poultry nutrition and health. Wageningen Academic Publishers, Wageningen, the Netherlands.

Surai, P.F., 2020. Vitagene in avian biology and poultry health. Wageningen Academic Publishers, Wageningen, The Netherlands.

Surai, P.F. (Ed.), 2021. Selenium in pig nutrition and health. Wageningen Academic Publishers, Wageningen, the Netherlands.

Surai, P.F., 2022. Silymarin as a vitagene modulator: effects on mitochondria integrity in stress conditions. In: Ostojik, S.M. (ed) Molecular nutrition and mitochondria. Elsevier, Academic Press, London, UK, pp. 535-559.

Surai, P.F., Earle-Payne, K. and Kidd, M.T., 2021. Taurine as a natural antioxidant: From direct antioxidant effects to protective action in various toxicological models. Antioxidants 10: 1876.

Surai, P.F., Kochish, I.I. and Kidd, M.T., 2020. Taurine in poultry nutrition. Animal Feed Science and Technology 260: 114339.

Surai, P.F., Kochish, I.I., Fisinin, V.I. and Velichko, O.A., 2018. Selenium in poultry nutrition: From sodium selenite to organic selenium sources. The Journal of Poultry Science 55: 79-93.

Tabandeh, M.R., Oryan, A., Mohhammad-Alipour, A. and Tabatabaei-Naieni, A., 2013. Silibinin regulates matrix metalloproteinase 3 (stromelysine1) gene expression, hexoseamines and collagen production during rat skin wound healing. Phytotherapy Research 27: 1149-1153.

Tanveer, A., Hussain, K., Tasneem, H., Arif, I., Rashid, M., Abbas, N., Shamim, R., Shah, P.A. and Bukhari, N.I., 2022. Prediction of CYP-mediated silybin A-losartan pharmacokinetic interactions using physiological based pharmacokinetic modeling. Journal of Pharmacokinetics and Pharmacodynamics 49: 311-323.

Tavanai, E., Mohammadkhani, G., Farahani, S. and Jalaie, S., 2019. Protective effects of silymarin against age-related hearing loss in an aging rat model. Indian Journal of Otolaryngology and Head and Neck Surgery 71: 1248-1257.

Thakare, V.N., Aswar, M.K., Kulkarni, Y.P., Patil, R.R. and Patel, B.M., 2017. Silymarin ameliorates experimentally induced depressive like behavior in rats: Involvement of hippocampal BDNF signaling, inflammatory cytokines and oxidative stress response. Physiology & Behavior 179: 401-410.

Thakare, V.N., Dhakane, V.D. and Patel, B.M., 2016. Potential antidepressant-like activity of silymarin in the acute restraint stress in mice: Modulation of corticosterone and oxidative stress response in cerebral cortex and hippocampus. Pharmacological Reports 68: 1020-1027.

Thakare, V.N., Patil, R.R., Oswal, R.J., Dhakane, V.D., Aswar, M.K. and Patel, B.M., 2018. Therapeutic potential of silymarin in chronic unpredictable mild stress induced depressive-like behavior in mice. Journal of Psychopharmacology 32: 223-235.

Tvrdý, V., Pourová, J., Jirkovský, E., Křen, V., Valentová, K. and Mladěnka, P., 2021. Systematic review of pharmacokinetics and potential pharmacokinetic interactions of flavonolignans from silymarin. Medicinal Research Reviews 41: 2195-2246.

Vargas-Mendoza, N., Ángeles-Valencia, M., Madrigal-Santillán, E.O., Morales-Martínez, M., Tirado-Lule, J.M., Solano-Urrusquieta, A., Madrigal-Bujaidar, E., Álvarez-González, I., Fregoso-Aguilar, T., Morales-González, Á. and Morales-González, J.A., 2020. Effect of silymarin supplementation on physical performance, muscle and myocardium histological changes, bodyweight, and food consumption in rats subjected to regular exercise training. International Journal of Molecular Sciences 21: 7724.

Vargas-Mendoza, N., Angeles-Valencia, M., Morales-González, Á., Morales-Martínez, M., Madrigal-Bujaidar, E., Álvarez-González, I., Fregoso-Aguilar, T., Delgado-Olivares, L., Madrigal-Santillán, E.O. and Morales-González, J.A., 2021. Effect of silymarin supplementation in lung and liver histological modifications during exercise training in a rodent model. Journal of Functional Morphology and Kinesiology 6: 72.

Vidlar, A., Vostalova, J., Ulrichova, J., Student, V., Krajicek, M., Vrbkova, J. and Simanek, V., 2010. The safety and efficacy of a silymarin and selenium combination in men after radical prostatectomy – a six month placebo-controlled double-blind clinical trial. Biomedical papers of the Medical Faculty of the University Palacky 154: 239-244.

Viktorová, J., Dobiasová, S., Řehořová, K., Biedermann, D., Káňová, K., Šeborová, K., Václavíková, R., Valentová, K., Ruml, T., Křen, V. and Macek, T., 2019. Antioxidant, anti-inflammatory, and multidrug resistance modulation activity of Silychristin derivatives. Antioxidants 8: 303.

Vimberg, V., Kuzma, M., Stodůlková, E., Novák, P., Bednárová, L., Šulc, M. and Gažák, R., 2015. Hydnocarpin-type flavonolignans: Semisynthesis and inhibitory effects on Staphylococcus aureus biofilm formation. Journal of Natural Products 78: 2095-2103.

Voruganti, S., Yamsani, S.K. and Yamsani, M.R., 2014. Effect of silibinin on the pharmacokinetics of nitrendipine in rabbits. European Journal of Drug metabolism and Pharmacokinetics 39: 277-281.

Vostálová, J., Tinková, E., Biedermann, D., Kosina, P., Ulrichová, J. and Rajnochová Svobodová, A., 2019. Skin protective activity of silymarin and its flavonolignans. Molecules 24: 1022.

Vostalova, J., Vidlar, A., Ulrichova, J., Vrbkova, J., Simanek, V. and Student, V., 2013. Use of selenium-silymarin mix reduces lower urinary tract symptoms and prostate specific antigen in men. Phytomedicine 21: 75-81.

Wang, H., Yan, T., Xie, Y., Zhao, M., Che, Y., Zhang, J., Liu, H., Cao, L., Cheng, X., Xie, Y., Li, F., Qi, Q., Wang, G. and Hao, H., 2015. Mechanism-based inhibitory and peroxisome proliferator-activated receptor α-dependent modulating effects of silybin on principal hepatic drug-metabolizing enzymes. Drug Metabolism and Disposition 43: 444-454.

Wang, L., Wang, Z., Xia, M.M., Wang, Y.Y., Wang, H.Y. and Hu, G.X., 2014. Inhibitory effect of silybin on pharmacokinetics of imatinib *in vivo* and *in vitro*. Canadian Journal of Physiology and Pharmacology 92: 961-964.

Wang, Q., Zou, L., Liu, W., Hao, W., Tashiro, S., Onodera, S. and Ikejima, T., 2011. Inhibiting NF-κB activation and ROS production are involved in the mechanism of silibinin's protection against D-galactose-induced senescence. Pharmacology, Biochemistry, and Behavior 98: 140-149.

Ward, J., Kapadia, K., Brush, E. and Salhanick, S.D., 2013. Amatoxin poisoning: case reports and review of current therapies. The Journal of Emergency Medicine 44: 116-121.

Wu, J.W., Lin, L.C. and Tsai, T.H., 2009. Drug-drug interactions of silymarin on the perspective of pharmacokinetics. Journal of Ethnopharmacology 121: 185-193.

Xie, Y., Zhang, D., Zhang, J. and Yuan, J., 2019. Metabolism, transport and drug-drug interactions of silymarin. Molecules 24: 3693.

Yamsani, S.K. and Yamsani, M.R., 2014. Effect of silymarin pretreatment on the bioavailability of domperidone in healthy human volunteers. Drug Metabolism and Drug Interactions 29: 261-267.

Yan, W.J., Tan, Y.C., Xu, J.C., Tang, X.P., Zhang, C., Zhang, P.B. and Ren, Z.Q., 2015. Protective effects of silibinin and its possible mechanism of action in mice exposed to chronic unpredictable mild stress. Biomolecules & Therapeutics 23: 245-250.

Yang, Z., Pan, Q., Zhang, D., Chen, J., Qiu, Y., Chen, X., Zheng, F. and Lin, F., 2019. Silibinin restores the sensitivity of cisplatin and taxol in A2780-resistant cell and reduces drug-induced hepatotoxicity. Cancer Management and Research 11: 7111-7122.

Ye, Y. and Liu, Z., 2018. Management of Amanita phalloides poisoning: A literature review and update. Journal of Critical Care 46: 17-22.

Yu, C., Pan, L., Wang, G., Cai, Z., Zhou, Y., Zheng, X., Chen, C. and Zhang, X., 2020. Silybin enhances the blood concentration of brexpiprazole in rats by downregulating expression of CYP3A4 and CYP2D6. Die Pharmazie 75: 198-200.

Zalat, Z.A.K., Elewa, H.A., Abdel-Latif, M., Alm El-Din, M.A. and Kohaf, N.A., 2020a. Evaluation of the cardioprotective effect of l-carnitine and silymarin in cancer patients receiving anthracycline-containing chemotherapy. Journal of Bioscience and Applied Research 6: 190-206.

Zalat, Z., El-Din, M.A., Kohaf, N.A.E.M., Abdel-Latif, M. and Elewa, H., 2020b. 292P Evaluation of the cardioprotective effects of l-carnitine and silymarin in cancer patients receiving anthracycline-containing chemotherapy. Annals of Oncology 31: S359.

Zhu, Z. and Sun, G., 2018. Silymarin mitigates lung impairments in a rat model of acute respiratory distress syndrome. Inflammopharmacology 26: 747-754.

Part V.

Practical applications of silymarin in poultry/animal industry

A cheerful heart is good medicine but not on an empty stomach

Chapter 17
Silymarin in poultry and farm animal nutrition and health

Don't count your chickens before they are hatched

Anton Surai[1] and Peter F. Surai[2-7]*
[1]Healthy Food Services, Bristol, UK; [2]Vitagene and Health Research Centre, Bristol, UK; [3]Department of Microbiology and Biochemistry, Faculty of Veterinary Medicine, Trakia University, Stara Zagora, Bulgaria; [4]Department of Animal Nutrition, Faculty of Agricultural and Environmental Sciences, Szent Istvan University, Hungary; [5]Saint-Petersburg State Academy of Veterinary Medicine, St. Petersburg, Russia; [6]Sumy National Agrarian University, Sumy, Ukraine; [7]Odessa National Academy of Food Technologies, Odessa, Ukraine
psurai@feedfood.co.uk

Abstract

Silymarin (SM) has received tremendous attention in medical science for the last few decades. In great contrast, research interest and practical applications of this phytochemical mixture in poultry and farm animal nutrition and health are quite limited and appeared mainly in last 5-10 years. Therefore, this chapter briefly summarises data on SM in poultry, pig and other farm animal nutrition. The presented data indicates that SM/Milk thistle showed some promising results as feed additives in poultry, pig and other farm animal nutrition. However, taking into account high price sensitivity of poultry (especially broiler) and pig feed it seems likely that direct usage of SM as a feed additive has a limited value, since it is not economically valuable. Sometimes usage of Milk thistle could be more economically valuable option, but variability in chemical composition which would affect its efficacy as well as possible presence of anti-nutritional factors would limit its usage in commercial broiler production. However, in layer and breeder nutrition and potentially in rearing bird nutrition MT could be a valuable product to be used. There are some promising results related to usage of SM in sow nutrition and this question warrants further investigations. The most important findings related to SM and Milk thistle are their protective effects under various stress conditions, including mycotoxin feed contamination and heat stress. Anti-stress and anti-toxic activities of SM put this phytochemical mixture into veterinary category of dietary supplements. Furthermore, it seems likely that a combined usage of SM with other nutrients having synergetic protective effects (e.g. carnitine, betaine, taurine, etc.) could be a way of further supplement development. There is a growing body of evidence indicating that beneficial effects of SM in human medicine can be translated into the development of the veterinary preparations supplied with feed or water.

Keywords: silymarin, poultry, chicken, pigs, farm animals

DOI:10.3920/978-90-8686-944-2_017,

17.1 Introduction

SM has received tremendous attention in medical science for the last few decades. In great contrast, research interest and practical applications of this phytochemical in poultry and farm animal nutrition and health are quite limited and appeared mainly in last 5-10 years. Therefore, the aim of this chapter to briefly summarise data on SM/MT in poultry, pig and other farm animal nutrition.

17.2 Silymarin in poultry

Based on multiple protective effects of SM shown above in various model systems one can expect its beneficial effect in commercial poultry production associated with stress conditions. Data on protective effects of SM and milk thistle seeds on poultry are shown in Table 17.1.

17.2.1 Broilers

MT, MTS and SM were tested during growth of chicks, including days 1-35 (Shanmugam *et al.*, 2022), 1-40 (Bagno *et al.*, 2021), 1-42 (Janocha *et al.*, 2021), 1-60 (Schiavone *et al.*, 2007), 7-42 (Bendowski *et al.*, 2022), 12 to day 37 (Statnik *et al.*, 2015) and 21 to day 91 days (Abdalla *et al.*, 2018). SM was used at various doses including 0.2, 0.4, 0.5, 0.6, 1.0 and 1.5 mg/kg, while MT or MTS were used at 1.25-3%. Interestingly, high doses of MT (5 and 15%) showed detrimental effects on growing chickens (Statnik *et al.*, 2015).

The main beneficial effects included improved final body weight (Abdalla *et al.*, 2018; Bendowski *et al.*, 2022, Janocha *et al.*, 2021; Shanmugam *et al.*, 2022), body weight gain and carcass weight (Bendowski *et al.*, 2022), FCR (Abdalla *et al.*, 2018; Janocha *et al.*, 2021), nutrient digestibility (Shanmugam *et al.*, 2022), meat quality including water holding capacity, and improved flavour, tenderness and palatability of meat (Janocha *et al.*, 2021) and decreased muscle fat (Schiavone *et al.*, 2007). MTS was also shown to improve the welfare (footpad dermatitis and gait index) of the chickens (Bendowski *et al.*, 2022), liver integrity and AO defences (Abdalla *et al.*, 2018) and increased muscles resistance to oxidative stress (Schiavone *et al.*, 2007). In general, in most cases under normal physiological conditions SM and its derivatives were shown to have little or no significant effects on broiler performance (Zaker-Esteghamati *et al.*, 2020). However, the authors indicated that SM could help maintaining and enhancing the sensory quality of broiler meat.

17.2.2 Protective effects of SM/MT on poultry under stressful conditions

Taking into account molecular mechanisms of protective effects of SM it seems likely that beneficial effects of this phytochemical would depend on the level of stress during chicken growth. Therefore, in Table 17.2 protective effects of MT/SM on broiler chicks under mycotoxin and other stress condition are summarised. In 7 chicken trials AFB1

Table 17.1. Effect of milk thistle (MT), milk thistle seeds (MTS) or SM on broiler chicks.

N	Experimental design	Effects of SM/MT/MTS	References
1	102 one-day-old male ROSS 308 chicks, 3 groups, Basal diet (BD), BD + 4.08 or 6.12 g MTS, which were added to 200 ml of water at 90 ◦C per each replicate for E1 and E2, respectively, and then applying the preparation to a bell drinker from 7 to 42 days of age	MTS improved body weight, body weight gain and carcass weight and decreased abdominal fat at higher dosage. No effect on meat quality. No effect on GSH, but decreased vit. C in breast muscles. MTS improved the welfare (footpad dermatitis and gait index) of the chickens	Bendowski *et al.*, 2022
2	1,088 one-day-old Ross 308 broiler chicks, 4 groups, BD, BD+ 0.02%, 0.04%, and 0.06% of SM for 35 days	SM linearly increased the final body weight, and the nutrient digestibility of dry matter, gross energy, and nitrogen and caecal *Lactobacillus* counts. Relative weights of breast muscle, bursa of Fabricius were increased, water holding capacity was enhanced and drip loss linearly decreased	Shanmugam *et al.*, 2022
3	300 one-day-old ISA F15 broiler, 6 groups, BD, BD+ 0.1; 0.5; 1; 1.5 and 2 mg MT extract/kg body weight for 40 days	MT increased the number of red blood cells, haemoglobin, white blood cells in the blood, and decreased the level of albumin and increased the content of γ-globulins in serum	Bagno *et al.*, 2021
4	120 Ross 308 broiler, (BD, MTS1 (MT seeds; 0/2% starter/grower), MTS2 (2/3% starter/grower) for 42 days	MTS improved body weight and FCR, decreased muscle fat, improved water holding capacity of breast muscle, improved flavour, tenderness and palatability of breast and leg muscles and improved juiciness of thigh muscle	Janocha *et al.*, 2021
5	125 Gimmizah cockerels from day 21 to day 91, 5 groups. BD, BD+Vit.E (150 mg VE/kg diet), BD+SM (0.5 g/kg diet), BD+ MT (12.5 g/kg diet, equal to 0.5 g SM), BD+ MT (25 g/kg diet, equal to 1 g SM)	SM improved body weight, body weight gain, FCR (days 21-63), liver integrity (blood AST and ALT), AO defences (GSH, TAC and MDA), but relative economic efficiency was lower (93.9%), than in control group. MT showed similar positive responses and 12.5 g MT/kg diet was most economically valuable (12% higher than in BD group)	Abdalla *et al.*, 2018
6	75 ROSS 308 cockerels, 3 groups, BD, BD+MT (5%) and BD+MT (15%) from day 12 to day 37	MT cake detrimentally affected feed consumption, FCR and broiler carcass yield	Statnik *et al.*, 2015
7	180 male chicks (ROSS 508), BD, BD +40 or 80 mg/kg SM, 60 days	Reduced lipid content of breast and thigh muscles, increased muscles resistance to oxidative stress	Schiavone *et al.*, 2007

Table 17.2. Protective effects of SM/MT/MTS on broiler chicks against mycotoxin and other stress condition.

N	Experimental design	Effects of SM/MT/MTS	References
1	300 one-day-old male chicks, 5 groups, including BD, BD+AFB1 (0.6 mg AFB1/kg); BD+AFB1+MT (10 g/kg) and 2 groups fed a toxin binder for 42 days	MT ameliorated AFB1-induces reduction in feed intake and body weight but did not affect FCR. MT prevented AFB1-associated liver weight and abdominal fat increase. MT also ameliorated some AFB1-induced liver damages (plasma AST) and decreased concentration of caecal Coliform bacteria	Feshanghchi *et al.*, 2022
2	240 1-day-old Cobb 500 chicks. 4 treatments: BD; BD+SM (100 mg/kg); BD+Mtx (0.05 mg/kg aflatoxin and 20 mg/kg fumonisin) and BD+Mtx+SM for 42 days	SM ameliorated Mtx-induced reduction in weight gain and prevented deterioration in FCR. No effects on gut integrity	Armanini *et al.*, 2021
3	160 one-day old chicks (Ross 308), 4 groups: BD, BD + mtx (aflatoxins 8.4 µg/kg + T2 toxin 24.3 µg/kg), BD+SM (0.5%), BD+mtx+SM for 35 days	SM improved body weight (BW) and weekly weight gain (WDG), increased feed intake. SM also ameliorated mtx-induced reduction in BW, WGG and feed intake and deterioration in FCR	Abdulwahid and Oleiwi, 2021
4	430 (7-day-old) Ross broiler chicks. 7 experimental groups with a 2 × 3 factorial arrangement, including two aflatoxin levels (0.5 and 2 mg/kg) and three levels of SM (0, 500 and 1,000 mg/kg) for 21 days	SM improved performance of AF-challenged birds by suppressing ileal bacteria and enhancing absorptive surface area	Jahanian *et al.*, 2017
5	216 broiler day-old chicks (Ross 308), 9 groups, BD, BD+ AFB1 (250 or 500 µg/kg) and MTS (0.5 or 1%) for 35 days	MTS partly ameliorated AFB1-induced decrease in villus length and the ratio of villus length to crypt depth, indicating improvement in gut morphology and absorptive capacity and improving protein digestibility	Hasheminejad *et al.*, 2015
6	216 one-d-old Ross 308 male broiler chicks, 9 groups, 250-500 µg/kg AFB1, 0.5 and 1% MTS	AFB1 disturbed metabolism of Ca, glucose and creatinine, increased AST activity (liver damage). MTS significantly reduced the effect of AFB1 on the above parameters	Amiridumari *et al.*, 2013
7	144 Ross 308 male broiler chicks, 4 groups: BD, BD+SM (1%), BD+OTA (3 mg/kg); BD+OTA+SM; from day 11 to day 42	SM partly ameliorated OTA-induced histopathological and biochemical detrimental changes in the liver and kidney	Stoev *et al.*, 2021
8	70 Ross 308 broiler chicks, 5 groups: BD, BD+OTA (5 mg/kg), BD+OTA+ *Silybum marianum* dry powder (SMDP; 1.1 g/kg); 2 other groups with herbal additives, from day 11 to day 42	SMDP partly ameliorated OTA-induced histopathological detrimental changes in the liver, lung, brain, kidney, gut and mitigated OTA-associated immunosuppression including decrease in immune organ pathology	Stoev *et al.*, 2019

Table 17.2. Protective effects of SM/MT/MTS on broiler chicks against mycotoxin and other stress condition.

N	Experimental design	Effects of SM/MT/MTS	References
9	240 one-day-old birds, 12 groups. BD, OTA (1 or 2 mg/kg), SM (10 g/kg), Vit. E (200 mg/kg) for 42 days	SM and Vit. E alone or in combination ameliorated the immunotoxic effects induced by 1.0 mg OTA/kg, no protection against 2.0 mg OTA/kg	Khatoon *et al.*, 2013
10	216 one-day-old broiler chicks (Ross 308), 9 groups, BD, BD+AFB1 (250 or 500 µg/kg) and MTS (0.5 or 1%) for 35 days	MTS partly ameliorated AFB1-induced decrease in feed consumption and body weight and mitigated AFB1-induced deterioration in FCR	Makki *et al.*, 2013
11	240 one-day-old broiler chicks, 4 groups. BD; BD+AFB (80-520 µg/kg of the feed); BD+AFB+MT (10 g/kg feed), BD+AFB+ Mycotoxin Binder	MT partly ameliorated AFB-induced decrease of feed consumption and weight gain and completely recovered AFB-compromised FCR and significantly decreased AFB-induced mortality	Chand *et al.*, 2011
12	Twenty one 14-day-old male commercial broilers, BD; DD+AFB1 at 0.8 mg/kg of feed and BD+AFB1 +SM phytosome, at 600 mg/kg of BW for 35 days	SM restored compromised by AFB1 daily gain and FCR to the control level and reduced hepatic histopathological changes induced by the toxin	Tedesco *et al.*, 2004a
13	240 one-day-old broilers, 4 groups. BD, SM 100 mg/kg BW, CCl4 1 ml/kg and SM+CCl4	CCl4 damaged liver and imposed oxidative stress by down-regulating CAT, GPx, and SOD2. SM showed protective effects by ameliorating those changes	Baradaran *et al.*, 2019
14	640 one-day-old broilers, 8 treatments including 2 concentrations (0 and 100 mg/kg BW) of SM or Nano-SM (NES) and CCl4 (0 and 1 ml/kg BW) for 42 days	Nano-SM more effectively than SM ameliorated CCl4-induced liver damages (decreased serum ALT), mitigated downregulation of SOD1 and upregulation of HSP47 caused by CCl4	Yousefdoost, *et al.*, 2019
15	120 broiler chicks, BD, BD+ milk thistle seeds (MTS): 5, 10 or 15 g/kg, 42 days	MTS at 15 g/kg decreased the negative effects of natural summer stress on broilers: Serum MDA↓, antibody titer against ND↑, improved FCR for weeks 2, 3, 4 and 5	Ahmad *et al.*, 2020
16	240 chicks (ROSS 308), BD and BD+100 mg/kg SM, 42 days, days 7-28, increased by 4°C temperature for 4 hours	SM improved performance, immunity and carcass characteristics and decreased the adverse effects of the heat stress	Morovat *et al.*, 2016
17	384 seven-day-old Ross broiler chicks, 8 groups: two microbial conditions (unchallenged and E. Coli challenged), and 4 supplementations (BD, BD+SM (500 or 1,000 mg/kg) for 5 weeks	In the E. coli-infected broiler chicks SM improved ADWG, FCR and gut health: increased both jejunal villi height and VH:CD ratio and reduced crypt depth	Jahanian *et al.*, 2021

was used in the feed at 0.08-2 mg/kg, in other trials a mixture of AFB1 8.4 μg/kg + T2 toxin 24.3 μg/kg, as well as OTA at 1or 2 mg/kg were used. In addition, CCl_4 intoxication and heat stress were also tested as stress factors imposing oxidative stress. SM and MT/MTS were used as protective additives to decrease detrimental effects of the aforementioned stress factors. In most cases SM or MT showed some protective effects, but very often did not return the markers of chicken health or oxidative stress to the control levels.

Aflatoxins are shown to be highly toxic for poultry. They are unavoidable natural contaminants produced by *Aspergillus flavus* and *Aspergillus parasiticus* being common fungal contaminants of nuts but are also found to be growing on a variety of feedstuff, including maize, wheat, rice, and cottonseed. Although 20 AFs have been identified, only four of them, namely AFB1, AFB2, AFG1, and AFG2 occur naturally and are significant contaminants of a wide variety of foods and feeds. AFB1 is considered to be the most toxic and carcinogenic compound of this group of mycotoxins. It is classified by the International Agency of Research on Cancer as Group 1 human carcinogen. AFs may be converted to more reactive, electrophilic epoxides by phase I metabolism occurring primarily in the liver. This group of mycotoxins also possesses high teratogenic, mutagenic, and immunosuppressive activities. The liver is the main target organ for AF toxicity and carcinogenicity. Aflatoxicosis can progress to potentially lethal acute hepatitis with vomiting, abdominal pain, hepatitis, and eventually death (Surai, 2006).

Therefore, in poultry AFs can compromise performance, including growth rate, FCR, gut health and immunocompetence, reduce egg production and hatchability, increase liver and kidney weight and impose tissue lesions. The protective effects of SM/MT in broilers fed on mycotoxin-contaminated diets included amelioration of mycotoxin/AFB-compromised production indexes including:

- feed intake (Abdulwahid and Oleiwi, 2021; Chand *et al.*, 2011; Feshanghchi *et al.*, 2022; Makki *et al.*, 2013);
- body weight (Abdulwahid and Oleiwi, 2021; Feshanghchi *et al.*, 2022; Makki *et al.*, 2013);
- weight gain (Abdulwahid and Oleiwi, 2021; Armanini *et al.*, 2021; Chand *et al.*, 2011);
- FCR (Armanini *et al.*, 2021; Chand *et al.*, 2011; Feshanghchi *et al.*, 2022; Makki *et al.*, 2013);
- mortality (Chand *et al.*, 2011);
- gut health (Hasheminejad *et al.*, 2015; Jahanian *et al.*, 2017);
- liver damage (Amiridumari *et al.*, 2013; Feshanghchi *et al.*, 2022; Tedesco *et al.*, 2004a);
- antioxidant defences in the liver of laying hens (Eid *et al.*, 2022) and ducklings (El-Sheshtawy *et al.*, 2021).

These data are in agreement with a conclusion from recent reviews (Alhidary *et al.*, 2017; Zaker-Esteghamati *et al.*, 2020) indicating that supplementing SM in diets containing aflatoxins can increase feed intake and performance due to improvement of poultry health. Interestingly, SM also showed protective effect against OTA in broilers (ameliorated immunosuppression; Khatoon *et al.*, 2013) and laying hens (mitigated OTA induced decreased body weight, egg production, egg weight and alleviated OTA-compromised FCR; Eid *et al.*, 2022). The protective effect of SM against CCl_4 toxicity in broilers was related to preservation of CCl_4-compromised AO defences (Baradaran *et al.*, 2019). Furthermore, SM and MT were protective against heat-stress-induced performance deterioration and immunosuppression in broilers (Ahmad *et al.*, 2020; Morovat *et al.*, 2016). In addition, in quail, MT and SM were reported to ameliorate Cd-induced compromised mortality, organ weights, spermatogenesis, and histopathological lesions (Saleemi *et al.*, 2019). High energy diet was also shown to be an important stress factor imposing oxidative stress in testes (MDA↑, GPx↓) and disturbed spermatogenesis in quails and MTS was reported to have protective effects against the aforementioned disturbances (Çeribaşı *et al.*, 2020). There are also some indications that SM could had positive effects on the microflora and intestinal integrity of broilers (Zaker-Esteghamati *et al.*, 2020).

17.2.3 SM/MT for laying hens, ducklings and quail

Data on effects of MT/SM on layers, ducklings and quail are shown in Table 17.3.

It was shown that dietary supplementation of 3% MTM improved FCR, reduced ileal *E. coli* enumeration and enhanced the villus height-to-crypt depth ratio in laying hens (Hashemi Jabali *et al.*, 2018). Furthermore, MTS (7%) was reported to increase feed consumption, laying intensity, number of eggs produced per group per day and improved Haugh units, but decreased eggshell strength (Šťastník *et al.*, 2019).

Lower dose of MTM (30 g/kg) was found to reduce hepatic lipid percentage, improved liver health (AST and ALT) and improved eggshell strength and thickness (Gholamalian *et al.*, 2022). Furthermore, in growing ducklings (from day 7 for 63 days) SM at 0.6 g/kg improved live body weight, body weight gain, FCR and carcass yield, liver integrity (serum AST and ALT), AO defences (SOD, GPx, GSH, MDA) and decreased abdominal fat percent. Increased SM doses did not show further improvement (Elnaggar *et al.*, 2021). Therefore, SM at a proper dosage can be used to increase the production performance in broilers and layers, stimulate the immune response, improve the carcass and enhance the intestinal health under commercial stress conditions (Abd El-Ghany, 2022).

17.3 Silymarin in farm animals

As mentioned above there is a range of publications showing various beneficial effects of SM/MT in poultry. There are also publications available describing results of SM/MT usage in animal nutrition including pigs/sows, cows and other animals.

Table 17.3. Effects of MT/SM on layers, ducklings and quail.

N	Experimental design	Effects of SM/MT/MTS	References
1	480 laying hens (Hy-Line W-36), 12 groups including 4 dietary fat sources (fish oil, sunflower oil, poultry oil and fat powder) and 2 levels of MT meal (MTM, 15 and 30 g/kg) for 70 days after 10 days of adaptation	MTM at 30 g/kg reduced hepatic lipid percentage, improved liver health (AST and ALT) and improved eggshell strength and thickness	Gholamalian *et al.*, 2022
2	300 local laying hens of 28 weeks of age, 4 groups. BD, BD+SM (1 g/kg), BD+OTA (1 mg/kg), BD+OTA+SM	SM ameliorated OTA induced decreased body weight, egg production, egg weight and ameliorated OTA-compromised FCR	Eid *et al.*, 2022
3	Seventy 80-weeks Lohmann LSL-Lite hens were allocated to 7 treatments for 12 weeks: BD; BD+SM (100 mg/kg BW); BD+SM (200 mg/kg BW); BD+nanoSM and BD+ lecithinized SM with the same doses	SM in all forms increased egg production, egg weight, and egg mass and improved FCR. Silymarin also improved Haugh units, nutrient digestibility, intestinal morphology, and pH of digesta	Faryadi *et al.*, 2021
4	Eighteen laying hens were allotted into 3 groups for 20 weeks: BD; BD+SM (200 mg/kg) and BD+SM (400 mg/kg)	SM at 200 mg/kg improved eggs laying rate (+2.91%) and FCR (-4.52%). No effect of SM at 400 mg/kg	Quarantelli *et al.*, 2009
5	30 Bovans Brown laying hens, 2 groups, BD and BD+MTS (7%) from the age 69 weeks to 80 weeks	MTS increased feed consumption, laying intensity, number of eggs produced per group per day, improved Haugh units, but decreased eggshell strength	Šťastník *et al.*, 2019
6	200 leghorn laying hens (Hy-Line W-36), 8 treatments. Four levels of milk thistle meal (0%, 15%, 30% and 60%) were used for 80 days	Dietary supplementation of 3% milk thistle meal improved FCR, reduced ileal *E. coli* enumeration and enhanced the villus height-to-crypt depth ratio	Hashemi Jabali *et al.*, 2018
7	120 one-day-old Pekin ducklings, four groups: BD, BD+AF (30 µg/kg), BD+AF+SM (600 mg/kg/ diet); BD+AF+ lycopene for 10 days	SM decreased MDA and the hepatic residue of AF, and improved AO defences in the liver (CAT, GST and MDA)	El-Sheshtawy *et al.*, 2021
8	200 7-day-old ducklings (Cairina Moschata Domestica), 4 groups, BD, BD+SM (0.6, 0.9 or 1.4 g/kg diet until day 70	SM at 0.6 g/kg improved live body weight, body weight gain, FCR and carcass yield, liver integrity (serum AST and ALT), T3 concentration and AO defences (SOD, GPx, GSH, MDA) and decreased abdominal fat percent. Increased SM doses did not show further improvement.	Elnaggar *et al.*, 2021
9	2 weeks old white, female, Hungarian ducks, 3 groups (n=6). BD; BD+ mtx (0.9 mg/kg DON and 0.66 mg/kg ZEA), BD+Mtx+MT (0.5) until day 47	MT partly ameliorated Mtx-induced vacuolar degeneration of hepatocytes cytoplasm, solitary hepatocyte necrosis and cell deaths. However, MT increased diene conjugates concentration	Egresi *et al.*, 2020

Table 17.3. Effects of MT/SM on layers, ducklings and quail.

N	Experimental design	Effects of SM/MT/MTS	References
10	120 male (15-day-old) Japanese quail chicks, 4 groups, BD, high energy diet (HD), milk thistle seeds (MTS, 1%), HD+MTS for 35 days	HD imposed oxidative stress in testes (MDA↑, GPx↓) and disturbed spermatogenesis; almost all the disturbances were ameliorated by MTS. MTS decreased body weight (alone or HD+MTS)	Çeribaşı *et al.*, 2020
11	144 quails, 9 groups, different combinations of Cd chloride (150 and 300 mg/kg feed), SM (250 mg/kg), and MT (10 g/kg) feed.	Supplementing MT and SM ameliorated mortality, organ weights, spermatogenesis, and histopathological lesions	Saleemi *et al.*, 2019

17.3.1 SM/MT for sows and growing piglets

The data on SM efficacy in pig nutrition are shown in Table 17.4.

In sows SM (0.05%, 0.1%, and 0.2%) was sown to increase (Zhang *et al.*, 2021):

- litter weight and litter weight gain;
- feed intake in week 1, week 2, and the entire lactation period;
- average daily milk yields during lactation;
- milk fat content;
- AO defences (SOD, GPX, CAT, GSH/GSSG).

Similarly, SM (40 g/day from day 108 of gestation to weaning) was reported to increase feed intake, milk yield and AO defences, enhanced protein metabolism and decreased inflammation. Furthermore, SM improved growth performance of sow's progeny offspring (Jiang *et al.*, 2020). Interestingly, SM at lower doses (1 or 8 g/day throughout a 20-day lactation) did not show any measurable effects on sows (Farmer *et al.*, 2017). In barrows MT (3%, from body weight 25 kg for 100 days) improved the average daily weight gains by 2%, while higher MT dose (6%) increased the gains by 3.8%. MT also improved meat quality (colour and water-holding capacity) and its oxidative stability with MT (6%) being more effective (Grela *et al.*, 2020). Lower dose of MT (0.7%) in fattener pigs showed limited benefits, including increased pH45 and pH24 values in the offal (Kropiwiec-Domańska *et al.*, 2022).

17.3.2 SM/MT for cows, ewes and rabbits

Some benefits of SM in other farm animals have been described (Table 17.5). Initially it was shown that SM (10 g/cow/day) had no effect on the liver of lactating cows (Tedesco *et al.*, 2004c). The same authors showed that SM (10 g SM daily as oral drenches) from 10 days prior to the calving date to 15 days after calving improved milk production throughout lactation with earlier peak of milk production. Furthermore,

Table 17.4. Effects of SM on pigs and sows.

N	Experimental design	Effects of SM	References
1	60 fattener pigs; BD and BD+ ground MT at 7 g/kg	Increased pH45 and pH24 values in the offal; decreased the weight of heart and lungs and increased the weight of liver and kidneys. Increased fat content in hearts, lungs and kidneys and decreased fat in the liver	Kropiwiec-Domańska *et al.*, 2022
2	140 crossed fattening pigs, four treatments: BD, BD + micelle silymarin (MS, 0.05%); BD+MS, 0.1%; and BD+MS 0.2% for 10 weeks	Dose-dependent improvement in the average daily gain (ADG) of pigs (during 5 to 10 weeks), the apparent total tract digestibility of nitrogen was enhanced (in week 5 and week 10) and meat quality improvement were observed	Zhang and Kim, 2022
3	Sixty pregnant sows (85 d), 3 groups, BD, BD+SM (250 mg/kg), BD+SM (500 mg/kg) for 46 days	SM increased the total feed intake and average daily feed intake, decreased serum MDA, plasma D-lactic acid and faecal isobutyric acid concentrations	Liangkai *et al.*, 2022
4	40 multiparous sows from the 109th prenatal day to the 21st postnatal day. Four groups; BD, BD+SM (0.05%, 0.1%, and 0.2%)	On weaning day, increased litter weight and litter weight gain were linearly improved; feed intake in week 1, week 2, and the entire lactation period was increased; increased average daily milk yields during lactation; increased milk fat content; improved AO defences (SOD, GPX, CAT, GSH/GSSG) of sows and their progeny	Zhang *et al.*, 2021
5	110 sows from day 108 of gestation to weaning, BD, BD+SM (40 g/day)	Increased feed intake and enhanced protein metabolism; increased milk yield; improved growth performance of their offsprings; improved AO defences (GPx and CAT) and decreased inflammation (IL-1β)	Jiang *et al.*, 2020
6	60 barrows (BW=25.0±0.5 kg), 3 groups, BD, BD+MT (3%), BD+MT (6%) for 100 days	MT (3%) improved the average daily weight gains by 2% and MT (6%) improved the gains by 3.8%. MT also improved meat quality (colour and water-holding capacity) and its oxidative stability with MT6% being more effective	Grela *et al.*, 2020
7	99 lactating sows, BD, BD+SM (1 g/day); BD+SM (8 g/day) throughout a 20-day lactation	No effect on circulating prolactin or urea, on oxidative damage to proteins or antioxidant potential in sows lactation feed intake, milk composition, backfat and BW of sows and piglet growth were not affected by treatment	Farmer *et al.*, 2017

Table 17.5. Effects of SM on cows, ewes and rabbits.

N	Experimental design	Effects of supplements	References
1	20 pregnant cows, BD and BD+ a mixture of SM (7.77 g/day/cow and lycopene 1.27 g/day/cow) from 7 days before the expected calving date to the first 14 days in milk	Increased energy corrected milk yield and milk fat yield over the first 21 days of lactation; lower mean log10 SCC compared to control cows and lower overall concentration of TBARS	Garavaglia *et al.*, 2015
2	30 pregnant cows, BD and BD+SM (10 g) daily as oral drenches, from 10 days prior to the calving date to 15 days after calving	Improved milk production than control cows throughout lactation; earlier the peak of milk production; better maintained body condition score after calving; increased plasma non-esterified fatty acids on day 7	Tedesco *et al.*, 2004b
3	20 pregnant dairy cows, BD and BD+SM (10 g) daily as oral drenches, from 10 days prior to the calving date to 15 days after calving	At the used dosage, SM had no adverse or positive effect on the liver of lactating cows	Tedesco *et al.*, 2004c
4	20 Greek mountain ewes, in second lactation, 2 groups, BD and BD+ 3% (w/w) milk thistle oil (MTSO).	MTSO significantly increased milk yield and affected fatty acid profile of milk fat	Karaiskou *et al.*, 2021
5	20 Sanjabi ewes, 2 groups, BD and BD+ SM (2g/kg) for 15 d after lambing	SM reduced postpartum body weight loss, increased the feed intake, stimulated earlier milk yield peak and improved antioxidant defences	Khamisabadi, 2020
6	36 New Zealand white does (rabbits), 4 groups, BD, BD+ 3 ml; 6 ml or 9 ml MT ethanolic extract (MTE); The trail lasted until kits weaning	Higher doses of MTE (6 and 9 ml) increased feed intake during pregnancy and lactation, milk production, litter weight at birth and weaning and litter size at birth and weaning	Refaie *et al.*, 2019
7	35 rabbit bucks, 5 groups, BD; BD+ MTS (5 mg/kg); BD+ MTS (10 mg/kg); BD+ Rosemary leaves (5 or 10 g/kg)	MTS improved the sperm concentration, total sperm output, live sperm, total live sperm, total motile sperm and enhanced fertility	Attia *et al.*, 2017
8	Eighty-four male New Zealand White bucks (1.75-2.0 kg), 7 groups: BD; BD + salinomycin (SMC 20 or 40 mg/kg); SM (6.5 or 13 mg/kg BW); BD+SMC+SM for 28 days	SM was shown to partly prevent and cure salinomycin-induced toxicity in rabbits	Ghonaim *et al.*, 2022

after calving, in SM-consuming cows better body condition score was maintained (Tedesco *et al.*, 2004b). Feeding a mixture of SM (7.77 g/day) and lycopene (1.27 g/day) to pregnant cows from 7 days before the expected calving date to the first 14 days in milk was found to increase energy corrected milk yield and milk fat yield over the first 21 days of lactation. Furthermore, lower mean log10 SCC compared to control cows and lower overall concentration of TBARS were observed (Garavaglia *et al.*, 2015).

In ewes SM (2 g/kg for 15 d after lambing) was reported to mitigate postpartum body weight loss, to increase the feed intake, stimulated earlier milk yield peak and improved antioxidant defences (Khamisabadi, 2020). Interestingly, milk thistle oil (3%) in ewe diets was shown to increase milk yield and affected fatty acid profile of milk fat (Karaiskou *et al.*, 2021). There are some indications that SM/MT could be effective in rabbit nutrition as well. For example, in rabbit bucks MTS (0.5 or 1%) improved sperm quality (concentration, total sperm output, live sperm, total live sperm, total motile sperm) and enhanced fertility (Attia *et al.*, 2017). In New Zealand white does MT extract (Refaie *et al.*, 2019):

- improved feed intake during pregnancy and lactation;
- enhanced milk production;
- increased litter weight at birth and weaning;
- increased litter size at birth and weaning.

17.4 Conclusions

As can be seen from data presented above SM/MT showed some promising results as feed additives in poultry, pig and other farm animal nutrition. However, taking into account high price sensitivity of poultry (especially broiler) and pig feed it seems likely that direct usage of SM as a feed additive has a limited value, since it is not economically valuable (Abdalla *et al.*, 2018). Sometimes usage MT/MTS could be more economically valuable option, but variability in chemical composition which would affect its efficacy as well as possible presence of anti-nutritional factors would limit its usage in commercial broiler production (Stastnik *et al.*, 2020). However, in layer and breeder nutrition and potentially in rearing bird nutrition MT could be a valuable product to be used. There are some promising results related to usage of SM in sow nutrition and this question warrants further investigations. In a recent review devoted to usage of milk thistle in farm and companion animals (Guerrini and Tedesco, 2023) it was concluded that in farm animals (poultry, pigs and ruminants) milk thistle/SM can improve the performance and product quality including support of liver function, improvement of gut health and morphology.

The most important findings related to SM and MT are their protective effects under various stress conditions, including mycotoxin feed contamination and heat stress. Anti-stress and anti-toxic activities of SM put this phytochemical into veterinary category of dietary supplements. Furthermore, it seems likely that a combined usage of SM with other nutrients having synergetic protective effects (e.g. carnitine, betaine, TAU, etc.) could be a way of further supplement development. There is a growing body of evidence indicating that beneficial effects of SM in human medicine can be translated in the development of the veterinary preparations supplied with feed or water.

References

Abdalla, A.A., Abou-Shehema, B.M., Hamed, R. and Elden, M.R., 2018. Effect of silymarin supplementation on the performance of developed chickens under summer conditions 1-during growth period. Egyptian Poultry Science Journal 38: 305-329.

Abd El-Ghany, W.A., 2022. The potential uses of silymarin, a milk thistle (*Silybum marianum*) derivative in poultry production system. Online Journal of Animal and Feed Research 12: 46-52.

Abdulwahid, M.T. and Oleiwi, A.F., 2021. Ameliorating effects of silymarin against mycotoxin and its effect on some production and hematological parameters of broilers. Journal of Genetic and Environmental Resources Conservation 9: 207-214.

Ahmad, M., Chand, N., Khan, R.U., Ahmad, N., Khattak, I. and Naz, S., 2020. Dietary supplementation of milk thistle (*Silybum marianum*): growth performance, oxidative stress, and immune response in natural summer stressed broilers. Tropical Animal Health and Production 52: 711-715.

Alhidary, I.A., Rehman, Z., Khan, R.U. and Tahir, M., 2017. Anti-aflatoxin activities of milk thistle (*Silybum marianum*) in broiler. World's Poultry Science Journal 73: 559-566.

Amiridumari, H., Sarir, H., Afzali, N. and Fanimakki, O., 2013. Effects of milk thistle seed against aflatoxin B1 in broiler model. Journal of Research in Medical Sciences 18: 786-790.

Armanini, E.H., Boiago, M.M., Cécere, B.G.O., Oliveira, P.V., Teixeira, C.J.S., Strapazzon, J.V., Bottari, N.B., Silva, A.D., Fracasso, M., Vendruscolo, R.G., Wagner, R., Gloria, E.M.D., Horn, V.W., Mendes, R.E., Baldissera, M.D., Vedovatto, M. and Da Silva, A.S., 2021. Protective effects of silymarin in broiler feed contaminated by mycotoxins: growth performance, meat antioxidant status, and fatty acid profiles. Tropical Animal Health and Production 53: 442.

Attia, Y.A., Hamed, R.S., Bovera, F., Abd El, A.E.H.E., Al-Harthi, M.A. and Shahba, H.A., 2017. Semen quality, antioxidant status and reproductive performance of rabbits bucks fed milk thistle seeds and rosemary leaves. Animal Reproduction Science 184: 178-186.

Bagno, O., Shevchenko, S., Shevchenko, A., Prokhorov, O., Shentseva, A., Vavin, G. and Ulrich, E., 2021. Physiological status of broiler chickens with diets supplemented with milk thistle extract. Veterinary World 14: 1319-1323.

Baradaran, A., Samadi, F., Ramezanpour, S.S. and Yousefdoust, S., 2019. Hepatoprotective effects of silymarin on CCl_4-induced hepatic damage in broiler chickens model. Toxicology Reports 6: 788-794.

Bendowski, W., Michalczuk, M., Jóźwik, A., Kareem, K.Y., Łozicki, A., Karwacki, J. and Bień, D., 2022. Using milk thistle (*Silybum marianum*) extract to improve the welfare, growth performance and meat quality of broiler chicken. Animals 12: 1085.

Çeribaşı, S., Türk, G., Özçelik, M., Doğan, G., Çeribaşı, A.O., Mutlu, S.İ., Erişir, Z., Güvenç, M., Güngören, G., Acısu, T.C., Akarsu, S.A., Kaya, Ş.Ö., Sönmez, M., Yüce, A., Çiftçi, M., Çambay, Z., Bağcı, E., Azman, M.A. and Şimşek, Ü.G., 2020. Negative effect of feeding with high energy diets on testes and metabolic blood parameters of male Japanese quails, and positive role of milk thistle seed. Theriogenology 144: 74-81.

Chand, N., Muhammad, D., Durrani, F.R., Qureshi, M.S. and Ullah, S.S., 2011. Protective effects of milk thistle (*Silybum marianum*) against aflatoxin B1 in broiler chicks. Asian-Australasian Journal of Animal Sciences 24: 1011-1018.

Egresi, A., Süle, K., Szentmihályi, K., Blázovics, A., Fehér, E., Hagymási, K. and Fébel, H., 2020. Impact of milk thistle (*Silybum marianum*) on the mycotoxin caused redox-homeostasis imbalance of ducks liver. Toxicon 187: 181-187.

Eid, Y.Z., Hassan, R.A., El-soud, S.A. and Eldebani, N., 2022. The protective role of silymarin to ameliorate the adverse effects of ochratoxin-A in laying hens on productive performance, blood biochemistry, hematological and antioxidants status. Brazilian Journal of Poultry Science 24: eRBCA-2021-1515.

Elnaggar, A.S., El-Said, E. and Ali, R., 2021. Physiological and immunological responses of ducks (Cairina moschata domestica) to silymarin supplementation. Egyptian Poultry Science Journal 40: 895-913.

El-Sheshtawy, S.M., El-Zoghby, A.F., Shawky, N.A. and Samak, D.H., 2021. Aflatoxicosis in Pekin duckling and the effects of treatments with lycopene and silymarin. Veterinary World 14: 788-793.

Faryadi, S., Sheikhahmadi, A., Farhadi, A. and Nourbakhsh, H., 2021. Effects of silymarin and nano-silymarin on performance, egg quality, nutrient digestibility, and intestinal morphology of laying hens during storage. Italian Journal of Animal Science 20: 1633-1644.

Farmer, C., Lapointe, J. and Cormier, I., 2017. Providing the plant extract silymarin to lactating sows: effects on litter performance and oxidative stress in sows. Animal 11: 405-410.

Feshanghchi, M., Baghban-Kanani, P., Kashefi-Motlagh, B., Adib, F., Azimi-Youvalari, S., Hosseintabar-Ghasemabad, B., Slozhenkina, M., Gorlov, I., Zangeronimo, M.G., Swelum, A.A., Seidavi, A., Khan, R.U., Ragni, M., Laudadio, V. and Tufarelli, V., 2022. Milk thistle (*Silybum marianum*), marine algae (Spirulina platensis) and toxin binder powders in the diets of broiler chickens exposed to aflatoxin-B1: Growth performance, humoral immune response and cecal microbiota. Agriculture 12: 805.

Garavaglia, L., Galletti, S. and Tedesco, D., 2015. Silymarin and lycopene administration in periparturient dairy cows: effects on milk production and oxidative status. New Zealand Veterinary Journal 63: 313-318.

Gholamalian, R., Mahdavi, A.H. and Riasi, A., 2022. Hepatic fatty acids profile, oxidative stability and egg quality traits ameliorated by supplementation of alternative lipid sources and milk thistle meal. Journal of Animal Physiology and Animal Nutrition 106: 860-871.

Grela, E.R., Świątkiewicz, M., Florek, M. and Wojtaszewska, I., 2020. Impact of milk thistle (*Silybum marianum* L.) seeds in fattener diets on pig performance and carcass traits and fatty acid profile and cholesterol of meat, backfat and liver. Livestock Science 239: 104180.

Ghonaim, A.H., Hopo, M.G., Ismail, A.K., AboElnaga, T.R., Elgawish, R.A., Abdou, R.H. and Elhady, K.A., 2022. Hepatoprotective and renoprotective effects of silymarin against salinomycin-induced toxicity in adult rabbits. Veterinary World 15: 2244-2252.

Guerrini, A. and Tedesco, D.E.A., 2023. Use of Milk Thistle in Farm and Companion Animals: A Review. Planta Medica 10.1055/a-1969-2440. https://doi.org/10.1055/a-1969-2440.

Hashemi Jabali, N.S., Mahdavi, A.H., Ansari Mahyari, S., Sedghi, M. and Akbari Moghaddam Kakhki, R., 2018. Effects of milk thistle meal on performance, ileal bacterial enumeration, jejunal morphology and blood lipid peroxidation in laying hens fed diets with different levels of metabolizable energy. Journal of Animal Physiology and Animal Nutrition 102: 410-420.

Hasheminejad, S.A., Makki, O.F., Nik, H.A. and Ebrahimzadeh, A., 2015. The effects of aflatoxin B1 and silymarin-containing milk thistle seeds on ileal morphology and digestibility in broiler chickens. Veterinary Science Development 5: 6017.

Jahanian, E., Mahdavi, A.H., Asgary, S. and Jahanian, R., 2017. Effects of dietary inclusion of silymarin on performance, intestinal morphology and ileal bacterial count in aflatoxin-challenged broiler chicks. Journal of Animal Physiology and Animal Nutrition 101: e43-e54.

Jahanian, E., Mahdavi, A.H. and Jahanian, R., 2021. Silymarin improved the growth performance via modulating the microbiota and mucosal immunity in Escherichia coli-challenged broiler chicks. Livestock Science 249: 104529.

Janocha, A., Milczarek, A. and Pietrusiak, D., 2021. Impact of milk thistle (*Silybum marianum* [L.] Gaertn.) seeds in broiler chicken diets on rearing results, carcass composition, and meat quality. Animals 11: 1550.

Jiang, X., Lin, S., Lin, Y., Fang, Z., Xu, S., Feng, B., Zhuo, Y., Li, J., Che, L., Jiang, X. and Wu, D., 2020. Effects of silymarin supplementation during transition and lactation on reproductive performance, milk composition and haematological parameters in sows. Journal of Animal Physiology and Animal Nutrition 104: 1896-1903.

Karaiskou, C., Kasapidou, E., Michailidis, G., Markantonatos, X. and Basdagianni, Z., 2021. Effect of dietary milk thistle (*Silybum marianum* L.) oil supplementation on animal performance and milk fatty acid composition in dairy ewes. Small Ruminant Research 203: 106493.

Khamisabadi, H., 2020. Effects of silymarin on milk production, liver enzymes, oxidative status and HSP70 gene expression in postparturient Sanjabi ewes. Cellular and Molecular Biology 66: 76-81.

Khatoon, A., Zargham Khan, M., Khan, A., Saleemi, M.K. and Javed, I., 2013. Amelioration of ochratoxin A-induced immunotoxic effects by silymarin and vitamin E in White Leghorn cockerels. Journal of Immunotoxicology 10: 25-31.

Kropiwiec-Domańska, K., Babicz, M., Kędzierska-Matysek, M., Szyndler-Nędza, M., Skrzypczak, E. and Woliński, B., 2022. Effect of milk thistle (*Silybum marianum*) supplementation on pork offal quality. Animals 12: 1526.

Liangkai, W., Gaifeng, H., Cimin, L., Fengming, C., Xinliang, B., Rui, L. and Yulong, Y., 2022. Dietary silymarin ameliorating reproductive and lactation performance of sows via regulating body antioxidant and metabolism. Digital Chinese Medicine 5: 286-294.

Makki, O.F., Afzali, N. and Omidi, A., 2013. Effect of different levels of silymarin (*Silybum marianum*) on growth rate, carcass variables and liver morphology of broiler chickens contaminated with aflatoxin B1. Poultry Science Journal 1: 105-116.

Morovat, M., Chamani, M., Zarei, A. and Sadeghi, A.A., 2016. Dietary but not in ovo feeding of *Silybum marianum* extract resulted in an improvement in performance, immunity and carcass characteristics and decreased the adverse effects of high temperatures in broilers. British Poultry Science 57: 105-113.

Refaie, A.M., Ghazal, M.N., Abo El-Azayem, E.H., El-maged, A. and Marwa, H., 2019. Impact of dietary supplementation of milk thistle (*Silybum marianum*) seed extract on doe rabbits performance. Egyptian Journal of Nutrition and Feeds 22: 375-382.

Saleemi, M.K., Tahir, M.W., Abbas, R.Z., Akhtar, M., Ali, A., Javed, M.T., Fatima, Z., Zubair, M., Bhatti, S.A. and Zahoor Ul Hassan, 2019. Amelioration of toxicopathological effects of cadmium with silymarin and milk thistle in male Japanese quail, Coturnix japonica. Environmental Science and Pollution Research International 26: 21371-21380.

Shanmugam, S., Park, J.H., Cho, S. and Kim, I.H., 2022. Silymarin seed extract supplementation enhances the growth performance, meat quality, and nutrients digestibility, and reduces gas emission in broilers. Animal Bioscience 35: 1215-1222.

Schiavone, A., Righi, F., Quarantelli, A., Bruni, R., Serventi, P. and Fusari, A., 2007. Use of *Silybum marianum* fruit extract in broiler chicken nutrition: influence on performance and meat quality. Journal of Animal Physiology and Animal Nutrition 91: 256-262.

Šťastník, O., Mrkvicová, E., Pavlata, L., Roztočilová, A., Umlášková, B. and Anzenbacherová, E., 2019. Performance, biochemical profile and antioxidant activity of hens supplemented with addition of milk thistle (*Silybum marianum*) seed cakes in diet. Acta Universitatis Agriculturae et Silviculturae Mendelianae Brunensis 67: 993-1003.

Statnik, O., Detvanova, L., Karasek, F., Stenclova, H., Kalhotka, L., Pavlata, L. and Mrkvicova, E., 2015. The influence of milk thistle seed cakes on broiler chickens performance parameters. Mendel Net 152-156.

Stastnik, O., Pavlata, L. and Mrkvicova, E., 2020. The Milk Thistle Seed Cakes and Hempseed Cakes are Potential Feed for Poultry. Animals 10: 1384.

Stoev, S., Mircheva, T., Denev, S., Chobanova, S. and Ivanov, V., 2021. The Protective Effect of Silymarin against Ochratoxin A Induced Histopathological and Biochemical Changes in Chicks. Journal of Advanced Veterinary Research 11: 1-8.

Stoev, S.D., Njobeh, P., Zarkov, I., Mircheva, T., Zapryanova, D., Denev, S. and Dimitrova, B., 2019. Selected herbal feed additives showing protective effects against ochratoxin A toxicosis in broiler chicks. World Mycotoxin Journal 12: 257-268.

Surai, P.F., 2006. Selenium in nutrition and health. Nottingham University Press, Nottingham, UK.

Tedesco, D., Domeneghini, C., Sciannimanico, D., Tameni, M., Steidler, S. and Galletti, S., 2004c. Silymarin, a possible hepatoprotector in dairy cows: biochemical and histological observations. Journal of Veterinary Medicine. A, Physiology, Pathology, Clinical Medicine 51: 85-89.

Tedesco, D., Steidler, S., Galletti, S., Tameni, M., Sonzogni, O. and Ravarotto, L., 2004a. Efficacy of silymarin-phospholipid complex in reducing the toxicity of aflatoxin B1 in broiler chicks. Poultry Science 83: 1839-1843.

Tedesco, D., Tava, A., Galletti, S., Tameni, M., Varisco, G., Costa, A. and Steidler, S., 2004b. Effects of silymarin, a natural hepatoprotector, in periparturient dairy cows. Journal of Dairy Science 87: 2239-2247.

Yousefdoost, S., Samadi, F., Jafari, S.M., Ramezanpour, S.S., Hassani, S. and Ganji, F., 2019. Application of nanoencapsulated silymarin to improve its antioxidant and hepatoprotective activities against carbon tetrachloride-induced oxidative stress in broiler chickens. Livestock Science 228: 177-186.

Zaker-Esteghamati, H., Seidavi, A.R. and Bouyeh, M., 2020. A review on the effect of *Silybum marianum* and its derivatives on broilers under healthy and aflatoxicosis conditions: part 1: Performance, carcass and meat characteristics, and intestinal microflora. World's Poultry Science Journal 76: 318-327.

Zhang, Q., Ahn, J.M. and Kim, I.H., 2021. Micelle silymarin supplementation to sows' diet from day 109 of gestation to entire lactation period enhances reproductive performance and affects serum hormones and metabolites. Journal of Animal Science 99: skab354.

Zhang, Q. and Kim, I.H., 2022. Micelle silymarin supplementation to fattening diet augments daily gain, nutrient digestibility, decreases toxic gas emissions, and ameliorates meat quality of fattening pigs. Czech Journal of Animal Science 67: 125-136.

Chapter 18
From hepatoprotection to general health of poultry

Prevention is better than cure

Anton Surai[1] and Peter F. Surai[2-7]*
[1]Healthy Food Services, Bristol, UK; [2]Vitagene and Health Research Centre, Bristol, UK; [3]Department of Microbiology and Biochemistry, Faculty of Veterinary Medicine, Trakia University, Stara Zagora, Bulgaria; [4]Department of Animal Nutrition, Faculty of Agricultural and Environmental Sciences, Szent Istvan University, Hungary; [5]Saint-Petersburg State Academy of Veterinary Medicine, St. Petersburg, Russia; [6]Sumy National Agrarian University, Sumy, Ukraine; [7]Odessa National Academy of Food Technologies, Odessa, Ukraine
psurai@feedfood.co.uk

Abstract

This chapter presents a recent view on the development of vitagene-modulating supplements (some of them contain SM) to deal with various problems in commercial poultry and animal production. By modulating vitagenes via supplying special nutrient mixtures with drinking water it is possible to develop a 'system of quick response', which can help nutritionist/technologist/veterinarian to deal with emergency situations in commercial poultry/animal production associated with various environmental, technological, nutritional or internal stresses. It appears that vitagene activation is an important approach helping decrease negative consequences of various stresses. It should be mentioned that the aim of the usage of the vitagene-modulating compositions is to help birds mobilise their internal resources/reserves to the maximum extent and usage of such nutritional supplements do not affect general nutrition or nutrient balance. These are additional 'instruments' in hands of nutritionists, technologists and veterinarians helping them with stress management. The data provided in this chapter proved that vitagene activation could be considered as an effective means/tool to deal with various stresses in poultry production. Therefore, the first vitagene-regulating nutrient composition (PerforMax/Magic Antistress Mix) was proven to be effective in those situations where oxidative stress takes place and vitagene activations was reported to improve bird's resistance to stresses and therefore maintain their productive and reproductive performance. Two other concepts (VitaTonic and ShellBone) also found its way to poultry industry and help poultry producers deal with liver health problems as well as with eggshell quality and bone integrity problems. The presented data are a good example of technology transfer from the laboratory research into the commercial chicken production. There are also indications that the vitagene concept and vitagene-regulating nutritional mixtures could be effective in fighting stresses in pig production as well as for health maintaining of other animals (calves and cattle, lambs and sheep, kids and goats, fur-animals, companion animals, zoo animals, fish, etc.) under various stress conditions.

DOI:10.3920/978-90-8686-944-2_018,

Keywords: silymarin, anti-stress supplement, poultry, chicken, vitagenes

18.1 Introduction

Nutrition plays a pivotal role in maintaining poultry health, productive and reproductive performance of commercially rearing and housing birds. It is proven that poultry production is associated with a range of stresses which are responsible for their decreased performance and compromised health. Initially, increased doses of vitamin E have been used in commercial poultry production under various stress condition, including heat stress with various efficiency and variable success (Surai, 1999; 2002; Surai *et al.*, 2019a). Similarly, other nutrients possessing antioxidant activities, including selenium (Surai, 2018a; 2021; Surai and Kochish, 2019), carotenoids (Surai, 2012a,b; Surai and Kochish, 2020; Surai *et al.*, 2011a; 2001b), polyphenols (Surai, 2014; 2015a; 2022) have been widely used to deal with commercially-relevant stresses. However, efficacy of dietary supplementation of various antioxidants beyond their nutritional needs greatly varies and their increased supplementation could be quite costly with low return on investment.

Recently developed the vitagene concept (Chapter 7) is based on understanding that there is a range of genes in poultry responsible for stress adaptation and they are called VITAGENES. Therefore, search for vitagene-regulating nutrients and development of vitagene-modulating supplements are considered to be important milestones in the development of the effective stress management under commercial stress conditions in poultry industry. The aim of this chapter is to present our view on the development of vitagene-modulating supplements, some of them contain SM, to deal with various problems in commercial poultry production.

18.2 Usage of drinking systems for vitagene-activating nutrient mixture delivery

At the beginning of the development of vitagene-modulating nutrient mixtures it was necessary to choose the best way of their delivery to birds (Surai *et al.*, 2018; Surai, 2020a). Traditional usage of various feed additives/supplements has many advantages, however, in stress conditions this system has several important limitations.

18.2.1 Low flexibility

For example, in commercial egg and meat production there are situations when nutrients/drugs are needed to be delivered to birds urgently. However, in traditional commercial poultry production, feed bins usually contain feed for few days and before that feed is used, it is technically impossible to add anything via feeding system.

18.2.2 Difficulties with precise dosing

It is well known that under stressful conditions feed consumption very often decreases. At the same time requirement in some nutrients, including antioxidants usually increases. Therefore, in such conditions precise dosing via feed is almost impossible. However, it is well known that under stressful conditions water consumption by commercial birds is usually increased. Even in situations when for some reasons birds refuse the feed, they are still drinking water. Therefore, a drinking system in a poultry house could be a system of choice for the delivery of vitagene-regulating nutrients.

18.2.3 Quick response system

By using drinking system in poultry house, it is possible to develop a quick response system. This could be explained in a practical situation. A veterinarian or nutritionist/technologist discovered a problem with 5-day-old birds in the poultry house – the birds look sleepy and there are about 30,000 birds in the shed. Therefore, to prevent further deterioration of the situation and possible mortality some management actions must be done reasonably quickly. However, there is a need for extra time for the specialists to evaluate a situation in detail, collect some samples of feed, blood, tissues, etc. and send them for analyses to various laboratories. Therefore, it could take a day or several days before the picture is clear and a diagnosis is available. That is exactly the time when vitagene upregulation by supplying some nutrients via drinking system could be a crucial factor 'to buy' some time for a proper diagnostics. Vitagene upregulation can help birds to survive a day or few days before the necessary treatment is available. Depending on the cause of the problem, birds might need extra vaccination, antibiotics or other drugs and this would be supplied after the diagnosis is confirmed in the lab. Therefore, supporting birds in this case would help prevent extra losses. In this case vitagene upregulation seems to be an important approach in poultry management.

18.2.4 Technological advances

Currently, drinking systems in poultry houses are widely used for vaccinations as well as for supplying some acidifiers, antibiotics, etc. The same drinking system can be used for urgent supply of some vitagene-activating nutrients. Various medicators/dosatrons (Figure 18.1) allow precise dosing of nutrients/preparations with drinking water and by upregulating the vitagenes it is possible to help stressed birds deal with stresses and improve their stress adaptability.

Of note, old poultry sheds could lack dosatrons and in this case usually there is a water tank installed and it can be used for the same purpose. Therefore, there are situations in commercial poultry production where chickens need immediate attention, and it is reasonable to use a drinking system to supply important vitagene-regulating nutrients in such conditions.

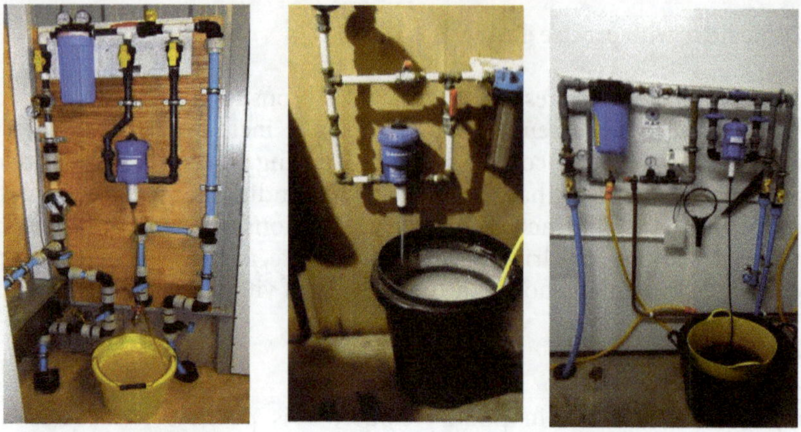

Figure 18.1. Dosatrons in poultry houses.

Our market analysis clearly showed that there has been a range of vitamin-mineral-amino acid mixtures produced for supplying to poultry via drinking system. Some of them are widely used in Eastern European countries. A closer look at the composition and history of the development of such mixtures indicate that they were developed 50-60 years ago when premix industry was still developing and there were cases of vitamin/mineral deficiency in commercial birds. Therefore, such nutritional mixtures helped nutritionist to balance various diets when premixes were of low quality/stability. However, since then the premix industry has made a great progress and today cases of vitamin and mineral/amino acid deficiencies in commercial conditions of many countries with the developed poultry industry are rather an exception, than the rule. It should be also taken into account that additional supplementation of most vitamins (especially B-vitamins), minerals or amino acids beyond their requirements, which are usually met by supplementing feed with commercial premixes at the stage of manufacturing, would not give any extras in terms of productive or reproductive performance but would increase cost of production of eggs or meat. Furthermore, vitamin and mineral doses supplied with premixes are substantially higher than minimal physiological requirement in those nutrients. Therefore, usage of such preparations in many cases is just a tribute to history and sometimes reflect a lack of knowledge in modern poultry nutritional standards.

In contrast to the aforementioned vitamin-mineral-amino acid mixtures, our new concept is based on the supplying to birds specific nutrient mixtures possessing vitagene-activating properties. This would increase expression of target genes (vitagenes) leading to improved ability of poultry to adapt to stress and increase stress resistance. In this case a unique composition of nutrients (a synergistic combination) is more important than concentrations of any individual compound in the preparation. Therefore, this mixture provides protective effects even if the diet is balanced in major nutrients. As a result of additional synthesis of protective molecules (HSP70, HO-1, SOD, Trx-system, GSH-system and sirtuins) the body/tissue/cell can maintain a healthy redox balance, providing optimal conditions for cell signalling and adaptation to stress, including environmental, technological, nutritional and internal stresses (Surai, 2019a,b; 2020a; Surai and Fisinin, 2012a,b; 2016a,b,d; Surai *et al.*, 2018; 2019b). Therefore, by mobilising internal reserves of the body to a greater extent, than without vitagene activation, the bird can withstand/resist increased stresses and overcome them with minimal loses.

18.3 VitaTonic concept development

Three applications of the vitagene concept were developed. Firstly, it was a combination of nutrients, including SM, called VitaTonic, possessing hepatoprotective properties, to support liver in growing broilers and rearing birds as well as in layers and breeders. Secondly, another combination of nutrients called ShellBone, targeting eggshell gland and eggshell quality as well as bone development in poultry was designed. Finally, a universal nutrient combination called Performax/Magic antistress mix to deal with major stresses in poultry production was developed.

18.3.1 From healthy liver to general health

The liver in birds is considered to be the main metabolic organ involved in a range of metabolic and homeostatic functions associated with the synthesis (amino-acids, proteins, lipids, coagulation factors, bile, immunoglobulins, etc.), metabolism (carbohydrates, proteins, lipids, vitamins, etc.), storage (vitamins A, D_3, B12, Fe and Cu), excretion, and detoxification processes (Figure18.2; Zaefarian *et al.*, 2019).

In poultry, lipid synthesis (lipogenesis) in the liver is shown to be very active being about 20-times greater than in adipose tissues. For example, in laying hens, major constituents of the egg yolk are synthesised in the liver and deposited in the egg. Since intensity of egg production in laying hens at the peak can exceed 98%, the liver works at the biological limit of its ability and under high metabolic stress. Therefore, process of lipid synthesis and release can easily be disturbed leading to various metabolic disorders. There are some anatomical and physiological features predisposing poultry to fat deposition in the liver: due to the direct entry into the portal blood system, portomicrons have to pass through the liver before they reach the rest of the circulation (Zaefarian *et al.*, 2019).

Furthermore, fat deposition in poultry liver depends on many nutritional and environmental factors, including (Fouad and El-Senousey, 2014; Zaefarian *et al.*, 2019):
- fat sources: PUFAs including omega-3 fatty acids usually decrease fat accumulation;
- feed restriction: re-feeding after feed restriction could increase fat accumulation in the liver;
- feed structure: fat synthesis and deposition can be increased by feeding crumbled or pelleted diets to broilers;
- nutrient density: affects lipid accumulation in the liver;

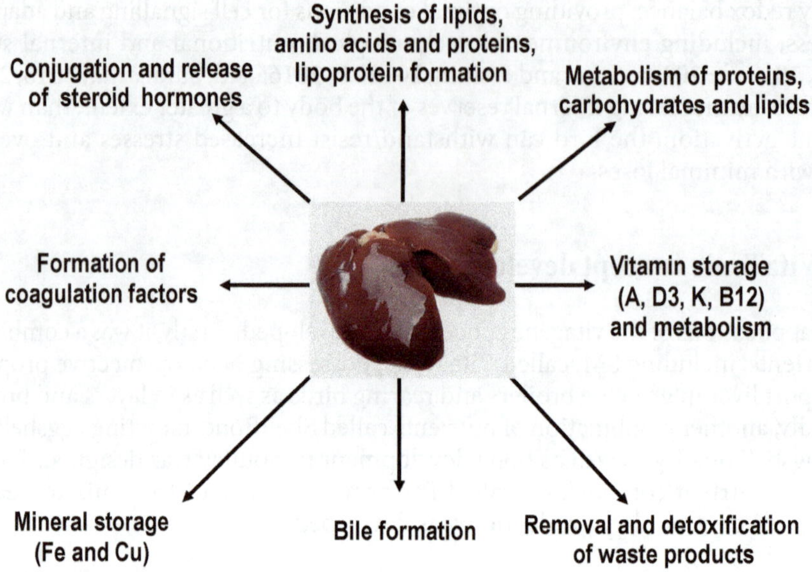

Figure 18.2. Main biological functions of the liver in poultry (adapted from Surai, 2020a).

- dietary fibre: affects microbiota and lipid accumulation in the liver;
- anti-nutritional factors: can disturb liver metabolism and increase lipid accumulation in the liver;
- various infectious agents and dietary toxins (mycotoxins, etc.): can disturb liver metabolism and increase lipid accumulation in the liver;
- biotin deficiency: predisposes birds to fatty liver;
- lack of exercise (cage housing): predisposes birds to fatty liver;
- positive energy balance: predisposes birds to fatty liver;
- hormonal (oestrogen) level: predisposes birds to fatty liver;
- heat stress: predisposes birds to fatty liver;
- other stresses: predispose birds to fatty liver.

In general, there is a range of pathological changes in the poultry liver due to the aforementioned factors, including fatty liver, hepatosis, necrosis, hepatitis and cholangitis (Zaefarian *et al.*, 2019), leading to decreased productive and reproductive performance of birds (Figure 18.3).

18.3.2 Fatty-liver haemorrhagic syndrome (FLHS)

Fatty-liver haemorrhagic syndrome (FLHS) is a sporadic disease occurring in commercial caged, high productive, often overweight laying hens in the latter half of the laying period leading to a fall in egg production in the affected flock (Ridell, 1991). The disease was first reported in 1956 by Couch who described it as fatty liver syndrome (Couch, 1956) and a more precise terminology 'fatty liver haemorrhagic

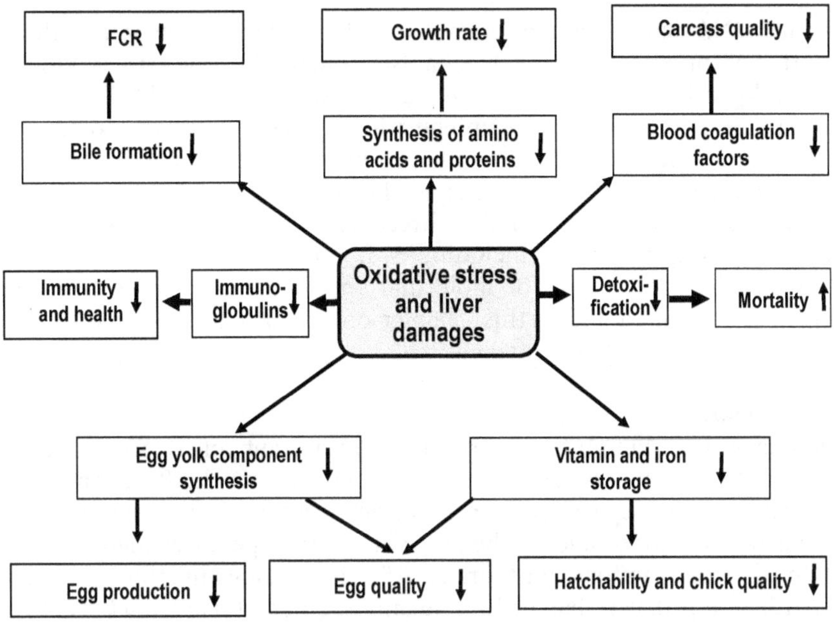

Figure 18.3. Effect of liver disturbance on productive and reproductive performance of poultry (adapted from Surai, 2020a).

syndrome' differentiating it from fatty, non-haemorrhagic livers was introduced by Wolford and Polin (1972). The disease usually increases flock mortality (Butler, 1976) and dead hens are characterised by large blood clots in the liver and abdominal cavities and the liver is usually from a golden yellow to pale yellow or very pale brown in colour (Fowler, 1990; Ridell, 1991) with very high (40-70%) fat content (Ivy and Nesheim, 1973). However, after more than 60 years of research in this field, the molecular mechanisms for the explanation of the hepatic necrosis and haemorrhage are still unknown. Squires and Leeson (1988) and Spurlock and Savage (1992) put forward a hypothesis suggesting that the liver haemorrhages may be caused by an excessive lipid peroxidation of the unsaturated fatty acids accumulated within the hepatocytes, leading to oxidative damage in the cell and organelle membranes.

This hypothesis was further developed with indication that oxidative stress, disruption of redox status, cell signalling and transcription factor (Nrf2 and NF- κB) are involved in the development of inflammation and FLHS (Surai, 2019c; 2020a; Surai *et al.*, 2018). There is a growing evidence indicating that oxidative stress is a leading cause of detrimental consequences of fatty liver and metabolic changes in the body (Elvira-Torales *et al.*, 2019; Gillessen and Schmidt, 2020; Nagashimada and Ota, 2019; Ore and Akinloye, 2019; Surai, 2019c; Surai *et al.*, 2018; Xu *et al.*, 2019).

Oxidative stress has been suggested as a conjoint pathological mechanism of FLHS, and it contributes to initiation and progression of liver injury, associated with lipid, protein and DNA damages and promotes several disorders of metabolic pathways and a disruption of antioxidant defence mechanisms and modulating pathways that control normal biological functions (Surai *et al.*, 2018). Therefore, the VitaTonic concept is based on usage of nutrient mixture upregulating vitagenes, decreasing oxidative stress in the liver and other tissues, showing hepatoprotective effect and maintaining liver health in commercial birds including laying hens under commercially-relevant stress conditions. The first choice includes three hepatoprotective nutrients possessing vitagene-activating properties including SM, carnitine and betaine. In previous chapters detailed description of molecular mechanisms of protective effects of SM has been presented and in this Chapter only information related to fatty liver prevention/treatment will be provided.

18.3.2.1 Silymarin

Detailed analysis of literature confirming an important role of SM in prevention/treatment of liver disorders have been presented in Chapter 12. Recent meta-analysis of studies devoted to usage of SM for prevention/treatment human non-alcoholic fatty liver confirmed an importance of the nutrient as a therapeutic element (Zhong *et al.*, 2017). In particular, antioxidant (Surai, 2015a; 2020a), anti-inflammatory (Lovelace *et al.*, 2015; Surai, 2020a; Chapter 10) and anti-apoptotic (Haddadi *et al.*, 2018; Surai *et al.*, 2021a) properties of SM are a background for its usage as a hepatoprotectant in poultry production (Saeed *et al.*, 2017a) and a combination of SM and carnitine was shown to be more effective than each of the nutrient used singly (Liu *et al.*, 2009; Mousa and Osman, 2016). The liver is a primary organ involved in biotransformation of food toxicants and drugs. Toxins absorbed from the intestinal tract first enter the liver resulting in tissue damages and a variety of liver disorders.

Hepatic disorders are mainly caused by toxic chemicals (alcohol), xenobiotics (carbon tetrachloride, chlorinated hydrocarbons), anticancer (doxorubicin, cisplatin), immunosuppressant (cyclosporine), analgesic anti-inflammatory (paracetamol, thioacetamide), anti-tubercular (isoniazid, rifampicin) drugs, radiations (gamma radiations), heavy metals (cadmium, arsenic), mycotoxins (aflatoxin, T-2 toxin, fumonisins, ochratoxins), galactosamine, lipopolysaccharides, etc. (Chapter 8) and SM was able to show substantial protective effects in the aforementioned model systems. Furthermore, hepatoprotective effects of SM were demonstrated in a range of various studies (Amiridumari *et al.*, 2013; Dumari *et al.*, 2014; Muhammad *et al.*, 2012; Tedesco *et al.*, 2004; Chapter 12). SM also decreased fat content of the chicken carcass and improved antioxidant defences in the chicken liver (Gengwu *et al.*, 2016).

SM was also shown to decrease hepatotoxicity of aflatoxin B1, as evidenced by positive effects on feed consumption, daily gain and liver morphology of growing broilers (Fani *et al.*, 2013) and improved gut microbiota, helped maintain absorptive capacity of the small intestine (Jahanian *et al.*, 2017) and maintained spleen integrity (Kalorey *et al.*, 2005; for more details see Chapter 9). Recently, hepatoprotective effects of SM have been shown in CCl_4 induced toxicity in broilers (Baradaran *et al.*, 2019; Malayeri *et al.*, 2014). In particular, the CCl_4-challenged birds revealed considerable hepatic injures, however, liver damages were amended by the SM treatment. Interestingly, a remarkable down-regulation in the expression of CAT, GPx, and SOD2 hepatic genes was detected in CCl_4-challenged birds, whereas SM prevented down-regulation of the aforementioned genes (Baradaran *et al.*, 2019). Similar hepatoprotective effects of SM were observed in CCl_4-treated rats (Abdel-Moneim *et al.*, 2015; Al-Rasheed *et al.*, 2016), but a combination of SM +TAU was more effective than single nutrient usage (Abdel-Moneim *et al.*, 2015). SM-mediated protection against maneb- and PQ-induced hepatotoxicity in rats was also shown (Ahmad *et al.*, 2013).

In general, SM functions in poultry are not restricted by hepatoprotection, it participates in regulation of many various physiological functions and biochemical pathways (Figure 18.4).

In particular, protective effects of SM on the chicken gut in various stress conditions described earlier (Chapter 11), as well as immunoprotective actions in the case of aflatoxin B (Chand *et al.*, 2011) and ochratoxin A (Khatoon *et al.*, 2013) in the chicken diet deserve more attention.

18.3.2.2 Carnitine

L-Carnitine (LC) is shown to transport long-chain fatty acids across the inner mitochondrial membrane during β-oxidation helping liver deal with lipid excess and may play an important role in reducing fat deposition in modern strains of broiler chickens (Zaefarian *et al.*, 2019). It is well known that LC is synthesised *in vivo* from lysine and methionine and obtained from animal-derived feed ingredients (Surai, 2015b,c,d). Protective effects of carnitine and its derivatives are most pronounced in

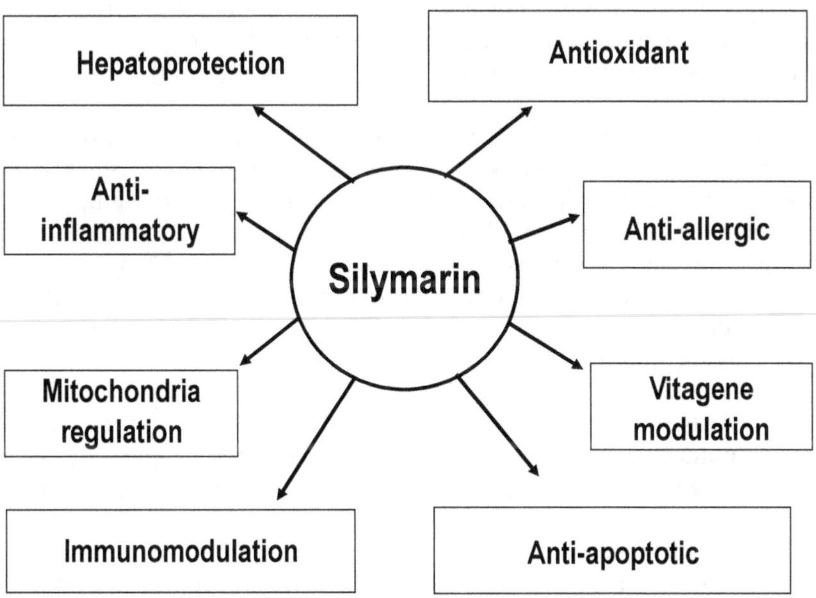

Figure 18.4. Biological functions of silymarin in poultry (adapted from Surai, 2020a).

various stress conditions. By decreasing negative consequences of stresses carnitine can improve productive and reproductive performance and general health of growing chickens, parent stock, and commercial layers (Arslan, 2006; Golzar Adabi *et al.*, 2011; Surai, 2018d; 2020a; Surai *et al.*, 2018). In a recent review of effects LC on poultry it was shown that under normal conditions in most cases there was no effect of this nutrient on productive and reproductive performance of growing broilers or layers (Ringseis *et al.*, 2018). However, effect of LC on lipid metabolism was confirmed in 7 from 25 trials reviewed: abdominal fat percentage was significantly reduced. Similarly, providing LC in drinking water was associated with a reduction of abdominal fat accumulation in Turkish native ducks and geese (Arslan *et al.*, 2003). It seems likely that protective effect of LC supplementation can be seen in various stress conditions when its requirement probably increases but internal synthesis decreases (Surai *et al.*, 2018). From the same 25 studies reviewed by Ringseis *et al.* (2018) in 3 studies LC reduced ascites mortality (Geng *et al.*, 2004; Wang *et al.*, 2013) and under high temperature conditions LC improved BW gain (Celik and Ozturkcan, 2003).

The same conclusion can be drawn from seven layer studies analysed by Ringseis *et al.* (2018): supplemental LC is able to prevent adverse effects of diet-induced oxidative stress on performance and lipid peroxidation in laying hens (Güçlü *et al.*, 2011). Protective effects of LC on laying hens were also observed at high ambient temperature (Celik *et al.*, 2004) as well as in layers of advanced (92 weeks) age (Kazemi-Fard *et al.*, 2015), whereas supplemental L-carnitine is largely ineffective under normal feeding conditions. It was observed that dietary LC in the breeder diet was transferred to egg yolk and hatching rate was increased from 83% to 87% and from 82.4% to 85.3% in groups supplemented with 50 and 100 mg LC, respectively (Leibetseder, 1995). It seems likely that LC has some epigenetic effects on poultry breeders. For example, feeding female broiler breeders a diet supplemented with 25 mg/kg LC was shown to reduce the carcass fat content of their progeny (Kidd *et al.*, 2005).

Protective effects of LC and its derivatives on the antioxidant systems of the body are shown in various models of oxidative stress/toxicity caused by CCl_4, cisplantin, ethanol, 3-Nitropropionic acid, valproate, diethylnitrosamine, doxorubicin, adriamycin, tamoxifen, indomethacin, APAP, Cd, aflatoxin, thioacetamide, methotrexate, etc. LC and its derivatives were effective in decreasing oxidative stress caused by neurotoxic agents such as glutamate, quinolinic acid or 3-nitropropionic acid, rotenone, dexamethasone, aminoglycosides, scopolamine, 1-methyl-4-phenyl-1,2,3,6-tetrahydropyridine, silver nano-particles, etc. (Surai, 2020a).

Carnitine was also effective in prevention of oxidative stress in the L-buthionine-sulfoximine-induced cataract model, selenite-induced cataractogenesis, LPS-treated rats, high dietary copper in laying hens, HFD in rats, fructose-fed rats, experimental glaucoma, acetic acid-induced colitis, atherosclerotic rats (Surai, 2020a). Carnitine showed clear antioxidant protective activities in caerulein-induced acute pancreatitis, adjuvant arthritis, and in hyperthyroid rats as well as in a mouse model of non-alcoholic steatohepatitis, in mice with familial amyotrophic lateral sclerosis, STZ-induced diabetes in rats, ifosfamide-induced Fanconi syndrome, chemically induced model of maple syrup urine disease and unilateral ureteral obstruction-induced oxidative stress. etc. (for references see Surai, 2020a).

Furthermore, carnitine was shown to be a more effective protectant in antioxidant mixtures than when it is used singly. Clearly, hepatoprotective properties of carnitine, together with its antioxidant and vitagene-regulating properties (Surai, 2020a; Surai *et al.*, 2018) make it an ideal component for the development of the vitagene-regulating nutrient mixture to maintain liver health in stress conditions of commercial egg and meat production. Immunomodulating properties of carnitine and protective effects of carnitine on immunity in stress condition, described by Surai (2020a) are additional bonuses for inclusion of this nutrient in an antistress vitagene-regulating mixture.

18.3.2.3 Betaine

Betaine is a naturally occurring trimethyl derivative of the amino acid glycine which can be found in relatively large quantities in aquatic invertebrates, sugar beets and their by-products (Metzler-Zebeli *et al.*, 2009). Biological functions of betaine are based on its action as osmoprotectant assisting in cellular water homeostasis and as a methyl group donor via transmethylation. There is also a range of other betaine activities contributing to its protective effect on the chicken liver, gut and immunity (Figure 18.5).

The significance of betaine in poultry nutrition was first shown in the early 1940s (Kidd *et al.*, 1997). Similar to other nutrients discussed above (e.g. SM and carnitine), supplemental betaine may be beneficial for poultry during certain physiologically

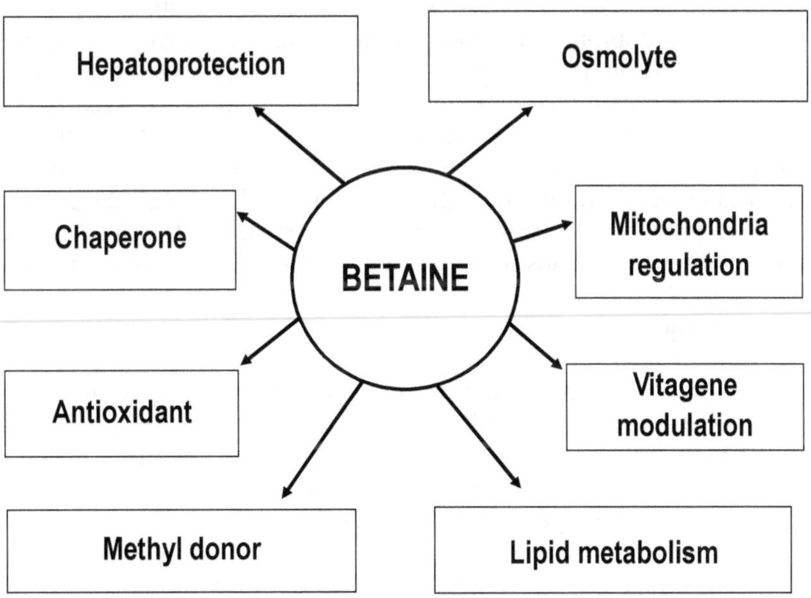

Figure 18.5. Biological functions of betaine (adapted from Surai, 2020a).

challenging conditions, including the high metabolic demand of rapid growth, various stresses (disease challenge, osmotic stress, heat stress, etc.; Kidd *et al.*, 1997; 2005). Betaine is shown to be involved in the protein and lipid (energy) metabolism and it has been often referred to as a 'carcass modifier'. There is a substantial evidence that betaine can significantly reduce abdominal fat pad and improve breast meat yield in broiler chickens, tom turkeys, and meat ducks (for review see Metzler-Zebeli *et al.*, 2009). The fat-lowering effect of betaine was proven in many different trials (Xing *et al.*, 2011; Zhan *et al.*, 2006). Betaine was shown to be effective in alleviating most of the disturbances in fatty liver disease in various animal models by reversing changes in fatty acid and lipid metabolism, relieving oxidative stress and restoring mitochondrial function (Day and Kempson, 2016). Furthermore, the mechanisms underlying hepatoprotective effects were also suggested to involve:

- the stimulation of lipolysis and inhibition of lipogenesis (via gene expression and subsequent activity of lipolytic-/lipogenic-related proteins);
- stimulation of autocrine/endocrine IGF-1 release;
- insulin receptor signalling pathways;
- stimulation of growth hormone secretion;
- increased creatine synthesis; and
- increases in protein synthesis (via intracellular hyper-hydration; Cholewa *et al.*, 2014).

Betaine antioxidant action (Alirezaei *et al.*, 2012; Chen *et al.*, 2020; Li *et al.*, 2019a; Wen *et al.*, 2019), vitagene-regulating properties (Surai *et al.*, 2017a; 2018) including HSP70 regulation (Dangi *et al.*, 2016; Surai, 2020a; Surai and Kochish, 2017), chaperone functions (Figueroa-Soto and Valenzuela-Soto, 2018; Roth *et al.*, 2012) and mitochondria-stabilising effects (Heidari *et al.*, 2018; Lee, 2015) could be of great importance for hepatoprotective actions of the nutrient. Protective effects of betaine under various stress conditions in poultry have been a topic of current research (Liu *et al.*, 2019; Ratriyanto and Mosenthin, 2018; Saeed *et al.*, 2017b; Wen *et al.*, 2019). Furthermore, gut protection under microbial stress (Hamidi *et al.*, 2009; Fetterer *et al.*, 2003), mycotoxin stress (Liew and Mohd-Redzwan, 2018; Surai and Fisinin, 2015) in chickens and immunomodulating properties (Chand *et al.*, 2017; Kidd, 2004; Zhan, 2001) in poultry made this nutrient an important addition into the antistress composition to prevent various stresses and to maintain liver integrity and health.

18.3.3 Practical applications

As it was shown above, combining 3 hepatoprotectors having similar protective activities as well as each of them adding some extras (activating liver regeneration by SM, osmotic protection by betaine, decreasing blood lipids by carnitine, etc.) made the protective activity of the mixture more comprehensive and unique in comparison to individual use of the compounds (Figure 18.6).

It was also important to add into the developed composition a mixture of B-vitamins, regulating lipid metabolism in the liver (B1, B5, B6 and B12), Zn, Mn and Mg (see

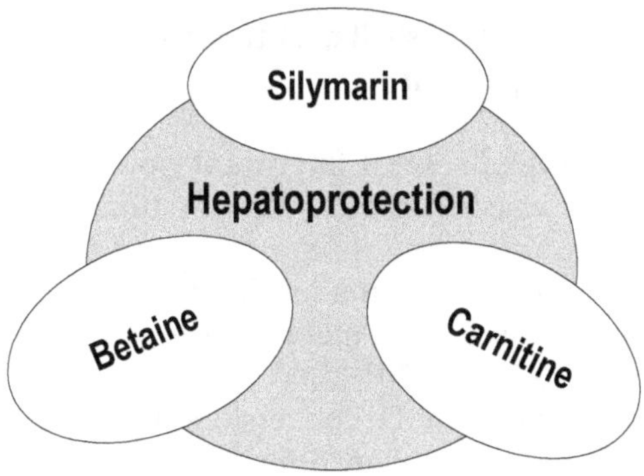

Figure 18.6. A synergistic mixture of hepatoprotectors (Surai, 2020a).

explanations in ShellBone discussions) and two organic acids to have extra protective effects on the gut.

18.4 ShellBone concept development

18.4.1 Egg production and eggshell quality

World's egg production exceeds 80 million metric tons and eggshell quality determines the success of egg industry. Eggshell is shown to have an unusual combination of mechanical properties providing suitable conditions for the developing chick, which must be stiff and rigid but also brittle enough to be broken at hatching (Taylor *et al.*, 2016). However, when eggs are produced for human consumption, compromised eggshell quality causes considerable economic losses for the egg industry. For example, about 7-10% eggs are broken during laying in battery and furnished cages, plus breakage during egg collection (2-4%), transportation (1.2-2.7%), grading and packing (1.5-3.4%) is added (Mertens *et al.*, 2006) leading to huge losses in the egg industry. On average, losses from damaged eggshells account for >10% of total egg production (Fathi *et al.* 2010; Van Mourik *et al.* 2017). Since there is a trend to house layers longer than 80 weeks eggshell breakage could reach >30%. In hens around half-way (49 weeks) through the production period, both shell quality and bone strength were shown to deteriorate (Wistedt *et al.*, 2019).

Since intact eggshell is an important barrier to various pathogens (Sá e Silva, *et al.*, 2016), including *Salmonella*, broken eggshell is an important risk factor for human egg consumption. On the other hand, eggshell cracks in hatching eggs can substantially decrease hatchability, especially in eggs stored before incubation (Nasri *et al.*, 2020). In particular hairline cracks in hatching eggs cause dramatic decrease in egg hatchability (Barnett *et al.*, 2004; Jabbar *et al.*, 2019) and create a lot of problems in egg producing industry (Surai, 2019d).

18.4.2 Molecular mechanisms of eggshell quality deterioration and a choice of nutrients to design a feed supplement

Our recent research identified several important points related to understanding molecular mechanisms of eggshell quality deterioration in aging birds. They could be summarised as follows:

- We believe that subclinical inflammation in the eggshell gland, associated with various commercial stresses, is a major cause of eggshell formation defects, including hairline cracks (Surai, 2019d).
- Decreased efficacy of vitamin D conversion into its active hormonal form 1,25(OH)$_2$D$_3$ in ageing birds contributes substantially to eggshell quality deterioration (Surai, 2018b,c).
- Decreased synthesis of organic matrix components in ageing birds (Surai, 2018e) is an important contributor to decreased eggshell elasticity leading to increased percentage of cracked eggs.

18.4.3 TAU and shell gland

The ShellBone concept was developed to address the aforementioned problems with eggshell and with bone quality. In particular, TAU is considered to be an important nutrient regulating inflammation via affecting such transcription factors as NF-κB and Nrf2 (Figure 18.7).

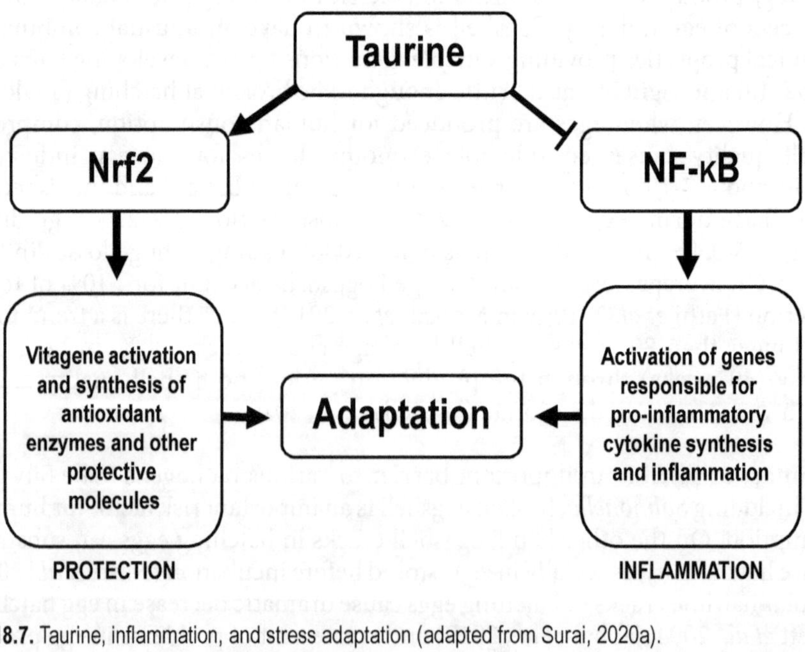

Figure 18.7. Taurine, inflammation, and stress adaptation (adapted from Surai, 2020a).

Furthermore, TAU also affects vitagenes leading to improved adaptability to stress and increased stress resistance (Surai, 2018d; 2020a; Surai *et al.*, 2020a; 2021b). There is growing evidence that vitamin D, especially its active hormonal form ($1,25(OH)_2D_3$) possesses strong anti-inflammatory properties. For example, $1,25(OH)_2D_3$ was found to be effective in attenuating ER stress and the NF-κB-driven inflammatory response in mammary epithelial (MCF-7) cells (Wen *et al.*, 2020). Furthermore, protective/inhibitory effects of $1,25(OH)_2D_3$ on the inflammation associated with mastitis were clearly shown (Lippolis *et al.*, 2011; Merriman *et al.*, 2017; 2018).

$1,25(OH)_2D_3$ was shown to exert its anti-inflammation effects through regulating the biosynthesis of pro-inflammatory molecules in the prostaglandin pathway or through NF-κB affecting cytokine production and inflammatory response (Li *et al.*, 2019b; Lin and Li, 2016).

18.4.4 Active vitamin D metabolites and eggshell formation

In laying hens, eggshell formation takes place daily in the hen's eggshell gland being one of the most rapid mineralisation processes known in nature. To produce the eggshell large amounts of $CaCO_3$ is required and the hen has to export about 2 g calcium comprising 10% of her total body calcium ach day (Nys and Le Roy, 2018). Eggshell calcium is derived from duodenal absorption and skeletal (medullary bone) stores. Importantly, duodenal calcium uptake was indicated to be increased 6-fold during shell formation, but efficiency of Ca absorption is age-dependent and declines from 37 weeks of age in layers (Al-Batshan *et al.*, 1994).

Important roles of vitamin D in Ca absorption and metabolism are well established. Vitamin D affects expression and synthesis of Ca-binding proteins being an essential regulator of eggshell and bone formation and their integrity maintenance. An understanding of molecular mechanisms controlling $1,25(OH)_2D_3$ production is of great importance in explaining how the layer intestine adapts to fluctuations in calcium requirement and provision. In poultry, dietary vitamin D_3 is shown to be absorbed in the small intestine and is transported via blood to the liver where it is converted into 25-hydroxycholecalciferol (25-OH-D_3), the major circulating form of vitamin D3. The next stage of vitamin D3 metabolism includes transport of 25-OH-D_3 to the kidneys where it is converted into 1,25-dihydroxycholecalciferol (calcitriol; $1,25(OH)_2D_3$), the most biologically active, hormonal metabolite of the vitamin (Waldenstedt, 2006). Essential roles of $1,25(OH)_2D_3$ in eggshell formation is well established and during layer maturation (transfer from immature pullets to laying birds) concentration of $1,25(OH)_2D_3$ in plasma increased more than 5-fold (Bar, 2009).

Furthermore, eggshell calcification is shown to be associated with a further 2-fold increase in the plasma level of $1,25(OH)_2D_3$ (Nys and Le Roy, 2018). However, with age, there is a progressive deterioration in the ability of the hen's liver to hydroxylate vitamin D_3 to 25-OH-D_3 (Soares *et al.*,1976) and reduced kidney 25-OH-D_3 hydroxylation resulted in inadequate production of $1,25(OH)_2D_3$ associated with decreased absorption of Ca (Stevens *et al.*, 1984) and decline in egg shell quality and deterioration in tibia strength with age.

Therefore, by using preformed $1.25(OH)_2D_3$ it is possible to design a product of 'fast response' which can be used to address vitamin D inadequacy issues during egg production and broiler growth. Stressful conditions, such as high bird density, heat stress, mycotoxicosis, enteritis, malabsorption syndromes, and certain immune disorders may impair absorption or liver hydroxylation of vitamin D_3, which is one rationale for the use of vitamin D_3 metabolites in layer/broiler feed. The expression of vitamin D receptor (VDR) was shown to decrease upon induction of ER stress and $1,25(OH)_2D_3$ was found to counter-regulates the inhibitory effect of ER stress on VDR expression in mammary epithelial cells (Wen *et al.*, 2020).

There is a range of publications confirming an important role of supplying $1,25(OH)_2D_3$ on eggshell and bone formation. For example, when $1,25(OH)_2D_3$ was the only source of vitamin D_3 in the layer diet increased feed consumption and egg production were observed, in comparison to non-supplemented diet (Frost *et al.*, 1990). The is a range of studies confirming that $1,25(OH)_2D_3$ supports egg production and eggshell mineralisation/quality and minimising eggshell breakage. For example, the effect of replacing dietary vitamin D_3 by $1,25(OH)_2D_3$ in 32-week-old White Leghorn laying hens over 9 weeks on eggshell quality and egg production was studied (Tsang *et al.*, 1990a). The authors showed that after 4 weeks of experimental feeding, laying hens fed on a diet supplemented with 5 μg $1,25(OH)_2D_3$/kg diet produced eggs with improved eggshell quality as indicated by significantly higher specific gravity and percentage of shell than eggs from control hens fed on a diet supplemented with 27.5 μg D_3/kg diet.

Interestingly, eggs obtained from hens fed on a diet without vitamin D_3 supplementation were characterised by very thin or soft shell, reflecting depletion of the birds' reserves of vitamin D_3 or its metabolites within 4-week period (Tsang *et al.*, 1990a). Therefore, an optimal dose of $1,25(OH)_2D_3$ in the layer diets was associated with the best eggshell quality and tibial weights relative to the control group supplemented with vitamin D3 (Tsang *et al.*, 1990b). Interestingly, doubling the level of vitamin D_3 supplementation in the control diet almost linearly increased the circulating concentration of 25-OH-D_3 but did not change the concentration of $1,25(OH)_2D_3$, Ca, or egg specific gravity (SG), while replacing vitamin D3 by the optimal concentration of $1,25(OH)_2D_3$ improved egg SG (Tsang and Grunder, 1993).

In Japanese quail dietary supplementation with $1,25(OH)_2D_3$ was associated with increased egg specific gravity, shell weight, percentage of shell, and egg breaking strength (Kaetzel and Soares, 1979). Furthermore, Bar *et al.* (1988) reported that the inclusion of $1,25(OH)_2D_3$ in the diet of aging hens decreased the rate of decline of shell weight and density in birds. In 56-week-old laying hens, the addition of $1,25(OH)_2D_3$ in the feed prevented a rapid decrease in egg production due to a *Mycoplasma gallisepticum* infection observed in hens fed the basal diet (Carlos, and Edward, 1998). Dietary supplementation with $1,25(OH)_2D_3$ (as *Cestrum diurnum* leaf) helped maintain higher (80%) egg production in comparison to the control group supplemented with vitamin D_3 (68%) or negative control without vitamin D supplementation (55%) at the end of production period (72 weeks; Chennaiah *et al.*, 2004). Feeding dried *Solanum glaucophyllum* (SG) plant material, as a source of 1,25$(OH)_2D_3$, to laying hens has been shown to lead to thicker eggshells (Azcona *et al.*, 1982; Morris, 1977).

It seems likely that 1,25$(OH)_2D_3$ is needed for normal chondrocyte metabolism (Boyanabc *et al.*,1999), therefore, affecting bone formation and metabolism. This is relevant not only to layer bone health maintenance (medullary bone is the major source of Ca for eggshell formation, providing about 40% of the Ca required) but also for commercially growing birds, where tibial dyschondroplasia (TD) is a substantial problem. TD, a bone deformity disease of rapidly growing birds, characterised by accumulation of non-mineral and avascular cartilage that leads to chondrocyte death due to lack of blood supply, could cause great economic losses in broiler production. There is a growing body of evidence indicating that TD can be prevented, or its incidence and severity reduced by using 1,25$(OH)_2D_3$ (Edwards, 1990; Edwards *et al.*, 1992; Rennie and Whitehead, 1996; Rennie *et al.*, 1993) suggesting that the metabolic conversion of vitamin D_3 to 1,25$(OH)_2D_3$ is not sufficient under some stressful conditions to meet the requirement for this metabolite for physiological bone development.

Interestingly, 1,25$(OH)_2D_3$ was shown to be effective not only in regulation of Ca absorption and metabolism, but also phosphorus utilisation in broilers can be improved by feeding 1,25$(OH)_2D_3$ (Edwards, 2002). Dietary supplementation of 1,25$(OH)_2D_3$ was reported to alleviate the incidence and severity of TD and rickets and increase bone mineralisation (Edwards *et al.*, 1992; Elliot and Edwards, 1997; Rennie *et al.*, 1993, 1995).

18.4.5 Manganese and eggshell quality

It has been shown that Mn plays an important role in maintaining structure and integrity of eggshell (Swiatkiewicz *et al.*, 2015; Xiao *et al.*, 2015). In particular, Mn dietary supplementation was shown to increase eggshell thickness and strength by improving eggshell structure, including changes in the mammillary layer of the eggshell (Leach and Gross, 1983; Xiao *et al.*, 2014; Zhang *et al.*, 2017a,b).

Eggshell is considered to be bio-ceramics composed of six layers: the uncalcified inner and outer shell membranes, irregular cones corresponding to the mammillary knob layer, the palisade layer, thin vertical crystal layer and the outer layer, the cuticle (Nys and Le Roy, 2018). In the phase of shell formation (five hours after ovulation) the egg enters the uterus (shell gland) and rotates with the linear deposition of calcium carbonate (0.33 g/h in laying hens) with the mammillary and palisade layers are sequentially formed (Nys *et al.*, 2004). During about 20 hours, in the shell gland, the egg acquires the shell, consisting of 95% (by weight) calcium carbonate ($CaCO_3$) and about 3.5% is represented by organic matrix consisting mainly of proteoglycans and glycoproteins in the calcified layers and fibrillar proteins with disulphide cross-links and collagen types I, V and X in the eggshell membranes (Nys *et al.*, 2004).

It is proven that the eggshell ultrastructure (e.g. calcite crystal size, shape and orientation and other parameters) determines its biomechanical properties (Ahmed *et al.*, 2005; Fathi *et al.*, 2016; Radwan, 2016; Radwan *et al.*, 2010). There is a positive correlation between calcite crystal size inside the eggshell, their orientation and thickness of cones of mammillary layer (Dunn *et al.*, 2012). The size, orientation and thickness of cones of mammillary knob layer determine major characteristics of commercial importance (e.g. strength) of the eggshell (Fernandez *et al.*, 2001; Nys *et al.*, 1999).

Formation of cones of mammillary knob layer takes place at the beginning of the eggshell formation (from 5.5 up to 10 h to ovulation) associated with initiation of aggregation and growth in nucleation points (Nys *et al.*, 2004). It was shown that chicken eggshell contains two main sulphated polymers (proteoglycans), referred to as mammillan and ovoglycan which are involved in nucleation and growth of the eggshell calcite crystals. Based on existing evidence the putative role of mammillan, a keratan sulphate proteoglycan, is in the nucleation of the first calcite crystals, while that of ovoglycan, a dermatan sulphate proteoglycan, is in the regulation of the growth and orientation of the later forming crystals of the chicken eggshell (Arias *et al.*, 2001).

Kinetics of CaCO3 crystal formation and their morphologic structure are affectively modulated by organic matrix components found in the liquid of eggshell gland (Gautron *et al.*, 1997; Nys *et al.*, 1999). Furthermore, Mn supplementation with feed or water can improve eggshell ultrastructure due to modulation of sulphated proteoglycans in membranes and in the calcified eggshell (Xiao *et al.*, 2014; Zhang *et al.*, 2017a). Dietary Mn supplementation is involved in the process of protein glycosylation and glycan metabolism and can improve the expression of genes encoding proteoglycans and glycoproteins in the eggshell gland, thus improving eggshell quality by increasing the mammillary-knob density during the initial deposition stage of shell formation (Zhang *et al.*, 2018).

Since Mn is an integral part of SOD, main enzyme of the antioxidant defence network (Surai, 2016; 2000b; 2020a), regulated at the vitagene level (Surai, 2020a, Surai *et al.*, 2019b), an additional supplementation of Mn could be an effective way to increase antioxidant defences (Pappas *et al.*, 2018; Surai, 2005) in the eggshell gland leading to decreased inflammation (Surai, 2019d) and improvement of eggshell quality (Surai *et al.*, 2018).

18.4.6 Zinc and eggshell quality

During eggshell formation many different enzymes take part in the process. For example, carbonic anhydrase (CA) is Zn-dependent enzyme responsible for reversible hydration of carbon dioxide and bicarbonate:

$$CO_2 + H_2O \leftrightarrow HCO_3^- + H^+$$

Furthermore, HCO_3^- is a precursor of $CaCO_3$, main structural constituent of the eggshell. More than 70 years ago it was shown that CA affected eggshell quality and is the most important enzyme in calcite formation (Gutowska and Mitchell, 1945). CA was indicated to contain 0.31-0.34% of Zn (Hove *et al.*, 1940). As expected, Zn deficiency is associated with decreased activity of a number of enzymes, including CA, in different animal species, including avian species (Ensminger *et al.*, 1990). Furthermore, partial or complete CA inhibition led to decreased eggshell quality (Holm *et al.*, 2006; Nys *et al.*, 1999), reduced eggshell thickness (Holm *et al.*, 2006), and mass (Nys, 2001) and production of shell-less or soft-shelled eggs (Benesch *et al.*, 1944; Diamant and Schluns, 1964; Lundholm, 1990). On the other hand, increased CA activity in laying hens by oestradiol was observed to increase eggshell quality at the second part of production period (Wistedt *et al.*, 2014). Interestingly, at 49 weeks of age, a dramatic reduction in duodenal CA activity, coinciding with decreased gland density in the eggshell gland was observed (Wistedt *et al.*, 2019).

Similar age-dependent decrease in CA activity in the shell gland of laying hens was observed (Snapir and Perek, 1070). Furthermore, increased Zn dietary supplementation for aged layers was shown to increase eggshell strength leading to decreased percentage of eggshell cracks and breakage (Zamani *et al.*, 2005) with simultaneous increased CA activity in the eggshell gland (Zhang *et al.*, 2017a). It seems likely that Zn can also improve eggshell quality as a result of direct regulation of eggshell formation by affecting growth stage of calcite crystals *in vitro* (Elzinga and Reeder, 2002). Interestingly, various combinations of Zn an Mn in the diet were shown to improve eggshell strength (Mabe *et al.*, 2003; Stefanello *et al.*, 2014; Swiatkiewicz and Koreleski, 2008).

18.4.7 Ascorbic acid and eggshell quality

About 80 years ago it was shown that poultry can synthesise ascorbic acid in their kidney (Grollman and Lehninger, 1957; Roy and Guha, 1958). However, under various stress conditions ascorbic acid synthesis could be compromised and dietary supplementation of this vitamin could have positive effects on productive and reproductive performance of poultry (McKee and Harrison, 1995). However, efficacy of such ascorbic acid dietary supplementation is condition-dependent and quite variable (Pardue and Thaxton, 1986; Scott, 1975). There is a range of publications claiming beneficial effects of ascorbic acid on egg shell strength (Balnave *et al.*, 1991; Bell and Marion, 1990; El-Boushy and van Albada, 1970; Orban *et al.*, 1993; Peebles and Brake, 1985; Perek and Kendler, 1963; Thornton and Moreng, 1958; Zapata and Gernat, 1995). However, molecular mechanisms of vitamin C effects on eggshell quality require further investigation. In particular, ascorbic acid participates in vitamin D metabolism in poultry (Weiser *et al.*, 1988a).

It was shown that decreased $1,25(OH)_2D_3$ concentration in chicken serum was associated with decreased eggshell quality (Castaldo and Maurice, 1990) and dietary supplementation of 1,25$(OH)_2D_3$ for layers at 71-weeks for 8 weeks decreased percentage of eggs with damaged/cracked eggshell, while additional usage of ascorbic acid in these conditions further improved eggshell quality (Weiser *et al.*, 1992). Therefore, participation of vitamin C in cholecalciferol hydroxylation (Weiser *et al.*, 1988b) and 1,25$(OH)_2D_3$ synthesis (Farquharson *et al.*, 1998) may be a background of synergistic action of these two vitamins. Furthermore, ascorbic acid dietary supplementation was indicated to increase egg production and hatchability (Balnave *et al.*, 1991; Bell and Marion, 1990; Orban *et al.*, 1993; Peebles and Brake, 1985; Zapata and Gernat, 1995), to decrease percentage of eggs with damaged eggshell (Weiser *et al.*, 1992) at the second part of the productive period.

It seems likely that vitamin C is especially effective in poultry flocks with comparatively low egg production (Peebles and Brake, 1985). As mentioned above, vitamin C efficacy in poultry nutrition depends on stress level and duration and combinations of other antioxidants included into the diet. For example, Whitehead *et al.* (1992) demonstrated that decreased feed consumption and egg production reduction by laying hens under heat stress (35 °C) were prevented by inclusion into the diet quite high (500 g/t) vitamin C levels. Interestingly, a combination of ascorbic acid and vitamin E was shown to significantly improve eggshell quality under heat stress (Chung *et al.*, 2005).

It should be mentioned that vitamin C dietary supplementation also showed positive effects on layer bone strength (Chung *et al.*, 2005). At the same time, dietary vitamin C can decrease detrimental effects caused by various drugs (Ali *et al.*, 1984), heavy metal contamination (Hill, 1979; Toussant and Latshaw, 1994), and increase resistance to various poultry diseases (Amakye-Anim *et al.*, 2000). As mentioned above, 1,25$(OH)_2D_3$ concentration in blood decreased in layers with eggshell problems (Castaldo and Maurice, 1990; Soares, 1984) and ascorbic acid dietary supplementation was reported to increase 1,25$(OH)_2D_3$ concentration and improve bone calcification in birds (Weiser *et al.*, 1988a). In general, vitamin C participates in bone formation by stimulating synthesis of hydroxyproline, an important amino acid in collagen synthesis. It should be taken into account that collagen fibrils comprise an important part of organic matrix of eggshell and bones (Weiser *et al.*, 1988b).

Therefore, ascorbic acid plays an important role in the formation and development of bones as a co-factor in transcription and enzymatic reactions which regulate early differentiation of osteoblasts as well as biosynthesis of various molecules of organic matrix of bones, including collagen. In particular, ascorbic acid was shown to inhibit osteoclast activity and reduce their number, simultaneously increase differentiation of osteoblast leading to enhancement of bone development (Gabbay *et al.*, 2010).

18.4.8 Practical approaches

Eggshell quality deterioration in ageing birds is a great problem in commercial poultry production. There is a range of publications indicating beneficial role of various nutrients on eggshell quality. For example, supplying ascorbic acid with feed or water in stress conditions was shown to have beneficial effects on eggshell and bone quality. It seems likely that a combination of ascorbic acid with other nutrients, including 1,25$(OH)_2D_3$, TAU and minerals may show higher protective efficacy than its single usage. In general, it should be stated that for improvement of eggshell quality and solving problems with bone quality, including deformity and TD the following nutrients are of great importance:

- **Taurine**
  - a major player in prevention of eggshell gland inflammation responsible for decreased eggshell quality, including hairline cracks;
  - activating vitagenes, responsible for stress adaptation and improved stress resistance.
- **1,25$(OH)_2D_3$**
  - an active hormonal form of vitamin D, regulating Ca absorption and metabolism;
  - possessing anti-inflammatory properties and helping TAU in eggshell gland protection;
  - regulating vitagenes and helping stress adaptation.
- **Mn**
  - an important co-factor of many enzymes, including those responsible for synthesis of organic matrix, determining eggshell composition and major properties, including strength and elasticity;
  - a cofactor of MnSOD, main antioxidant enzyme, regulated at vitagene level and helping stress adaptation.
- **Zn**
  - a cofactor of CA, main enzymes of CaCO3 formation in the eggshell;
  - an essential part of Cu/ZnSOD, cytosolic form of the SOD, regulated at the vitagene level;
  - a vitagene activator, helping stress adaptation.
- **Ascorbic acid**
  - natural antioxidant regulating antioxidant defences;
  - an essential element of organic matrix of the bone and eggshell formation;
  - a vitagene activator, helping stress resistance building.

Therefore, the ShellBone concept is based on usage of the combination of the aforementioned nutrients supplied with drinking water to improve eggshell quality and bone health in commercial poultry. In general, anti-inflammatory properties of ShellBone and VitaTonic (Figure 18.8) related to the regulation of transcription factors (NF-κB and Nrf2) as well as vitagenes (HSP70, HO-1, SOD, thioredoxin- and glutathione systems, and sirtuins), provide an effective protection to the liver and shell gland as well as maintain gut health and high immunocompetence.

18.5 The development of multi-nutrient mixture for vitagene activation and increasing stress resistance of poultry

From the data presented in Chapter 7 it is clear that there is a range of vitagene-regulating nutrients and in many cases a combination of several nutrients were shown to be more

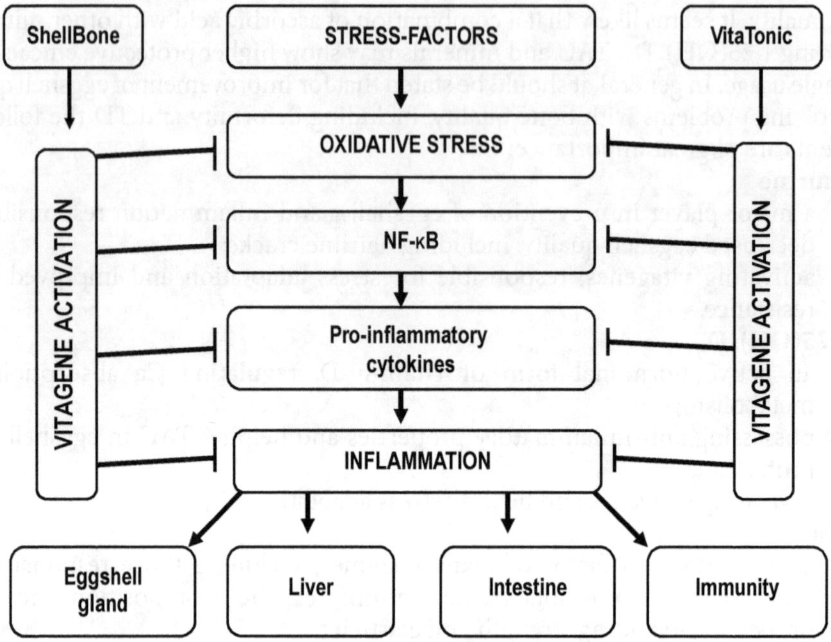

Figure 18.8. Protective effects of ShellBone and VitaTonic (adapted from Surai, 2020a).

effective that any single nutrient. Therefore, when developing a vitagene-regulating nutrient mixture for improving chicken adaptability to stresses several points need to be taking into account.

- **Vitagene-regulating nutrients.** To upregulate vitagenes nutrient composition should include carnitine, betaine, TAU, ascorbic acid, vitamins A, D_3, E, Se and possibly other nutrients in optimal proportions. In this case an optimal combination of nutrients seems to be more important than concentrations of any of the individual compound (Fisinin and Surai, 2011a,b; Surai, 2011; 2015e; Surai and Boroday, 2010; Surai and Fisinin, 2012a,b; Surai and Fotina, 2010a; 2011a; 2012a,b,c,d; Surai *et al.* 2017a; 2018).
- **Vitamin E recycling.** To further upregulate antioxidant defences in stress conditions it is necessary to provide nutrients taking part in vitamin E recycling. Reported data suggest that, if the recycling of vitamin E from its oxidised form is effective, even comparatively low vitamin E concentrations can provide optimal protection of biological membranes (Surai, 1999; 2002; 2006; 2018a; 2020a; 2021; Surai *et al.*, 2018; 2019a). Ascorbic acid, selenium (as a part of TrxR), vitamins B1 and B2 are essential elements of vitamin E recycling (Figure 18.9).

As a result of antioxidant action of vitamin E, tocopheroxyl radical is formed. This radical can be reduced back to an active form of α-tocopherol by coupling with ascorbic acid oxidation. Ascorbic acid can be regenerated back from the oxidised form by recycling with GSH which can receive a reducing potential from NADPH,

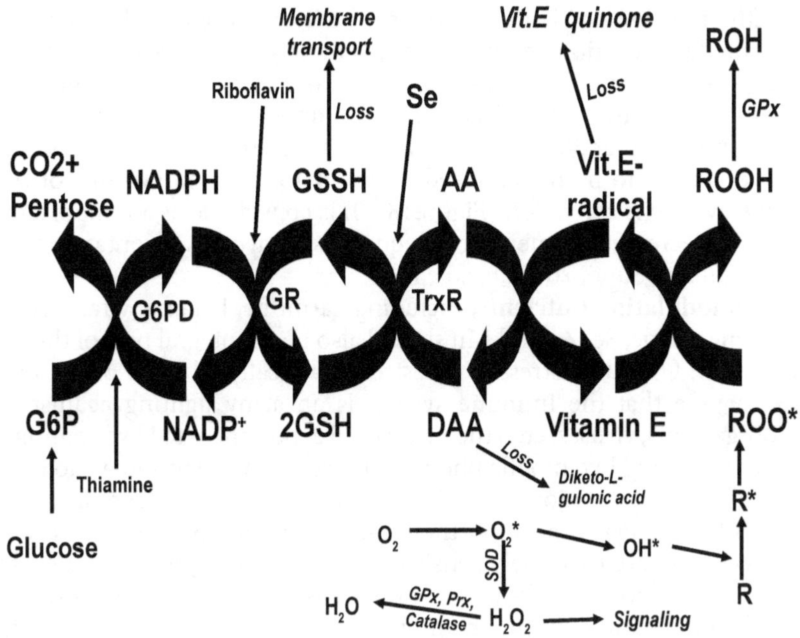

Figure 18.9. Redox cycle of vitamin E (adapted from Surai, 2020a).

synthesised in the pentose phosphate cycle of carbohydrate metabolism. Enzymes involved in vitamin E recycling are as follows: 1. TrxR; 2. GR; 3. Glucose-6-phosphate dehydrogenase. Due to incomplete regeneration (the efficiency of recycling is usually less than 100%) in biological systems, the antioxidants have to be obtained from the diet (e.g. vitamin E) or synthesised in the tissues (ascorbic acid and GSH).

- **Osmolytes.** Osmotic stress is considered to be an important part of intracellular changes observed in stress conditions. Betaine is considered to be an effective osmolyte providing protection against cellular dehydration (osmotic shock), regulating water balance and exerting a stabilising effect on tissue metabolism under various stress conditions (Ratriyanto and Mosenthin, 2018). This is especially important in the chicken gut. Betaine also can upregulate some vitagenes and it is also a source of methyl groups and showing a range of protective effects in the case of various stresses including heat stress, mycotoxin stress and others (Surai *et al.*, 2018).
- **Liver and gut supporting nutrients.** Since mycotoxins are considered to be main feed-derived stressors, and it is practically impossible to avoid mycotoxin feed contamination (Surai and Dvorska, 2005; Surai *et al.*, 2010), it is important to use nutrients supporting liver and gut, main sites of mycotoxin detoxification in the body (Surai *et al.*, 2018). There is evidence that major mycotoxins, including T-2 toxin, ochratoxins, aflatoxin, fumonisins, etc. are detoxified in the liver (Fisinin and Surai, 2012a,b,c,d) and DON is mainly detoxificated by gut microbiota (Fisinin and Fisinin, 2012e,f). Therefore, carnitine, betaine, vitamin E, Se, lysine

and methionine are nutrients supporting the liver and gut of the chicken to help mycotoxin detoxification and minimise liver and gut damage (Surai *et al.*, 2018). It is important to mention that even when the diet contains some mycotoxin binders the problem is not solved, since it is impossible to bind all mycotoxin at the level of more that 50-60% of their presence in the diet. The rest of unbound mycotoxins have to be metabolised by the detoxification systems of the body. Therefore, vitagene activation (Figure18.10) is considered as an important step in prevention/decrease detrimental consequences of mycotoxin contamination of the diet (Fisinin and Surai, 2012a,b,c,d,e,f).

- **Immunomodulating nutrients**, including carnitine, betaine, vitamins E and C, methionine, lysine, Se, Zn and Mn should also be an integral part of the antistress composition. Oxidative stress can destroy practically all parts of the immunity. If we imagine that the immune system is an army fighting against invaders (microorganisms, viruses, etc.) then we would expect them to have communicating devices, something like mobile phones, to receive and send signals to each other. Remarkably enough, major immune cells (macrophages, neutrophils/heterophils, T- and B-lymphocytes) have on their surface 'mobile phones' called receptors. Those receptors are extremely sensitive to communicating molecules, but they are also sensitive to free radicals and can be easily downregulated or damaged. In such a situation without proper communication all those huge armies of immune cells would become useless. They also can start fighting each other, as well as eventually destroying immunocompetence and causing autoimmune reactions. There is fast growing evidence that communication between all types of immune cells (Surai, 2002; 2006; 2018; 2020; 2021) is a key for high immunocompetence. If immune cells are soldiers using chemical weapon to kill the enemy, then special gear protecting them from their own weapon would be a crucial for effective battle. In the case of immune cells, such a gear is represented by natural antioxidants synthesised under vitagene governance, including HSP70, GSH, GPx, Trx, TrxR, sirtuins, etc. Some recent studies suggest that if not properly protected from their own weaponry, phagocyte functions could be compromised, including initial overproduction of free radicals with consecutive damages to specific enzymatic systems resulting in decreasing efficiency of oxidative burst and apoptosis. Based on the presented model it is clear that antioxidant defence is a crucial factor of immune defence in the body and vitagenes play a central role in this defence. In fact, protective molecules, like HSP70, can 'cover up' receptors at time of stress helping immune-communication and maintaining immunocompetence in stress conditions (Fisinin and Surai, 2011c; 2013a), including gut immunity (Fisinin and Surai, 2013b). This is the case in heat stress, mycotoxin stress and a range of other commercially relevant stresses (Surai *et al.*, 2018).
- **Trace elements** are of great importance in antioxidant defences (Pappas *et al.*, 2018; Surai, 2005). As mentioned above Mn is an integral part of the MnSOD, main mitochondrial AO enzyme. Furthermore, Zn is a part of Cu,ZnSOD, located in cytosol. Selenium is an integral part of at least 25 selenoproteins and more than half of them are involved in AO defence and redox balance maintenance (Surai, 2018; 2021; Surai and Kochish, 2019). It is proven that Mg deficiency

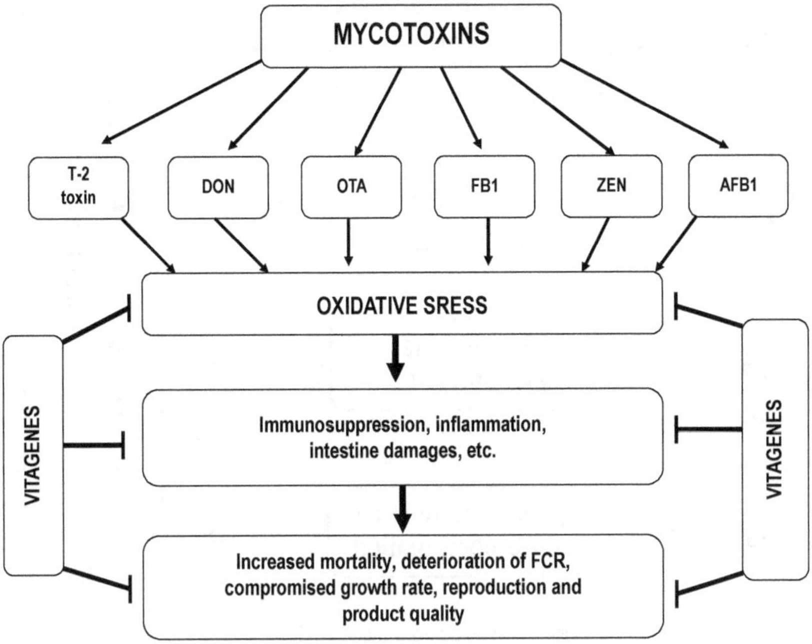

Figure 18.10. Mycotoxins, oxidative stress and vitagenes.

affects appetite and recently Mg is considered to be involved in activation of CAT (Estevez and Petrucci, 2019) and in coordination of antioxidant defences (Monteiro *et al.*, 2016).

Therefore, a choice of minerals for an antioxidant composition to fight stresses should includes Mn, Zn, Se and Mg (Figure 18.11).

- **Essential amino acids** participate in various protective pathways in stress conditions. In particular, methionine (Met), a sulphur-containing amino acid, participates in the initiation and prolongation step of protein synthesis, trans-methylation reactions, the synthesis of cysteine and cystine, being an important component of antioxidant systems (Mastrototaro *et al.*, 2016). Met participates in synthesis of GSH and carnitine and activates MsrA, to counteract oxidative stress (Martinez *et al.*, 2017). Another essential amino acid playing important roles in carnitine synthesis and supporting growth and development of farm animals/poultry is lysine (Surai, 2020a). Therefore, a combine supplementation of methionine and lysine in stress conditions, when their requirements are increased, while consumption could be compromised due to feed consumption reduction, is an additional option during an effective antioxidant mixture development.
- **Organic acids** are shown to enhance poultry performance via regulation of microbiome and other mechanisms affecting the morphology and physiology of the gut and the immune system (Dittoe *et al.*, 2018). This is especially important in the case of feed grade antibiotic prohibition in many countries worldwide with

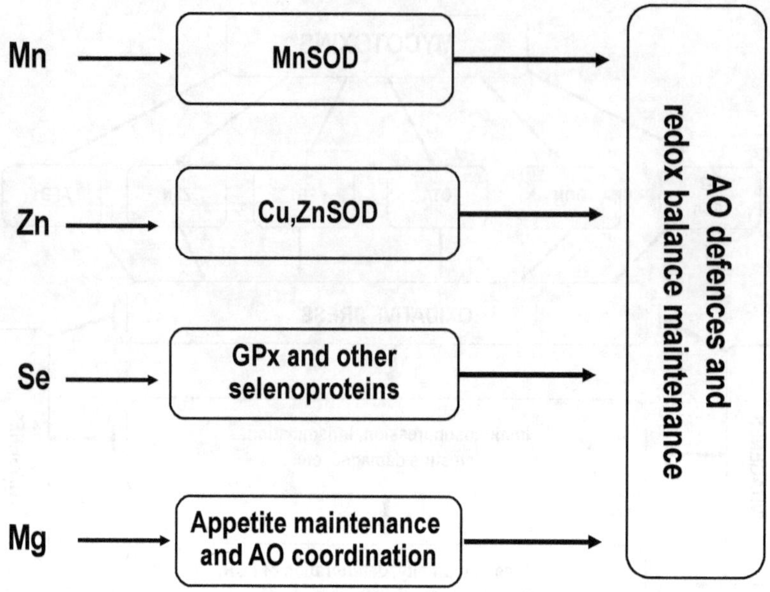

Figure 18.11. Minerals for AO composition (adapted from Surai, 2020a).

developed poultry production. Therefore, adding an effective mixture of organic acids into the antioxidant composition would be also beneficial for birds and for the product/supplement quality maintenance.

- **Electrolytes.** It is known that the bird's survivability during heat stress depends on the water consumption, which depends directly on bird's age and on electrolyte balance of the diet (Ahmad and Sarwar, 2006). Under heat stress, the loss of carbon dioxide (CO_2) through respiration and bicarbonate ions through urine can disturb the acid-base balance. Therefore, electrolyte supplementation, either through drinking water or feed, was shown to help correcting blood acid-base balance having beneficial effects for broilers under different heat stress regimens (Ahmad and Sarwar, 2006; Mushtaq *et al.*, 2013). An optimal electrolyte balance and its correction in the body via water/feed supplementation were shown to have protective effects during transport stress (Schaefer *et al.*, 1997) and other stress situations (Olanrewaju *et al.*, 2007). Therefore, inclusion of electrolytes into an antioxidant composition for fighting stresses could help not only in heat stress conditions, but also in other stresses, including transportation stress and chicken placement.

The first commercial product based on the aforementioned concept of the development of the effective antioxidant-related, vitagene-regulating mixture was developed, successfully tested and now can be found on the market in different countries worldwide. Since such a product (Magic antistress mix/PerforMax) containing carnitine, betaine, vitamins, minerals, electrolytes, organic acids and amino acids was first introduced in Ukrainian and Russian markets (Fotina *et al.*, 2011; Grigorieva *et al.*, 2017; Shatskikh *et al.*, 2015a; 2016c; Velichko *et al.*, 2013), major research publications related to the results of the product testing in the university trials and in commercial poultry settings were published in Russian/Ukrainian peer reviewed journal and they will be briefly reviewed below.

18.6 Effect of the vitagene-regulating anti-stress composition on rearing birds, layer and broiler breeders

The importance and efficacy of using the anti-stress composition (PerforMax/Magic Antistress Mix) for rearing birds and adult egg-type parent stock (Hy-Line) at one of the biggest egg producing farms in Russia (Borovskaya poultry farm, Tumen region) have been described recently and below there is a summary of major findings. The study was conducted with rearing birds as well as with adult laying hens and cockerels of the parent stock (Hy Line Brown, line SD). There were two poultry trials, two physiological trials and a big commercial trial. In total 53,400 birds were used with the major results were presented in the PhD thesis (Latipova, 2014a).

In the first phase of the experiment, the effect of Magic Antistress Mix (PerforMax) on the rearing birds was studied. There were a control and an experimental group with 2,000 females and 400 males in each group. The control group was fed in accordance with Hy Line recommendations with the diet formulated to meet all requirements in major nutrients and energy. The experimental group had an additional antistress supply via drinking water at the level of 100 g/100 L of drinking water during days 1-5, 9-13, 21-25, 27-31, 45-49, 63-67 and 75-79 which were related to stresses imposed by vaccinations, grading, and transfer to the breeding houses. The experiment lasted for 105 days (Shatskikh and Latipova, 2014b). In general, growth and development of chickens were similar in both groups with slight increase in body weight (1,242 g vs 1,200 g) at 15 weeks of age in the experimental female birds. Furthermore, usage of the antistress composition was shown to improve birds uniformity at age of 15 weeks (Shatskikh *et al.*, 2016c; Figure 18.12).

Therefore, the experimental birds were closer to target body weight (1,230 g) than the control birds. The usage of the antistress composition positively affected testes development of 15-week-old cockerels (2.47 g vs 1.05 g, $P<0.05$; Shatskikh and Latipova, 2014b). It is interesting to note that in the experimental cockerels testes weight was also improved at 26 and 56 weeks of age (Shatskikh and Latipova, 2013). The liver of experimental birds was characterised by a significant increase in vitamin A content at various ages. There was an increase in Ca content of the bones of female birds at 15 weeks indicating better Ca reserves for future egg production. Results of balance experiments indicated that females and males of the experimental group were characterised by significantly improved usage of nitrogen, calcium and phosphorus from the diet. Usage of the antistress composition with water in period of chicken stress positively affected experimental birds (Shatskikh and Latipova, 2014a,b).

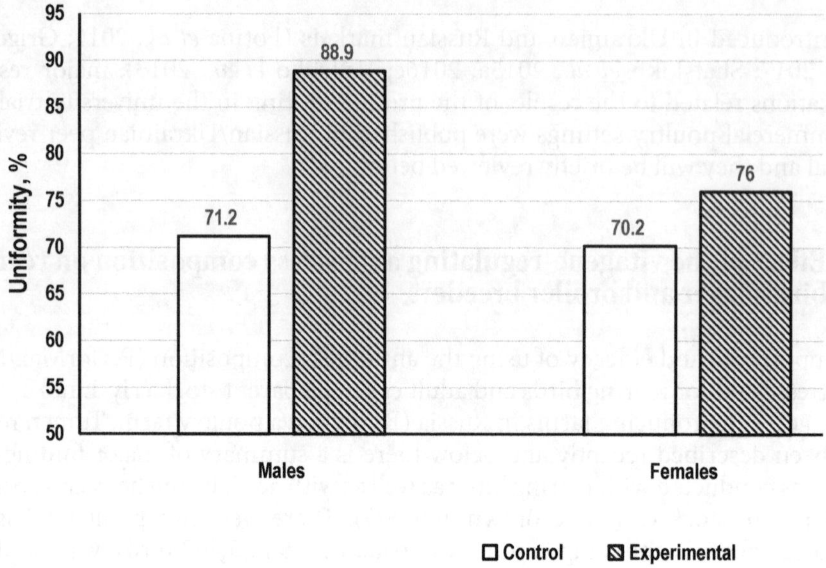

Figure 18.12. Uniformity of rearing birds at 15 weeks, % (adapted from Shatskikh *et al.*, 2016c).

The second phase of the experiment was a continuation of the first phase and lasted from day 106 until day 448 and similar to a previous experiment PerforMax (Magic Antistress Mix) was used with water at 100 g/100 L of drinking water at days 106-107, 109-111, 148-157 and 238-246 associated with increased stresses of vaccinations, first egg laying, active egg production growth and peak of egg production (Latipova, 2014a). The main results of egg production are shown in the Table 18.1. As can be seen from the presented data, usage of the antistress composition with drinking water at specific periods of the increased stress can improve breeder's performance. In particular, there was an increase by 2% of the egg peak production and peak plato lasted about 50 days longer than that in the control birds. It is interesting to note that hen housed egg production in the control group (260.8 eggs) was higher than the target for the line (253.4 eggs) and in the experimental group it was increased by 6 eggs. Improved egg production was associated with increased weight of the oviduct in the experimental layers (Shatskikh and Latypova, 2013). It is also important to mention that FCR (feed per 10 eggs) was also improved by usage of the antistress composition and was better than the target for the line.

As a result, more than 12,000 additional eggs were obtained in the experimental group (Latipova and Shatskikh, 2014d). It is interesting to note that eggshell strength at age 26, 36 and 56 weeks was improved in the experimental group by 2.8, 5.6 and 5.6% respectively (Figure 18.13). The most interesting finding was related to a significant increase in carotenoid level in the egg yolk of the experimental birds. Since carotenoids were not supplied with the antistress composition this increase could be due to improved absorption of nutrients resulted from antistress composition usage. This can also explain improved FCR in the experimental birds. Vitamin A level in

Table 18.1. Egg production of Hy Line parent laying hens per 64 weeks (Latipova and Shatskikh, 2014d; Shatskikh *et al.*, 2016c).

Parameter[1]	Group	
	Control	Experimental
Total egg produced	504,958	517,200
Age of the first egg laid, days	108	106
Age of achieving 50% laying, days	143	142
Peak of egg production, %	94.3	96,9
Age of achieving egg peak production, days	180	172
Plato of peak production, days	59	110
Egg production intensity, %	86.5	87.0
Eggs per hen housed (T – 253,4 eggs)	260.8	266.9
Eggs per hen day (T – 259,5 eggs)	263.6	268.1
Feed per 10 eggs, kg (T – 1,35 kg)	1.36	1.33

[1] T = target for Hy Line Brown.

the egg yolk from the experimental layers was also increased probably reflecting its transfer from the antistress composition. Antistress composition usage was associated with improved fertility at 16, 40, 48 and 56 weeks by 2.5; 2.7; 2.8 and 3.7% respectively. In the same experimental group, the hatch of condition chickens improved at 26, 32, 40, 48 and 56 weeks by 3.6; 2.1; 3.4; 4.9 and 4.3% respectively (Figure 18.14 and Figure 18.15; Latipova, 2014b).

Furthermore, vitamin A concentration in the liver of newly hatched chick from the experimental group was significantly increased. Epigenetic effects could have important role in the poultry production, but there is a lack of scientific studies in this area.

The aim of the present study was to evaluate a possible effect of supplying an antistress composition, containing vitagene-activating nutrients (carnitine, betaine, vitamins, etc.; PerforMax/Magic Antistress Mix) at 100 g/100 L drinking water to Hy Line breeders on their progeny chicks with specific emphasis to chick uniformity as an important determinant of rearing birds quality (Shatskikh *et al.*, 2016b,c). There were 1,938 layers and 176 cockerels in control and experimental groups and the experiment lasted from day 106 until day 448. The obtained data indicate that supplying the antistress composition to breeders was associated with a significant improvement of the uniformity (at day 28) in progeny chicks obtained from breeders of various ages: 26 weeks (81.3 vs 67.3%), 32 weeks (85.5 vs 76.8%), 40 weeks (83.2 vs 68.8%), 48 weeks (75.5 vs 68%) and 56 weeks (73.7 vs 62%) (Figure 18.16).

It is interesting to note that there was no difference in weight of day-old chicks between groups independent on breeder's age. Therefore, it seems likely that changes

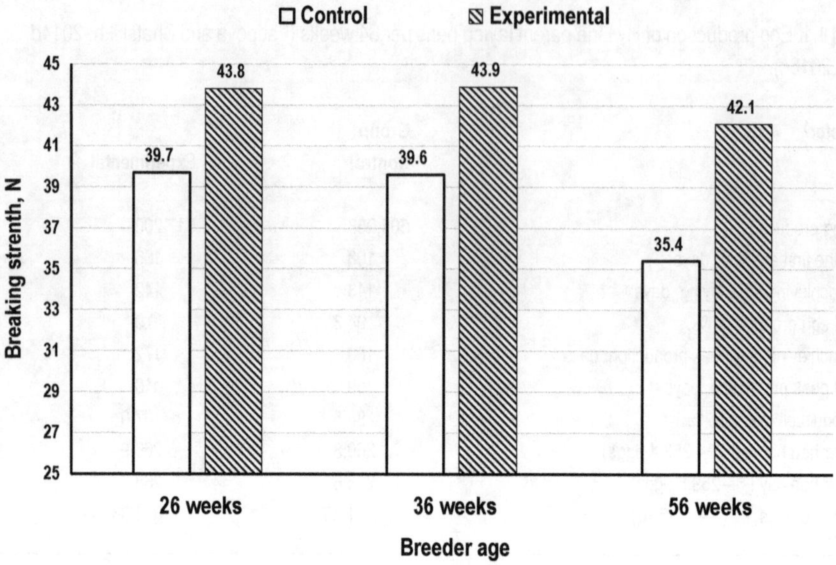

Figure 18.13. Egg shell breaking strength, N (adapted from Shatskikh *et al.*, 2016c).

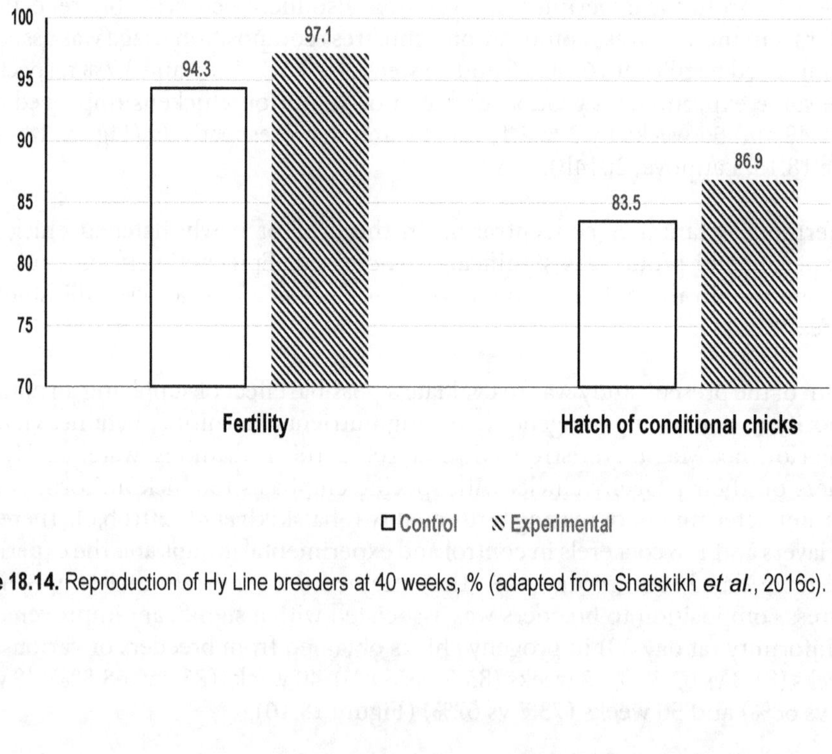

Figure 18.14. Reproduction of Hy Line breeders at 40 weeks, % (adapted from Shatskikh *et al.*, 2016c).

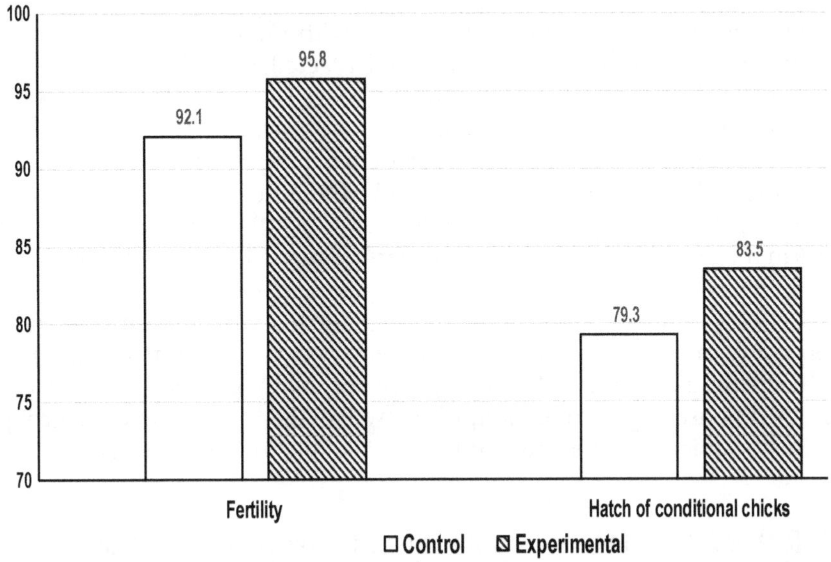

Figure 18.15. Reproduction of Hy Line breeders at 56 weeks, % (adapted from Shatskikh *et al.*, 2016c).

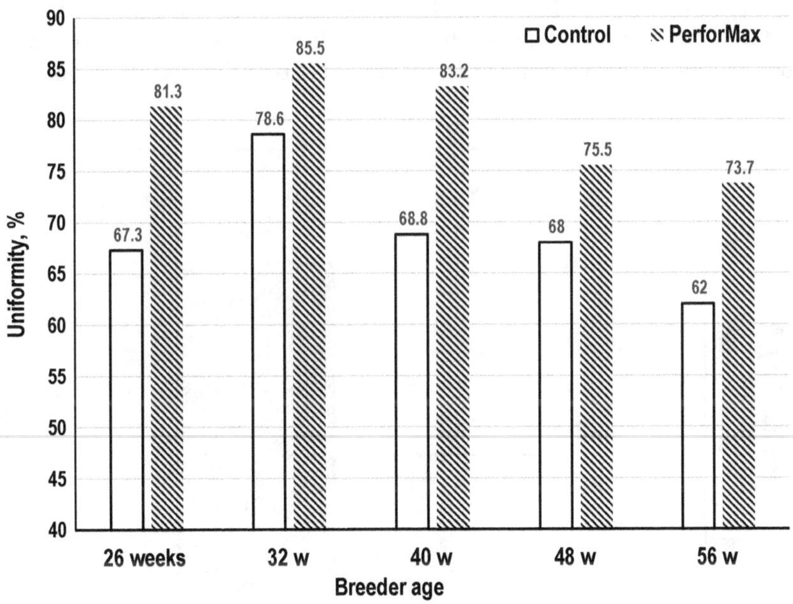

Figure 18.16. Day 28 uniformity of the chicks obtained from the eggs laid by hens of different ages, % (adapted from Shatskikh *et al.*, 2016c).

in egg composition due to supplying breeders with important nutrients, including methyl donors (betaine, methionine, vitamin B12, etc.), could have epigenetic effects of the progeny chick. A positive effect of the usage of PerforMax/Magic Antistress Mix was confirmed in a big commercial trial and it was proven that the antistress composition supplied with water can improve hatching egg production efficacy and is an economically valuable tool to be used in the industry (Latipova *et al.*, 2014). Hatching egg production profitability increased from 19.7% in the control group up to 29.3% in the experimental group of breeders (Figure 18.17; Shatskikh *et al.*, 2016c).

Positive effects of using vitagene-regulating nutrient mixture shown with layer breeders above can be transferred to the broiler breeders. Experimental data indicates that by decreasing commercially relevant stresses in broiler breeders it is possible to increase hen housed egg production, which was higher in experimental group than that in Ross standard for the line (Surai *et al.*, 2017b; 2018; Figure 18.18).

18.7 Effects of the vitagene-regulating anti-stress composition on broilers

The experiment was conducted at the poultry farm AO Prodo Tyumen Broiler (Tumen region, Russia) in a poultry house equipped for conducting experimental trials and measuring growth parameters weekly (Grigorieva *et al.*, 2017). Twelve thousand and four hundred newly hatched Arbor Acres chicks were divided into two equal groups with four replicates in each group and placed in a poultry house.

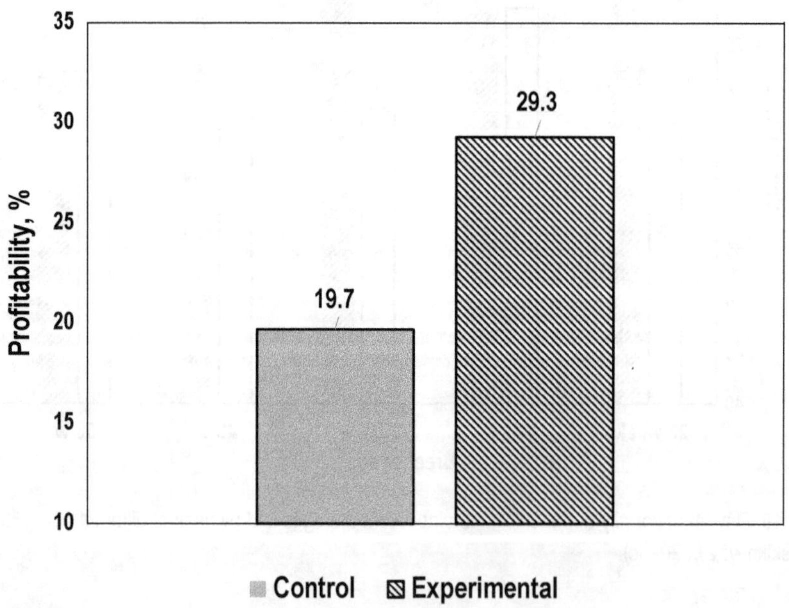

Figure 18.17. Hatching egg production profitability, %, (adapted from Shatskikh *et al.*, 2016c).

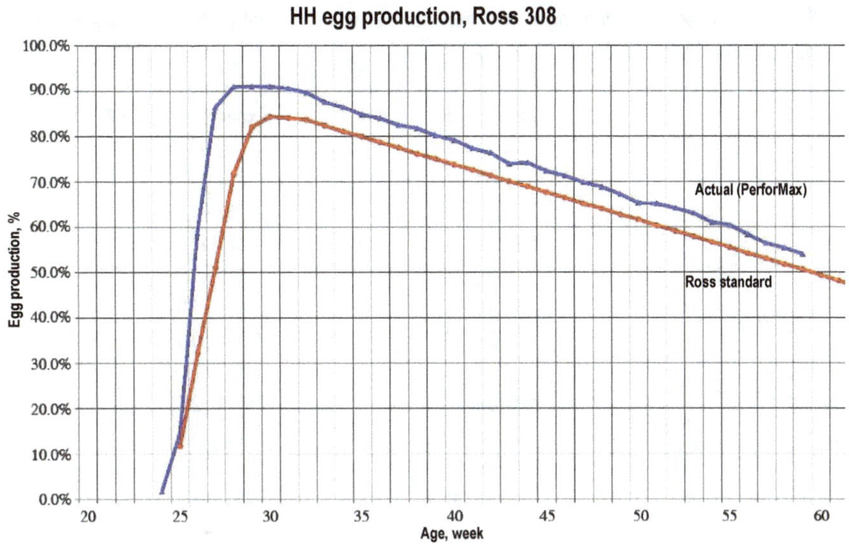

Figure 18.18. Effect of vitagene-regulating nutrient mixture on egg production in Ross breeders (adapted from Surai *et al.*, 2017b; 2018).

Temperature, light and other parameters of chicken growth were maintained in accordance with recommendations of Arbor Acres accepted at the poultry farm. The diet was balanced in all major nutrients in accordance with the same Arbor Acres recommendations accepted at the poultry farm. In additional to the balanced diet the experimental birds were supplemented with Magic Antistress Mix/PerforMax with drinking water at a dose of 1 g/L in stressful period of chicken growth in accordance with recommendations of the preparation developer (Feed-Food Ltd., UK). Chickens were grown up to 35 days and information was collected weekly. Body weight and daily gain (g), mortality (%), daily feed consumption (g) and FCR were assessed in three growth periods (15-21 days, 22-28 days and 29-35 days) and for whole growth period (1-35 days). To compare broiler growth results the European Production Efficiency Factor (EPEF) is used. At the end of the experiment intestinal weight was assessed and internal organ examination was conducted to check for nephritis, enteritis and intestinal atony. Efficacy of vaccination against infectious bursitis was assessed by ELISA in accordance with recommendations of test system producer (Bio-Tek Instruments, Inc., USA). Vaccination Index (VI) was calculated as a ratio of average antibody titre by ELISA to variation coefficient (Cv, %). During statistical analysis, average parameters (*M*) and the standard errors (±SEM) were determined. Significance of differences with Control was assessed by *t*-test by using ANOVA, differences were considered to be significant at $P<0.05$.

Chicken viability (Table 18.2) in both groups was within standards for the poultry farm. However, the mortality for 35 days in the control group (3.8%) was numerically higher in comparison to the experimental group (2.3%). In commercial conditions

Table 18.2. Effect of usage with drinking water of vitagene-stimulating additive on growth and development of broilers (adapted from Grigorieva *et al.*, 2017).

Parameter	Control (n=6,200)	Experimental (n=6,200)
15-21 days of age		
Body weight, g	935.5±8.75	926.0±19.5
Daily gain, g	68.6±2.4	68.3±1.6
Mortality, %	0.40±0.04	0.30±0.05
Feed consumption, g/chicken	101.4±1.8	99.5±1.9
FCR	1.48±0.03	1.46±0.03*
22-28 days of age		
Body weight, g	1,457.5±6.5	1,457.8±29.8
Daily gain, g	74.6±0.6	76.1±3.0
Mortality, %	0.50±0.05	0.3±0.08*
Feed consumption, g/chicken	119.6±1.40	116.5±3.7
FCR	1.61±0.02	1.54±0.04*
29-35 days of age		
Body weight, g	2,019.0±7.50	2,007.5±27.5
Daily gain, g	80.2±0.80	78.6±2.8
Mortality, %	1.90±1.30	0.9±0.2
Feed consumption, g/chicken	132.4±3.30	126.7±2.7
FCR	1.65±0.04	1.62±0.04
1-35 days of age		
Body weight, g	2,019.0±7.50	2,007.5±27.5
Daily gain, g	56.5±0.20	56.2±0.8
Feed consumption, kg/chicken	3.15±0.07	3.02±0.02*
Viability, %	96.2±1.2	97.7±0.5
FCR	1.56±0.04	1.50±0.02*
EPEF	356.8±10.8	372.8±9.6**

[1] *, ** differences with Control are statistically significant at $P<0.05$ and $P<0.01$, respectively.

such a difference could be significant for a meat producer. Usage of Magic Antistress Mix/PerforMax with drinking water was associated with decrease number of enteritis, nephritis and intestinal atony as well as pododermatitis. For the first two weeks of the experimental period data in the control and experimental groups were not different. Later (Table 18.2) there was an improvement in FCR in the experimental group in comparison to the control group resulting in decreased feed consumption per week.

There was no difference in body weight and daily gain between the control and experimental groups. Therefore, the main advantage of usage of the vitagene activating composition for growing broilers was associated with improvement of FCR, which in the experimental group (1.50) was significantly better than that in the control group (1.56).

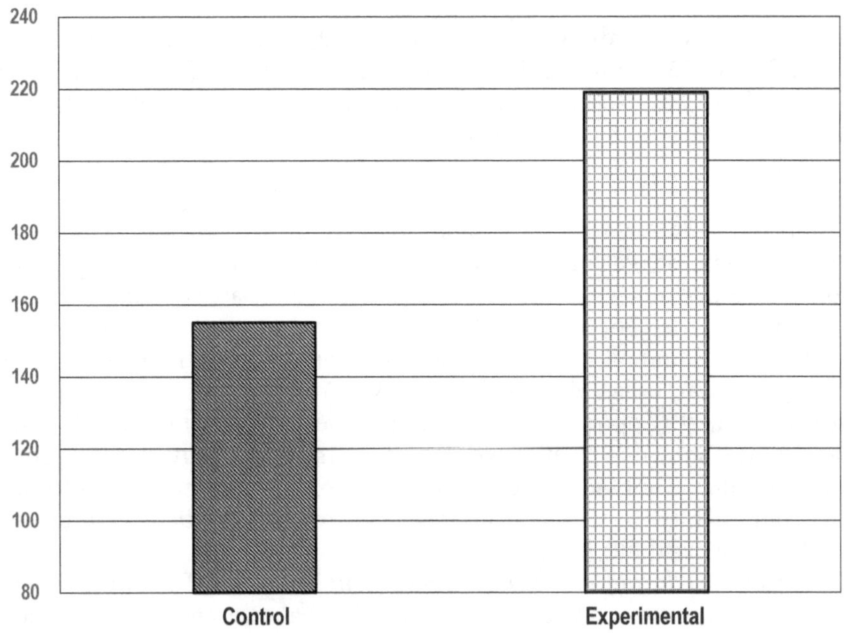

Figure 18.19. Vaccination index in the 35-day old chickens (adapted from Grigorieva *et al.*, 2017).

Taking into account all data of the chicken growth and development for 5 weeks EPEF in the control group was shown to be 356.8, while in the experimental group it was 372.8, being comparable at the time with an efficacy of broiler production at the best farms in Russia and abroad. It is important to mention that in experimental chickens at day 35 intestinal weight was higher (by 5%) in comparison to the control chickens. Obtained data indicate that average antibody titre in 35 days old chickens was 4,500 in the control group and 5,258 in the experimental group. It is interesting that *Cv* in the experimental group (24%) was lower than that in the control group (29%). As a result, the vaccination index in the experimental group was significantly higher than that in the control group (Figure 18.19).

As a result of FCR improvement due to water application of the antistress composition economics of meat production was improved (Table 18.2). Due to the PerforMax application an additional income per kg of meat production comprises 1.66 roubles. An earlier study conducted at the same poultry farm showed that supplying the antistress vitagene-activating composition with drinking water improved bird's performance. The biggest positive effect of such a supplementation was seen at the FCR: 1st week1.44 vs 1.55; 2nd week: 1.60 vs 1.66; 3rd week 1.70 vs 1.72; 4th week 1.83 vs 2.06 and for the whole growth period (39 days) 1.85 vs 2.04 and daily gain was improved by 1.85 g. The mortality was the same in both groups (3.0 vs 2.8%).

By using the vitagene-regulating composition the cost of production of 1 kg of broiler body weight decreased by 13 cents (Velichko *et al.*, 2013; Velichko and Surai, 2014).

At small university trial the same vitagene-regulating additive supplied to broilers improved FCR (1.75 vs 1.88) and increased daily gain by 3 g (55.7 vs 52.7 g; Fotina *et al.*, 2011). There was also a commercial trial with caged broilers comparing 2 control and 3 experimental (supplemented with the same vitagene-regulating mixture) sheds (Table 18.3).

The results of the commercial trial (Table 18.3) confirmed previous results showing beneficial effects of PerforMax supplementation on the broiler growth and development. Since molecular mechanisms of the stresses are similar in monogastric animals, the vitagene concept of fighting stresses was successfully applied for ducks (Surai *et al.*, 2012) and pigs as well (Surai and Litvinov, 2017; Surai and Melnichuk, 2012). In particular, usage of PerforMax (Magic Antistress Mix) for piglets to fight stresses at weaning (Gaponov *et al.*, 2011) and heat stress (Surai, 2017; Surai and Fotina, 2013a) is shown to be effective. Therefore, the technology of stress protection in poultry production, based on directed activation of vitagenes allows to increase adaptive ability of birds to commercially-relevant stresses. In particular, the technology can be effectively used for:

- *Chicken support during and after their placement in the shed.* This is a critical period of time when antioxidant defences and redox balance are crucial for effective development of the gut and immunity.
- *Vaccination.* Vitagene activation before and after vaccination is considered to be an effective means of reduction of vaccination stress and improvement of vaccination efficacy.
- *Nutritional stresses* (for example, mycotoxin feed contamination). Support of the liver and gut, main sites of mycotoxin detoxification and metabolism are of great importance to decrease detrimental consequences of mycotoxin toxicity consequences.
- *Heat or cold stress.* Reduction of detrimental consequences of temperature stress could help prevent/decrease growth deterioration, immunosuppression and mortality.

Table 18.3. Effect of PerforMax on broiler growth and development (Adapted from Surai, 2020a).

Shed, chicken number	Days of growth	Body weight, kg	Daily gain, g	FCR	Survival, %	EPEF[1]
Control, 22605	41	2.302	55.2	1.88	92.2	275
Control, 22585	40	2.271	55.8	1.92	93.4	276
PerforMax, 22620	40	2.503	61.6	1.80	95.2	331
PerforMax, 22603	41	2.594	62.3	1.85	94.8	324
PerforMax, 22621	42	2.584	60.6	1.81	95.1	323
PerforMax/Control		+274 g	+6 g	-0.08	+2.2%	+50

[1] EPEF = European production efficiency factor.

- *Technological stresses.* Protection against technological stresses (e.g. problems with equipment, etc.) could help maintaining high productive and reproductive performance.
- *Rearing bird transfer to breeder houses.* Improved antioxidant defences and maintenance of the redox balance during this stressful period are of great importance to prevent feather pecking and stimulate egg production.
- *Thinning.* Vitagene activation during this stressful procedure could prevent detrimental consequences of the stress.
- *Peak of egg production.* This is the most demanding period of egg production and vitagene activation can help achieving higher peak of egg production and increasing its duration.
- *Any other stressful period of bird's growth, development and production/reproduction.*

Protective effects of PerforMax in poultry production are summarised in the Figure 18.20. Activation of vitagenes by the specific nutrient mixture (PerforMax) is shown to be an effective strategy to maintain good health and high productive and reproductive performance of birds in commercial stressful conditions.

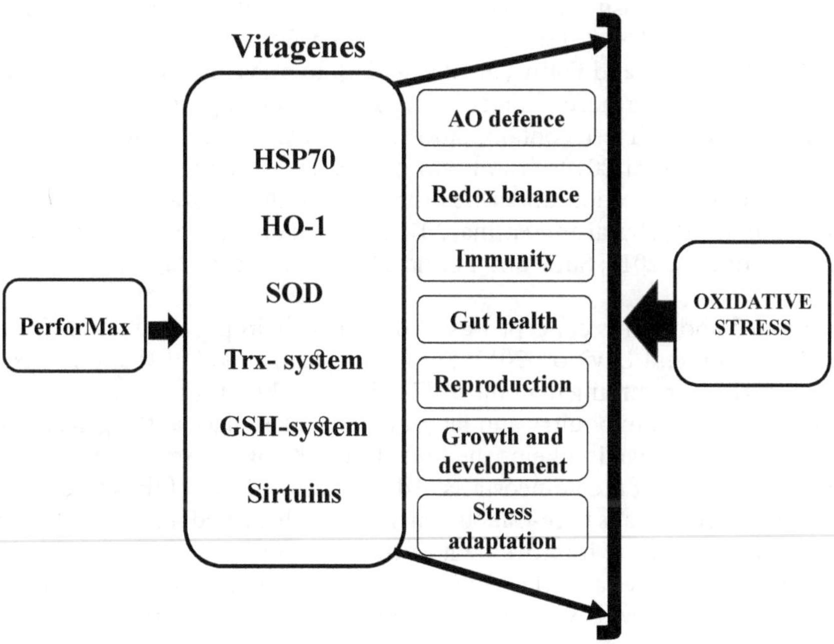

Figure 18.20. Protective effects of PerforMax in poultry production (Surai, 2020a).

18.8 Vitagene activation as an important strategy in stress prevention/alleviation

Our research for the last 10 years allowed to transfer the vitagene concept from medical science to poultry sciences (Fisinin and Surai, 2011a,b; Surai, 2011; 2015e; 2016; 2019a,b,c,d; 2020a,c; Surai and Earle-Payne, 2022; Surai and Fisinin, 2012a,b; 2014; 2015; 2016a,b,c,d,e; Surai and Fotina, 2010a; 2011a; 2012a,b,c,d; Surai and Kochish, 2017; 2018; Surai *et al.*, 2017a,b; 2018; 2019b; 2020b; 2021a,b,c). Practical aspects of usage of the concept for effective protection against various stresses in commercial stressful conditions have been considered above. The vitagene concept is proved to be effective in broiler production (Fotina *et al.*, 2011; 2014; Grigorieva *et al.*, 2017; Velichko and Surai, 2014; Velichko *et al.*, 2013), in nutrition and management of rearing birds, egg breeders and meat breeders (Latipova, 2014a,b; Latipova and Shatskikh, 2014a,b,c,d; Latipova *et al.*, 2014; 2016; Shatskikh and Latipova, 2013; 2014a,b; Shatskikh *et al.*, 2015a,b; 2016a,b,c; Surai, 2020a; Surai *et al.*, 2017b; 2018).

The vitagene-regulating mixture was also effective for improvement of hatchability and chick quality (Fisinin and Surai, 2012g,h; Surai and Fisinin, 2013), at chicken placement (Surai and Fisinin, 2012h; 2015), for support of high immunocompetence (Fisinin and Surai, 2011c; 2013a,b; Surai and Fotina, 2012e; 2013b; Surai *et al.*, 2012), eggshell quality (Surai and Fotina, 2010b; 2011b), to prevent/restrict feather pecking (Surai, 2012c). Furthermore, vitagene activation is an important strategy to fight stresses associated with feed contamination by T-2 toxin (Fisinin and Surai, 2012c,d), DON (Fisinin and Surai, 2012e,f) and ochratoxins (Fisinin and Surai, 2012a,b), as well as showing protective action under heat stress in poultry (Surai and Fotina, 2013c) and pigs (Surai, 2017; Surai and Fotina, 2013a) as well under other stressful situations (Surai and Boroday, 2010; Surai and Fotina, 2010a; 2011a; 2012a,b,c,d).

As mentioned above, this concept was also applicable in pig production (Gaponov *et al.*, 2012; Surai and Litvinov, 2017; Surai and Melnichuk, 2012) and is associated with maternal programming in poultry (Fisinin *et al.*, 2016). Therefore, it was proven that stress adaptation in poultry and farm animals takes place at the gene (vitagene) level and vitagene activation helps the body to use its own reserves more efficiently for re-establishment of the homeostasis. Additional synthesis of the aforementioned protective molecules leads to re-establishment of the disturbed redox balance and cell signalling with following improvement of the stress resistance. Therefore, vitagene activation helps improve adaptive ability of poultry to various stress conditions. The vitagene interactions with various transcription factors, including Nrf2 и NF-κB deserves further research.

18.9 Conclusions

The vitagene concept successfully found its applications in poultry production and the development of 3 vitagene-regulating compositions described above confirmed its validity. Therefore, by modulating vitagenes via supplying special nutrient mixtures with drinking water it is possible to develop a 'system of quick response', which can help nutritionist/technologist/ veterinarian to deal with emergency situations in commercial poultry production associated with various environmental, technological, nutritional or internal stresses. It appears that vitagene activation is an important approach helping decrease negative consequences of various stresses. It should be mentioned that the aim of the usage of the aforementioned compositions is to help birds mobilise their internal resources/reserves to the maximum extent and usage such nutritional supplements do not affect general nutrition or nutrient balance.

On the one hand, PerforMax is considered as a generic antistress supplement which can deal with most low to moderate stresses of the commercial egg and meat production. On the other hand, when stress consequences are more severe, including eggshell problems or fatty liver problems, ShellBone and VitaTonic can be used. These are additional 'instruments' in hands of nutritionists, technologists and veterinarians helping them with stress management. As can be seen from the data provided above vitagene activation could be considered as an effective means to deal with various stresses in poultry production. It is well accepted that commercial poultry production is associated with a range of stresses starting from laying eggs by breeders, their collection and incubation, continuing with chicken placement, vaccinations and growth and finalising at bird transportation to slaughtering.

Therefore, the first vitagene-regulating nutrient composition (PerforMax/Magic Antistress Mix) was proven to be effective in those situations where oxidative stress takes place and vitagene activations was reported to improve bird's resistance to stresses and therefore maintain their productive and reproductive performance. Two other concepts (VitaTonic and ShellBone) also found its way to poultry industry and help poultry producers deal with liver health problems as well as with eggshell quality and bone integrity problems. The aforementioned data are a good example of technology transfer from the laboratory research into the commercial chicken production. There are also indications that the vitagene concept and vitagene-regulating nutritional mixtures could be effective in fighting stresses in pig production as well as for health maintaining of other animals (calves and cattle, lambs and sheep, kids and goats, fur-animals, companion animals, zoo animals, fish, etc.) under various stress conditions (Surai, 2020; Surai *et al.*, 2018).

References

Abdel-Moneim, A.M., Al-Kahtani, M.A., El-Kersh, M.A. and Al-Omair, M.A., 2015. Free radical-scavenging, anti-inflammatory/anti-fibrotic and hepatoprotective actions of taurine and silymarin against CCl4 induced rat liver damage. PLoS One 10: e0144509.

Ahmad, I., Shukla, S., Kumar, A., Singh, B.K., Kumar, V., Chauhan, A.K., Singh, D., Pandey, H.P. and Singh, C., 2013. Biochemical and molecular mechanisms of N-acetyl cysteine and silymarin-mediated protection against maneb-and paraquat-induced hepatotoxicity in rats. Chemico-Biological Interactions 201: 9-18.

Ahmad, T. and Sarwar, M., 2006. Dietary electrolyte balance: implications in heat stressed broilers. World's Poultry Science Journal 62: 638-653.

Ahmed, A.M.H., Rodríguez-Navarro, A.B., Vidal, M.L., Gautron, J., García-Ruiz, J.M. and Nys, A.Y., 2005. Changes in eggshell mechanical properties, crystallographic texture and in matrix proteins induced by moult in hens. British Poultry Science 46: 268-279.

Al-Batshan, H.A., Scheideler, S.E., Black, B.L., Garlich, J.D. and Anderson, K.E., 1994. Duodenal calcium uptake, femur ash, and eggshell quality decline with age and increase following molt. Poultry Science 73: 1590-1596.

Ali, B.H., Homeida, A.M. and Knifton, A., 1984. The effect of furazolidone on fertility of male chickens. Comparative Biochemistry and Physiology Part C: Comparative Pharmacology 78: 43-47.

Alirezaei, M., Gheisari, H.R., Ranjbar, V.R. and Hajibemani, A., 2012. Betaine: a promising antioxidant agent for enhancement of broiler meat quality. British Poultry Science 53: 699-707.

Al-Rasheed, N., Faddah, L., Al-Rasheed, N., Bassiouni, Y.A., Hasan, I.H., Mahmoud, A.M., Mohamad, R.A. and Yacoub, H.I., 2016. Protective effects of silymarin, alone or in combination with chlorogenic acid and/or melatonin, against carbon tetrachloride-induced hepatotoxicity. Pharmacognosy Magazine 12: S337-S345.

Amakye-Anim, J., Lin, T.L., Hester, P.Y., Thiagarajan, D., Watkins, B.A. and Wu, C.C., 2000. Ascorbic acid supplementation improved antibody response to infectious bursal disease vaccination in chickens. Poultry Science 79: 680-688.

Amiridumari, H., Sarir, H., Afzali, N. and Fanimakki, O., 2013. Effects of milk thistle seed against aflatoxin B1 in broiler model. Journal of Research in Medical Sciences 18: 786-790.

Arias, J.I., Jure, C., Wiff, J.P., Fernández, M.S., Fuenzalida, V. and Arias, J.L., 2001. Effect of sulfate content of biomacromolecules on the crystallization of calcium carbonate. MRS Online Proceedings Library Archive 711: 243-248.

Arslan, C., 2006. L-carnitine and its use as a feed additive in poultry feeding a review. Revue de Médecine Vétérinaire 157: 134-142.

Arslan, C., Citil, M. and Saatci, M., 2003. Effects of L-carnitine administration on growth performance, carcass traits, blood serum parameters and abdominal fatty acid composition of ducks. Archives of Animal Nutrition 57: 381-388.

Azcona, J.O., Bonino, M.F., Schang, S.J., Gallego, S.E. and Boland, R.L., 1982. Effect of calcinogenic substances from Solanum malacoxylon on eggshell thickness and performance of laying hen. Zootechnica International, February,12-13.

Balnave, D., Zhang, D. and Moreng, R.E., 1991. Use of ascorbic acid to prevent the decline in eggshell quality observed with saline drinking water. Poultry Science 70: 848-852.

Bar, A., 2009. Calcium transport in strongly calcifying laying birds: mechanisms and regulation. Comparative Biochemistry and Physiology Part A: Molecular & Integrative Physiology 152: 447-469.

Bar, A., Striem, S., Rosenberg, J. and Hurwitz, S., 1988. Egg shell quality and cholecalciferol metabolism in aged laying hens. The Journal of Nutrition 118: 1018-1023.

Baradaran, A., Samadi, F., Ramezanpour, S.S. and Yousefdoust, S., 2019. Hepatoprotective effects of silymarin on CCl4-induced hepatic damage in broiler chickens model. Toxicology Reports 6: 788-794.

Barnett, D.M., Kumpula, B.L., Petryk, R.L., Robinson, N.A., Renema, R.A. and Robinson, F.E., 2004. Hatchability and early chick growth potential of broiler breeder eggs with hairline cracks. Journal of Applied Poultry Research 13: 65-70.

Bell, D.E. and Marion, J.E., 1990. Vitamin C in laying hen diets. Poultry Science 69: 1900-1904.

Benesch, R., Barron, N.S. and Mawson, C.A., 1944. Carbonic anhydrase, sulphonamides and shell formation in the domestic fowl. Nature 153: 138-139.

Boyanabc, B.D., Sylvia, V.L., Dean, D.D., Pedrozo, H., Del Toro, F., Nemere, I., Posner, G.H. and Schwartz, Z., 1999. 1, 25-(OH) 2D3 modulates growth plate chondrocytes via membrane receptor-mediated protein kinase C by a mechanism that involves changes in phospholipid metabolism and the action of arachidonic acid and PGE2. Steroids 64: 129-136.

Butler, E.J., 1976. Fatty liver diseases in the domestic fowl – A review. Avian Pathology 5: 1-14.

Carlos, A.B. and Edwards Jr, H.M., 1998. The effects of 1, 25-dihydroxycholecalciferol and phytase on the natural phytate phosphorus utilization by laying hens. Poultry Science 77: 850-858.

Castaldo, D.J. and Maurice, D.V., 1990. Plasma calcitriol in chickens producing strong and weak egg shells and the response of hens to exogenous calcitriol. International Journal for Vitamin and Nutrition Research 60: 320-323.

Celik, L. and Öztürkcan, O., 2003. Effects of dietary supplemental L-carnitine and ascorbic acid on performance, carcass composition and plasma L-carnitine concentration of broiler chicks reared under different temperature. Archives of Animal Nutrition 57: 27-38.

Celik, L.B., Tekeli, A. and Öztürkcan, O., 2004. Effects of supplemental l-carnitine in drinking water on performance and egg quality of laying hens exposed to a high ambient temperature. Journal of Animal Physiology and Animal Nutrition 88: 229-233.

Chand, N., Muhammad, D., Durrani, F.R., Qureshi, M.S. and Ullah, S.S., 2011. Protective effects of milk thistle (*Silybum marianum*) against aflatoxin B1 in broiler chicks. Asian-Australasian Journal of Animal Sciences 24: 1011-1018.

Chand, N., Naz, S., Maris, H., Khan, R.U., Khan, S. and Qureshi, M.S., 2017. Effect of betaine supplementation on the performance and immune response of heat stressed broilers. Pakistan Journal of Zoology 49: 1857-1862.

Chen, R., Wen, C., Gu, Y., Wang, C., Chen, Y., Zhuang, S. and Zhou, Y., 2020. Dietary betaine supplementation improves meat quality of transported broilers through altering muscle anaerobic glycolysis and antioxidant capacity. Journal of the Science of Food and Agriculture 100: 2656-2663.

Chennaiah, S., Qadri, S.S.Y.H., Rao, S.R., Shyamsunder, G. and Raghuramulu, N., 2004. Cestrum diurnum leaf as a source of 1,25(OH)2 Vitamin D3 improves egg shell thickness. The Journal of Steroid Biochemistry and Molecular Biology 89: 589-594.

Cholewa, J.M., Guimaraes-Ferreira, L. and Zanchi, N.E., 2014. Effects of betaine on performance and body composition: a review of recent findings and potential mechanisms. Amino Acids 46: 1785-1793.

Chung, M.K., Choi, J.H., Chung, Y.K. and Chee, K.M., 2005. Effects of dietary vitamins C and E on egg shell quality of broiler breeder hens exposed to heat stress. Asian-Australasian Journal of Animal Sciences 18: 545-551.

Couch, J.R., 1956. Fatty livers in laying hens – a condition which may occur as a result of increased strain. Feedstuffs 28: 46-54.

Dangi, S.S., Dangi, S.K., Chouhan, V.S., Verma, M.R., Kumar, P., Singh, G. and Sarkar, M., 2016. Modulatory effect of betaine on expression dynamics of HSPs during heat stress acclimation in goat (Capra hircus). Gene 575: 543-550.

Day, C.R. and Kempson, S.A., 2016. Betaine chemistry, roles, and potential use in liver disease. Biochimica et Biophysica Acta-General Subjects 1860: 1098-1106.

Diamants, T., and Schluns, J., 1964. Lokalisation und bedeutung der karboanhydrase im uterus von legehennen. Acta Histochemica 19: 296-302.

Dittoe, D.K., Ricke, S.C. and Kiess, A.S., 2018. Organic acids and potential for modifying the avian gastrointestinal tract and reducing pathogens and disease. Frontiers in Veterinary Science 5: 216.

Dumari, M.A., Sarir, H., Makki, O.F. and Afzali, N., 2014. Effect of milk thistle (*Silybum marianum* l.) on biochemical parameters and immunity of broiler chicks fed aflatoxin b1 after three weeks. Iranian Journal of Toxicology 8: 1098-1103.

Dunn, I.C., Rodríguez-Navarro, A.B., Mcdade, K., Schmutz, M., Preisinger, R., Waddington, D., Wilson, P.W. and Bain, M.M., 2012. Genetic variation in eggshell crystal size and orientation is large and these traits are correlated with shell thickness and are associated with eggshell matrix protein markers. Animal Genetics 43: 410-418.

Edwards Jr, H.M., 1990. Efficacy of several vitamin D compounds in the prevention of tibial dyschondroplasia in broiler chickens. The Journal of Nutrition 120: 1054-1061.

Edwards Jr, H.M., 2002. Studies on the efficacy of cholecalciferol and derivatives for stimulating phytate utilization in broilers. Poultry Science 81: 1026-1031.

Edwards, H.M., Elliot, M.A. and Sooncharernying, S., 1992. Effect of dietary calcium on tibial dyschondroplasia. Interaction with light, cholecalciferol, 1, 25-dihydroxycholecalciferol, protein, and synthetic zeolite. Poultry Science 71: 2041-2055.

El-Boushy, A.R. and Van Albada, M., 1970. The effect of vitamin C on egg shell quality under high environmental temperatures. Netherlands Journal of Agricultural Science 18: 62-71.

Elliot, M.A. and Edwards JNR, H.M., 1997. Effect of 1,25-dihydroxycholecalciferol, cholecalciferol and fluorescent lights on the development of tibial dyschondroplasia and rickets in broiler chickens. Poultry Science 76: 570-580.

Elvira-Torales, L.I., García-Alonso, J. and Periago-Castón, M.J., 2019. Nutritional importance of carotenoids and their effect on liver health: A review. Antioxidants 8: 229.

Elzinga, E.J. and Reeder, R.J., 2002. X-ray absorption spectroscopy study of Cu2+, and Zn2+, adsorption complexes at the calcite surface: Implications for site-specific metal incorporation preferences during calcite crystal growth. Geochimica et Cosmochimica Acta 66: 3943-3954.

Ensminger, M.E., Oldfield, J.E. and Heinemann, W.W., 1990. Feeds and nutrition. Second Revised Ed. The Ensminger Publishing Co. Clovis, CA, USA.

Estevez, M. and Petracci, M., 2019. Benefits of magnesium supplementation to broiler subjected to dietary and heat stress: Improved redox status, breast quality and decreased myopathy incidence. Antioxidants 8: 456.

Fani, M.O., Afzali, N. and Omidi, A., 2013. Effect of different levels of silymarin (*Silybum marianum*) on growth rate, carcass variables and liver morphology of broiler chickens contaminated with aflatoxin B1. Poultry Science Journal 1: 105-116.

Farquharson, C., Berry, J.L., Mawer, E.B., Seawright, E. and Whitehead, C.C., 1998. Ascorbic acid-induced chondrocyte terminal differentiation: the role of the extracellular matrix and 1, 25-dihydroxyvitamin D. European Journal of Cell Biology 76: 110-118.

Fathi, M.M., El-Dlebshany, A.E., Bachine El-Deen, M., Radwan, L.M. and Rayan, G.N., 2016. Effect of long-term selection for egg production on eggshell quality of Japanese quail (Coturnix japonica). Poultry Science 95: 2570-2575.

Fathi, M.M., Afifi, Y.K. and El-Safty, A.S., 2010. Ultrastructural diversity of eggshell quality in some Egyptian local breeds of chicken. Egyptian Poultry Science 30: 813-827.

Fernandez, M.S., Moya, A., Lopez, L. and Arias, J.L., 2001. Secretion pattern, ultrastructural localization and function of extracellular matrix molecules involved in eggshell formation. Matrix Biology 19: 793-803.

Fetterer, R.H., Augustine, P.C., Allen, P.C. and Barfield, R.C., 2003. The effect of dietary betaine on intestinal and plasma levels of betaine in uninfected and coccidia-infected broiler chicks. Parasitology Research 90: 343-348.

Figueroa-Soto, C.G. and Valenzuela-Soto, E.M., 2018. Glycine betaine rather than acting only as an osmolyte also plays a role as regulator in cellular metabolism. Biochimie 147: 89-97.

Fisinin, V.I. and Surai, P.F., 2011a. Effective protection against stresses in poultry production: from vitamins to vitagenes. Ptitsa i Pitseproducti (Poultry and Poultry Products, Moscow) 5: 23-26.

Fisinin, V.I. and Surai, P.F., 2011b. Effective protection against stresses in poultry production: from vitamins to vitagenes. Ptitsa i Pitseproducti (Poultry and Poultry Products, Moscow) 6: 10-13.

Fisinin, V.I. and Surai, P.F., 2011c. Immunity in modern animal and poultry production: New discoveries and prospects. Zhivotnovodstvo Sjogodni (Today's Animal Production, Ukraine) 9: 40-47.

Fisinin, V.I. and Surai, P.F., 2012a. Mycotoxins and antioxidants: Uncompromised fighting (Ochratoxin A). Part 1., Kombikorma (Moscow) 3: 55-60.

Fisinin, V.I. and Surai, P.F., 2012b. Mycotoxins and antioxidants: Uncompromised fighting (Ochratoxin A). Part 2., Kombikorma (Moscow) 4: 59-60.

Fisinin, V.I. and Surai, P.F., 2012c. Mycotoxins and antioxidants: Uncompromised fighting (T-2 toxin – metabolism and toxicity). Ptitsa i Pitseproducti (Poultry and Poultry Products, Moscow) 3: 38- 41.

Fisinin, V.I. and Surai, P.F., 2012d. Mycotoxins and antioxidants: Uncompromised fighting (T-2 toxin – mechanisms of toxicity and protection). Ptitsa i Pitseproducti (Poultry and Poultry Products, Moscow) 4: 36-39.

Fisinin, V.I. and Surai, P.F., 2012e. Properties and toxicity of deoxynivalenol (DON). Part 1. Zhivotnovodstvo Rossiyi (Russian Animal Production, Moscow) 5: 11-16.

Fisinin, V.I. and Surai, P.F., 2012f. Properties and toxicity of deoxynivalenol (DON). Part 2. Zhivotnovodstvo Rossiyi (Russian Animal Production, Moscow) 6: 3-5.

Fisinin, V.I. and Surai, P.F., 2012g. First days of chicken life: From stress prevention to effective adaptation. Ptitsevodstvo (Moscow) 2: 11-15.

Fisinin, V.I. and Surai, P.F., 2012h. Chicken early nutrition and muscle development. Ptitsevodstvo (Moscow) 3: 9-12.

Fisinin, V.I. and Surai, P.F., 2013a. Immunity in modern animal and poultry production: from theory to practice of immunomodulation. Ptitsevodstvo (Moscow) 5: 4-10.

Fisinin, V.I. and Surai, P.F., 2013b. Gut immunity in birds: facts and thoughts. Agricultural Biology (Moscow) 4: 1-25.

Fisinin, V.I., Shatskikh, E.V., Latipova, E.N. and Surai, P.F., 2016. Maternal effects in poultry production – from vitamins to vitagenes and epigenetics. Ptitsa i Pitseproducti (Poultry and Poultry Products, Moscow) 1: 29-33.

Fotina, A., Fotina, T.I. and Surai, P., 2014. Effect of a water-soluble antistress composition on broiler chickens. Proceedings of the XIVth European Poultry Conference. Stavenger, Norway 23-27 June, 2014, p. 555.

Fotina, A.A., Fotina, T.I. and Surai, P.F., 2011. Effect of antistress preparation 'Feed Food Magic Antistress Mix' on growing chickens. Annals of Sumy Agrarian University, Veterinary Medicine Series 2: 158-162.

Fouad, A.M. and El-Senousey, H.K., 2014. Nutritional factors affecting abdominal fat deposition in poultry: a review. Asian-Australasian Journal of Animal Sciences 27: 1057-1068.

Fowler, N.G., 1990. Nutritional disorders. In: Jordan, F.T.W. (ed) Poultry diseases, London, UK, pp. 297-319.

Frost, T.J., Roland Sr, D.A. and Untawale, G.G., 1990. Influence of vitamin D3, 1α-Hydroxyvitamin D3, and 1, 25-Dihydroxyvitamin D3 on eggshell quality, tibia strength, and various production parameters in commercial laying hens. Poultry Science 69: 2008-2016.

Gabbay, K.H., Bohren, K.M., Morello, R., Bertin, T., Liu, J. and Vogel, P., 2010. Ascorbate synthesis pathway: dual role of ascorbate in bone homeostasis. Journal of Biological Chemistry 285: 9510-19520.

Gaponov, I.V., Fotina, T.I. and Surai, P.F., 2012. Physiological and technological stresses at time of piglet weaning. Protective effect of the antistress preparation. Svinatstvo Ukraini (Pig Production of Ukraine, Kiev) 6: 6-9.

Gautron, J., Hincke, M.T. and Nys, Y., 1997. Precursor matrix proteins in the uterine fluid change with stages of eggshell formation in hens. Connective Tissue Research 36: 195-210.

Geng, A., Guo, Y. and Yuan, J., 2004. Effects of dietary L-carnitine and coenzyme Q10 supplementation on performance and ascites mortality of broilers. Archives of Animal Nutrition 58: 473-482.

Gengwu, G., Ming, J., Fan, W., Wei, L., Juan, T. and Changgeng, Y., 2016. Effects of dietary silymarin on growth performance, enzymes of hepatic lipid metabolism and antioxidant ability in GIFT Oreochromis niloticus. Journal of Fisheries of China 40: 1309-1320.

Gillessen, A. and Schmidt, H.H., 2020. Silymarin as supportive treatment in liver diseases: A narrative review. Advances in Therapy 37: 1279-1301.

Golzar Adabi, S., Cooper, R.G., Ceylan, N. and Corduk, M., 2011. L-carnitine and its functional effects in poultry nutrition. World's Poultry Science Journal 67: 277-296.

Grigorieva, M.A., Velichko, O.A., Shabaldin, S.V., Fisinin, V.I. and Surai, P.F., 2017. Vitagene regulation as a new strategy to fight stresses in poultry production. Agricultural Biology (Moscow) 52: 716-730.

Grollman, A.P. and Lehninger, A.L., 1957. Enzymic synthesis of L-ascorbic acid in different animal species. Archives of Biochemistry and Biophysics 69: 458-467.

Güçlü, B.K., Kara, K., Çakır, L., Çetin, E. and Kanbur, M., 2011. Carnitine supplementation modulates high dietary copper-induced oxidative toxicity and reduced performance in laying hens. Biological Trace Element Research 144: 725-735.

Gutowska, M.S. and Mitchell, C.A., 1945. Carbonic anhydrase in the calcification of the egg shell. Poultry Science 24: 159-167.

Haddadi, R., Nayebi, A.M. and Brooshghalan, S.E., 2018. Silymarin prevents apoptosis through inhibiting the Bax/caspase-3 expression and suppresses toll like receptor-4 pathway in the SNc of 6-OHDA intoxicated rats. Biomedicine & Pharmacotherapy 104: 127-136.

Hamidi, H., Pourreza, J. and Rahimi, H., 2009. Dietary betaine affect duodenal histology of broilers challenged with a mixed coccidial infection. Pakistan Journal of Biological Sciences 12: 291-295.

Heidari, R., Niknahad, H., Sadeghi, A., Mohammadi, H., Ghanbarinejad, V., Ommati, M.M., Hosseini, A., Azarpira, N., Khodaei, F., Farshad, O. and Rashidi, E., 2018. Betaine treatment protects liver through regulating mitochondrial function and counteracting oxidative stress in acute and chronic animal models of hepatic injury. Biomedicine & Pharmacotherapy 103: 75-86.

Hill, C.H., 1979. Studies on the ameliorating effect of ascorbic acid on mineral toxicities in the chick. The Journal of Nutrition 109: 84-90.

Holm, L., Blomqvist, A., Brandt, I., Brunström, B., Ridderstråle, Y. and Berg, C., 2006. Embryonic exposure to o, p′-DDT causes eggshell thinning and altered shell gland carbonic anhydrase expression in the domestic hen. Environmental Toxicology and Chemistry 25: 2787-2793.

Hove, E., Elvehjem, C.A. and Hart, E.B., 1940. The relation of zinc to carbonic anhydrase. Journal of Biological Chemistry 136: 425-434.

Ivy, C.A. and Nesheim, M.C., 1973. Factors influencing the liver fat content of laying hens. Poultry Science 52: 281-291.

Jabbar, A., Hameed, A., Yousaf, A., Riaz, A. and Ditta, Y.A., 2019. The influence of hairline crack eggs on hatchery parameters and performance of chicks. World Veterinary Journal 9: 76-83.

Jahanian, E., Mahdavi, A.H., Asgary, S. and Jahanian, R., 2017. Effects of dietary inclusion of silymarin on performance, intestinal morphology and ileal bacterial count in aflatoxin-challenged broiler chicks. Journal of Animal Physiology and Animal Nutrition 101: e43-e54.

Kaetzel Jr, D.M. and Soares Jr, J.H., 1979. Effects of cholecalciferol steroids on bone and egg shell calcification in Japanese quail. The Journal of Nutrition 109: 1601-1608.

Kalorey, D.R., Kurkure, N.V., Ramgaonkar, J.S., Sakhare, P.S., Warke, S. and Nigot, N.K., 2005. Effect of polyherbal feed supplement. Asian-Australasian Journal of Animal Sciences 18: 375-383.

Kazemi-Fard, M., Yousefi, S., Dirandeh, E. and Rezaei, M., 2015. Effect of different levels of L-carnitine on the productive performance, egg quality, blood parameters and egg yolk cholesterol in laying hens. Poultry Science Journal 3: 105-111.

Khatoon, A., Zargham Khan, M., Khan, A., Saleemi, M.K. and Javed, I., 2013. Amelioration of ochratoxin A-induced immunotoxic effects by silymarin and vitamin E in white Leghorn cockerels. Journal of Immunotoxicology 10: 25-31.

Kidd, M.T., 2004. Nutritional modulation of immune function in broilers. Poultry Science 83: 650-657.

Kidd, M.T., Ferket, P.R. and Garlich, J.D., 1997. Nutritional and osmoregulatory functions of betaine. World's Poultry Science Journal 53: 125-139.

Kidd, M.T., McDaniel, C.D., Peebles, E.D., Barber, S.J., Corzo, A., Branton, S.L. and Woodworth, J.C., 2005. Breeder hen dietary L-carnitine affects progeny carcase traits. British Poultry Science 46: 97-103.

Latipova, E.N., 2014a. Efficacy of usage of antistress preparations 'Vitaminocid' and 'Magic Antistress Mix' in poultry farming. PhD Thesis. Orenburg, Russia.

Latipova, E.N., 2014b. Reproductive parameters of layer breeders and progeny quality as a result of antistress preparation usage. Agrarniy Vestnik Urala (Agricultural Ural Journal) 120: 24-31.

Latipova, E.N. and Shatskikh, E.V., 2014a. Reproductive performance of egg breeders as a result of usage of 'Vitaminocid' and 'Magic Antistress Mix'. Glavniy Zootechnik (Chief Zootechnician, Moscow) 4: 34-40.

Latipova, E.N. and Shatskikh, E.V., 2014b. Reproductive parameters of layer breeders and progeny quality as affected by antistress preparation usage. Agrarniy Vestnik Urala (Agricultural Ural Journal) 120: 24-31.

Latipova, E.N. and Shatskikh, E.V., 2014c. Development of breeding birds and incubation egg quality as a result of usage antistress preparations. Bio 164: 4-8.

Latipova, E.N. and Shatskikh, E.V., 2014d. 'Vitaminocid' and 'Magic Antistress Mix' in the diet of the egg breeders. Agrarniy Vestnik Urala (Agricultural Ural Journal) 119: 36-40.

Latipova, E.N., Shatskikh, E.V. and Surai, P.F., 2016. Effect of an antistress dietary supplement on the reproductive performance of layer breeders. The Proceedings of the XXV Worlds Poultry Congress. 2016. Abstracts, S1-0137.

Latipova, E.N., Shatskikh, E.V., Nesvet, E.G., Surai, P.F. and Zelenskaya, O.V. (2014). Usage of antistress preparations 'Vitamonocid' and 'Magic Antistres Mix' in poultry farming: research and practical advice. Ural Agricultural University, Ekaterinburg, Russia.

Leach Jr, R.M. and Gross, J.R., 1983. The effect of manganese deficiency upon the ultrastructure of the eggshell. Poultry Science 62: 499-504.

Lee, I., 2015. Betaine is a positive regulator of mitochondrial respiration. Biochemical and Biophysical Research Communications 456: 621-625.

Leibetseder, J., 1995. Effects of L-carnitine in poultry. Archiv fur Tierernahrung 48: 97-108.

Li, C., Wang, Y., Li, L., Han, Z., Mao, S. and Wang, G., 2019a. Betaine protects against heat exposure-induced oxidative stress and apoptosis in bovine mammary epithelial cells via regulation of ROS production. Cell Stress and Chaperones 24: 453-460.

Li, H., Li, W. and Wang, Q., 2019b. 1, 25-dihydroxyvitamin D 3 suppresses lipopolysaccharide-induced interleukin-6 production through aryl hydrocarbon receptor/nuclear factor-κB signaling in oral epithelial cells. BMC Oral Health 19: 236.

Liew, W.P.P. and Mohd-Redzwan, S., 2018. Mycotoxin: its impact on gut health and microbiota. Frontiers in Cellular and Infection Microbiology 8: 60.

Lin, Z. and Li, W., 2016. The roles of vitamin D and its analogs in inflammatory diseases. Current Topics in Medicinal Chemistry 16: 1242-1261.

Lippolis, J.D., Reinhardt, T.A., Sacco, R.A., Nonnecke, B.J. and Nelson, C.D., 2011. Treatment of an intramammary bacterial infection with 25-hydroxyvitamin D(3). PloS One 6: e25479.

Liu, W., Yuan, Y., Sun, C., Balasubramanian, B., Zhao, Z. and An, L., 2019. Effects of dietary betaine on growth performance, digestive function, carcass traits, and meat quality in indigenous yellow-feathered broilers under long-term heat stress. Animals 9: 506.

Liu, Z., Shen, H. and Zhang, J., 2009. Clinical effect of silymarin combined with levocarnitine on non-alcoholic fatty liver disease. China Modern Medicine 7: R575.

Lovelace, E.S., Wagoner, J., MacDonald, J., Bammler, T., Bruckner, J., Brownell, J., Beyer, R.P., Zink, E.M., Kim, Y.M., Kyle, J.E. and Webb-Robertson, B.J.M., 2015. Silymarin suppresses cellular inflammation by inducing reparative stress signaling. Journal of Natural Products 78: 1990-2000.

Lundholm, C.E., 1990. The eggshell thinning action of acetazolamide; relation to the binding of Ca2+ and carbonic anhydrase activity of the shell gland homogenate. Comparative Biochemistry and Physiology. C. Comparative Pharmacology 95: 85-89.

Mabe, I., Rapp, C., Bain, M.M. and Nys, Y., 2003. Supplementation of a corn-soybean meal diet with manganese, copper, and zinc from organic or inorganic sources improves eggshell quality in aged laying hens. Poultry Science 82: 1903-1913.

Malayeri, M.R.M., Tehrani, A.D. and Rezaei, A., 2014. Preventive effects of silymarin extract on carbon tetrachloride-induced hepatotoxicity in broilers. Journal of Veterinary Clinical Pathology 8: 445-459.

Martínez, Y., Li, X., Liu, G., Bin, P., Yan, W., Más, D., Valdivié, M., Hu, C.A.A., Ren, W. and Yin, Y., 2017. The role of methionine on metabolism, oxidative stress, and diseases. Amino Acids 49: 2091-2098.

Mastrototaro, L., Sponder, G., Saremi, B. and Aschenbach, J.R., 2016. Gastrointestinal methionine shuttle: Priority handling of precious goods. IUBMB life 68: 924-934.

McKee, J.S. and Harrison, P.C., 1995. Effects of supplemental ascorbic acid on the performance of broiler chickens exposed to multiple concurrent stressors. Poultry Science 74: 1772-1785.

Merriman, K.E., Poindexter, M.B., Kweh, M.F., Santos, J.E. and Nelson, C.D., 2017. Intramammary 1, 25-dihydroxyvitamin D3 treatment increases expression of host-defense genes in mammary immune cells of lactating dairy cattle. The Journal of Steroid Biochemistry and Molecular Biology 173: 33-41.

Merriman, K.E., Powell, J.L., Santos, J.E. and Nelson, C.D., 2018. Intramammary 25-hydroxyvitamin D3 treatment modulates innate immune responses to endotoxin-induced mastitis. Journal of Dairy Science 101: 7593-7607.

Mertens, K., Bamelis, F., Kemps, B., Kamers, B., Verhoelst, E., De Ketelaere, B., Bain, M., Decuypere, E. and De Baerdemaeker, J., 2006. Monitoring of eggshell breakage and eggshell strength in different production chains of consumption eggs. Poultry Science 85: 1670-1677.

Metzler-Zebeli, B.U., Eklund, M. and Mosenthin, R., 2009. Impact of osmoregulatory and methyl donor functions of betaine on intestinal health and performance in poultry. World's Poultry Science Journal 65: 419-442.

Monteiro, C.P., Matias, C.N., Bicho, M., Santa-Clara, H. and Laires, M.J., 2016. Coordination between antioxidant defences might be partially modulated by magnesium status. Magnesium Research 29: 161-168.

Morris, K.M.L., 1977. The effect on eggshell thickness of the inclusion of the calcinogenic plant Solanum malacoxylon in the diet of laying hens. The Veterinary Record 101: 502-504.

Mousa, M.A. and Osman, A.S., 2016. The implication of L-carnitine and silymarin supplementation on growth performance and some blood parameters of broilers. Assiut Veterinary Medical Journal 62: 132-138.

Muhammad, D., Chand, N., Khan, S., Sultan, A. and Mushtaq, M., 2012. Hepatoprotective role of milk thistle (*Silybum marianum*) in meat type chicken fed aflatoxin B1 contaminated feed. Pakistan Veterinary Journal 32: 443-446.

Mushtaq, M.M.H., Pasha, T.N., Mushtaq, T. and Parvin, R., 2013. Electrolytes, dietary electrolyte balance and salts in broilers: an updated review on growth performance, water intake and litter quality. World's Poultry Science Journal 69: 789-802.

Nagashimada, M. and Ota, T., 2019. Role of vitamin E in nonalcoholic fatty liver disease. IUBMB life 71: 516-522.

Nasri, H., van den Brand, H., Najjar, T. and Bouzouaia, M., 2020. Egg storage and breeder age impact on egg quality and embryo development. Journal of Animal Physiology and Animal Nutrition 104: 257-268.

Nys, Y., 2001. Recent developments in layer nutrition for optimising shell quality. In: Proceedings of the 13th European symposium on poultry nutrition. Blankenberge, Belgium, pp. 42-52.

Nys, Y., Gautron, J., Garcia-Ruiz, J.M. and Hincke, M.T., 2004. Avian eggshell mineralization: biochemical and functional characterization of matrix proteins. Comptes Rendus Palevol 3: 549-562.

Nys, Y., Hincke, M.T., Arias, J.L., Garcia-Ruiz, J.M. and Solomon, S.E., 1999. Avian eggshell mineralization. Poultry and Avian Biology Reviews 10: 143-166.

Nys, Y. and Le Roy, N., 2018. Calcium homeostasis and eggshell biomineralization in female chicken. In: Feldman, D. (ed.) Vitamin D, 4 Ed., Academic press, Cambridge, UK, pp. 361-382.

Olanrewaju, H.A., Thaxton, J.P., Dozier III, W.A. and Branton, S.L., 2007. Electrolyte diets, stress, and acid-base balance in broiler chickens. Poultry Science 86: 1363-1371.

Orban, J.I., Roland, D.A., Cummins, K. and Lovell, R.T., 1993. Influence of large doses of ascorbic acid on performance, plasma calcium, bone characteristics, and egg shell quality in broilers and laying hens. Poultry Science 72: 691-700.

Ore, A. and Akinloye, O.A., 2019. Oxidative stress and antioxidant biomarkers in clinical and experimental models of non-alcoholic fatty liver disease. Medicina 55: 26.

Pardue, S.L. and Thaxton, J.P., 1986. Ascorbic acid in poultry: a review. World's Poultry Science Journal 42: 107-123.

Pappas, A.C., Godiewska, K. and Surai, P.F., 2018. Dietary food and feed supplements with trace elements. In: Chojnacka, K. and Saeid, A. (eds) Recent advances in trace elements. John Willey & Sons Ltd., Hoboken, USA, pp. 421-441.

Peebles, E.D. and Brake, J., 1985. Relationship of dietary ascorbic acid to broiler breeder performance. Poultry Science 64: 2041-2048.

Perek, M. and Kendler, J., 1963. Ascorbic acid as a dietary supplement for White Leghorn hens under conditions of climatic stress. British Poultry Science 4: 191-200.

Radwan, L.M., 2016. Eggshell quality: a comparison between Fayoumi, Gimieizah and Brown Hy-Line strains for mechanical properties and ultrastructure of their eggshells. Animal Production Science 56: 908-912.

Radwan, L.M., Fathi, M.M., Galal, A. and El-Dein, A.Z., 2010. Mechanical and ultrastructural properties of eggshell in two Egyptian native breeds of chicken. International Journal of Poultry Science 9: 77-81.

Ratriyanto, A. and Mosenthin, R., 2018. Osmoregulatory function of betaine in alleviating heat stress in poultry. Journal of Animal Physiology and Animal Nutrition 102: 1634-1650.

Rennie, J.S. and Whitehead, C.C., 1996. Effectiveness of dietary 25-and 1-hydroxycholecalciferol in combating tibial dyschondroplasia in broiler chickens. British Poultry Science 37: 413-421.

Rennie, J.S., McCormack, H.A., Farquharson, C., Berry, J.L., Mawer, E.B. and Whitehead, C.C., 1995. Interaction between dietary 1, 25-dihydroxycholecalciferol and calcium and effects of management on the occurrence of tibial dyschondroplasia, leg abnormalities and performance in broiler chickens. British Poultry Science 36: 465-477.

Rennie, J.S., Whitehead, C.C. and Thorp, B.H., 1993. The effect of dietary 1, 25-dihydroxycholecalciferol in preventing tibial dyschondroplasia in broilers fed on diets imbalanced in calcium and phosphorus. British Journal of Nutrition 69: 809-816.

Ridell, C., 1991. Developmental, metabolic, and miscellaneous disorders. In: Calnek, B.W., Barnes, H.J., Beard, C.W., Reid, W.M. and Yofer, H.W. (eds) Diseases of poultry. Iowa State University Press, Ames, USA, pp. 827-862.

Ringseis, R., Keller, J. and Eder, K., 2018. Basic mechanisms of the regulation of L-carnitine status in monogastrics and efficacy of L-carnitine as a feed additive in pigs and poultry. Journal of Animal Physiology and Animal Nutrition 102: 1686-1719.

Roth, S.D., Schüttrumpf, J., Milanov, P., Abriss, D., Ungerer, C., Quade-Lyssy, P., Simpson, J.C., Pepperkok, R., Seifried, E. and Tonn, T., 2012. Chemical chaperones improve protein secretion and rescue mutant factor VIII in mice with hemophilia A. PloS One 7: e44505.

Roy, R. and Guha, B., 1958. Species differences in regard to the biosynthesis of ascorbic acid. Nature 182: 319-320.

Sá e Silva, M., Susta, L., Moresco, K. and Swayne, D.E., 2016. Vaccination of chickens decreased Newcastle disease virus contamination in eggs. Avian Pathology 45: 38-45.

Saeed, M., Babazadeh, D., Arif, M., Arain, M.A., Bhutto, Z.A., Shar, A.H., Kakar, M.U., Manzoor, R. and Chao, S., 2017a. Silymarin: a potent hepatoprotective agent in poultry industry. World's Poultry Science Journal 73: 483-492.

Saeed, M., Babazadeh, D., Naveed, M., Arain, M.A., Hassan, F.U. and Chao, S., 2017b. Reconsidering betaine as a natural anti-heat stress agent in poultry industry: a review. Tropical Animal Health and Production 49: 1329-1338.

Schaefer, A.L., Jones, S.D.M. and Stanley, R.W., 1997. The use of electrolyte solutions for reducing transport stress. Journal of Animal Science 75: 258-265.

Scott, M.L., 1975. Environmental influences on ascorbic acid requirements in animals. Annals of the New York Academy of Sciences 258: 151-168.

Shatskikh, E.V. and Latipova, E.N., 2013. Effect of antistress preparations on the growth and development of egg type breeder birds. Agrarniy Vestnik Urala (Agricultural Ural Journal) 117: 33-37.

Shatskikh, E.V. and Latipova, E.N., 2014a. Development of internal organs in egg type rearing birds as a result of usage of antistress additives. Agrarniy Vestnik Urala (Agricultural Ural Journal) 122: 35-42.

Shatskikh, E.V. and Latipova, E.N., 2014b. Effect of antistress preparations on the development of rearing birds. Ptitsevodstvo (Moscow) 1: 22-27.

Shatskikh, E.V., Surai, P.F. and Latipova, E.N., 2015a. Morphological characteristics of blood of egg type birds as a result of usage of antistress additives. Agrarniy Vestnik Urala (Agricultural Ural Journal) 131: 44-48.

Shatskikh, E., Latypova, E., Fisinin, V., Denev, S. and Surai, P., 2015b. Molecular mechanisms and new strategies to fight stresses in egg-producing birds. Agricultural Science and Technology 7: 3-10.

Shatskikh, E.V., Latipova, E.N. and Surai, P.F., 2016a. Supplying an antistress composition with water to decrease negative consequences of commercially-relevant stresses in rearing birds. The Proceedings of the XXV Worlds Poultry Congress. 2016. Abstracts, S1-0140.

Shatskikh, E.V., Latipova, E.N., Fisinin, V.I. and Surai, P.F., 2016b. Epigenetic effects of an antioxidant composition in layer breeder diet. The Proceedings of the XXV Worlds Poultry Congress. 2016. Abstracts, S1-0142.

Shatskikh, E.V., Latipova, E.N., Nesvet, E.G. and Koburneev, I.V., 2016c. Usage of anti-stress preparations in poultry production. Ural State University. Russia, Ekaterinburg, Russia.

Snapir, N. and Perek, M., 1970. Distribution of calcium, carbonic anhydrase and alkaline phosphatase activities in the uterus and isthmus of young and old white leghorn hens. Poultry Science 49: 1526-1531.

Soares, J.H. Jr., McLonghlin, C.M., Swerdel, M.R. and Bossard, E., 1976. Effect of hydroxy vitamin D metabolites on the mineralization of eggshell and bones, in: Proceedings of the Maryland nutrition conference, College Park, MD, USA, pp. 85-92.

Soares, J.H., Jr., 1984. Calcium metabolism and its control – a review. Poultry Science 63: 2075-2083.

Spurlock, M.E. and Savage, J.E., 1992. Research note: Antioxidant activity of Japanese quail liver cytosol in the absence and presence of reduced glutathione. Poultry Science 71: 928-931.

Squires, E.J. and Leeson, S., 1988. Aetiology of fatty liver syndrome in laying hens. British Veterinary Journal 144: 602-609.

Stefanello, C., Santos, T., Murakami, A., Martins, E., and Carneiro, T. 2014. Productive performance, eggshell quality, and eggshell ultrastructure of laying hens fed diets supplemented with organic trace minerals. Poultry Science 93:104-113.

Stevens, V.I., Blair, R. and Salmon, R.E., 1984. Influence of maternal vitamin D3 carry-over on kidney 25-hydroxyvitamin D3-l-hydroxylase activity of poults. Poultry Science 63: 765-774.

Surai, P.F., 1999. Vitamin E in avian reproduction. Poultry Avian Biology Reviews 10: 1-60.

Surai, P.F., 2002. Natural antioxidants in avian nutrition and reproduction. Nottingham University Press, Nottingham, UK.

Surai, P.F., 2005. Minerals and antioxidants. In: Tucker, L.A. and Taylor-Pickard, J.A. (eds) Redefining mineral nutrition. Nottingham University Press, Nottingham, UK, pp. 147-177.

Surai, P.F., 2006. Selenium in nutrition and health. Nottingham University Press, Nottingham, UK.

Surai, P.F., 2011. Stresses in poultry production: from understanding mechanisms to the development of protection methods. Agrarnoye Resheniye (Russia) 4: 42-46.

Surai, P.F., 2012a. The antioxidant properties of canthaxanthin and its potential effects in the poultry eggs and on embryonic development of the chick. Part 1. World's Poultry Science Journal 68: 465-476.

Surai, P.F., 2012b. The antioxidant properties of canthaxanthin and its potential effects in the poultry eggs and on embryonic development of the chick. Part 2. World's Poultry Science Journal 68: 717-726.

Surai, P.F., 2012c. New approaches in fighting stresses decrease cannibalism in chickens. Korma I Facti (Feed and Facts, Kiev) 2: 7-8.

Surai, P.F., 2014. Polyphenol compounds in the chicken/animal diet: from the past to the future. Journal of Animal Physiology and Animal Nutrition 98: 19-31.

Surai, P.F., 2015a. Silymarin as a natural antioxidant: An overview of the current evidence and perspectives. Antioxidants 4, 204-247.

Surai, P.F., 2015b. Carnitine enigma: From antioxidant action to vitagene regulation. Part 1. Absorption, metabolism and antioxidant activities. Journal of Veterinary Science & Medicine 3, 2: 14.

Surai, P.F., 2015c. Carnitine enigma: From antioxidant action to vitagene regulation. Part 2. Transcription factors and practical applications. Journal of Veterinary Science & Medicine 3, 2: 17.

Surai, P.F., 2015d. Antioxidant action of carnitine: Molecular mechanisms and practical applications. EC Veterinary Science 2.1: 66-84.

Surai, P.F., 2015e. Stresses in poultry production: from understanding mechanisms of development to the development of protection. Zhivotnovodstvo Rossii (Russian Animal Production, Moscow;), Special issue: 30-31.

Surai, P.F., 2016. Antioxidant systems in poultry biology: Superoxide dismutase. Journal of Animal Nutrition 1: 8.

Surai, P.F., 2017. What happens with pig under the heat stress and how to protect them from the stress. Korma I Facti (Feed and Facts, Kiev) 6-7: 35-37.

Surai, P.F., 2018a. Selenium in poultry nutrition and health. Wageningen Academic Publishers, Wageningen, The Netherlands.

Surai, P.F., 2018b. Egg shell and carcass quality in birds at the second part of production period. Vitamin D role. Ptakhivnitstvo.ua (Ukrainian Poultry Science, Kiev) 9: 6-11.

Surai, P.F., 2018c. Egg shell and carcass quality in birds at the second part of production period. Vitamin D role. Part 2. Ptakhivnitstvo.ua (Ukrainian Poultry Science, Kiev) 10: 16-17.

Surai, P.F., 2018d. Taurine and carnitine in poultry production: from vitagene activation to chicken health maintenance. Ptakhivnitstvo.ua (Ukrainian Poultry Science, Kiev) 1-2: 12-17.

Surai, P.F., 2018e. Egg shell and carcass quality in birds at the second part of production period. Organic matrix role. Ptakhivnitstvo.ua (Ukrainian Poultry Science, Kiev) 11: 6-9.

Surai, P.F., 2019a. Vitagenes in poultry production: stresses and antioxidants. Suchasne Ptakhivnitstvo (Modern Poultry Science, Ukraine) 9-10: 24-27.

Surai, P.F., 2019b. Vitagenes in poultry production: adaptation to commercially relevant stresses. Suchasne Ptakhivnitstvo (Modern Poultry Science, Ukraine) 7-8: 28-32.

Surai, P.F., 2019c. From healthy liver to general health and high productivity of poultry. Ptaknivnitstvo.ua 1-2: 4-7.

Surai, P.F., 2019d. Decreasing eggshell hairline cracks: from vitagenes to a ShellBone concept ShellBone. Ptaknivnitstvo.ua 5: 24-27.

Surai, P.F., 2020a. Vitagene in avian biology and poultry health. Wageningen Academic Publishers, Wageningen, The Netherlands.

Surai, P.F., 2020b. Superoxide dismutase as a new entrant into the vitagene family in animals/poultry. EC Nutrition 15.3: 01-03.

Surai, P.F., 2020c. Antioxidants in poultry nutrition and reproduction: An update. Antioxidants 9, 2: 105.

Surai, P.F. (Ed.), 2021. Selenium in pig nutrition and health. Wageningen Academic Publishers, Wageningen, The Netherlands.

Surai, P.F., 2022. Silymarin as a vitagene modulator: effects on mitochondria integrity in stress conditions. In: Ostojik, S.M. (ed) Molecular nutrition and mitochondria. Elsevier, Academic Press, London, UK, pp. 535-559.

Surai, P.F. and Boroday, V.P., 2010. Stresses in poultry production: from understanding of mechanisms of development to the development of methods of protection. Suchasne Ptakhivnitstvo (Modern Poultry Science, Ukraine) 7-8: 31- 36.

Surai, P.F. and Dvorska, J.E., 2005. Effects of mycotoxins on antioxidant status and immunity. In: Diaz, D. (ed) The mycotoxins blue book. Nottingham University Press, Nottingham, UK, pp. 93-137.

Surai, P.F. and Earle-Payne, K., 2022. Antioxidant defences and redox homeostasis in animals. Antioxidants 11: 1012.

Surai, P.F., Earle-Payne, K. and Kidd, M.T., 2021b. Taurine as a natural antioxidant: From direct antioxidant effects to protective action in various toxicological models. Antioxidants 10: 1876.

Surai, P.F. and Fisinin, V.I., 2012a. The modern antistress technologies in poultry: From antioxidants to vitagenes. Agricultural Biology (Moscow) 4: 3-13.

Surai, P.F. and Fisinin, V.I., 2012b. Modern methods for fighting stresses in poultry production: from antioxidants to sirtuins and vita-genes. Effectivne Ptakhivnitstvo (Effective Poultry Production, Ukraine) 8: 8-13.

Surai, P.F. and Fisinin, V.I., 2013. Natural antioxidants in hen's embryogenesis and antioxidant defence in postnatal development. Agricultural Biology (Moscow) 2: 3-17.

Surai, P.F. and Fisinin, V.I., 2014. Antioxidant systems of the body: From vitamin E to polyphenols and beyond. Proceedings of the 35th western nutrition conference. September 24-25, 2014, Edmonton, Alberta, pp. 265-277.

Surai, P.F. and Fisinin, V.I., 2015. Antioxidant-prooxidant balance in the intestine: Applications in chick placement and pig Weaning. Journal of Veterinary Science & Medicine 3: 16.

Surai, P.F. and Fisinin, V.I., 2016a. Vitagenes in poultry production. Part 1. Technological and environmental stresses. World's Poultry Science Journal 72: 721-733.

Surai, P.F. and Fisinin, V.I., 2016b. Vitagenes in poultry production. Part 2. Nutritional and internal stresses. World's Poultry Science Journal 72: 761-772.

Surai, P.F. and Fisinin, V.I., 2016c. Vitagenes in poultry production. Part 3. Vitagene concept development. World's Poultry Science Journal 72: 793- 804.

Surai, P.F. and Fisinin, V.I., 2016d. Natural antioxidants and stresses in poultry production: from vitamins to vitagenes. Proc. XXV world poultry congress, invited lecture papers, Beijing, China, 5-9 September, 2016, pp. 116-121.

Surai, P.F. and Fisinin, V.I., 2016e. Antioxidant system regulation: from vitamins to vitagenes. In: Watson, R.R and De Meester, F. (eds) Handbook of cholesterol. Wageningen Academic Publishers, Wageningen, the Netherlands, pp. 451-481.

Surai, P.F., Fisinin, V.I., Shatskikh, E.V and Latipova, E.N., 2017b. Modern methods of fighting stresses in poultry and pig production: Vitagene concept in action. Sfera 2: 40-43.

Surai, P.F. and Fotina, T.I., 2010a. Once more about stresses. From changes in gene expression to usage with drinking water of antistress premix. Effectivne Ptakhivnitstvo (Effective Poultry Production, Ukraine) 8: 20-25.

Surai, P.F. and Fotina, T.I., 2010b. Eggshell quality in egg production. What is new in modern science? Korma I Facti (Feed and Facts, Ukraine) 4: 6-10.

Surai, P.F. and Fotina, T.I., 2011a. New approaches in fighting stresses in poultry production. From vitamins to vitagenes and sirtuins. Agrarnoye Resheniye (Russia) 9-10: 34-39.

Surai, P.F. and Fotina, T.I., 2011b. Eggshell quality in egg production: introduction of innovative technologies into industry. Ptakhivnitstvo.ua (Modern Poultry Production, Ukraine) 1: 8-12.

Surai, P.F. and Fotina, T.I., 2012a. Vitagenes – next step after nutrigenomics: Lessons for poultry production. Ptakhivnitstvo (Kiev) 68: 429-435.

Surai, P.F. and Fotina, T.I., 2012b. Stresses in poultry production. Molecular mechanisms. Propozhizia (Ukraine) 9: 130-132.

Surai, P.F. and Fotina, T.I., 2012c. Stresses in poultry production. Methods of prevention. Propozhizia, Ukraine 10: 132-134.

Surai, P.F. and Fotina, T.I., 2012d. In order to prevent stresses. Nashe Ptakhivnitstvo (Our Poultry Production, Ukraine) 3: 72-74.

Surai, P.F. and Fotina, T.I., 2012e. Molecular mechanisms of immunosuppression: is there light at the end of the tunnel? Part 1. Suchasna Veterinarna Madicina (Modern Veterinary Medicine, Ukraine) 6: 22-25.

Surai, P.F. and Fotina, T.I., 2013a. Physiological mechanism and practical measures to decrease negative consequences of heat stress in pig production. Svinarstvo Ukraini (Pig Production of Ukraine, Kiev) 6: 12-15.

Surai, P.F. and Fotina, T.I., 2013b. Molecular mechanisms of immunosuppression. Is there light at the end of the tunnel? Part 2. Suchasna Veterinarna Medicina (Modern Veterinary Medicine, Ukraine) 1: 26-27.

Surai, P.F. and Fotina, T.I., 2013c. Physiological mechanisms of the development of heat stress in poultry production. Tvarinnitstvo Syogodni (Today's Animal Production, Ukraine) 6: 54-60.

Surai, P.F., Fotina, A.A and Fotina, T.I., 2012. Effect of Feed-Food Magic Antistress Mix on natural resistance of ducklings. Proceedings of Sumy National Agrarian University 7: 58-61.

Surai, P.F. and Kochish, I.I., 2017. Antioxidant systems and vitagenes in poultry biology: Heat shock proteins. In: Asea, A.A.A. and Kaur, P. (eds) Heat shock proteins in veterinary. Springer, Cham, Switzerland, pp. 123-177.

Surai, P.F. and Kochish, I.I., 2018. Oxidative damage of biological molecules on animal metabolism and physiology. Proc. of the 2018 animal nutritional conference of Canada. 2-3 May, 2018, Edmonton, Canada, pp. 234-251.

Surai, P.F. and Kochish, I.I., 2019. Nutritional modulation of the antioxidant capacities in poultry: the case of selenium. Poultry Science 98: 4231-4239.

Surai, P.F. and Kochish, I.I., 2020. Carotenoids in aviculture. In: Jacob-Lopes, E., Queiroz, M.I. and Zepka, L.Q. (eds) Pigments from microalgae handbook. Springer Nature Switzerland, Cham, Switzerland, pp. 515-540.

Surai, P.F., Kochish, I.I., and Fisinin, V.I., 2017a. Antioxidant systems in poultry biology: Nutritional modulation of vitagenes. European Journal of Poultry Science 81: 1612-9199.

Surai, P.F., Kochish, I.I., Fisinin, V.I., Grozina, A.A. and Shatskikh E.V., 2018. Molecular mechanisms of chicken gut health maintenance: role of microbiota. Agricultural Technologies, Moscow, Russia.

Surai, P.F., Kochish, I.I., Fisinin, V.I., and Kidd, M.T., 2019b. Antioxidant defence systems and oxidative stress in poultry biology: An update. Antioxidants 8, 7: 235.

Surai, P.F., Kochish, I.I., and Kidd, M.T., 2020a. Taurine in poultry nutrition. Animal Feed Science and Technology 260: 114339.

Surai, P.F., Kochish, I.I., and Kidd, M.D., 2020b. Natural antioxidants in redox balance maintenance and animal health protection. In: Kidd, M.D. (ed) Branched-chain amino acids: Metabolism, benefits and role in disease. Nova Science Publishers, New York, USA, pp. 31-76.

Surai, P.F., Kochish, I.I., and Kidd, M.T., 2021a. Redox homeostasis in poultry: Regulatory roles of NF-κB. Antioxidants 10: 186.

Surai, P.F., Kochish, I.I., and Fisinin, V.I., 2021c. Vitagenes in avian biology: protective functions of sirtuins. In: Maise, K. (ed) Sirtuin biology in medicine. Academic Press, UK, USA, pp. 353-372.

Surai, P.F., Kochish, I.I., Romanov, M.N. and Griffin, D.K., 2019a. Nutritional modulation of the antioxidant capacities in poultry: the case of vitamin E. Poultry Science, 98: 4030-4041.

Surai, P.F. and Litvinov, A., 2017. From vitamins to vitagenes. Modern method to fight stresses in pig production. Svinovodstvo (Pig Produuction, Russia) 3: 56- 58.

Surai, P.F. and Melnichuk, S.D., 2012. Mechanisms of protection from stresses in pig production: from vitamins to vitagenes. Svinarstvo Ukraini (Pig Production of Ukraine, Kiev) 2: 10-15.

Surai, P.F., Mezes, M., Fotina, T.I. and Denev, S.D., 2010. Mycotoxins in human diet: a hidden danger. In: De Meester, F., Zibadi, S. and Watson R.R. (eds) Modern dietary fat intakes in disease promotion. Humana Press, New York, USA, pp. 275-303.

Surai, P.F., Speake, B.K. and Sparks, N.H.C., 2001a. Carotenoids in avian nutrition and embryonic development. 1. Absorption, availability and levels in plasma and egg yolk. The Journal of Poultry Science 38: 1-27.

Surai, P.F., Speake, B.K. and Sparks, N.H.C., 2001b. Carotenoids in avian nutrition and embryonic development. 2. Antioxidant properties and discrimination in embryonic tissues. The Journal of Poultry Science 38: 38: 117-145.

Swiatkiewicz, S. and Koreleski, J., 2008. The effect of zinc and manganese source in the diet for laying hens on eggshell and bones quality. Veterinarni Medicina 53: 555-563.

Świątkiewicz, S., Arczewska-Włosek, A., Krawczyk, J., Puchała, M. and Jozefiak, D., 2015. Dietary factors improving eggshell quality: an updated review with special emphasis on microelements and feed additives. World's Poultry Science Journal 71: 83-94.

Taylor, D., Walsh, M., Cullen, A. and O'Reilly, P., 2016. The fracture toughness of eggshell. Acta Biomaterialia 37: 21-27.

Tedesco, D., Steidler, S., Galletti, S., Tameni, M., Sonzogni, O. and Ravarotto, L., 2004. Efficacy of silymarin-phospholipid complex in reducing the toxicity of aflatoxin B1 in broiler chicks. Poultry Science 83: 1839-1843.

Thornton, P.A. and Moreng, R.E., 1958. The effect of ascorbic acid on egg quality factors. Poultry Science 37: 691-698.

Toussant, M.J. and Latshaw, J.D., 1994. Evidence of multiple metabolic routes in vanadium's effects on layers. Ascorbic acid differential effects on prepeak egg production parameters following prolonged vanadium feeding. Poultry Science 73: 1572-1580.

Tsang, C.P., Grunder, A.A. and Narbaitz, R., 1990a. Optimal dietary level of 1 alpha,25-dihydroxycholecalciferol for eggshell quality in laying hens. Poultry Science 69: 1702-1712.

Tsang, C.P.W., Grunder, A.A., Soares, J.H. and Narbaitz, R., 1990b. Effect of 1α, 25-dihydroxycholecalciferol on egg shell quality and egg production. British Poultry Science 31: 241-247.

Tsang, C.P.W. and Grunder, A.A., 1993. Effect of dietary contents of cholecalciferol, 1α, 25-dihydroxycholecalciferol and 24, 25-dihydroxycholecalciferol on blood concentrations of 25-hydroxycholecalciferol, 1α, 25-dihydroxycholecalciferol, total calcium and eggshell quality. British Poultry Science 34: 1021-1027.

Van Mourik, S., Alders, B.P.G.J., Helderman, F., van de Ven, L.J.F. and Groot Koerkamp, P.W.G., 2017. Predicting hairline fractures in eggs of mature hens. Poultry Science 96: 1956-1962.

Velichko, O. and Surai, P.F., 2014. Effect of an antistress composition supplied with water on chick growth and development. Proceedings of the XIVth European Poultry Conference. Stavenger, Norway 23-27 June, 2014, p. 551.

Velichko, O.A., Shbaldin, S.V. and Surai, P.F., 2013. Practical aspects of usage of a vitagene concept in poultry production. Ptitsa I Ptitseproducti (Poultry and Poultry Products, Moscow) 4: 42-45.

Waldenstedt, L., 2006. Nutritional factors of importance for optimal leg health in broilers: A review. Animal Feed Science and Technology 126: 291-307.

Wang, Y.W., Ning, D., Peng, Y.Z. and Guo, Y.M., 2013. Effects of dietary L-carnitine supplementation on growth performance, organ weight, biochemical Parameters and Ascites Susceptibility in Broilers Reared Under Low-temperature Environment. Asian-Australasian Journal of Animal Sciences 26: 233-240.

Weiser, H., Schlachter, M. and Fenster, R., 1988a. The importance of vitamin C for the metabolism of vitamin D3 in poultry. In: Proceedings of the 18th World Poultry Congress, Nagoya, Japan. p. 831.

Weiser, H., Schlachter, M. and Bachmann, H., 1988b. The importance of vitamin C for hydroxylation of vitamin D3 to 1,25(OH)2D3 and of 24R,25(OH)2D3 to a more active metabolite. In: Noeman, A.W., Schaefer, K., Grigolet, H.G. and Herrath, D. (eds) Vitamin D: Molecular, cellular and clinical endocrinology. Walter de Gruyter, Berlin, Germany, pp. 644-653.

Weiser, H., Schlachter, M., Probst, H.P. and Korman, A.W., 1992. The relevance of ascorbic acid for bone metabolism. Proceedings of the 2nd symposium on ascorbic acid in domestic animals. Kratause Ittingen, Switzerland, pp. 73-95.

Wen, C., Chen, Y., Leng, Z., Ding, L., Wang, T. and Zhou, Y., 2019. Dietary betaine improves meat quality and oxidative status of broilers under heat stress. Journal of the Science of Food and Agriculture 99: 620-623.

Wen, G., Eder, K. and Ringseis, R., 2020. 1, 25-hydroxyvitamin D3 decreases endoplasmic reticulum stress-induced inflammatory response in mammary epithelial cells. Plos One 15: 0228945.

Whitehead, C.C., Mitchell, M.A. and Njoku, P.C., 1992. Effects of ascorbic acid on egg yolk and shell precursor in heat-stressed laying hens. Proceedings of the 2nd symposium on ascorbic acid in domestic animals. Kratause Ittingen, Switzerland, pp. 262-269.

Wistedt, A., Ridderstråle, Y., Wall, H. and Holm, L., 2014. Exogenous estradiol improves shell strength in laying hens at the end of the laying period. Acta Veterinaria Scandinavica 56: 34.

Wistedt, A., Ridderstråle, Y., Wall, H. and Holm, L., 2019. Age-related changes in the shell gland and duodenum in relation to shell quality and bone strength in commercial laying hen hybrids. Acta Veterinaria Scandinavica 61: 14.

Wolford, J.H. and Polin, D., 1972. Lipid accumulation and hemorrhage in livers of laying chickens. A study on fatty liver-hemorrhagic syndrome (FLHS). Poultry Science 51: 1707-1713.

Xiao, J.F., Wu, S.G., Zhang, H.J., Yue, H.Y., Wang, J., Ji, F. and Qi, G.H., 2015. Bioefficacy comparison of organic manganese with inorganic manganese for eggshell quality in Hy-Line Brown laying hens. Poultry Science 94: 1871-1878.

Xiao, J.F., Zhang, Y.N., Wu, S.G., Zhang, H.J., Yue, H.Y. and Qi, G.H., 2014. Manganese supplementation enhances the synthesis of glycosaminoglycan in eggshell membrane: a strategy to improve eggshell quality in laying hens. Poultry Science 93: 380-388.

Xing, J., Kang, L. and Jiang, Y., 2011. Effect of dietary betaine supplementation on lipogenesis gene expression and CpG methylation of lipoprotein lipase gene in broilers. Molecular Biology Reports 38: 1975-1981.

Xu, D., Xu, M., Jeong, S., Qian, Y., Wu, H., Xia, Q. and Kong, X., 2019. The role of Nrf2 in liver disease: Novel molecular mechanisms and therapeutic approaches. Frontiers in Pharmacology 9: 1428.

Zaefarian, F., Abdollahi, M.R., Cowieson, A. and Ravindran, V., 2019. Avian liver: the forgotten organ. Animals 9: 63.

Zamani, A., Rahmani, H.R. and Pourreza, J., 2005. Supplementation of a corn-soybean meal diet with manganese and zinc improves eggshell quality in laying hens. Pakistan Journal of Biological Sciences 8: 1311-1317.

Zapata, L.F. and Gernat, A.G., 1995. The effect of four levels of ascorbic acid and two levels of calcium on eggshell quality of forced-molted White Leghorn hens. Poultry Science 74: 1049-1052.

Zhan, X., 2001. Effects of betaine on immune responses of Newcastle disease in broiler chicks. Chinese Journal of Veterinary Science 21: 99-102.

Zhan, X.A., Li, J.X., Xu, Z.R. and Zhao, R.Q., 2006. Effects of methionine and betaine supplementation on growth performance, carcase composition and metabolism of lipids in male broilers. British Poultry Science 47: 576-580.

Zhang, Y.N., Zhang, H.J., Wu, S.G., Wang, J. and Qi, G.H., 2018. Dietary manganese supplementation affects mammillary knobs of eggshell ultrastructure in laying hens. Poultry Science 97: 1253-1262.

Zhang, Y.N., Wang, J., Zhang, H.J., Wu, S.G. and Qi, G.H., 2017a. Effect of dietary supplementation of organic or inorganic manganese on eggshell quality, ultrastructure, and components in laying hens. Poultry Science 96: 2184-2193.

Zhang, Y.N., Zhang, H.J., Wang, J., Yue, H.Y., Qi, X.L., Wu, S.G. and Qi, G.H., 2017b. Effect of dietary supplementation of organic or inorganic zinc on carbonic anhydrase activity in eggshell formation and quality of aged laying hens. Poultry Science 96: 2176-2183.

Zhong, S., Fan, Y., Yan, Q., Fan, X., Wu, B., Han, Y., Zhang, Y., Chen, Y., Zhang, H. and Niu, J., 2017. The therapeutic effect of silymarin in the treatment of nonalcoholic fatty disease: A meta-analysis (PRISMA) of randomized control trials. Medicine 96: e9061.

Chapter 19
Looking ahead: silymarin and health

All is well that ends well

Peter F. Surai[1-6] and Anton Surai[7]*
[1]Vitagene and Health Research Centre, Bristol, UK; [2]Department of Microbiology and Biochemistry, Faculty of Veterinary Medicine, Trakia University, Stara Zagora, Bulgaria; [3]Department of Animal Nutrition, Faculty of Agricultural and Environmental Sciences, Szent Istvan University, Hungary; [4]Saint-Petersburg State Academy of Veterinary Medicine, St. Petersburg, Russia; [5]Sumy National Agrarian University, Sumy, Ukraine; [6]Odessa National Academy of Food Technologies, Odessa, Ukraine; [7]Healthy Food Services, Bristol, UK
psurai@feedfood.co.uk

Abstract

This final chapter of the book gives an updated summary of the health-promoting effects of silymarin (SM). Major molecular mechanisms of protective action of SM were considered in previous chapters of the book. Additional mechanisms of SM action presented in this chapter include oestrogen receptor regulation, modulation of peroxisome proliferator-activated receptors (PPAR) and modulation of other transcription factors. The general conclusion from previous 18 chapters of the book is presented in this chapter. Accumulating scientific evidence indicates that SM is characterised by a wide range of protective pharmacological activities including: hepatoprotective, neuroprotective, anti-diabetic, cardio-protective, anti-inflammatory, immune-modulatory, anti-viral, anti-cancer and anti-toxic/chemo-preventive activities. SM can affect redox homeostasis regulation at different levels. This includes reduction of RONS production by stabilising mitochondria, main source of RONS production, and improving efficacy of phagocyte action, the second major source of RONS; affecting stress-response programs and making AO system alert and be ready for protective actions; modulating transcription factors, including Nrf2, a master-regulator of AO system and NF-κB, main driver of pro-inflammatory cytokine synthesis and inflammation; activating vitagenes and inducing synthesis of a range protective molecules participating in re-establishment of the redox homeostasis and stress adaptation. SM in cooperation with other natural antioxidants is involved in gut health and immunocompetence maintenance helping human and animals to adapt to stress and overcome it with minimal damages. It is just a matter of time before full potential of this enigmatic phytochemical mixture can be realised in human and veterinary medicine and nutrition.

Keywords: silymarin, oestrogen receptor, PPAR, redox homeostasis, vitagenes

DOI:10.3920/978-90-8686-944-2_019,

19.1 Introduction

Silymarin is being extensively studied for its:
- hepatoprotective (Chapter 12);
- neuroprotective (Chapter 13);
- anti-diabetic (Chapter 14);
- cardio-protective (Chapter 15);
- anti-inflammatory (Chapter 10);
- immune-modulatory (Chapter 9);
- anti-viral (Ferraz *et al.*, 2021; Liu *et al.*, 2019);
- anti-cancer (Fallah *et al.*, 2021; Koltai and Fliegel, 2022; Wadhwa *et al.*, 2022); and
- anti-toxic/chemo-preventive (Chapter 8) effects.

Molecular mechanisms of protective SM action include:
- antioxidant activities (Chapter 4);
- mitochondria preservation/stabilisation and decreased ROS production (Surai, 2022);
- vitagene modulation and improved stress adaptation (Chapter 7);
- Nrf2 activation and additional synthesis of a range of antioxidants and redox homeostasis maintenance (Chapter 5);
- NF-κB and pro-inflammatory cytokine down-regulation leading to anti-inflammatory action (Chapter 6);
- ER regulation (see below);
- modulation of PPAR (see below); and
- modulation of other transcription factors (see below).

In the following sections additional relevant information will be considered to explain protective properties of SM/SB against various disorders/diseases in human and veterinary medicine and prospects and limitation of its usage will be also addressed.

19.2 Silymarin and oestrogen receptor regulation

The oestrogen receptors (ERs) are members of the family of the steroid and nuclear receptor superfamily, which consists of 60 distant receptors, including five vertebrate steroid receptors groups such as androgen receptors, mineralocorticoid receptors, ERs, glucocorticoid receptors, and progesterone receptors. The major ERs include ERα (known as ESR1) and ERβ (known as ESR2; Khan *et al.*, 2022). Recently, novel G-protein-coupled oestrogen receptor 1 (GPER1) have also been identified as a prominent ER (Chen *et al.*, 2022). Some important characteristics of the ERs are shown in Table 19.1.

ERα was discovered in the 1960s, while ERβ was discovered only in 1996 and they consist of five domains (A/B, DNA-binding; D, ligand-binding; and F (Yu *et al.*, 2022) and are encoded by different genes (ESR1 and ESR2), located on nonhomologous human chromosomes: 6 and 14, respectively (Tang *et al.*, 2019). Interestingly, GPER1

Table 19.1. Major characteristics of ERα and ERβ (adapted from Chen *et al.*, 2022 and Khan *et al.*, 2022).

ER characteristics	ERα	ERβ
Category	Nuclear steroid hormone receptor superfamily	Nuclear steroid hormone receptor superfamily
Size	595 amino acids	530 amino acids
Numbers of isoforms	3	5
Major isoforms	ERα46, ERα36	ERβ2, ERβ3, ERβ4, ERβ5
Location	Nucleus	Nucleus
Distribution in tissues[1]	Hypothalamus, hippocampus, testes, ovary, endometrium, uterus, prostate, kidney, liver, breast, epididymis, muscle, adipose tissue	Testes, ovary, prostate, vascular endothelium, bladder, colon, adrenal gland, pancreas, muscle, adipose tissue
Type of expression	Constitutive	Constitutive
Subcellular localisation	Nucleus, cell membrane, cytoplasm	Nucleus, cytoplasm
Selective agonists	17-oestradiol, estriol, xenooestrogens, phytoestrogens	17-oestradiol, estrone, xenoestrogens, phytoestrogens

[1] GPER1 is shown to be widely distributed and expressed in the skeletal muscle, vascular endothelium, neurons and various immune cells including T cell, B cell, mononuclear, macrophage, and neutrophils (Chen *et al.*, 2022).

was identified using molecular cloning techniques in 2012 (Chen *et al.*, 2022; Filardo and Thomas, 2012). As can be seen from Table 19.1, ERα and ERβ, as well as GPER1, are expressed in various tissues and are involved in control of different critical physiological functions by activating target genes through signal transduction and transcription factors (Khan *et al.*, 2022). Ligand activation is associated with dissociation from the chaperone (Hsp90), dimerization of the monomer and translocation of cytosolic receptors to the nucleus. It is believed that ERs act as homologous dimers and/or heterodimers in transcription in association with various coregulators and combining them with oestrogen response elements (EREs; Figure 19.1).

It is reported that through combining with transcription factors, activated ERs can also indirectly bind to DNA. Furthermore, transcription can be regulated by post-translational modification in the absence of a ligand (Heger *et al.*, 2013; Ye *et al.*, 2018). Indeed, ERs regulate the expression of a great number of genes, both positively and negatively, depending on conditions (e.g. ligand, tissue, etc.). For example, in human osteosarcoma cells, of the approximately 100 E2-regulated (up-regulated or down-regulated more than 2-fold) genes were described, some were stimulated by E2 equally through ERα and ERβ, whereas others were selectively stimulated via ERα or ERβ.

Interestingly, 56% of all genes commonly regulated through ERα and ERβ were shown to encode proteins associated with cytokine/immune response (e.g. NK cell lectin-type receptors (NKG family), IL-8, COX2, CD34 antigen, defensin β1, IL-13 receptor 2, phospholipase A2, selenoprotein P1, and sialomucin/CD164), signal transduction, and cell motility and cytoskeleton regulation. Several ER-selective genes were shown to be associated with nucleic acid processing (Stossi *et al.*, 2004). ERα and ERβ, are known to be involved in regulating a variety of physiological processes (Yu *et al.*, 2022).

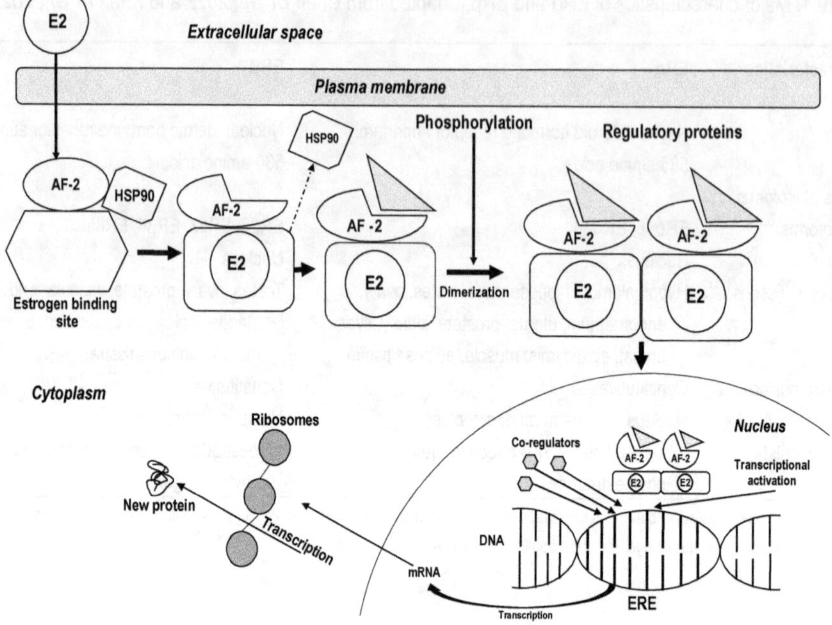

Figure 19.1. Scheme of basic molecular biological way of ERs function (adapted from Heger *et al.*, 2013; Ye *et al.*, 2018). CoR = coregulators; E2 = oestradiol; ER = oestrogen receptor; ERE = oestrogen response element; HSP 90 = heat shock protein 90.

ERα and ERβ, are recognised to have regulatory actions in a variety of physiological processes relevant to glucose metabolism and diabetes (See Chapter 14), cardioprotection and anti-cancer action. SB as the natural agonist of ERβ is believed to plays an immunosuppressive role being a potential therapeutic tool in the treatment of autoimmune diseases, including rheumatoid arthritis. SB is reported to upregulate ERβ expression, to induce apoptosis, to inhibit proliferation, and to reduce expression of the pro-inflammatory cytokines IL-17 and TNF-α, through ERβ binding, in T lymphocytes from healthy donors and patients with active RA (Dupuis *et al.*, 2018).

In a model system based on the rat pancreatic β-cell line, INS-1, damaged with pro-inflammatory cytokines, TNF-α or IL-1β, it was shown that SB was able to protect the suppression in the expression of both ERα and ERβ that were involved in insulin synthesis and release, respectively. Furthermore, it seems likely that SB can ameliorate the loss of critical INS-1 cells by regulating autophagy and preventing apoptosis (Yang *et al.*, 2018).

SB (15 μM) is found to protects rat pancreatic β-cell through up-regulation of oestrogen receptors' signalling including ERs phosphorylation that depresses ROS/RNS generation in amylin/A$\beta_{1\text{-}42}$-treated INS-1 cells (Yang *et al.*, 2019a). SB (15 μM) was reported to protect INS-1 cells from amylin-induced apoptosis through activation of glucagon-like peptide-1 receptor (GLP-1R)/ protein kinase A (PKA) signalling. Interestingly, SB inhibition of the toxic effects of $A\beta_{1\text{-}42}$ was reported to be independent of GLP-1R/PKA pathway (Yang *et al.*, 2019b). The ERs are considered to be key regulators of glucose and lipid metabolism.

It was shown that SB (10 μM) can upregulate ERα signalling pathway. In fact, ERα-specific inhibitors were reported to abolish the anti-lipotoxic effect of SB. Indeed, SB protects INS-1 cells against apoptosis and mitochondrial damage through upregulation of ERα pathway (Sun *et al.*, 2019). SB was found to up-regulate both ERα and Erβ pathways in UVB-treated dermal HFF cells and epidermal HaCaT cells, resulting in protection of skin from UVB-damage (Liu *et al.*, 2021). SB treatment was indicated to protect human skin cells from UVB injury through upregulation of ERs (Liu *et al.*, 2021). ERs were also shown to be involved in the neuroprotective effect of SB in $A\beta_{1\text{-}42}$-treated rats (Song *et al.*, 2018).

Altering ER machinery, together with maintaining redox homeostasis, reducing oxidative stress, inflammatory cytokines, affecting cellular apoptosis machinery and β-amyloid aggregation are considered to be major mechanisms that are responsible for neuroprotection by SM/SB (Borah *et al.*, 2013; Ullah and Khan, 2018). ERβ up-regulation was observed to be involved in SB-induced growth inhibition of human breast cancer MCF-7 cells (Zheng *et al.*, 2016). ERα and ERβ were shown to be involved in the protective effects of SB in pancreatic β cell line INS-1 (Chu *et al.*, 2020; Yang *et al.*, 2018; 2019a). SB was found to increase L-cell mass and function through an ER-mediated antioxidant pathway. Preincubation of GLUTag cells with SB induced Nrf2 pathway, while the protective antioxidant effect of SB was shown to be blocked by the selective ERα antagonist MPP or ERβ antagonist PHTPP in the cells (HFD).

Importantly, in contrast to other studies showing stimulating effects of SM/SB on ERs, SB (50 μM) was also established to promote the migration and myogenic differentiation of murine C2C12 myoblasts via modulation of ROS generation and down-regulation of ERα expression (Long *et al.*, 2020). Similarly, in a rat model of Zearalenone-induced hepatotoxicity and reproductive toxicity in rats SM (100, 200, or 500 mg SM/kg for 6 wk.) was reported to decrease expression of oestrogen receptor 1 (a gene expressed ERα) in ovaries and the uterus (Gao *et al.*, 2018). Furthermore, ERα down-regulation was reported to play a fundamental role in SB-induced autophagy and apoptosis in human breast cancer MCF-7 cells (Zheng *et al.*, 2015).

19.3 Silymarin and transcription factors PPARs

The peroxisome proliferator-activated receptors (PPARs) are a group of three nuclear receptor isoforms, PPARγ, PPARα, and PPARδ/β, discovered in the 1990s in rodents, were named after their property of peroxisome proliferation (Kota *et al.*, 2005). PPARs are known to be ligand-regulated transcription factors controlling gene expression and affecting various important cellular events including proliferation, differentiation, and apoptosis (Berger and Moller, 2002). PPARs are reported to form a heterodimer with retinoid-X receptor (RXR) and bind a peroxisome proliferator response element (PPRE) on target genes (Nakamura *et al.*, 2014). It is shown that PPARs control expression of various genes that are essential for lipid and carbohydrate metabolism being 'master' transcriptional regulators of nutrient metabolism and energy homeostasis (Berger *et al.*, 2005).

In particular, PPARγ is considered to be the master transcription factor for adipogenesis, while PPARα is mainly expressed in the tissues with a high efficiency of mitochondrial fatty acid oxidation including the liver, whereas PPARβ/δ is highly expressed in the small intestine and keratinocyte (Neels and Grimaldi, 2014). It is believed that expression levels of PPARs are regulated by diets and nutrient status in a tissue-dependent manner and the activities of PPARα and PPARγ are regulated by phosphorylation (Juge-Aubry *et al.*, 1999). It is also evident that the three PPAR members share a high degree of homology, however, they are shown to substantially differ in tissue distribution, ligand specificity, and physiological roles (Berger and Moller, 2002). There is considerable evidence that all three PPARs play crucial roles in lipid and fatty acid metabolism as a result of direct binding to and modulating genes involved in lipid metabolism (Fan and Evans, 2015).

Recently, a great number of papers have reviewed PPARs functions and importance in regulation of various physiological and biochemical processes within the body (Scheggi *et al.*, 2022; Sobolev *et al.*, 2022; Wagner and Wagner, 2022; Ye *et al.*, 2022; Zhou *et al.*, 2022) and impact of phytochemicals on PPAR receptors and its implications for disease prevention and treatments have been evaluated (Enayati *et al.*, 2022). The evolutionary pattern and regulation characteristics of PPARs have also been described (Zhou *et al.*, 2015). It is shown that PPARα is activated by adiponectin and could inhibit NF-κB pathway, while PPARγ improves insulin action, FFA oxidation, adiponectin secretion, and suppresses secretion of proinflammatory cytokines (Musso *et al.*, 2010).

It is generally accepted that PPAR signalling is an important part of the body's antioxidant system playing a fundamental role in various stress conditions. For instance, the antioxidant effect of PPARα has been demonstrated and PPAR-responsive elements have been identified in the promoter regions of several antioxidant genes, including main antioxidant enzymes, namely, Cu/ZnSOD and CAT. Therefore, PPARα can bind to PPREs to promote the expression of antioxidants to inhibit oxidative stress (Kim and Yang, 2013; Khoo *et al.*, 2013; Li *et al.*, 2012; Liu *et al.*, 2012) having a regulatory effect on the production of oxidative, proinflammatory and profibrotic mediators (Diep *et al.*, 2002). Furthermore, induction of PPARα by its agonist WY14643 treatment was found to ameliorate the oxidative stress and severity of liver injury and restored expression of stress-altered genes as a due to ethanol treatment (Kong *et al.*, 2011).

SM treatment significantly reduced the high fructose diet-induced increase expression of PPARα and PPARγ in the rat liver (Prakash *et al.*, 2014). Interestingly, isosilybin a from milk thistle seeds was identified as an agonist of PPARγ (Pferschy-Wenzig *et al.*, 2014). Results of the molecular docking, reporter gene assay, and the targeting gene expression analysis indicated that SB is a weak agonist of PPARα (Wang *et al.*, 2015). In rat hepatoma FaO cells loaded with lipids and exposed to 0.75 mmol/l oleate/palmitate, SB was demonstrated to increase PPARα and PPARδ, but decreased PPARγ (Vecchione *et al.*, 2016). The PPARγ protein expression was increased upon SB exposure in Human Hepatic Stellate LX-2 cells (Ezhilarasan *et al.*, 2016). A combination of SM and curcumin was shown to ameliorate a paracetamol-induced decrease in PPARγ expression in rat liver (Ahmad *et al.*, 2019). In a mouse model of experimental non-alcoholic steatohepatitis SB was indicated to mitigate increased expression of PPARγ (Suguro *et al.*, 2020). In a model of chemically induced renal carcinogenesis in male Wistar rats *Silybum marianum* total extract, SM or SB were shown to ameliorate decreased expression PPARγ and Nrf2 and mitigate increased expression of NF-κB in the kidney tissue (Yassin *et al.*, 2021).

Interestingly, SM/SB was shown to modulate other transcription factors, including:

- hypoxia-inducible Factor-1 (HIF-1; Jung *et al.*, 2009; Lin *et al.*, 2013; Wang *et al.*, 2012);
- signal transducer and activation of transcription (STAT; Agarwal *et al.*, 2007; Hou *et al.*, 2010; Tyagi *et al.*, 2012; Verdura *et al.*, 2021);
- E2F1 (Moshtaghion *et al.*, 2013);
- runt-related transcription factor 2 (RUNX2; Yin *et al.*, 2013);
- the pancreatic and duodenal homeobox-1 (Pdx1) transcription factor (Chen *et al.*, 2014; Soto *et al.*, 2014a);
- homeobox protein NKX6.1 (Lovelace *et al.*, 2015; Soto *et al.*, 2014b);
- Activating Transcription Factor 4 (ATF-4; Lovelace *et al.*, 2015);
- forkhead box (FOXO) transcription factors (Lovelace *et al.*, 2015; Prakash *et al.*, 2014; Zhang *et al.*, 2015);
- p53 (Shafiei-Roudbari *et al.*, 2017);
- the microphthalmia-associated transcription factor (MITF; Uto *et al.*, 2022).

Oxidation-reduction (redox) based regulation of gene expression is considered to be a fundamental regulatory mechanism in cell biology acting at the cell-signalling level (Surai, 2020a). Since excessive ROS production is damaging to many biological molecules, the antioxidant system network is responsible for prevention of the damages. However, a basal level of ROS is essential for cell communication, adaptation and survival. Therefore, a moderate level of ROS can create adaptive responses and improve adaptive ability to stressful challenges/conditions by alerting/turning protective mechanisms (Surai, 2020a; Surai and Earle-Payne, 2022). In animals, redox signalling pathways use ROS as signalling molecules to activate vitagenes responsible for regulation of various functions including growth, differentiation, proliferation and apoptosis leading to effective stress adaptation. Furthermore, the antioxidant defence system network is also under regulation by various transcription factors. These protective pathways operate in coordinated manner being critically important for animal adaptation to various stresses. In particular, transcription factors involved in redox status regulation include Nrf2, NF-κB, FOXO, p53, HSF1, HIF-1, STATs and others (Surai, 2020a).

HIF proteins are known to constitute a family of transcriptional regulators playing a crucial role in regulating gene expression under conditions of low oxygen (Chu *et al.*, 2022). STATs comprising seven intracellular transcription factors, the STAT1, STAT2, STAT3, STAT4, STAT5a, STAT5b, and STAT6 are reported to be involved in multiple biological processes, such as immunoregulation, haematopoiesis, cell proliferation, differentiation and apoptosis (Tsiogka *et al.*, 2022). The transcription factor E2F1 is shown to be a central player in regulation of cell cycle progression, DNA-damage response, and apoptosis (Denechaud *et al.*, 2017). Runt-related transcription factor 2 (RUNX2) is believed to be a key transcription factor for bone development associated with osteoblast differentiation (Komori, 2022). The pancreatic and duodenal homeobox-1 (Pdx1) transcription factor is shown to play a central role in pancreatic development and in insulin gene expression (Jennings *et al.*, 2020).

Homeobox protein NKX6.1 is known to be a transcription factor and a crucial regulator of pancreatic β cell growth, development, identity, and proliferation (Aigha *et al.*, 2020). Activating Transcription Factor 4 (ATF-4) is known to participate in a variety of cellular responses to specific environmental stresses, intracellular derangements, or growth factors (Ebert *et al.*, 2022).

Forkhead box (FOXO) transcription factors participate in several signalling pathways related to human health and diseases and are considered to be crucial for maintaining cardiomyocyte metabolism and cell survival, and the functions of the FOXO family proteins are known to be modulated by a wide variety of post-translational modifications including phosphorylation, ubiquitination, acetylation, arginine methylation, and O-glycosylation (Han *et al.*, 2022). p53 is a transcription factor that is known to suppress tumour growth through regulation of a number of target genes with diverse biological functions (Sullivan *et al.*, 2018). MITF has emerged as a key coordinator of many aspects of melanocyte and melanoma biology participating in a range of biological processes including cell survival, differentiation, proliferation, metabolism, invasion, senescence, and DNA damage repair (Goding and Arnheiter, 2019).

Therefore, it seems likely that protective properties of SM/SB in various model systems, including anti-toxic effects (Chapter 8), hepatoprotective (Chapter 12), neuroprotective (Chapter 13), anti-diabetic (Chapter 14) actions, protection against arthritis and other diseases (Chapter 15), as well as immunomodulating (Chapter 9), gut-modulating (Chapter 11) properties and anti-inflammatory action (Chapter 10) are associated with the aforementioned molecular mechanisms. On the one hand, direct antioxidant action of SM/SB is unlikely to occur in biological systems because of its comparatively low availability and low active concentrations in target tissues. On the other hand, activation of various transcription factors and vitagenes could be a leading molecular mechanism of SM/SB protective actions and this area of research need further expanding.

Furthermore, in most of cases a combination of various described mechanisms would be involved to provide optimal redox status and lead to optimal stress adaptation. In normal physiological conditions under minimal stress, the body can easily deal with

ROS production and use some of them, including H_2O_2, for cell signalling. However, under various stress conditions a role of adaptogens, such as SM/SB, is significantly increased. The restoration of the redox homeostasis is the main task for such adaptogens. This complex process involves a range of regulatory factors from stress sensing to creating an adequate response and by modulating transcription factors and vitagenes SM/SB help dealing with homeostasis disturbances and providing adequate protection (Figure 19.2).

Mitochondria and phagocyte cells are major sources of reactive oxygen and nitrogen species (RONS). There are also various stress conditions in commercial animal and poultry production associated with increasing RONS production. It is well proven that RONS play important roles as signalling molecules; however, in the case of RONS overproduction leading to their concentration to exceed threshold level, they can cause damage to main biological molecules, including lipids, proteins, and DNA/RNA. As a result of RONS excess, a stress response program (Oxidative stress response, OSR) is activated. Since oxidative stress can cause a range of damages to various molecules,

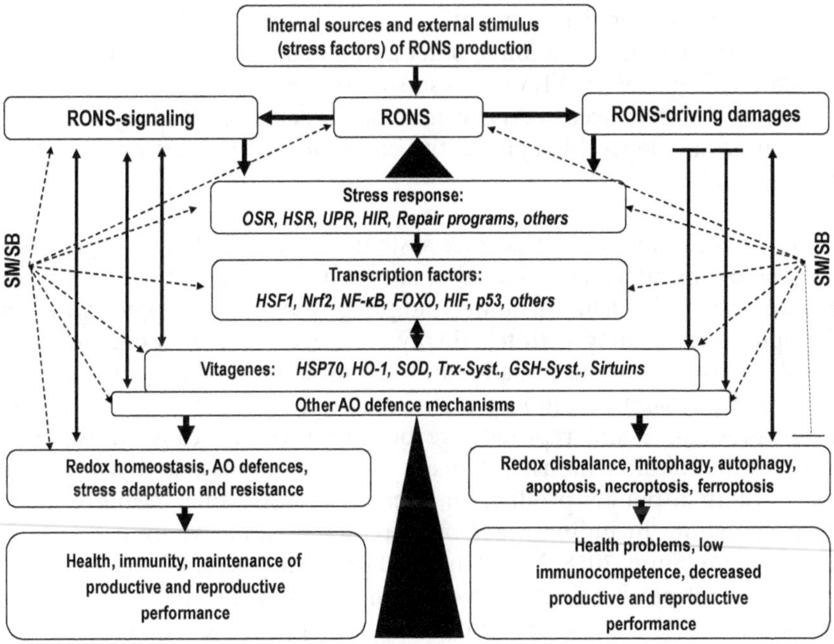

Figure 19.2. Protective roles of SM/SB in animals (adapted from Surai, 2020b). FOXO = transcription factors; GSH-syst. = glutathione system(glutathione/ glutathione reductase/glutaredoxin/ glutathione peroxidase); HIF = hypoxia-inducible transcription factor; HIR = hypoxia-induced response; HO-1 = heme oxygenase 1; HSF1 = heat shock factor; HSP70 = heat shock protein 70; HSR = heat shock response; NF-κB = transcription factor; Nrf2 = transcription factor; OSR = oxidative stress response; p65 = transcription factor; RONS = reactive oxygen and nitrogen species; SOD = superoxide dismutase; Trx-Syst. = thioredoxin system (thioredoxin/thioredoxin peroxidase (peroxiredoxins)/sulfiredoxin/thioredoxin reductase); UPR = unfolded protein response.

in addition to OSR, other stress response programs, including heat shock response (HSR), unfolded protein response (UPR), hypoxia-induced response (HIR), and DNA damage response, are also activated. This leads to induction of expression of various transcription factors, including HSF1, Nrf2, NF-κB, FOXO, HIF, p53, and others.

The upregulation of transcription factors leads to activation of various genes, including vitagenes. Activation of HSF increased production of HSP70, Nrf2 activation increased synthesis of SOD, HO-1, elements of thioredoxin and glutathione systems; and FOXO activation would cause increased expression of sirtuins. There is a complex system of interplay between vitagenes and transcription factors. Most remarkably, some vitagenes, like SOD, are affected by several transcription factors including Nrf2, NF-κB, p53, etc. Since SOD is responsible for production of H_2O_2, major signalling ROS, control of its concentration is of paramount importance. Furthermore, products of vitagene activation, e.g. sirtuins, would affect expression and activity of some transcription factors, including Nrf2, NF-κB, FOXO, etc. Some vitagenes can be activated directly without transcription factor involvement. This includes transcriptional regulation of SOD in response to ROS as well as activation of sirtuins by changes in NAD+/NADH ratio. In general, redox homeostasis plays an important role in the regulation of antioxidant defences. RONS are also responsible for adaptive production/activation of other antioxidants, which are not included into vitagene family (e.g. CoQ, CAT, various selenoproteins, etc.) and they responsible for redox balance maintenance, stress resistance and adaptation leading to good health, high immunocompetence, high productive and reproductive performance of poultry and farm animals.

However, when the antioxidant defence system, together with the vitagene network, are not able to prevent or repair damages imposed by RONS to biological molecules, other protective mechanisms including mitophagy, autophagy, apoptosis, necroptosis, and ferroptosis are dealing with terminally damaged molecules, organelles or cells. As a result of disrupted redox balance and accumulation of damages in cells/tissues, health-related problems, including low immunocompetence, appear. In addition, decreased productive and reproductive performance can cause heavy economic losses for animal/poultry industry. Since it is almost impossible to avoid stresses in commercial animal/poultry production, a search for nutritional means of antioxidant system modulation, including usage of increased doses of vitamin E (Surai *et al.*, 2019a), selenium (Surai, 2018; 2021; Surai and Kochish, 2019), TAU (Surai *et al.*, 2020; 2021a) and carnitine (Surai, 2015a,b,c), is on the agenda of many research groups world-wide and SM/SB can also contribute to AO system regulation.

Therefore, from the aforementioned in previous chapters data it is clear that SM/SB can affect redox balance regulation at different levels (Figure 19.2), including:

- reduction of RONS production by stabilising mitochondria, main source of RONS production, and improving efficacy of phagocyte action, the second major source of RONS (Surai, 2015d; 2022);
- affecting stress-response programs and maintaining AO system alert and ready for protective actions (Surai, 2015d);

- modulating transcription factors, including Nrf2, a master-regulator of AO system (Surai *et al.*, 2019b), and NF-κB, main driver of pro-inflammatory cytokine synthesis and inflammation (Surai *et al.*, 2021b);
- activating vitagenes and inducing synthesis of a range protective molecules participating in re-establishment of the redox homeostasis and stress adaptation (Surai, 2020a).

Therefore, SM/SB in cooperation with other natural antioxidants is involved in gut health and immunocompetence maintenance helping animals to adapt to stress and overcome it with minimal damages.

19.4 Increasing silymarin availability is a way forward

Important limitations of SM/SB usage in clinical practise include poor aqueous solubility leading to limited intestinal absorption resulted in its low bioavailability (Kesharwani *et al.*, 2020) and difficulties in obtaining a preparation of SM with a defined, stable and reproducible composition (Lorenzo *et al.*, 2020). The availability issues are related to chemical structures of SM constituents and nanotechnology-based approaches in formulation development could help is solving those problems (Di Costanzo and Angelico, 2019; Piazzini *et al.*, 2019). The authors considered solid nanoparticles, polymeric nanoparticles, inorganic nanoparticles, solid lipid nanoparticles, nanostructured lipid carriers, inclusion complexation, nanomicelles, nanoemulsions and liposomes as new important carriers for SM/SB. In addition, encapsulating SM in liposomes, forming complexes with phospholipids, cyclodextrins and hydroxyapatite were also considered in detail (Paltinean *et al.*, 2022). Liposomes, transfersomes, niosomes, and ethosomes are also potential nanocarriers for phytochemicals. Furthermore nano-phytosomes, recently developed lipid-based vesicles to improve the transport of plant-based nutraceuticals, including SM/SB, seem to be an important contribution to the field (Barani *et al.*, 2021).

However, it will take some time before commercial production of new formulations will be available. On the other hand, the chemical composition of any plant extract is always variable since it depends on conditions of plant growth (climate, fertilisers, age, etc.), extraction techniques, storage conditions, analytical advances, etc. Some of those parameters (e.g. variations in climate conditions, including temperature, humidity, etc.) are quite changeable and difficult to be stabilised leading to variability in chemical composition of plant tissues including fruits and their extracts (Chambers *et al.*, 2017).

19.5 Conclusions

From the data presented in 19 chapters of this book it is clear that SM possesses many beneficial properties, including its anti-toxic effects, which make this supplement unique in terms of its protective effects in various human disorders/diseases. Indeed, SM/SB is a very useful tool in complimentarily medicine.

Main points for the future are as follows:

- It is known that most drugs available for human disease treatment have some side effects and drug toxicity is an important limitation in drug usage, for example, in cancer therapy. For instance, SM has recently been shown to reduce hepatic side effects of fingolimod in patients with relapsing-remitting multiple sclerosis (Ghiasian *et al.*, 2021). SM is shown to be important in the management of antiepileptic drug induced liver injury (Asgarshirazi *et al.*, 2017). Similarly, in patients with acne SM prevented liver damage caused by isotretinoin and the authors suggested to use SM as an effective, low-cost, and low-complication treatment in clinical practice (Mirnezami *et al.*, 2020). SM can also decrease CS nephrotoxicity in various chemotherapy regimens in cancer patients (Momeni *et al.*, 2015). Therefore, anti-toxic complimentary/adjuvant therapy by SM deserves more attention. Oral administration of SM has been demonstrated to significantly reduce hepatotoxicity severity after 1 month of treatment in non-metastatic breast cancer patients treated with doxorubicin/cyclophosphamide-paclitaxel regimen (Moezian *et al.*, 2022). Furthermore, SM could be an important part of complimentary/adjuvant therapy in cases where other drugs failed to correct the situation related to oxidative-stress related disorders with redox disbalance and inflammation involved. In addition, SM was recently indicated to show immunoregulatory effects on inflammatory response and liver function in multiple sclerosis patients (Abbasirad *et al.*, 2021). Interestingly, the 4-week adjuvant treatment with oral SM was shown to result in an improved wound recovery in patients with second degree-burn (Mahmoodi-Nesheli *et al.*, 2018).
- SM usage in sport medicine to support athletes and at horse racing to support animals under extreme physical load awaits more developments (Boukazoula and Ayari, 2022; Dockalova *et al.*, 2022). It seems likely that simultaneous aerobic training and SM supplementation could have interactive effects on reducing glycaemic indices and improving liver integrity in men with type 2 diabetes (Ghalandari *et al.*, 2023).
- Cosmetic industry can use SM/SB in topical application with various creams to keep healthy skin, including sunscreen applications (Iraji *et al.*, 2022; Jowkar *et al.*, 2020; Mohanty *et al.*, 2022; Rajnochová Svobodová *et al.*, 2016). SM topical application was also shown to reduce the severity of acute radiodermatitis in breast cancer patients (Karbasforooshan *et al.*, 2019). Prophylactic topical application of SM was reported to significantly reduce the severity of capecitabine-induced hand-foot syndrome in patients with gastrointestinal cancer (Elyasi *et al.*, 2017). Prophylactic administration of SM was found to significantly decrease the severity of radiotherapy induced mucositis and delay its occurrence in patients with head and neck cancer (Elyasi *et al.*, 2016).
- Milk thistle as well as SM/SB may be included into various functional food products (Zhang *et al.*, 2022), including yoghurt (Ismael *et al.*, 2014) to improve their quality and to be delivered to the body by different routes.

- SM is approved for its hepato-protective action in several countries, including India, Europe, Australia, and Canada with doses ranging from 70 to 240 mg thrice a day (Ralli *et al.*, 2021). SM is used as prescription medicines (Italy), a new drug (India), non-prescription drug (Germany and France), and as over-the-counter medicines, self-medication, herbal medicine, dietary supplements, health foods and functional foods in other countries (Ralli *et al.*, 2021). It seems likely that quickly accumulating evidence on beneficial effects of SM and its protective effects in various clinical settings would change its status in various countries.
- SM is considered to be an important tool for controlling complications related to various diseases including T2D, ulcerative colitis, rhinitis, osteoarthritis, beta-thalassemia (Ralli *et al.*, 2021) and other diseases.

Major part of research work conducted on SM/SB using various animal models and clinical trials was related to human health. Hepatoprotection and neuroprotection by SM/SB is well described in scientific literature. Furthermore, anti-diabetic and anti-arthritis as well as immunomodulation, gut health maintenance and anti-inflammatory properties of SM/SB are also of great importance. There are also interesting data on anti-cancer properties of SM/SB. However, in contrast to very encouraging and promising results obtained in experimental research using various *in vitro* and *in vivo* animal models, unfortunately, clinical trial results of SM/SB usage are not as convincing as animal studies. In fact, only a few well-designed clinical studies on SM/SB in human have been conducted and still little is known about its clinical efficiency (Marmouzi *et al.*, 2021). For example, a systematic review and meta-analysis of randomised controlled trials studying protective effects of SM in T2D (Voroneanu *et al.*, 2016) indicated limitations of such an analysis, to draw an adequately powered conclusion regarding SM clinical efficacy. This includes:

- small number of studies, small sample size and short-term follow-up and the absence of pharmacokinetic/pharmacodynamic tests prior to study commitment (Kadoglou *et al.*, 2022);
- elevated heterogeneity of the studies, including various SM products, different dosage regimens, treatment durations, and endpoints used in different studies;
- it is quite difficult to take into account the effect of the changes in types and dosages of other medications during the study period (Kadoglou *et al.*, 2022; Wah Kheong *et al.*, 2017).

The authors suggested that further clinical studies are necessary before a firm conclusion can be made (Voroneanu *et al.*, 2016). The same is true for other trials devoted to protective effects of SM/SB in liver diseases; while various *in vitro* and *in vivo* studies have shown that SM has various beneficial effects on the liver, including anti-inflammatory, anti-oxidant, and antifibrotic effects (Hupa *et al.*, 2017), the effect of SM in patients remains inconclusive (Navarro *et al.*, 2019; Wah Kheong *et al.*, 2017). Since in many clinical trials SM showed good safety and tolerability (Wah Kheong *et al.*, 2017), including safety in pregnancy (Soleimani, *et al.*, 2019), with minimal side effects, it has a great potential in treatment of patients with various disorders, but larger well-designed clinical trials are needed to confirm beneficial effects of SM in clinical management of various diseases (Hupa *et al.*, 2017).

In poultry production and avian veterinary medicine Milk Thistle and SM can be used as adaptogens to deal with commercially-relevant stresses and to maintain healthy liver. It seems likely that combinations of SM with other protective nutrients is a way forward in development of health protection programs (Surai *et al.*, 2018). Clearly, more research devoted to roles of SM/SB in transcription factor modulation and vitagene activation under various stress conditions is needed.

Therefore, accumulating scientific evidence indicates that SM/SB is characterised by a wide range of protective pharmacological activities (Antika and Dewi, 2021; see previous chapters), including: hepatoprotective, neuroprotective, anti-diabetic, cardio-protective, anti-inflammatory, immune-modulatory, anti-viral, anti-cancer and anti-toxic/chemo-preventive activities. Molecular mechanisms of protective SM/SB action include antioxidant activities, mitochondria preservation/stabilisation and decreased ROS production, vitagene modulation and improved stress adaptation, Nrf2 activation and additional synthesis of a range of antioxidants and redox homeostasis maintenance, NF-κB and pro-inflammatory cytokine down-regulation leading to anti-inflammatory action, ER regulation, modulation of PPAR and other transcription factors, etc.

It is just a matter of time before full potential of this enigmatic phytochemical can be realised in human and veterinary medicine and nutrition.

References

Abbasirad, F., Shayganneja d, V., Hosseininasab, F., Mirmosayyeb, O., Mahaki, B., Moayedi, B. and Esmaeil, N., 2021. Significant immunomodulatory and hepatoprotective impacts of silymarin in MS patients: A double-blind placebo-controlled clinical trial. International Immunopharmacology 97: 107715.

Agarwal, C., Tyagi, A., Kaur, M. and Agarwal, R., 2007. Silibinin inhibits constitutive activation of Stat3, and causes caspase activation and apoptotic death of human prostate carcinoma DU145 cells. Carcinogenesis 28: 1463-1470.

Ahmad, M.M., Rezk, N.A., Fawzy, A. and Sabry, M., 2019. Protective effects of curcumin and silymarin against paracetamol induced hepatotoxicity in adult male albino rats. Gene 712: 143966.

Aigha, I.I. and Abdelalim, E.M., 2020. NKX6.1 transcription factor: a crucial regulator of pancreatic β cell development, identity, and proliferation. Stem Cell Research & Therapy 11: 459.

Antika, L.D. and Dewi, R.M., 2021. The pharmacological properties of silymarin and its constituents. Natural Product Sciences 27: 68-77.

Asgarshirazi, M., Shariat, M. and Sheikh, M., 2017. Comparison of efficacy of folic acid and silymarin in the management of antiepileptic drug induced liver injury: a randomized clinical trial. Hepatobiliary & Pancreatic Diseases International 16: 296-302.

Barani, M., Sangiovanni, E., Angarano, M., Rajizadeh, M.A., Mehrabani, M., Piazza, S., Gangadharappa, H.V., Pardakhty, A., Mehrbani, M., Dell'Agli, M. and Nematollahi, M.H., 2021. Phytosomes as innovative delivery systems for phytochemicals: A comprehensive review of literature. International Journal of Nanomedicine 16: 6983-7022.

Berger, J. and Moller, D.E., 2002. The mechanisms of action of PPARs. Annual Review of Medicine 53: 409-435.

Berger, J.P., Akiyama, T.E. and Meinke, P.T., 2005. PPARs: therapeutic targets for metabolic disease. Trends in Pharmacological Sciences 26: 244-251.

Borah, A., Paul, R., Choudhury, S., Choudhury, A., Bhuyan, B., Das Talukdar, A., Dutta Choudhury, M. and Mohanakumar, K.P., 2013. Neuroprotective potential of silymarin against CNS disorders: insight into the pathways and molecular mechanisms of action. CNS neuroscience & Therapeutics 19: 847-853.

Boukazoula, F. and Ayari, D., 2022. Effect of milk thistle (*Silybum marianum*) supplementation on the serum levels of oxidative stress markers in male half marathon athletes. Biomarkers 27: 461-469.

Chen, K., Zhao, L., He, H., Wan, X., Wang, F. and Mo, Z., 2014. Silibinin protects β cells from glucotoxicity through regulation of the Insig-1/SREBP-1c pathway. International Journal of Molecular Medicine 34: 1073-1080.

Chen, P., Li, B. and Ou-Yang, L., 2022. Role of estrogen receptors in health and disease. Frontiers in Endocrinology 13: 839005.

Chambers, C.S., Holečková, V., Petrásková, L., Biedermann, D., Valentová, K., Buchta, M. and Křen, V., 2017. The silymarin composition … and why does it matter???. Food Research International, 100: 339-353.

Chu, C., Gao, X., Li, X., Zhang, X., Ma, R., Jia, Y., Li, D., Wang, D. and Xu, F., 2020. Involvement of estrogen receptor-α in the activation of Nrf2-antioxidative signaling pathways by silibinin in pancreatic β-cells. Biomolecules & Therapeutics 28: 163-171.

Chu, Q., Gu, X., Zheng, Q. and Zhu, H., 2022. Regulatory mechanism of HIF-1α and its role in liver diseases: a narrative review. Annals of Translational Medicine 10: 2.

Denechaud, P.D., Fajas, L. and Giralt, A., 2017. E2F1, a novel regulator of metabolism. Frontiers in Endocrinology 8: 311.

Di Costanzo, A. and Angelico, R., 2019. Formulation strategies for enhancing the bioavailability of silymarin: the state of the art. Molecules 24: 2155.

Diep, Q.N., Amiri, F., Touyz, R.M., Cohn, J.S., Endemann, D., Neves, M.F. and Schiffrin, E.L., 2002. PPARalpha activator effects on Ang II-induced vascular oxidative stress and inflammation. Hypertension 40: 866-871.

Dockalova, H., Baholet, D., Batik, A., Zeman, L. and Horky, P., 2022. Effect of milk thistle (*Silybum marianum*) seed cakes by horses subjected to physical exertion. Journal of Equine Veterinary Science 113: 103937.

Dupuis, M.L., Conti, F., Maselli, A., Pagano, M.T., Ruggieri, A., Anticoli, S., Fragale, A., Gabriele, L., Gagliardi, M.C., Sanchez, M., Ceccarelli, F., Alessandri, C., Valesini, G., Ortona, E. and Pierdominici, M., 2018. The natural agonist of estrogen receptor β silibinin plays an immunosuppressive role representing a potential therapeutic tool in rheumatoid arthritis. Frontiers in Immunology 9: 1903.

Ebert, S.M., Rasmussen, B.B., Judge, A.R., Judge, S.M., Larsson, L., Wek, R.C., Anthony, T.G., Marcotte, G.R., Miller, M.J., Yorek, M.A., Vella, A., Volpi, E., Stern, J.I., Strub, M.D., Ryan, Z., Talley, J.J. and Adams, C.M., 2022. Biology of activating transcription factor 4 (ATF4) and its role in skeletal muscle atrophy. The Journal of Nutrition 152: 926-938.

Elyasi, S., Shojaee, F., Allahyari, A. and Karimi, G., 2017. Topical silymarin administration for prevention of capecitabine-induced hand-foot syndrome: A randomized, double-blinded, placebo-controlled clinical trial. Phytotherapy Research 31: 1323-1329.

Elyasi, S., Hosseini, S., Niazi Moghadam, M.R., Aledavood, S.A. and Karimi, G., 2016. Effect of oral silymarin administration on prevention of radiotherapy induced mucositis: A randomized, double-blinded, placebo-controlled clinical trial. Phytotherapy Research 30: 1879-1885.

Enayati, A., Ghojoghnejad, M., Roufogalis, B.D., Maollem, S.A. and Sahebkar, A., 2022. Impact of phytochemicals on PPAR receptors: Implications for disease treatments. PPAR Research 2022: 4714914.

Ezhilarasan, D., Evraerts, J., Brice, S., Buc-Calderon, P., Karthikeyan, S., Sokal, E. and Najimi, M., 2016. Silibinin inhibits proliferation and migration of human hepatic stellate LX-2 cells. Journal of Clinical and Experimental Hepatology 6: 167-174.

Fallah, M., Davoodvandi, A., Nikmanzar, S., Aghili, S., Mirazimi, S., Aschner, M., Rashidian, A., Hamblin, M.R., Chamanara, M., Naghsh, N. and Mirzaei, H., 2021. Silymarin (milk thistle extract) as a therapeutic agent in gastrointestinal cancer. Biomedicine & Pharmacotherapy 142: 112024.

Fan, W. and Evans, R., 2015. PPARs and ERRs: molecular mediators of mitochondrial metabolism. Current Opinion in Cell Biology 33: 49-54.

Ferraz, A.C., Almeida, L.T., da Silva Caetano, C.C., da Silva Menegatto, M.B., Souza Lima, R.L., de Senna, J., de Oliveira Cardoso, J.M., Perucci, L.O., Talvani, A., Geraldo de Lima, W., de Mello Silva, B., Barbosa Reis, A., de Magalhães, J.C. and Lopes de Brito Magalhães, C., 2021. Hepatoprotective, antioxidant, anti-inflammatory, and antiviral activities of silymarin against mayaro virus infection. Antiviral Research 194: 105168.

Filardo, E.J. and Thomas, P., 2012. Minireview: G protein-coupled estrogen receptor-1, GPER-1: its mechanism of action and role in female reproductive cancer, renal and vascular physiology. Endocrinology 153: 2953-2962.

Gao, X., Xiao, Z.H., Liu, M., Zhang, N.Y., Khalil, M.M., Gu, C.Q., Qi, D.S. and Sun, L.H., 2018. Dietary silymarin supplementation alleviates zearalenone-induced hepatotoxicity and reproductive toxicity in rats. The Journal of Nutrition 148: 1209-1216.

Ghalandari, K., Shabani, M., Khajehlandi, A. and Mohammadi, A., 2023. Effect of aerobic training with silymarin consumption on glycemic indices and liver enzymes in men with type 2 diabetes. Archives of Physiology and Biochemistry 129: 76-81.

Ghiasian, M., Nafisi, H., Ranjbar, A., Mohammadi, Y. and Ataei, S., 2021. Antioxidative effects of silymarin on the reduction of liver complications of fingolimod in patients with relapsing-remitting multiple sclerosis: A clinical trial study. Journal of Biochemical and Molecular Toxicology 35: e22800.

Goding, C.R. and Arnheiter, H., 2019. MITF-the first 25 years. Genes & Development 33: 983-1007.

Han, R., Huang, H., Xia, W., Liu, J., Luo, H., Tang, J. and Xia, Z., 2022. Perspectives for Forkhead box transcription factors in diabetic cardiomyopathy: Their therapeutic potential and possible effects of salvianolic acids. Frontiers in Cardiovascular Medicine 9: 951597.

Heger, Z., Zitka, O., Krizkova, S., Beklova, M., Kizek, R. and Adam, V., 2013. Molecular biology of beta-estradiol-estrogen receptor complex binding to estrogen response element and the effect on cell proliferation. Neuro Endocrinology Letters 34: 123-129.

Hou, Y.C., Liou, K.T., Chern, C.M., Wang, Y.H., Liao, J.F., Chang, S., Chou, Y.H. and Shen, Y.C., 2010. Preventive effect of silymarin in cerebral ischemia-reperfusion-induced brain injury in rats possibly through impairing NF-κB and STAT-1 activation. Phytomedicine 17: 963-973.

Hupa, K.L., Jaeckel, E. and Manns, M.P., 2017. Silymarin for treatment of nonalcoholic steatohepatitis-A new kid on the block?. Clinical Gastroenterology and Hepatology 15: 1863-1865.

Iraji, F., Sharif Makhmalzadeh, B., Abedini, M., Aghaei, A. and Siahpoush, A., 2022. Effect of herbal cream containing Fumaria officinalis and silymarin for treatment of eczema: A randomized double-blind controlled clinical trial. Avicenna Journal of Phytomedicine 12: 155-162.

Ismael, S.M., Farahat, A.M., Ebrahim, Y.M. and Gohari, S.T., 2014. Functional and nutritional properties of stirred yoghurt supplemented with silymarin and its impact on chronic hepatic damage. World Journal of Dairy & Food Sciences 9: 36-50.

Jennings, R.E., Scharfmann, R. and Staels, W., 2020. Transcription factors that shape the mammalian pancreas. Diabetologia 63: 1974-1980.

Jowkar, F., Godarzi, H. and Parvizi, M.M., 2020. Can we consider silymarin as a treatment option for vitiligo? A double-blind controlled randomized clinical trial of phototherapy plus oral *Silybum marianum* product versus phototherapy alone. The Journal of Dermatological Treatment 31: 256-260.

Juge-Aubry, C.E., Hammar, E., Siegrist-Kaiser, C., Pernin, A., Takeshita, A., Chin, W.W., Burger, A.G. and Meier, C.A., 1999. Regulation of the transcriptional activity of the peroxisome proliferator-activated receptor alpha by phosphorylation of a ligand-independent trans-activating domain. The Journal of Biological Chemistry 274: 10505-10510.

Jung, H.J., Park, J.W., Lee, J.S., Lee, S.R., Jang, B.C., Suh, S.I., Suh, M.H. and Baek, W.K., 2009. Silibinin inhibits expression of HIF-1alpha through suppression of protein translation in prostate cancer cells. Biochemical and Biophysical Research Communications 390: 71-76.

Kadoglou, N., Panayiotou, C., Vardas, M., Balaskas, N., Kostomitsopoulos, N.G., Tsaroucha, A.K. and Valsami, G., 2022. A Comprehensive review of the cardiovascular protective properties of silibinin/silymarin: A new kid on the block. Pharmaceuticals 15: 538.

Karbasforooshan, H., Hosseini, S., Elyasi, S., Fani Pakdel, A. and Karimi, G., 2019. Topical silymarin administration for prevention of acute radiodermatitis in breast cancer patients: A randomized, double-blind, placebo-controlled clinical trial. Phytotherapy Research 33: 379-386.

Kesharwani, S.S., Jain, V., Dey, S., Sharma, S., Mallya, P. and Kumar, V.A., 2020. An overview of advanced formulation and nanotechnology-based approaches for solubility and bioavailability enhancement of silymarin. Journal of Drug Delivery Science and Technology 60: 102021.

Khan, M., Uzair, M., Nazli, A. and Chen, J.Z., 2022. An overview on estrogen receptors signaling and its ligands in breast cancer. European Journal of Medicinal Chemistry 241: 114658.

Khoo, N.K., Hebbar, S., Zhao, W., Moore, S.A., Domann, F.E. and Robbins, M.E., 2013. Differential activation of catalase expression and activity by PPAR agonists: implications for astrocyte protection in anti-glioma therapy. Redox Biology 1: 70-79.

Kim, T. and Yang, Q., 2013. Peroxisome-proliferator-activated receptors regulate redox signaling in the cardiovascular system. World Journal of Cardiology 5: 164-174.

Koltai, T. and Fliegel, L., 2022. Role of silymarin in cancer treatment: Facts, hypotheses, and questions. Journal of Evidence-Based Integrative Medicine 27: 2515690X211068826.

Komori, T., 2022. Whole aspect of Runx2 functions in skeletal development. International Journal of Molecular Sciences 23: 5776.

Kong, L., Ren, W., Li, W., Zhao, S., Mi, H., Wang, R., Zhang, Y., Wu, W., Nan, Y. and Yu, J., 2011. Activation of peroxisome proliferator activated receptor alpha ameliorates ethanol induced steatohepatitis in mice. Lipids in Health and Disease 10: 246.

Kota, B.P., Huang, T.H. and Roufogalis, B.D., 2005. An overview on biological mechanisms of PPARs. Pharmacological Research 51: 85-94.

Li, J.L., Wang, Q.Y., Luan, H.Y., Kang, Z.C. and Wang, C.B., 2012. Effects of L-carnitine against oxidative stress in human hepatocytes: involvement of peroxisome proliferator-activated receptor alpha. Journal of Biomedical Science 19: 32.

Lin, C.H., Li, C.H., Liao, P.L., Tse, L.S., Huang, W.K., Cheng, H.W. and Cheng, Y.W., 2013. Silibinin inhibits VEGF secretion and age-related macular degeneration in a hypoxia-dependent manner through the PI-3 kinase/Akt/mTOR pathway. British Journal of Pharmacology 168: 920-931.

Liu, C.H., Jassey, A., Hsu, H.Y. and Lin, L.T., 2019. Antiviral activities of silymarin and derivatives. Molecules 24: 1552.

Liu, W., Wang, F., Li, C., Otkur, W., Hayashi, T., Mizuno, K., Hattori, S., Fujisaki, H., Onodera, S. and Ikejima, T., 2021. Silibinin treatment protects human skin cells from UVB injury through upregulation of estrogen receptors. Journal of Photochemistry and Photobiology. B, Biology 216: 112147.

Liu, X., Jang, S.S., An, Z., Song, H., Kim, W.D., Yu, J.R. and Park, W.Y., 2012. Fenofibrate decreases radiation sensitivity via peroxisome proliferator-activated receptor α-mediated superoxide dismutase induction in HeLa cells. Radiation Oncology Journal 30: 88-95.

Long, X., Gao, Y., Liu, W., Liu, X., Hayashi, T., Mizuno, K., Hattori, S. and Ikejima, T., 2020. Natural flavonoid silibinin promotes the migration and myogenic differentiation of murine C2C12 myoblasts via modulation of ROS generation and down-regulation of estrogen receptor α expression. Molecular and Cellular Biochemistry 474: 243-261.

Lorenzo, J.M., Putnik, P., Kovačević, D.B., Petrović, M., Munekata, P.E., Gómez, B., Marszałek K., Roohinejad, S. and Barba, F.J., 2020. Silymarin compounds: Chemistry, innovative extraction techniques and synthesis. Studies in Natural Products Chemistry 64: 111-130.

Lovelace, E.S., Wagoner, J., MacDonald, J., Bammler, T., Bruckner, J., Brownell, J., Beyer, R.P., Zink, E.M., Kim, Y.M., Kyle, J.E., Webb-Robertson, B.J., Waters, K.M., Metz, T.O., Farin, F., Oberlies, N.H. and Polyak, S.J., 2015. Silymarin suppresses cellular inflammation by inducing reparative stress signaling. Journal of Natural Products 78: 1990-2000.

Mahmoodi-Nesheli, M., Alizadeh, S., Solhi, H., Mohseni, J. and Mahmoodi-Nesheli, M., 2018. Adjuvant effect of oral silymarin on patients' wound healing process caused by thermal injuries. Caspian Journal of Internal Medicine 9: 341-346.

Mirnezami, M., Jafarimanesh, H., Rezagholizamenjany, M., Alimoradian, A. and Ranjbaran, M., 2020. The effect of silymarin on liver enzymes in patients taking isotretinoin: A randomized clinical trial. Dermatologic Therapy 33: e13236.

Moezian, G., Javadinia, S.A., Sales, S.S., Fanipakdel, A., Elyasi, S. and Karimi, G., 2022. Oral silymarin formulation efficacy in management of AC-T protocol induced hepatotoxicity in breast cancer patients: A randomized, triple blind, placebo-controlled clinical trial. Journal of Oncology Pharmacy Practice 28: 827-835.

Mohanty, S., Badhei, L., Pal, A. and Panda, P., 2022. Novel cosmeceutical formulations: A better approach to photoprotection. International Journal of Applied Pharmaceutics 14: 9-17.

Momeni, A., Hajigholami, A., Geshnizjani, S. and Kheiri, S., 2015. Effect of silymarin in the prevention of Cisplatin nephrotoxicity, a clinical trial study. Journal of Clinical and Diagnostic Research 9: OC11-OC13.

Nakamura, M.T., Yudell, B.E. and Loor, J.J., 2014. Regulation of energy metabolism by long-chain fatty acids. Progress in Lipid Research 53: 124-144.

Navarro, V.J., Belle, S.H., D'Amato, M., Adfhal, N., Brunt, E.M., Fried, M.W., Reddy, K.R., Wahed, A.S., Harrison, S. and Silymarin in NASH and C Hepatitis (SyNCH) Study Group, 2019. Silymarin in non-cirrhotics with non-alcoholic steatohepatitis: A randomized, double-blind, placebo controlled trial. PloS One 14: e0221683.

Marmouzi, I., Bouyahya, A., Ezzat, S.M., El Jemli, M. and Kharbach, M., 2021. The food plant *Silybum marianum* (L.) Gaertn.: Phytochemistry, ethnopharmacology and clinical evidence. Journal of Ethnopharmacology 265: 113303.

Moshtaghion, S.M., Malekinejad, H., Razi, M. and Shafie-Irannejad, V., 2013. Silymarin protects from varicocele-induced damages in testis and improves sperm quality: evidence for E2f1 involvement. Systems Biology in Reproductive Medicine 59: 270-280.

Musso, G., Gambino, R. and Cassader, M., 2010. Non-alcoholic fatty liver disease from pathogenesis to management: an update. Obesity Reviews 11: 430-445.

Neels, J.G. and Grimaldi, P.A., 2014. Physiological functions of peroxisome proliferator-activated receptor β. Physiological Reviews 94: 795-858.

Paltinean, G.A., Tomoaia, G., Riga, S., Mocanu, A. and Tomoaia-Cotisel, M., 2022. Silymarin Based complexes – a mini review. Academy of Romanian Scientists Annals Series on Biological Sciences 11: 146-166.

Pferschy-Wenzig, E.M., Atanasov, A.G., Malainer, C., Noha, S.M., Kunert, O., Schuster, D., Heiss, E.H., Oberlies, N.H., Wagner, H., Bauer, R. and Dirsch, V.M., 2014. Identification of isosilybin a from milk thistle seeds as an agonist of peroxisome proliferator-activated receptor gamma. Journal of Natural Products 77: 842-847.

Piazzini, V., D'Ambrosio, M., Luceri, C., Cinci, L., Landucci, E., Bilia, A.R. and Bergonzi, M.C., 2019. Formulation of nanomicelles to improve the solubility and the oral absorption of silymarin. Molecules 24: 1688.

Prakash, P., Singh, V., Jain, M., Rana, M., Khanna, V., Barthwal, M.K. and Dikshit, M., 2014. Silymarin ameliorates fructose induced insulin resistance syndrome by reducing de novo hepatic lipogenesis in the rat. European Journal of Pharmacology 727: 15-28.

Rajnochová Svobodová, A., Zálešák, B., Biedermann, D., Ulrichová, J. and Vostálová, J., 2016. Phototoxic potential of silymarin and its bioactive components. Journal of Photochemistry and Photobiology. B, Biology 156: 61-68.

Ralli, T., Kalaiselvan, V., Tiwari, R., Shukla, S. and Kholi, K., 2021. Clinical and regulatory status of silymarin. Applied Drug Research, Clinical Trials and Regulatory Affairs 8: 104-111.

Scheggi, S., Pinna, G., Braccagni, G., De Montis, M.G. and Gambarana, C., 2022. PPARα signaling: A candidate target in psychiatric disorder management. Biomolecules 12: 723.

Shafiei-Roudbari, S.K., Malekinejad, H., Janbaz-Aciabar, H. and Razi, M., 2017. Crosstalk between E2F1 and P53 transcription factors in doxorubicin-induced DNA damage: evidence for preventive/protective effects of silymarin. The Journal of Pharmacy and Pharmacology 69: 1116-1124.

Sobolev, V.V., Tchepourina, E., Korsunskaya, I.M., Geppe, N.A., Chebysheva, S.N., Soboleva, A.G. and Mezentsev, A., 2022. The role of transcription factor PPAR-γ in the pathogenesis of psoriasis, skin cells, and immune cells. International Journal of Molecular Sciences 23: 9708.

Soleimani, V., Delghandi, P.S., Moallem, S.A. and Karimi, G., 2019. Safety and toxicity of silymarin, the major constituent of milk thistle extract: An updated review. Phytotherapy Research 33: 1627-1638.

Song, X., Liu, B., Cui, L., Zhou, B., Liu, L., Liu, W., Yao, G., Xia, M., Hayashi, T., Hattori, S., Ushiki-Kaku, Y., Tashiro, S.I. and Ikejima, T., 2018. Estrogen receptors are involved in the neuroprotective effect of silibinin in $A\beta_{1-42}$-treated rats. Neurochemical Research 43: 796-805.

Soto, C., Raya, L., Juárez, J., Pérez, J. and González, I., 2014a. Effect of silymarin in Pdx-1 expression and the proliferation of pancreatic β-cells in a pancreatectomy model. Phytomedicine 21: 233-239.

Soto, C., Raya, L., Pérez, J., González, I. and Pérez, S., 2014b. Silymarin induces expression of pancreatic Nkx6.1 transcription factor and β-cells neogenesis in a pancreatectomy model. Molecules 19: 4654-4668.

Stossi, F., Barnett, D.H., Frasor, J., Komm, B., Lyttle, C.R. and Katzenellenbogen, B.S., 2004. Transcriptional profiling of estrogen-regulated gene expression via estrogen receptor (ER) alpha or ERbeta in human osteosarcoma cells: distinct and common target genes for these receptors. Endocrinology 145: 3473-3486.

Suguro, R., Pang, X.C., Yuan, Z.W., Chen, S.Y., Zhu, Y.Z. and Xie, Y., 2020. Combinational application of silybin and tangeretin attenuates the progression of non-alcoholic steatohepatitis (NASH) in mice via modulating lipid metabolism. Pharmacological Research 151: 104519.

Sullivan, K.D., Galbraith, M.D., Andrysik, Z. and Espinosa, J.M., 2018. Mechanisms of transcriptional regulation by p53. Cell Death and Differentiation 25: 133-143.

Sun, Y., Yang, J., Liu, W., Yao, G., Xu, F., Hayashi, T., Onodera, S. and Ikejima, T., 2019. Attenuating effect of silibinin on palmitic acid-induced apoptosis and mitochondrial dysfunction in pancreatic β-cells is mediated by estrogen receptor alpha. Molecular and Cellular Biochemistry 460: 81-92.

Surai, P.F., 2015a. Carnitine enigma: From antioxidant action to vitagene regulation. Part 1. Absorption, metabolism and antioxidant activities. Journal of Veterinary Science & Medicine 3, 2: 14.

Surai, P.F., 2015b. Carnitine enigma: From antioxidant action to vitagene regulation. Part 2. Transcription factors and practical applications. Journal of Veterinary Science & Medicine 3, 2: 17.

Surai, P.F., 2015c. Antioxidant action of carnitine: Molecular mechanisms and practical applications. EC Veterinary Science 2.1: 66-84.

Surai, P.F., 2015d. Silymarin as a natural antioxidant: An overview of the current evidence and perspectives. Antioxidants 4: 204-247.

Surai, P.F., 2018. Selenium in poultry nutrition and health. Wageningen Academic Publishers, Wageningen, the Netherlands.

Surai, P.F. (Ed.), 2021. Selenium in pig nutrition and health. Wageningen Academic Publishers, Wageningen, the Netherlands.

Surai, P.F., 2020a. Vitagene in avian biology and poultry health. Wageningen Academic Publishers, Wageningen, The Netherlands.

Surai, P.F., 2020b. Antioxidants in poultry nutrition and reproduction: An update. Antioxidants 9: 105.

Surai, P.F., 2022. Silymarin as a vitagene modulator: effects on mitochondria integrity in stress conditions. In: Ostojik, S.M. (ed) Molecular nutrition and mitochondria. Elsevier, Academic Press, London, UK, pp. 535-559.

Surai, P.F. and Earle-Payne, K., 2022. Antioxidant defences and redox homeostasis in animals. Antioxidants 11: 1012.

Surai, P.F., Earle-Payne, K. and Kidd, M.T., 2021a. Taurine as a natural antioxidant: From direct antioxidant effects to protective action in various toxicological models. Antioxidants 10: 1876.

Surai, P.F. and Kochish, I.I., 2019. Nutritional modulation of the antioxidant capacities in poultry: the case of selenium. Poultry Science 98: 4231-4239.

Surai, P.F., Kochish, I.I. and Kidd, M.T., 2021b. Redox homeostasis in poultry: Regulatory roles of NF-κB. Antioxidants 10: 186.

Surai, P.F., Kochish, I.I., Fisinin, V.I., Grozina, A.A. and Shatskikh, E.V., 2018. Molecular mechanisms of gut health support in poultry: Role of microbiota. Monograph. Agricultural Technologies: Moscow, Russia.

Surai, P.F., Kochish, I.I., Fisinin, V.I., and Kidd, M.T., 2019b. Antioxidant defence systems and oxidative stress in poultry biology: An update. Antioxidants 8: 235.

Surai, P.F., Kochish, I.I., and Kidd, M.T., 2020. Taurine in poultry nutrition. Animal Feed Science and Technology 260: 114339.

Surai, P.F., Kochish, I.I., Romanov, M.N. and Griffin, D.K., 2019a. Nutritional modulation of the antioxidant capacities in poultry: the case of vitamin E. Poultry Science, 98: 4030-4041.

Tang, Z.R., Zhang, R., Lian, Z.X., Deng, S.L. and Yu, K., 2019. Estrogen-receptor expression and function in female reproductive disease. Cells 8: 1123.

Tsiogka, A., Kyriazopoulou, M., Kontochristopoulos, G., Nicolaidou, E., Stratigos, A., Rigopoulos, D. and Gregoriou, S., 2022. The JAK/STAT pathway and its selective inhibition in the treatment of atopic dermatitis: A systematic review. Journal of Clinical Medicine 11: 4431.

Tyagi, A., Agarwal, C., Dwyer-Nield, L.D., Singh, R.P., Malkinson, A.M. and Agarwal, R., 2012. Silibinin modulates TNF-α and IFN-γ mediated signaling to regulate COX2 and iNOS expression in tumorigenic mouse lung epithelial LM2 cells. Molecular Carcinogenesis 51: 832-842.

Ullah, H. and Khan, H., 2018. Anti-Parkinson potential of silymarin: Mechanistic insight and therapeutic standing. Frontiers in Pharmacology 9: 422.

Uto, T., Ohta, T., Katayama, K. and Shoyama, Y., 2022. Silibinin promotes melanogenesis through the PKA and p38 MAPK signaling pathways in melanoma cells. Biomedical Research 43: 31-39.

Vecchione, G., Grasselli, E., Voci, A., Baldini, F., Grattagliano, I., Wang, D.Q., Portincasa, P. and Vergani, L., 2016. Silybin counteracts lipid excess and oxidative stress in cultured steatotic hepatic cells. World Journal of Gastroenterology 22: 6016-6026.

Verdura, S., Cuyàs, E., Ruiz-Torres, V., Micol, V., Joven, J., Bosch-Barrera, J. and Menendez, J.A., 2021. Lung cancer management with silibinin: A historical and translational perspective. Pharmaceuticals 14: 559.

Voroneanu, L., Nistor, I., Dumea, R., Apetrii, M. and Covic, A., 2016. Silymarin in type 2 diabetes mellitus: A systematic review and meta-analysis of randomized controlled trials. Journal of Diabetes Research 2016: 5147468.

Wadhwa, K., Pahwa, R., Kumar, M., Kumar, S., Sharma, P.C., Singh, G., Verma, R., Mittal, V., Singh, I., Kaushik, D. and Jeandet, P., 2022. Mechanistic insights into the pharmacological significance of silymarin. Molecules 27: 5327.

Wagner, N. and Wagner, K.D., 2022. Peroxisome proliferator-activated receptors and the hallmarks of cancer. Cells 11: 2432.

Wah Kheong, C., Nik Mustapha, N.R. and Mahadeva, S., 2017. A randomized trial of silymarin for the treatment of nonalcoholic steatohepatitis. Clinical Gastroenterology and Hepatology 15: 1940-1949.

Wang, C., Wang, Z., Zhang, X., Zhang, X., Dong, L., Xing, Y., Li, Y., Liu, Z., Chen, L., Qiao, H., Wang, L. and Zhu, C., 2012. Protection by silibinin against experimental ischemic stroke: up-regulated pAkt, pmTOR, HIF-1α and Bcl-2, down-regulated Bax, NF-κB expression. Neuroscience Letters 529: 45-50.

Wang, H., Yan, T., Xie, Y., Zhao, M., Che, Y., Zhang, J., Liu, H., Cao, L., Cheng, X., Xie, Y., Li, F., Qi, Q., Wang, G. and Hao, H., 2015. Mechanism-based inhibitory and peroxisome proliferator-activated receptor α-dependent modulating effects of silybin on principal hepatic drug-metabolizing enzymes. Drug Metabolism and Disposition 43: 444-454.

Wang, J., Zhang, L., Cao, H., Shi, X., Zhang, X., Gao, Z., Ikeda, K., Yan, T., Jia, Y. and Xu, F., 2022. Silibinin improves L-cell mass and function through an ER-mediated antioxidative mechanism. Phytomedicine 99: 154022.

Yang, J., Sun, Y., Xu, F., Liu, W., Hayashi, T., Onodera, S., Tashiro, S.I. and Ikejima, T., 2018. Involvement of estrogen receptors in silibinin protection of pancreatic β-cells from TNFα- or IL-1β-induced cytotoxicity. Biomedicine & Pharmacotherapy 102: 344-353.

Yang, J., Sun, Y., Xu, F., Liu, W., Hayashi, T., Hattori, S., Ushiki-Kaku, Y., Onodera, S., Tashiro, S.I. and Ikejima, T., 2019a. Silibinin protects rat pancreatic β-cell through up-regulation of estrogen receptors' signaling against amylin- or $A\beta_{1-42}$-induced reactive oxygen species/reactive nitrogen species generation. Phytotherapy Research 33: 998-1009.

Yang, J., Sun, Y., Xu, F., Liu, W., Mai, Y., Hayashi, T., Hattori, S., Ushiki-Kaku, Y., Onodera, S., Tashiro, S.I. and Ikejima, T., 2019b. Silibinin ameliorates amylin-induced pancreatic β-cell apoptosis partly via upregulation of GLP-1R/PKA pathway. Molecular and Cellular Biochemistry 452: 83-94.

Yassin, N., AbouZid, S.F., El-Kalaawy, A.M., Ali, T.M., Elesawy, B.H. and Ahmed, O.M., 2021. Tackling of renal carcinogenesis in Wistar rats by *Silybum marianum* total extract, silymarin, and silibinin via modulation of oxidative stress, apoptosis, Nrf2, PPARγ, NF-κB, and PI3K/Akt signaling pathways. Oxidative Medicine and Cellular Longevity 2021: 7665169.

Ye, H., Dudley, S.Z. and Shaw, I.C., 2018. Intimate estrogen receptor-α/ligand relationships signal biological activity. Toxicology 408: 80-87.

Ye, X., Zhang, T. and Han, H., 2022. PPARα: A potential therapeutic target of cholestasis. Frontiers in Pharmacology 13: 916866.

Ying, X., Sun, L., Chen, X., Xu, H., Guo, X., Chen, H., Hong, J., Cheng, S. and Peng, L., 2013. Silibinin promotes osteoblast differentiation of human bone marrow stromal cells via bone morphogenetic protein signaling. European Journal of Pharmacology 721: 225-230.

Yu, K., Huang, Z.Y., Xu, X.L., Li, J., Fu, X.W. and Deng, S.L., 2022. Estrogen receptor function: impact on the human endometrium. Frontiers in Endocrinology 13, 827724.

Zhang, M., Liu, Y., Gao, Y. and Li, S., 2015. Silibinin-induced glioma cell apoptosis by PI3K-mediated but Akt-independent downregulation of FoxM1 expression. European Journal of Pharmacology 765: 346-354.

Zhang, Z., Li, X., Sang, S., McClements, D.J., Chen, L., Long, J., Jiao, A., Wang, J., Jin, Z. and Qiu, C., 2022. A review of nanostructured delivery systems for the encapsulation, protection, and delivery of silymarin: An emerging nutraceutical. Food Research International 156: 111314.

Zheng, N., Liu, L., Liu, W., Zhang, P., Huang, H., Zang, L., Hayashi, T., Tashiro, S., Onodera, S., Xia, M. and Ikejima, T., 2016. ERβ up-regulation was involved in silibinin-induced growth inhibition of human breast cancer MCF-7 cells. Archives of Biochemistry and Biophysics 591: 141-149.

Zheng, N., Zhang, P., Huang, H., Liu, W., Hayashi, T., Zang, L., Zhang, Y., Liu, L., Xia, M., Tashiro, S., Onodera, S. and Ikejima, T., 2015. ERα down-regulation plays a key role in silibinin-induced autophagy and apoptosis in human breast cancer MCF-7 cells. Journal of Pharmacological Sciences 128: 97-107.

Zhou, S., You, H., Qiu, S., Yu, D., Bai, Y., He, J., Cao, H., Che, Q., Guo, J. and Su, Z., 2022. A new perspective on NAFLD: Focusing on the crosstalk between peroxisome proliferator-activated receptor alpha (PPARα) and farnesoid X receptor, FXR. Biomedicine & Pharmacotherapy 154: 113577.

Zhou, T., Yan, X., Wang, G., Liu, H., Gan, X., Zhang, T., Wang, J. and Li, L., 2015. Evolutionary pattern and regulation analysis to support why diversity functions existed within PPAR gene family members. BioMed Research International 2015: 613910.

www.ingramcontent.com/pod-product-compliance
Lightning Source LLC
LaVergne TN
LVHW080801011026
849160LV00015B/1502

9789086863914